IBANISES

S0-AYT-828

Springer
Berlin
Heidelberg
New York
Barcelona
Budapest
Hong Kong
London
Milan
Paris
Santa Clara
Singapur
Tokyo

H.-Harald Sedlacek
Tarik Möröy

Immune Reactions

Headlines, Overviews,
Tables and Graphics

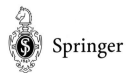 Springer

Prof. Dr. H.-HARALD SEDLACEK
Leiter Strategische Planung Therapeutika
Behringwerke AG
Emil-von-Behring-Str. 76
35001 Marburg

Prof. Dr. TARIK MÖRÖY
Institut für Molekularbiologie
und Tumorforschung
Emil-Mannkopf-Str. 2
35037 Marburg

CIP data applied for

Die Deutsche Bibliothek – CIP-Einheitsaufnahme

Sedlacek, Hans Harald:
Immune reactions : headlines, overviews, tables and graphics /
H.-Harald Sedlacek ; Tarik Möröy. – Berlin ; Heidelberg ; New
York ; Barcelona ; Budapest ; Hong Kong ; London ; Milan ;
Paris ; Tokyo : Springer, 1995
    ISBN 3–540–58957–0
NE: Möröy, Tarik:

ISBN 3-540-58957-0 Springer-Verlag Berlin Heidelberg New York

The use of general descriptive names, registered names, trademarks, etc. in this publication does not imply, even in the absence of a specific statement, that such names are exempt from the relevant protective laws and regulations and therefore free for general use.

Product Liability: The publisher can give no guarantee for information about drug dosage and application thereof contained in this book. In every individual case the respective user must check in accuracy by consulting other pharmaceutical literature.

Typesetting: Storch GmbH, Wiesentheid
Printing and Binding: Appl, Wemding
27/3136   SPIN 10482042 – Printed on acid free paper

Preface

This book represents a summary of structures and interactions of the immune system in forms of tables, figures and schematic diagrms. As current knowledge in the field of immunology expands very rapidly, the actual presentation is only an attempt to be exhaustive and is certainly incomplete; indeed information about antiinfective vaccines is not included, as very many very illustrative books already exist that cover this topic.

This book is based on the lectures of the authors at the Medical School and in the graduate program "Human Biology" at the Department of Medicine of the Philipps University in Marburg, Germany. The main goal of this book is to provide advanced medical and graduate students in immunology as well as researchers and instructors working in the field rapid access to information about complicated structures and networks in immunology which is not covered by the main textbooks without the need to consult the primary literature.

The book is organized in 26 chapters; each is introduced by a short overview. A detailed table of contents guides through the chapters and the different topics. In addition, a list of references is given at the end of the book for those readers interested in further details.

We are indebted to Ms. Manuela Rogala for her excellent assistance in organizing and editing the different chapters and for her excellent typing and computer graphics.

Marburg, Juli 1995
H.-HARALD SEDLACEK
TARIK MÖRÖY

Contents

1 Cytokines, Growth Factors and Their Receptors

1.1 Overview

Cytokines are growth factors which regulate proliferation, differentiation and function of cells of the blood and the immune system.

Cytokines are mainly secreted by cells of the blood and the immune system. Thus, these cells are able to control themselves in an autocrine and a paracrine way.

For their function cytokines have to bind to and to activate specific receptors on the membrane of the target cells. By regulation of the number of receptors on their membrane the target cells are able to control the effect of cytokines.

The various cytokines act differently and synergistically in a hierarchical system. Pluripotent cytokines are followed by cytokines specific for cell lineages and their function. The concentration and the combination of cytokines acting on a cell are decisive for its proliferation, differentiation and function.

1.1.1 Cytokines in Hematopoiesis

Cytokines Affecting Hematopoiesis (Proliferation and Differentiation)

Megakaryocytic cell line
SCF, IL-1, IL-2, IL-3, IL-4, IL-6, LIF, IL-7, IL-11, G-CSF, GM-CSF, M-CSF, erythropoietin, thrombopoietin

Erythropoiesis
SCF, IL-4, IL-6, IL-13, erythropoietin

Monocytopoiesis, macrophages
IL-1, IL-2, IL-3, IL-4, IL-6, LIF, IL-10, IL-11, IL-13, GM-CSF, G-CSF, M-CSF, IFN-γ, erythropoietin

Lymphopoiesis
NK-cells
SCF, IL-1, IL-2, IL-4, IL-12, IFN-γ
T-cells
SCF, IL-1, IL-2, IL-3, IL-4, IL-5, IL-6, IL-7, IL-10, IL-12, IFN-γ
B-cells
SCF, IL-1, IL-2, IL-3, IL-4, IL-5, IL-6, IL-7, IL-10, IL-11, IL-13, IFN-γ

Granulocytopoiesis
SCF, IL-1, IL-6, IL-11, GM-CSF, G-CSF, LIF, M-CSF, IFN-γ, erythropoietin
Neutrophils
IL-3, IL-4, IL-6, IL-8, GM-CSF, G-CSF

The Effect of Cytokines in Hematopoiesis

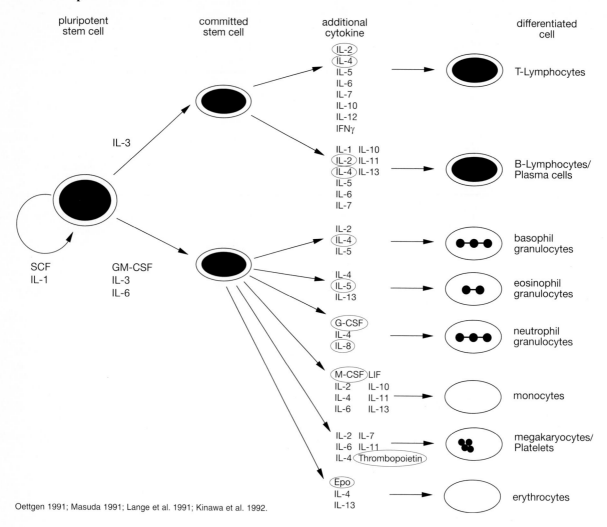

Oettgen 1991; Masuda 1991; Lange et al. 1991; Kinawa et al. 1992.

Eosinophils
   IL-3, IL-4, IL-5, IL-13, GM-CSF, G-CSF
Basophils
   IL-2, IL-3, IL-4, IL-5, GM-CSF, G-CSF
Mast cells
   SCF, IL-3, IL-4, IL-10, GM-CSF

Cytokines Involved in Immune Regulation and Hematopoietic Blood Cell Development	Family	Molecules	Synonyms	Chromosomal localization of encoding gene	MW (kDa)
	Growth factors	multi-CSF	IL-3	5q23–q31	14–28
		GM-CSF	CSF-α	5q23–q31	14–35
		G-CSF	CSF-β	17q11–q22	18–22
		M-CSF	CSF-1	5q33.1	47–74
		Epo		7q11–q22	34–39
		SCF			
		thrombopoietin	cMpl-ligand		38
	Interleukins	IL-1	hematopoietin-1	2q13–q21	31, 17
		IL-2	TCGF	4q26–q27	15
		IL-3	multi-CSF	5q23–q31	14–28
		IL-4	BSF-1	5q23–q32	15–20
		IL-5	BDGF-II, TRF	5q23–q32	12–18
		IL-6	BSF-2	7p15–p21	24
		IL-7	lymphopoietin-1	8p12–p13	17
		IL-8	NCF/NAP		10
		IL-9	p40		40
		IL-10			
		IL-11			
		IL-12	NKSF/CLMF		75
		IL-13			
	Interferons	IFN-α	leukocyte IFN	9p22–p13	18–20
		IFN-β	fibroblast IFN	9p22	23
		IFN-γ	immune IFN	12q24.1	20–25
	Tumor necrosis factors	TNF-α	cachectin	6p21.3	17
		TNF-β	lymphotoxin	6p21.3	25
	Others	PDGF			30–35
		TGF-α		2p13	
		TGF-β		19q13.1–q13.2	25
		LIF	HILDA	22q12	24
		FGF			

SCF, stem cell factor; TCGF, T-cell growth factor; BSF, B-cell stimulatory factor, BCGF, B-cell growth factor; TRF, T-cell replacing factor; NCF/NAP, neutrophil chemotactic factor/neutrophil-activating protein; PDGF, platelet-derived growth factor; TGF, transforming growth factor; LIF, leukemia-inhibiting factor; FGF, fibroblast growth factor; NKSF, natural killer cell stimulatory factor; CLMF, cytotoxic lymphocyte maturation factor.

1.1.2 Classification of Growth Factors

Growth factor family	Source	Target cells	Major effect
Epidermal growth factor family (characterized by cysteine-rich domain, transmembrane precursor molecules are activated by proteolytic cleavage)			
Epidermal growth factor (EGF)	epithelial cells	epithelial, mesenchymal cells	mitogen
Transforming growth factor-α (TGF α)	tumor-derived transformed cell lines	epithelial, mesenchymal cells	mitogen, transforming for fibroblasts
Amphiregulin (AP)	carcinoma cell lines	epithelial, mesenchymal cells	mitogen for fibroblasts, inhibits breast carcinoma cell growth, binds to single, double stranded DNA
Schwannoma-derived growth factor (SDGF)	Schwann cells	astrocytes, fibroblasts, Schwann cells	mitogen
gp30	breast carcinoma cells	c-*erbB2*-positive cells	mitogen
Cripto	teratocarcinoma cells	epithelial cells	mitogen
Vaccinia virus growth factor	vaccinia virus	epithelial cells	mitogen
Heparin-binding growth factor family (inactive ECM bound forms are activated by extracellular proteinases and heparinases)			
Acidic-fibroblast growth factor (aFGF)	ubiquitous	ubiquitous	mitogen, angiogenesis, neurotrophic
Basic fibroblast growth factor (bFGF)	ubiquitous	ubiquitous	mitogen, motility factor
int-2 oncoprotein (FGF-3)	embryonic cells	fibroblasts	mitogen
hst oncoprotein (FGF-4)	embryonic cells	fibroblasts	mitogen
Fibroblast growth factor-5 (FGF-5)	fibroblasts	fibroblasts	mitogen
Keratinocyte growth factor (KGF)	stromal cells	keratinocytes	mitogen, angiogenesis
Vascular endothelial cell growth factor (VEGF)	monocytes macrophages	vascular endothelial cells	mitogen, angiogenesis, vascular permeability factor
Platelet-derived growth factor family (dipeptides, homo- or heterodimers)			
Platelet-derived growth factor (PDGF)			
αα	mesenchymal cells platelets	mesenchymal cells	mitogen
ββ			
αβ			
v-*sis* viral oncoprotein	simian sarcoma virus	fibroblasts	mitogen

Massague et al. 1987; Pusztai et al. 1993.

Growth factor family	Source	Target cells	Major effect

Insulin-like growth factor family (structural and functional similarity to Proinsulin)

Insulin-like growth factor-I (IGF-I, somatomedin I)	ubiquitous	ubiquitous	mediates growth hormone activity, insulin-like effects
Insulin-like growth factor-II	ubiquitous	ubiquitous	insulin-like effects

Nerve growth factor family (cysteine-rich domains form the core structure, variable domains determine neuronal specificity)

Nerve growth factor (NGF)	Schwann cell, neurons melanocytes, cholinergic neurons in brain	peripheral neurons,	neurotrophic increases ACh synthesis
Brain-derived neurotrophic factor (BDNF)	neurons, glial cells	dopaminergic neurons in brain	neurotrophic
Neurotrophin-3 (NT-3)	many cell types	peripheral proprio-ceptive neurons	neurotrophic

Transforming growth factor-β family (homodimeric proteins, secreted precursor molecules are activated by serine proteases)

Transforming growth factor (TGF) – β_1 – β_2 – β_3 – β_4	ubiquitous	ubiquitous	mitogen for fibroblasts, inhibits proliferation of many cell types, angiogenesis
Müllerian inhibiting substance (MIS)	genital organs	genital organs	organogenesis
Bone morphogenic protein (MBP)			organogenesis

Growth factors not included in the above families

Hepatocyte growth factor (HGF)	many cell types	hepatocytes, epithelial cells	mitogen
Platelet-derived endothelial growth factor (PDEGF)	platelets	endothelial cells	angiogenesis, mitogen
Endothelin-1	many cell types	endothelial mesenchymal cells	vasoconstriction mitogen
Gro (melanocyte growth factor)	many cell types	melanocytes inflammatory cells	mitogen, proinflammatory

Pusztai et al. 1993; Massague et al. 1987

1.1.3 Receptors for Cytokines

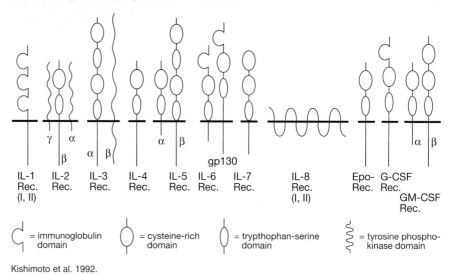

Kishimoto et al. 1992.

Cytokine Receptors

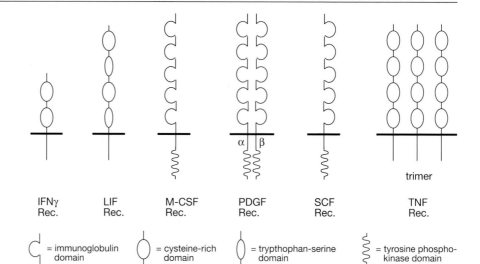

1.1.4 Receptors for Growth Factors

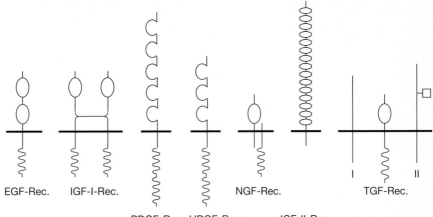

EGF-Rec. IGF-I-Rec. PDGF-Rec. HBGF-Rec. NGF-Rec. IGF-II-Rec. TGF-Rec.

Pusztai et al. 1993.

1.1.5 Characteristics of Chemokines

Factor	Size and structure	Origin	Function	References
RANTES (regulated upon activation, normal T expressed and secreted) (synonym MCP-2)	8 kDa, 68 aa 4 cysteins nonglycosylated	normal T-cells (nonactivated)	chemotaxis for CD4[+] and CD26[+] memory T-cells and monocytes histamine liberating factor (basophils, mast cells)	Schall et al. 1988, 1990
MCAF (monocyte chemotactic and activating factor) (synonym MCP-1)	8,5 kDa, 76 aa 1N-glycosylation site	monocytes lymphocytes fibroblasts endothelial cells after activation	activation of monocytes (inhibitable by glucocorticosteroids)	Zachariae et al. 1990 Rollins et al. 1991 Furutami et al. 1989 Mukaida et al. 1991 Sica et al. 1990
MIP-1 alpha (LD78) MIP-1 beta (ACT-2) (macrophage inflammatory protein-1)	8 kDa, 69 aa MIP-1α: 0-glycosylated MIP-1β: 0- and N-glycosylated	activated macrophages T-cells, B-cells mast cells and fibroblasts GM-CSF	chemotaxis and activation of T-cells, B-cells, macrophages, mast cells and fibroblasts MIP-1 beta: synergy with G-CSF, MIP-1 alpha: inhibition of GM-CSF, M-CSF histamine-liberating factor	Wolpe et al. 1987, 1989 Sherry et al. 1988 Broxmeyer et al. 1991 Oh et al. 1991 Graham et al. 1990
IL-8 (monocyte derived neutrophil chemotactic factor, neutrophil activating protein 1, NAP-1)	8 kDa, 77 aa, 72 aa, 70 aa or 69 aa 4 cystein residues 2 intrachain disulfide bridges active as dimer	activated T-cells monocytes fibroblasts endothelial cells keratinocytes chondrocytes	stimulation of neutrophil granulocytes	Schroder et al. 1987 Lindley et al. 1988 Clore et al. 1990 Lotz et al. 1992
MGSA/Gro	8 kDa 73 aa	melanoma cells epidermal cells fibroblasts (after PDGF stimulation)	chemotaxis and activation of neutrophils mitogenesis of melanoma cells	Walz et al. 1991 Cross et al. 1991
NAP-2 (neutrophil activating protein)	8 kDa 70 aa	thrombocytes	chemotaxis and activation of neutrophils	Walz 1991
β-Thromboglobulin		platelets other cells	antiangiogenic (binding of FGF) complex formation with TGFβ	Good et al. 1990 Averill et al. 1992 Murphy-Ullrich et al. 1992
Platelet factor 4		platelets	histamine release from human basophils enhancement of IgE receptors on eosinophils chemotactic for granulocytes and monocytes	McManus et al. 1979 Brindley et al. 1983 Denel et al. 1981
IP10	8,5 kDa	T-cells (DTH response)	chemotaxis of monocytes, lymphocytes	Walz 1991

1.1.6 Neutrophil Activating Peptides

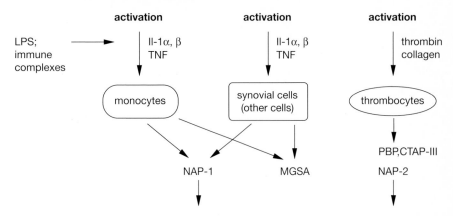

Function of NAP-1, -2:
   * strong activation of neutrophil granulocytes leading to
       – Ca^{++} increase (intracellular)
       – increase of chemotaxis
       – increase of exocytosis
       – increase of O$_2$ generation
       – upregulation of complement receptors (CR-1, CR-2)
       – diapedesis and tissue infiltration
   * only weak activity on monocytes, eosinophils and basophils
   * slight activation of lymphocytes
   * no species specificity (NAP-1)

MGSA, melanoma growth stimulatory activity; CTAP, connective tissue activating peptide; NAP, neutrophil activating peptide; PBP, platelet basic protein

Walz 1991.

1.2 Characteristics of Mediators, Receptors

1.2.1 SCF, IL-1

Stem Cell Factor (SCF)

Synonyms: C-kit ligand; mast cell growth factor, MGF

Size and structure:
- glycoprotein: 30 kDa, 164 aa (secreted soluble form)
- noncovalently linked dimer
- 2 intrachain disulfide bonds
- highly glycosylated with both N-linked and O-linked sugars (glycosylation not essential for activity)

Origin:
- expressed by bone marrow stromal cells, fibroblasts and fetal liver cells
- soluble, secreted form is believed to arise from proteolytic digestion of the membrane form (alternative splicing of the initial mRNA transcript either into soluble or membrane bound form may also be possible)

Function:
- multilineage growth factor effective on
  * hematopoietic cells, mast cells
  * melanocytes
  * developing primordial germ cells
- synergizes with
  * EPO (erythroid lineage)
  * IL-3, IL-6, IL-11, GM-CSF or G-CSF (early and late myeloid cells)
  * IL-6, IL-3 or IL-11 (megakaryopoiesis)
  * IL-7 (B-cells)
  * IL-2, IL-7 (T-cells)
  * IL-3 (mast cells)

Witte et al. 1990, Williams et al. 1992, Lu et al. 1991, Carow et al. 1991, Martin et al. 1990, Brandt et al. 1992, Tsuji et al. 1992, Avraham et al. 1992, Tsai et al. 1991.

SCF Receptor

Domains:

Extracellular	497 aa
Transmembrane	23 aa
Intracellular	433 aa

Molecular weight:
145 kDa

Distribution:
pluripotent hematopoietic stem cells, lymphoid precur-sors, myeloid precur-sors, megakaryocyte precursors, erythroid progenitors, B-cell progenitors, mast cells

The normal SCF-receptor is encoded by the c-*kit* protooncogene.

Receptors/cell:
100–1000

Affinity (Kd):
0,1–1 pM
Signal transduction:
SCF binding induces dimerization of receptors followed by modulation of phosphoinositide metabolism, rise of intracellular free calcium and activation of intrinsic TPK, auto-phosphorylation and phosphorylation of cellular proteins including c-*raf*, PLC-γ, PI-3 kinase and MAP kinase.

Chabot et al. 1988, Ogawa et al. 1991, Reith et al. 1991, Miyazawa et al. 1991, Okuda et al. 1992.

Human Interleukin-1 (IL-1)

Synonyms: lymphocyte activating factor LAF; endogenous pyrogen, EP

Size and structure:
IL-1α:
polypeptide; 17.5 kDa, 159 aa (precursor 31 kDa, 271 aa); IEP 5,3 cell-associated, involved in antigen presentation
IL-1β:
polypeptide; 17,5 kDa, 153 aa (precursor 31 kDa, 269 aa); IEP 7,3 secreted by proteolytic cleavage from precursor molecule, detectable in blood and serum
– free cysteine residues (not involved in disulfide bridges)
– share only 26% sequence homology
– lack glycosylation despite exhibiting consensus sequence for N-glycosylation
– bind to the same receptor
Origin:
– synthesis by macrophages, endothelial cells, keratinocytes, neutrophils, B-lymphocytes, fibroblasts, epithelial cells, dendritic cells
Function:
– IL-1α and IL-1β share the same biological properties (as far as tested)
– no species specificity, but intensity of responses is species-specific
In vitro:
– growth factor for haematopoietic stem cells
– initiating autocrine and paracrine activation cascades
  * enhancement of proliferation of T-cells together with mitogens (induction of IL-2 synthesis and IL-1 receptor expression)
  * stimulation of pre-B-cell differentiation
  * activation of macrophages, granulocytes, fibroblasts, osteoclasts, keratinocytes, NK-cells, endothelial cells (secretion of cytokines, prostaglandins, exocytosis of lysosomal enzymes, phagocytosis, cell adhesion, chemotaxis, upregulation of cytokine receptors)
In vivo:
– cytostatic for tumor cells (melanoma)
– increase of release of β-endorphins and increasing the number of opiate-like receptors in the brain (attenuation of pain)

- endogenous pyrogen by stimulation of local release of prostaglandins in the anterior hypothalamus
- release of ACTH
- induction of anorexia by acting on the central satiety centre
- induction of hypotension by release of PGI2, EDRF (NO) and EDHF from endothelial cells
- increase of production and release of acute phase proteins
- protection against the effects of lethal irradiation
- induction of arthritis similar to human rheumatoid arthritis when injected into the joint
- aggravation of EAE disease in rats after systemic application
- induction of diseases similar to septic shock when applied in combination with TNF

Walli et al. 1991; Fenton 1992; Stephan et al. 1987; Mizel 1982; Dinarello 1982; Hill et al. 1992; Pettipher et al. 1986; Okusawa et al. 1988; Oppenheim et al. 1986; Dower et al. 1987; Iwasaki et al. 1992; Herberlin et al. 1992; Kaushansky et al. 1988; Herrmann et al. 1988.

IL-1β Is Activated by IL-1β Converting Enzyme

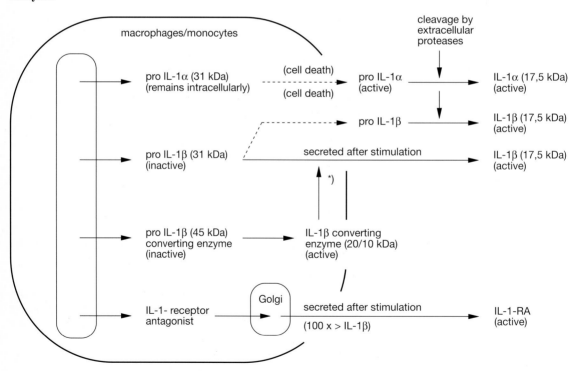

*) IL-1β converting enzyme is a Thiol (cysteine) protease specific for cleavage of pro IL-1β at the Asp (116)–Ala (117) bond.

Miller et al. 1993.

IL-1 Receptor Antagonist (IL-1 RA)

Size and structure:
- 17,5 kDa; 153 aa polypeptide; variable glycosilation in position 84
- sequence homology to IL-1α (19%) and IL-1IL-1β (26–30%)

Origin:
- produced by cultured monocytes, endothelial cells, keratinocytes, neutrophils, B-lymphocytes

Function:
species specific
Receptor binding:
- Kd: ≈0,2 nM (IL-1 receptor typ I)
- no difference to IL-1 (α,β) in affinity of binding to IL-1 receptor (type I, II) Kd: ≈0,2 nM
- association to and dissociation from IL-1 receptor (type I, II) is slower compared to IL-1 (α,β)
- binding does not activate IL-1 receptor (type I, II)
- competitive inhibition of binding to and activation of IL-1 receptor (type I, II) by IL-1 (α,β)
- for competitive inhibition IL-1 RA has to be in at least 100-fold excess

Cell biology:
- has no biological activity
- is a pure antagonist for IL-1 (α,β), inhibits IL-2 induction
  * growth of hematopoietic stem cells
  * T-cell proliferation and function
  * release of PGE_2 from fibroblasts
  * adhesion of PMN to endothelial cells
- to be antagonistic, IL-1 RA has to be present in more than 100× excess compared to IL-1 (α,β)

In vivo activity: IL-1 RA inhibits activity of IL-1 (α,β) in various animal models
- Blockage of intradermal activity of IL-1 (mouse, rabbit, pavian) in mixture with IL-1 RA. Complete blockage possible with ≥100× excess of IL-1 RA
- Reduction of inflammatory cell infiltration and tissue necrosis (ED_{50} ≥ 0,5 mg/kg twice daily) in
  * Experimental ulcerative colitis (Cominelli model)
  * Chronic bowel inflammation induced by streptococcal polysaccharides
  * Experimental rheumatoid arthritis (induced by streptococcus polysaccharide)
- Inhibition of bone resorption (activation of osteoclasts) after IL-1 treatment
- Reduction of death rate in experimental septic shock

Pharmacodynamic:
- IL-1 RA is secreted simultaneously with IL-1 (α,β) by monocytes and lymphocytes after activation (LPS, anti-CD3 MAb, immunocomplexes).
- Detectable in serum (level is higher for IL-1 RA than for IL-1) of pavians treated with LPS or *E. coli*.
- Most likely IL-1 RA is the natural inhibitor of IL-1 (α,β), whereby a considerable excess (100–1000×) of IL-1 RA has to be present for optimal activity.
- IL-1 RA does not seem to be immunosuppressive. IL-1 RA does not affect antibody response (IgM, IgG) to synthetic (TNP-KLH) or cellular (SRBC)

antigens or cellular immunoreaction (CTL, MLC) to allogeneic cells. Neither IL-1β nor IL-1 RA stimulate NK-cells, both increase, however, activation by IL-1.

  – The main activity of IL-1 RA seems to be inhibition of inflammations by inhibition of IL-1 mediated accumulation and activation of granulocytes and macrophages.

Clinical activity:

  – Clinical development is in progress for septic shock (phase III, NDA is planned for 1993 in the US); rheumatoid arthritis, GvHD, asthma and inflammatory bowel diseases (phase I/II).
  – Activity in allergic eye disease is going to be evaluated (phase I).
  – Results from controlled phase II study, (33 patients/group) in septic shock show a dose-dependent reduction of the death rate from 44% (control) to 25% or maximal 16% (infusion 67 mg/h or 133 mg/h, highest cumulative dose 10–30 g/patient).
  – Results from phase III study in septic shock (893 patients) show reduction in mortality from 34% (placebo) to 31% (67 mg/h) and 29% (133 mg/h).

Conti et al. 1992; Thompson et al. 1992; Hannum et al. 1990; Granowitz et al. 1992; Synergen press release 1993.

IL-1 Receptor	*Domains:*	Type I	Type II	Soluble IL-Rec.
	Extracellular	319 aa	330 aa	330 aa
	Transmembrane	20 aa	26 aa	
	Intracellular	213 aa	29 aa	
	Molecular weight:	≈ 80 kDA	60–68 kDa	46 kDa
	Distribution:	T-cells, B-cells, fibroblasts, endothelial cells, keratinocytes synovial cells	(T-cells), B-cells monocytes, macrophages, granulocytes, neutrophils, megakaryocytes	
	Receptors/cell:	25–1000	200–8000	
	Affinity (Kd):	IL-1α 0,05–0,5 nM	0,3–30 nM	
		IL-1β 0,5–10 nM	4–5 nM	
	Signal transduction:	via activation of a phosphorylation cascade involves an intrinsic G-protein-like activation		
	Internalization:	yes		
	Sequence homology:	extracellular domains of immunoglobulin superfamily		

Nicola 1991; Chizzonite et al. 1989; Bomsztyk et al. 1989; Hannum et al. 1990; Sims et al. 1989; Bomalaski et al. 1992; McMahan et al. 1991.

Recombinant IL-1 *Molecular weight:*   80 kDa (membrane bound)   59 kDa recombinant, soluble
Receptor Type I   *Affinity:*   IL-1α: 0,05–0,5 nM
(IL-1 RI)   IL-1β: 0,5–10 nM

Function:

  In vivo:

  – prophylactic activity on adjuvant arthritis in rats
  – prophylactic and therapeutic activity (dose: 25 µg/day daily for 5 days) on
    SLE (occurrence of disease, survival rate; normalization of T-cell response
    to polyclonal activation) in (lpr, lpr) mice
  – reduction of neutrophil granulocytes in bronchial lavage after intranasal
    application on IL-1 RI as mixture with bacteria or LPS
  – reduction of EAE disease in rats
  – prolongation of survival time of allogeneic heart transplants and reduction
    of lymphnode swelling in response to allogeneic cells injected; can be
    abrogated by simultaneous application of IL-1β

Fanslow et al. 1990; Jacobs et al. 1991; Schorlemmer et al. 1992.

1.2.2 IL-2

Interleukin-2 (IL-2)   Synonyms: T-cell growth factor, TCGF; killer helper factor, KHF; T-cell replac-
                          ing factor, TRF

Size and structure:
  – core protein 15 kDa, 133 aa, glycoprotein 14–16 kDa
  – monomer protein
  – 1×0-glycosylation site, glycosylation not necessary for function
  – two intrachain cysteine residues

Origin:
  secreted by T-cells after antigen specific stimulation of and co-stimulation with
  IL-1

Function:
  stimulates the proliferation of:
    short-term culture: (< 48 h)
       NK-cells
    long-term culture: (> 48 h)
       T-cells
       NK-cells
       B-cells
    in vivo: increase of PBMC from 10% to 60–80% after 12 weeks of therapy
  stimulates the secretion from:
    NK-cells:
       IFN gamma
       GM-CSF
       TNFα/β

T-cells: (B-cells)
  IL-2
  IL-1-Rec.
  TNFα/β
  IFN gamma
monocytes:
  IL-1, IL-6, IL-8, TNF
B-cells:
  Ig-production
basophils:
  histamine
stimulates
  NK-cells for cytolytic activity (cytolytic granules)
  T-cells for differentiation [help for T DTH T CTL cooperation (B-cells)
  memory T-cells]

Ritz et al. 1988; Voss et al. 1990; Lin et al. 1989; Smith 1988; Blackmen et al. 1986; Ehlers et al. 1991; Morgan et al. 1976; Sykora et al. 1984; Shows et al. 1984; Seigel et al. 1984; Ceuppens et al. 1985; White et al. 1992.

Capillary leak syndrome (CLS) provoked by IL-2, i.e. increase of generalized vascular permeability with egress of intra-vascular fluid (mainly in the lung)

Model:
  – normal mice injected with human IL-2 (dose related CLS)
Mechanism:
  – mediated via T-cells or LAK-cells interacting with or killing endothelial cells
    * athymic mice (nu/nu) or irradiated mice do not respond to IL-2 but to IL-2 + LAK-cells
    * CLS cannot be influenced by antihistamins (in humans) or serotonin agonists (mice)
    * LAK culture supernatant, IL-1, IL-2, IL-3, IL-4, IL-6, TNFα, GM-CSF, M-CSF or IFN gamma do not increase permeability of an endothelial cell monolayer; LAK-cells however, do.
  – interaction between T-cells or LAK-cells and endothelial cells may occur via secretion of lymphokines with direct vasoactive activity (lymphnode permeability factor; skin reactive factor; vascular permeability factor; TNFα)
Synergism:
  – IFNα enhances CLS induced by IL-2 (IFN gamma; TNFα is not effective; IL-1 or TNFα may even protect against IL-2 induced CLS)

Siegel et al. 1991; Krejci et al. 1989; Pick et al. 1972; Maillard 1972; Rosenstein 1986; Fairman 1987; Ettinghausen 1988; Damle 1987, 1989; Aronson 1988; Sondel 1986; Krejci 1989; Cortran 1988; Pari 1989.

Toxicities of IL-2   frequency

Heart	arrhythmias ischemia myocarditis hypocontractility	$\approx 10\%$
Kidney	azotemia oliguria reduction in sodium excretion elevated plasma renin hypotension	$\geq 50\%$
Lung	oedema	$\approx 20\%$
Gastrointestinal system	nausea vomiting diarrhea anorexia stomatitis haemorrhage intrahepatic cholestasis	$\geq 50\%$
Endocrine system	hypothyroidism increase of corticosteroids	
Dermis	macular erythema puritus psoriasis dermatomyositis	$\geq 50\%$
CNS	agitation somnolence coma	$\geq 50\%$
Blood	anemia leukopenia thrombocytopenia infections	10–50%

Siegel et al. 1991

IL-2-Receptor

Domains:	α-Subunit	β-Subunit	γ-Subunit	Soluble receptor
Extracellular	219 aa	214 aa	232 aa	219 aa
Transmembrane	19 aa	25 aa	29 aa	
Intracellular	13 aa	286 aa	86 aa	
Molecular weight:	55 kDA	75 kDa	130 kDa	45 kDa
Distribution:	T-cells after activation		resting T-cells, increase after activation	
	thymocytes myeloid precursors monocytes activated B-cells dendritic cells			
Receptors/cells:	25–1000			
Affinity (Kd):	10 nM	1 nM	1 nM	

10 pM

10 pM

| Signal transduction: | no signal transduction | phosphorylation of the beta-unit and other specific protein substrates with involvement of a protein kinase C-dependent pathway | | |
| Internalization: | – | – | | – |

yes (the gamma chain is the responsible subunit)

Smith 1989; Robb et al. 1981; Wang et al. 1987; Hatekeyama et al. 1989, 1991; Zmuidzinas et al. 1991; Gaulton et al. 1986; Saltzman et al. 1988, 1990; Asao et al. 1990; Reed et al. 1986; Stern et al. 1986; Williams et al. 1991; Minami et al. 1992.

IL-2 Receptor-Mediated Signaling

IL-2 mediates activation of T-cells, generation of lymphokine activated killer cells, augmentation of natural killer cells, growth and differentiation of B-cells, but can also act negatively in regulating cell growth and programming mature T-cells for apoptosis.

IL-2 acts by binding to the IL-2 receptor, which consists of three polypeptide chains (α, β and γ).

Binding of IL-2 to its receptor results in phosphorylation of cellular substrates including the β-chain of the receptor.

Several members of the src family of protein kinases associate with the IL-2 receptor, the most prominent being p56lck.

There are two regions in the IL-2 receptor β-chain that are responsible for the mediation of signals: the serine rich region (S) that does not require the association of src family kinases and the acidic region (A) that acts through association with the N-terminal part of p56lck.

The signals that are mediated upon binding of IL-2 to its receptor provoke among others the upregulation of the nuclear transcription factors c-*myc*, c-*myb* and c-*fos*.

Both the acidic and the serine rich regions of the IL-2 receptor are necessary for induction of *fos*.

Other signal transduction pathways as the PKC or the PKA pathway or Ca++ mobilization are not involved in IL-2 mediated signaling.

The activation of the cytoplasmic kinase *raf* is possibly involved in IL-2 mediated signaling.

Minami et al. 1992.

IL-2 Receptor Signaling

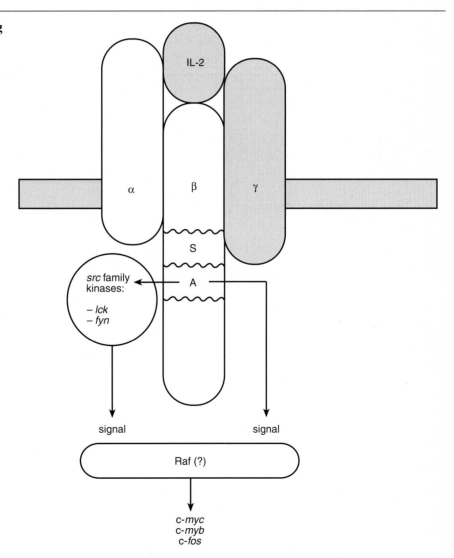

IL-2 Gene Promotor

AP1 is implicated in IL-2 gene regulation and consists of a heterodimer of *jun* and *fos*.

Phosphorylation of both *jun* and *fos* is necessary for full transactivation capacity of AP1.

Cyclosporin A blocks the activity and the promotor binding of NF-AT and NF-kB through inhibition of the phosphatase calcineurin and thus downregulates IL-2 expression.

Action of AP1 is probably not affected by cyclosporin A.

NF-kB is released from its inhibitor I-kB and translocated into the nucleus upon TCR activation and signal transduction.

NF-kB is part of the *rel* related family of transcription factors. Other members of the rel family may bind to NF-kB binding sites and can either activate or repress promotor activity.

IL-2 gene promotor contains two octamer motifs. The TCR activation induced complex that binds to these sites contains the POU transcription factor Oct-1 and another yet uncharacterized 40 kDa protein.

Fraser et al. 1993.

IL-2 Gene Transcriptional Regulation

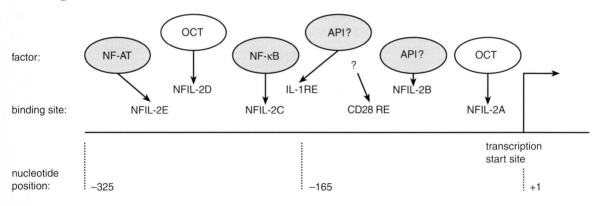

Fraser et al. 1993.

1.2.3 IL-3, IL-4, IL-5, IL-6

Interleukin-3 (IL-3)   Synonyms: colony forming unit stimulating activity, FU-SA; burst promoting activity; histamine producing cell stimulating factor; mast cell growth factor

Size and structure:
  15–25 kDa; 133 aa
    – glycoprotein; varying glycosidation results in size heterogeneity
    – one intrachain disulfide bond
Origin:
    – secreted by:
          PHA-stimulated T-cells
          CD4[+] T-helper cells
          mast cells
          keratinocytes
          thymic epithelial cells
Function:
    – species specific
    – stimulates proliferation of:
        * mast cells
        * neutrophils, basophils, eosinophils
        * macrophages
        * megakaryocytes
        * lymphocytes (T-, B-)
    activates:
        * eosinophils, basophils
        * macrophages, antigen presenting cells
          phagocytosis
          MHC-II expression
          secretion of IL-1 (synergy of IL-3 with LPS)
          secretion of IL-6, TNFα
    increases:
          expression of LFA-1 (synergy with IFN gamma, GM-CSF)
Side effects:
    fever, bone pain, headache, neck stiffnes

Ginsbury and Sachs 1963; Cerney 1974; Wagemaker et al. 1990; Luger et al. 1985; Ihle et al. 1983; Ganser et al. 1991; Frendl 1992; Oster et al. 1992; Otsuka et al. 1988; Clark-Lewis et al. 1988; Schrader et al. 1983; Shannon et al. 1987; Hauck-Freudsch et al. 1988; Cannistra et al. 1988.

IL-3 Receptor

Domains:	α-Subunit	β-Subunit	Dimer
Extracellular	287 aa	422 aa	
Transmembrane	20 aa	26 aa	
Intracellular	53 aa	433 aa	
Molecular weight:	70 kDa	120 kDa	190 kDa

Distribution: myeloid precursors, basophils, mast cells, macrophages, megakaryocytes

Receptors/cell: 100–1000

Affinity: (Kd)   10–100 nM   –   50–200 pM

Signal transduction:
– internalization of IL-3 upon binding and promotion

    of glucose uptake
– induction of translocation of protein kinase C
    from the cytosol to the plasma membrane,
    hydrolysis of phosphoinositide and generation
    of diacylglycerol
– upregulation of c-*jun* and/or activation
– of the c-*ras* protooncogene product

Sequence homology: –   IL-5-Rec.   –
                                    GM-CSF-Rec.

Palaszynski et al. 1984, Kitamura et al. 1991, Nicola et al. 1991, Farrar et al. 1985, Mufsin et al. 1992, Satoh et al. 1992.

Interleukin-4 (IL-4)

Size and structure:
    18–20 kDa; 130 aa
    – glycoprotein; three glycosylation sites; variable glycosylation gives variability in molecular weight
    – deglycosylated protein active
    – six cysteine residues

Origin:
    activated T-cells

Function:
    species-specific
    – "B-cell stimulatory" factor
    – provokes isotype switching in B-cells to IgE
    – increase in expression of Fc ε RI (mast cells, basophils) and Fc ε RII (B-cells, macrophages, eosinophils)
    – stimulates proliferation of
        lymphocytes (T-cells (TH$_2$), B-cells)
        monocytes, granulocytes, mast cells
        NK-cells
        fibroblasts
        endothelial cells
        erythrocyte progenitors and megakaryocytes
        (in synergy with G-CSF, EPO, IL-1)

- increase of cytotoxic activity of IL-2 pretreated T-cells, LAK-cells
- inhibition of cytotoxic activity of T-cells, LAK-cells in the absence of IL-2
- inhibition of release of IL-1, TNF, IL-6 and IL-8 by macrophages
- inhibition of cytotoxic activity of macrophages
- increase of surface MHC-I/II expression APC, B-cells
- inhibition of dendritric cells, induction of apoptosis
- inhibition of superoxide production in and release of oxygen radicals by macrophages

te Velde et al. 1990; Abramson et al. 1990; Becker 1992; Gauchat et al. 1992; Van Vlasselaer et al. 1992; Paul 1991; Howard et al. 1982; Spits et al. 1987; Kawakami et al. 1988, 1989; Crawford et al. 1987; Mule et al. 1987; Smith et al. 1987; Treisman et al. 1990; Littmann et al. 1989; Nishioka et al. 1991; Paul 1991; Park et al. 1987; Sideras et al. 1988; Snapper et al. 1988; Vercelli et al. 1988; Peschel et al. 1987; Kupper et al. 1987; Zlotnik et al. 1987; Koch et al. 1992.

**Biological Activity
of IL-4**

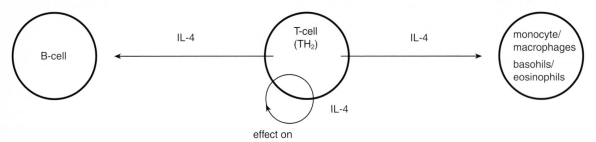

B-cell ← IL-4 → T-cell (TH₂) → IL-4 → monocyte/macrophages basohils/eosinophils

IL-4 effect on

B-cells

– proliferation (together with co-stimulation)
  (anti CD40, LPS, *Staphylococcus aureus,*
  anti IgM antibodies)
– inhibition of proliferative activity of IL-2
– maturation into mature B-cells
  by expression of
  * Fcε receptors (inhibited by IFNalpha, γ)
  * soluble IgM
  * LFA-1, -3
  * MHC-II
– increase in IgM and IgG secretion
– increase in IgE secretion in presence of
  T-cells or second signal (i.e. EBV)
  (blockage by IFN gamma)
– increase in IL-6 and TNF secretion

T-cells

– proliferation (CD4 + CD8)
  synergism with IL-2)
– enhancement of generation of CTL
– blockage of IFN gamma secretion by
  activated T-cells

effect on NK-cells

– reduction of TNF and serine protease
  secretion
– blockage of induction of LAK-cells
  by IL-2

Monocyte/macrophages

– increase in expression of
  * MHC-II
  * Fc ε receptors
  * M-CSF, G-CSF, GM-CSF
– inhibition of the secretion of
  * IL-1, TNFalpha, IL-6, IL-8, PGE2

basophils/eosinophils

differentiation from progenitors into
  basophils and eosinophils
– reduction of expression of Fc gamma
  receptors
– increase of Fc ε RI-receptors

bone marrow culture

– synergy with G-CSF, Epo in stimulation
  of proliferation

Banchereau et al. 1991; Baskar et al. 1990; Coffmann et al. 1986; Damle et al. 1989; Defrance et al. 7,8,9,10; Essner et al. 1989; Favre et al. 1990; Gordon et al. 1988; Hoffman e tal. 1988; Horokov et al. 1988; Howard et al. 1982; Isakson 1982; Kawakami et al. 1988; Rousset et al. 1989, 1998; Shields et al. 1989; Spits et al. 1988, 1987; Typhronitis et al. 1989; VallÇ et al. 1989; Vercelli et al. 1989, 1988; Wieser et al. 1989; Yokota et al. 1988, 1986; Dean et al. 1992.

IL-4-Receptor

Domains: Soluble IL-4-Rec.

    Extracellular   207 aa   207 aa (by alternative splicing)

    Transmembrane   24 aa

    Intracellular   569 aa

Molecular weight: 140 kDa   40 kDa

Distribution: T-cells, B-cells, monocytes, macrophages, NK-cells, granulocytes, mast cells, megakaryocytes, erythroid progenitors, fibroblasts, endothelial cells, muscle cells, brain, liver cells, bone marrow stromal cells

Receptors/cell: 100–5000

affinity (Kd):   0,05–1 nM

Signal transduction: involvement of serine and proline rich regions of the intracellular domain and cellular TPK

Cabrillat et al. 1987; Park et al. 1987; Galizzi et al. 1990; Idzerda et al. 1990; Seder et al. 1992; Rodriguez et al. 1992.

Interleukin-5 (IL-5)

Synonyms: eosinophil differentiating factor, EDF; T-cell replacing factor, TRF; B-cell growth factor, BCGF; IgA-enhancing factor, IgA-EF

Size and structure:
- glycoprotein: 45 kDa, 134 aa, core protein 12,4 kDa
- three intrachain cysteine residues
- three N-glycosylation sites
- disulfide linked dimer

Origin:
- activated T-cells

Function:
- high degree of species cross-reactivity
- differentiation, activation and chemotaxis of eosinophils
- stimulates proliferation and differentiation of B-cells
  * induction of IL-2 responsiveness
  * stimulation of IgM secretion and isotype switch to IgA
  * cooperation with IL-4 in increasing IgE secretion and CD23 expression
- cooperation with IL-2 to stimulate differentiation of T-cells into CTL, upregulation of IL-2 receptors on T-cells
- activation of basophil granulocytes

Sanderson 1990; Sanderson et al. 1988; Yokota et al. 1987; Takatsu et al. 1988; Tominaga et al. 1988, 1991; Azuma et al. 1986; Desreumaux et al. 1992; Nakanishi et al. 1987; Rasmussen et al. 1988; Bischoff et al. 1990; Takatsu et al. 1987; Pene et al. 1988; Harriman et al. 1988; Murray et al. 1987; Murahami et al. 1988; Swain et al. 1988.

IL-5-Receptor

Domains:	α-Subunit	β-Subunit (gp 130)	Dimer	Soluble rec.(a)
Extracellular	322 aa	422 aa		322 aa
Transmembrane	22 aa	26 aa		
Intracellular	54 aa	433 aa		
Molecular weight:	60 kDa	130 kDa	190 kDa	
Distribution:	B-cells, eosinophil granulocytes, basophil granulo-cytes, thymocytes			
Receptors/cell:	500–1000	–	7500–10000	
Affinity (Kd):	2–30 nM		10–100 pM	
Signal transduction:	possible involvement of proline rich cluster of intra-cellular domain and TPK			
Sequence homology:	β-subunit shared with IL-3-Rec. and GM-CSF-Rec.			

Devos et al 1991, Nicola et al. 1991, Mita et al. 1989, Desreumaux et al. 1992.

Interleukin-6 (IL-6)

Synonyms: IFNβ$_2$, B-cell stimulating factor, BSF-2; hepatocyte-stimulating factor, HSF

Size and structure:
 – glycoprotein 22–29 kDa, 213 aa
 – two intrachain disulfide bonds
 – several O- and N-linked glycosylation sites
 – variable glycosylation may affect activity
 – sequence homology to growth factors (G-CSF, chicken-myelomonocytic GF) and to inhibitory factors (oncostatin M; leukemia inhibitory factor, LIF)

Origin:
 – produced in:
  macrophages, T-cells, B-cells, fibroblasts, bone marrow stromal cells, endo-thelial cells, epidermal cells, microglia cells, chondrocytes, osteocytes
 – induced by:
  TPA, virus infection, leukotriene B$_4$, DNA damaging (UV-B light, ionizing radiation), endotoxins
 – suppression by:
  IL-1, TNF alpha (TNFβ, OSM, PDGF), TGFβ, IL-4, IFN gamma

Function:
 – high degree of species cross-reactivity
 – dependent on degree of glycosylation
 – action on
  * B-cells:
   initiation of IgM-IgG synthesis (synergy with IL-1) (no stimulation of B-cell proliferation)
  * T-cells:
   activation (in cooperation with IL-2 and other cytokines), induction of differentiation to CTL

* stem cells:
  proliferation of G-CSFU, M-CSFU, Meg-CSFU, E-CSFU co-stimulatory with M-CSF, G-CSF, GM-CSF or IL-4
  differentiation: Meg-CFU (in cooperation with IL-3) erythropoiesis (in cooperation with IL-4, Epo) B-cells (IgM-IgG synthesis)
* endothelial cells:
  angiogenesis (ovary, uterus)
* liver cells:
  increase in production of: amyloid A, CRP (α_1-AT, α_2-MG, haptoglobin, fibrinogen)
  decrease in production of: albumin, α_1-I3
* neurites:
  growth
- weak antiviral activity
- some of the immunosuppressive effects of glucocorticoids can be ascribed to their inhibition of IL-6 production by monocytes and fibroblasts
- estrogens inhibit IL-6 production by bone marrow stromal cells and may act antiosteoporotic by this pathway

Kishimoto et al. 1989; Brack et al. 1992; Biliau et al. 1987; Gauldie et al. 1987; Wong et al. 1988; Walther et al. 1988; Roodmann et al. 1992; Frei et al. 1989; van Snick et al. 1986, 1988; Ishibashi et al. 1989; Planck et al. 1992; Taga et al. 1987; Hagan et al. 1992; Girasole et al. 1992.

Elevated Levels of IL-6 in Diseases

Disease	IL-6 increase found in	References
Meningitis (bacterial, viral)	cerebrospinal fluid	Houssian et al. 1988
Amniotic infections	amniotic fluid	Romero et al. 1990
General infections (acute)	serum	Bauer et al. 1991
		Helfgott et al. 1989
HIV infection (AIDS)	serum	Breen et al. 1990
Chronic rheumatory arthritis	synovia (chondrocytes)	Hirano et al. 1988
Chronic inflammatory bowel disease	serum	Andus et al. 1991
Psoriasis	keratocytes	Grossmann et al. 1989
Glomerulonephritis	mesangial cells	Schlöndorff
		(Brack et al. 1992)
Transplant rejection	serum	Oers et al. 1988
Lymphoma (Castleman)	germinal centers	Villinger et al. 1991
Dementia (Alzheimer)	cortical plaques	Bauer et al. 1991
Osteodystrophia (Paget)	serum, bone marrow	Roodman et al. 1992
Multiple myeloma	serum, bone marrow	Bataille et al. 1989
		Klein et al. 1990
AML	leukemic cells	Oster et al. 1989
CML, CMML	leukemic cells	Everson et al. 1989
		Klein et al. 1990
Carcinoma (cervix, kidney, keratocytes, bladder, dendrites, smooth muscle)	tumor cells	Brack et al. 1992
Sarcoma (Kaposi)	tumor cells	Miles et al. 1990

The increase of IL-6 may be cause or consequence of the disease.

IL-6-Receptor	*Domains:*	IL-6-Rec.	GP-130 subunit	Complex	Soluble IL-6-Rec.
	Extracellular	339 aa	597 aa		339 aa
	Transmembrane	28 aa	22 aa		
	Intracellular	82 aa	277 aa		
	Molecular weight:	80 kDa	130 kDa	210 kDa	
	Distribution:	T-cells, B-cells, monocytes, fibroblasts, megakaryocytes, hepatocytes, keratinocytes, mesangial cells			
	Receptors/cells:	50–2000	–	50–2000	
	Affinity (Kd):	1–10 nM		40–70 pM	
	Signal transduction:	gp 130 does not bind IL-6 but mediates signal transduction via cellular tyrosine kinase and protein kinase and increased expression of the c-*fos* and c-*myc* protooncogenes			
	Sequence homology:	homology with LIF			

Kishimoto et al. 1989; Yamasaki et al. 1988; Taga et al. 1989; Hibi et al. 1990; Matsuda et al. 1988; Hirano 1991; Simpson et al. 1988; Hirano et al. 1992; Korholz et al. 1992; Honda et al. 1992.

1.2.4 LIF, IL-7, IL-8

Leukemia Inhibitory Factor (LIF)

Synonyms: differentiation-inducing factor, D-factor; differentiation-inhibitory factor, DIA; osteoclast activating factor, OAF

Size and structure:
 – glycoprotein 50-58 kDa, 179 aa, monomer
 – O- and N-linked glycosylation
 – approx. 50% of weight oligosaccharides, not essential for function
 – three intrachain disulfide bonds

Origin:
 – bone marrow stromal cells (after activation by IL-1α, -β, TGF-β or TNF)
 – thymic epithelial cells
 – carcinoma cells

Function:
 – shares many activities with IL-6
  * regulation of proliferation and differentiation of hematopoietic cells
  * enhancement of megakaryopoiesis in synergy with GM-CSF and IL-3
  * stimulation of osteoblasts, bone formation and calcification
 – inhibition of lipoprotein lipase activity in adipocytes *(induction of Cachexia)*
 – induction of myoblast proliferation
 – inhibition of angiogenesis
 – inhibition of stem cell differentiation

Metcalf et al. 1991, Rose et al. 1991, Le et al. 1990, Gascan et al. 1990, Wetzler et al. 1991, Bhatt et al. 1991, Leary et al. 1990, Bard et al. 1991, Smith et al. 1988.

LIF-Receptor   *Domains:*   LIF-rec.   complex with second subunit
                                                                        (no disulfide bonds)

                              Extracellular   789 aa
                              Transmembrane   26 aa
                              Intracellular   238 aa
                              Molecular weight: 250 kDa   370 kDa
                              Distribution: haematopoietic stem cells, megakaryocyte
                                                      progenitors, osteoblasts, neurons, myoblasts,
                                                      adipose cells, embryonic stem cells, hepatocytes,
                                                      kidney, epithelial cells, placental tissue
                                                      (not on lymphocytes, NK-cells, granulocytes, platelets)
                              Receptors/cell: 1000–6000   150–500
                              Affinity (Kd):   1–3 nM   10–300 pM
                              Signal transduction: activation of cellular TPK and protein phosphorylation
                              Sequence homology: IL-6 receptor (GP 130)

Hilton et al. 1988, Godard et al. 1992, Ferrera et al. 1992.

Interleukin-7 (IL-7)   Synonym: lymphopoietin-1, LP-1

                              Size and structure:
                                  – glycoprotein 22-25 kDa, 152 aa, core protein: 17,4 kDa
                                  – three N-glycosylation sites
                              Origin:
                                  – bone marrow stromal cells
                              Function:
                                  – moderate species specificity
                                  – stimulates growth and differentiation of precursor B-lymphocytes
                                  – stimulates proliferation of early T-cell progenitors (in synergy with SCF)
                                  – stimulates proliferation of T-cells (independent from IL-2)
                                  – differentiation factor for CD8[+] T-cells to become CTL (in synergy with
                                    IL-2 and IL-6)
                                  – increases expression of ICAM-1 on melanocytes and melanoma cells
                                  – supports megakaryocyte maturation

Namen et al. 1988, Goodwin et al. 1989, Morrisey et al. 1989, Grabstein et al. 1990, Hickman
et al. 1990, Kirnbauer et al. 1992.

IL-7-Receptor	*Domains:*	High-affinity receptor	Soluble receptor	Low affinity receptor
	Extracellular	219 aa	219 aa (by alternate splicing)	?
	Transmembrane	25 aa		
	Intracellular	195 aa		
	Molecular weight:	75–80 kDa	≈ 40 kDa	62–70 kDa
	Distribution:	B-cell progenitors, thymocytes, T-cells, CTL, LAK-cells, bone marrow macrophages	B-cell progenitors monocytes, other?	
	Receptors/cells:	250–750	1500–10000	
	Affinity (Kd):	10–100 pM	10–100 nM	
	Signal transduction:	via cellular TPK tyrosine phosphorylation of at least five major cytoplasmic proteins and transcriptional activation of the N-*myc* and c-*myc* protooncogenes	Unknown	

Touw et al. 1990, Goodwin et al. 1990, Armitage et al. 1992, Roifman et al. 1992, Morrow et al. 1992.

Interleukin-8 (IL-8)

Synonyms: leukocyte-adhesion inhibitor, LAI; neutrophil activation protein, NAP-1; neutrophil chemotactic factor, NCF

Size and structure:
– protein: 8 kDa, precursor: 10 kDa, 99 aa 4 variants: 77 aa, 72 aa, 70 aa, 69 aa generated from a common precursor of 99 aa by proteases, 72 aa is most active
– no glycosylation site
– four cysteine residues
– two intrachain disulfide bonds
– sequence homology (cysteine-X-cysteine family) to platelet factor 4, β-thromboglobulin
– in solution IL-8 exists as a dimer, and shows structural resemblance with the α_1/α_2 domains of human MHC-class I

Origin: monocytes, synovial cells, activated T-cells, fibroblasts, epithelial cells, chondrocytes, endothelial cells, keratinocytes, mesothelial cells

Function:
– activation of neutrophil granulocytes leading to
  * chemotactic behaviour towards IL-8
  * augmentation of exocytosis of lysosomal enzymes
  * upregulation of adhesion molecule (Mac-1) and complement receptor (CR-1) expression
  * inhibition of adhesion of PMN to endothelial cells

van Damme et al. 1989, Schroder et al. 1987, Yoshimura et al. 1987, Gregory et al. 1988, Lindley et al. 1988, Clore et al. 1990, Baldwin et al. 1990, Lotz et al. 1992, Farina et al. 1989, Paccaud et al. 1990, Lee et al. 1992, Beall et al. 1992.

IL-8-Receptor

Domains:	Type I	Type II	MCAF-Rec.
Extracellular	4×	4×	
	(39 aa, 13 aa,	(40 aa, 14 aa,	
	29 aa, 27 aa)	23 aa, 17 aa)	
Transmembrane	7×	7×	
	(28 aa, 23 aa,	(27 aa, 26 aa,	
	22 aa, 20 aa,	22 aa, 26 aa,	
	23 aa, 22 aa,	24 aa, 23 aa,	
	38 aa)	25 aa)	
Intracellular	4×	5×	
	(8 aa, 21 aa,	(8 aa, 17 aa,	
	16 aa, 38 aa)	23 aa, 19 aa,	
		44 aa)	
Molecular weight:	58 kDa	67 kDa	≈ 40 kDa
Distribution:	neutrophils, basophils,		Monocytes
	T-cells, monocytes		
Receptors/cells:	20 000–50 000	1000–2000	10 000–20 000
Ligands:	only IL-8	IL-8,	MCAF
		MGSA/GRO,	
		NAP-2	
Affinity (Kd):	0,1–4 nM	0,3–2 nM	2–25 nM
Signal transduction:	coupled to and via G-proteins		?
	activation of protein kinase C,		
	internalization of receptors		
	and recycling back to cell surface		

Holmes et al. 1991, Murphy et al. 1991, Grob et al. 1990, Samanta et al. 1990.

1.2.5 IL-10, IL-11, IL-12, IL-13

Interleukin-10 (IL-10)

Synonym: cytokine synthesis inhibiting factor

Size and structure:
  – protein 18 kDa, 179 aa (leader sequence 18 aa)
  – monomer, not glycosylated
  – sequence homology to BCRF1 of EBV
Origin:
  B-lymphocytes, EBV-positive B-cell lines, T-lymphocytes (TH2), monocytes
  (LPS-activated)
Function:
  species specific
  on T-cells (TH$_1$):
    * inhibition of cytokine synthesis (IFN gamma, IL-2, others)

on B-cells:
* stimulation of proliferation and differentiation
* inducing MHC-class II antigen expression but (in contrast to IL-4) no increase of CD23 expression
* cooperation with $TGF\beta_1$ to induce IgA synthesis, blockage of IL-4 induced isotype switch to IgE

on thymocytes:
* increase of proliferation (in synergy with IL-2, IL-4)

on macrophages:
* inhibition of secretion of IL-1, IL-3, $TNF\alpha$, GM-CSF, IFN gamma
* inhibition of IL-1α, -β, GM-CSF, IL-3, IL-6, IL-8, $TNF\alpha$, IFN gamma production
* upregulation of IL-1RA expression
* downregulation of MHC-class II expression

on mast cells:
* increase of proliferation (synergy with IL-3 or IL-4)

in lymphomas (positive for HIV + EBV):
autocrine growth factor

Emilie et al. 1992, Thomas 1992, Fiorentino et al. 1989, Suda et al. 1990, O'Garra et al. 1990, Go et al. 1990, Thompson-Snipes et al. 1991, Bogdan et al. 1991, Waal Melafyt et al. 1991, Benjamin et al. 1992, Vieira et al. 1991.

Interleukin-11 (IL-11)   *Size and structure:*
protein 23 kDa, 199 aa
Origin:
– bone marrow stromal fibroblast cells
– fetal fibroblast cells
– mesenchymal adherent cells
Function:
– stimulation of (T-cell dependent) development of B-cells
– stimulation of megakaryocytopoiesis in synergy with IL-3 (IL-11 alone does not stimulate)
– support of proliferation of committed macrophage progenitors

---

Paul et al. 1990, Thomas et al. 1992, Teramura et al. 1992.

Interleukin-12 (IL-12)   Synonyms: natural killer cell stimulatory factor, NKSF; cytotoxic lymphocyte
                               maturation factor, CLMF

Size and structure:
  glycoprotein 75 kDa
  disulfide linked heterodimeric;
  light chain 35 kDa
      (197 aa, 7 cysteine residues, 3 potential glycosylation sites)
  heavy chain 40 kDa
      (306 aa, 10 cysteine residues, 4 potential N-linked glycosylation sites)
      sequence homology mouse/man 70% (p40) or 60% (p35)
Origin:
  B-cells (EBV transformed)
Function: in vitro activity:
  cooperates with IL-2 in the generation and proliferation of
  – cytotoxic T-cells
  – NK-cells
  – LAK-cells
  increases the cytotoxic activity of
  – NK-cells
  induces IFN gamma production and secretion in T-cells, NK-cells
  inhibits IL-4 induced IgE secretion (inhibition of switching to IgE) in B-cells
  induces primarily a TH1 response in vitro and in vivo

Kiniwa et al. 1992; Gubler et al. 1991; Wolf et al. 1991; Kobayashi et al. 1989; Gately et al. 1991;
Chan et al. 1991; Plant et al. 1989; Stern et al. 1990; Wong et al. 1988; Naume et al. 1992; Hsieh
et al. 1993.

Interleukin-13 (IL-13)   *Size and structure:*
  – protein 10 kDa, 132 aa, not glycosylated
  – protein sequence ≈ 30 % homologous to IL-4; no homology with other cyto-
    kines
  – mouse and human IL-13 ≈ 58 % identical
Origin:
  – TH2 cells
Function:
  – induction of differentiation of
    * monocytes into macrophages
    * B-cells into plasma cells
  – induction of Fc ε RII (CD23) expression on B-cells, macrophages and
    eosinophils
  – in B-cells stimulation of
    * synthesis of mRNA
    * IgG4–IgE switching
    * secretion of (IgM) IgG4; IgE
  – activity is independent of IL-4 (no inactivation by MAb anti IL-4, no bind-
    ing to IL-4-Rec.)

Mc Kenzie et al. 1993; Punnonen et al. 1993.

1.2.6 GM-CSF, G-CSF, M-CSF, Erythropoietin, Thrombopoitein, IFN-γ

Granulocyte-Macro-phage Colony-Stimulating Factor (GM-CSF)

Size and structure:
- core protein 14,7 kDa, 127 aa
- four cysteine residues forming intrachain disulfide bonds
- glycoprotein 13–30 kDa

Origin:
   activated T-cells, macrophages, mast cells, endothelial cells, fibroblasts, osteoblasts

Function:
- species-specific
- stimulation of colony formation in semisolid medium (enter of S phase of cell cycle) of
  * granulocytes and macrophages (at low concentrations)
  * eosinophil, megakaryocytes and erythroblasts, multipotential hematopoietic cells (GEMM) (at higher concentrations)
  * continuous stimulation is needed
- activation of neutrophils, eosinophils, basophils, macrophages, endothelial cells, dendritic cells
- synergy with G-CSF or M-CSF
- suppression of proliferation of leukemic cells

Metcalf 1986; Gasson et al. 1984, 1991; Wong et al. 1985; Lee et al. 1985; Dunlop et al. 1991.

GM-CSF Receptors

Domains:	α-Subunit	β-Subunit	Dimer	Soluble α-subunit
Extracellular	297 aa	422 aa		297 aa
Transmembrane	27 aa	26 aa		
Intracellular	54 aa	433 aa		
Molecular weight:	84 kDa	120 kDa	205 kDa	

Distribution: myeloid precursors, monocytes, macrophages, eosinophils, neutrophils, megakaryocytes, endo-thelial cells, osteoblasts, Langerhans cells

Receptors/cell: 100–500

Affinity (Kd): 1–8 nM   –   3–100 pM

Signal transduction:
– via activation of G-protein and cellular TPK
– ligand receptor is recycled to the cell membrane
  (10% of receptor occupancy sufficient
  for stimulation of target cell)

Sequence homology:
– β-subunit shared with IL-3-Rec. and IL-5-Rec.
– binding of GM-CSF to its receptor downmodulates
  expression of receptors for G-CSF and M-CSF

Gearing et al. 1989; Metcalf 1990; Gasson et al. 1986; DiPersio et al. 1988; Dunlop et al. 1991.

GM-CSF Has Broad Biological Functions

Effect of GM-CSF

Cell type	Prolife-ration	Function
Bone marrow	+	
Neutrophils	+	– inhibition of migration
		– increase in
		* formation of radical oxygen
		* cytokine secretion
		* phagocytosis
		* exocytosis
		* arachidonic acid release, leukotriene and PAF synthesis
		* cytotoxicity (ADCC)
		* recruitment
		– changes in expression of adhesion molecules
Eosinophils	+	– increase in
		* cytotoxicity (ADCC)
		* leukotriene synthesis
Basophils	+	– provokes histamine release
Macrophages	+	– increase in
		* formation of radical oxygen
		* cytokine expression
		* cytotoxicity
		* adherence
Dendritic cells		– maturation
		– increases APC function
Endothelial cells	+	– activation

Gasson 1991.

Granulocyte Colony-Stimulating Factor (G-CSF)

Size and structure:
- core protein 18,6 kDa
- glycoprotein 20–24 kDa
- intrachain disulfide bridges

Origin:
activated T-cells, macrophages, endothelial cells, melanomas

Function:
- limited species specificity
- stimulation of colony formation in semisolid medium (enter of S phase of cell cycle) of
  * granulocytes (at low concentration)
  * macrophages (at high concentrations)
  * continuous stimulation is needed
- inhibition of maturation and activation
- suppression of proliferation of leukemic cells

Metcalf 1986, 1990.

G-CSF Receptor

Domains:	Monomer	Oligomer
Extracellular	603 aa	
Transmembrane	26 aa	
Intracellular	130 or 183 aa	
Molecular weight:	150 kDa	
Distribution:	granulocytes, pluripotent stem cells, myeloid progenitors, T-cells, fibroblasts, endothelial cells	
Receptors/cell:	50–500	
Affinity (Kd):	2–4 nM	0,05–0,4 nM
Signal transduction:	– activation of cellular TPK (10% of receptor occupancy sufficient for stimulation of target cell)	
	– binding of G-CSF to its receptor down-modulates the expression of receptors for GM-CSF and M-CSF	

Metcalf 1990, Dunlop et al. 1991.

Macrophage Colony-Stimulating Factor (M-CSF)

Size and structure:
- core protein 21 kDa
- glycoprotein 70–90 kDa
- intrachain disulfide bridges
- dimer with two equal subunits

Origin:
   monocytes, endothelial cells, fibroblasts

Function:
- stimulation of colony formation in semisolid medium (enter of S phase of cell cycle) of
  * macrophages (at low concentration)
  * granulocytes (at higher concentrations)
  * continuous stimulation is needed
  * synergy with GM-CSF
- commitment of bipotential progenitor cell to differentiate to macrophage progenitors
- initiation of maturation and activation

Metcalf 1974, 1986, 1990; Kawasaki et al. 1985; Das et al. 1982.

M-CSF Receptor

Domains: Soluble receptor
    Extracellular   512 aa   ≈ 500 aa
    Transmembrane   25 aa
    Intracellular   435 aa
Molecular weight: 165 kDa   100 kDa
Distribution: monocytes, macrophages and their committed precursors
                          placental trophoblasts
Receptors/cell: 1000–2000
Affinity (Kd):   0,2–0,4 nM
Signal transduction: M-CSF binding initiates dimerization of
                          receptors; activation of intrinsic TPK,
                          autophosphorylation and phosphorylation of
                          cellular proteins
                          binding of M-CSF to its receptor downmodulates
                          the expression of G-CSF and GM-CSF receptors

Sherr et al. 1985, 1990; Metcalf 1990.

Erythropoietin (Epo)

Size and structure:
  – glycoprotein 27–60 kDa, 166 aa
  – core protein 18 kDa
  – three sites for N-glycosylation, 1 site for O-glycosylation
  – carbohydrate composition ≈ 29%
    (sialic acid ≈ 7,7%, hexose 13%, *N*-acetylglucosamine 8,9%)
  sialic acid residues and N-linked oligosaccharides at Asp-24 and Asp-38 are
    important for biological activity
Origin:
  juxtoglomerular cells of the kidney, fetal liver cells
Function:
  – stimulation of proliferation of and differentiation into
    * pluripotent stem cells
    * granulocyte-erythrocyte-monocyte-megakaryocyte-CFU (GEMM-CFU)
    * erythrocyte-CFU (E-CFU)
    * erythroblasts
  – stimulation of denucleation of erythrocytes
  – acts at some point in G_1 as a cell cycle progression factor

Miyake et al. 1977, Goldwasser et al. 1975, Lin et al. 1985, Espada et al. 1972, Dube et al. 1988, Glass t al. 1975, Gallagher et al. 1962, Paul et al. 1973, Tsuda et al. 1989.

Erythropoietin	*Domains:*	Epo Rec.	G130 subunit	Complex
Receptor	Extracellular	225 aa	597 aa	
	Transmembrane	22 aa	22 aa	
	Intracellular	236 aa	277 aa	
	Molecular weight:	66 kDa	130 kDa	66 kDa + 130 kDa
	Sequence homology:	β-chain of IL-2 receptor		
	Distribution:	erythroid progenitors, megakaryocytes		
	Receptors/cell:	100–1000	–	
	Affinity (Kd):	200 pM	–	100 pM

Signal transduction:
– possibly via complex formation with the
  subunit GP 130
– changes in the phosphorylation level of
  both proteins, changes in the expression
  of the c-*myc* and c-*myb* protooncogenes and
  increase in intracellular free calcium ions

D'Andrea et al. 1989, Yoshimura et al. 1992, Choi et al. 1991, Quelle et al. 1991, Chern et al. (1991).

Thrombopoietin

Synonym: c-*mpl*-ligand)

Size and structure:
– glycoprotein $\approx$ 38 kDa, 332 aa
– 23% identity between the N-terminal region (153 aa) of the thrombopoietin
  and erythropoietin (including conservative substitutions $\approx$ 50% homology)
– four cysteins, two cysteins form disulfide bonds
– six potential N-linked glycosylation sites located in the C-terminal half of
  the protein

Origin:
liver cells (fetal, adult), kidney cells (adult)

Function:
species specific (limited)
– stimulation of proliferation of megakaryocytes (Meg-CSF activity)
– maturation of megakaryocytes (thrombopoietin activity)
– activity superior to IL-3 and other cytokines

Receptors/cell:
c-*mpl*
expressed only on primitive stem cells, megakaryocytes and platelets

de Sauvage et al. 1994.

Interferon γ   Synonym: immune interferon
(IFN gamma)
                          Size and structure:
                          – glycoprotein 20–25 kDa, 166 aa (signal peptide 23 aa)
                          – core protein 17 kDa
                          – two glycosylation sites
                          – N-terminal pyroglutamate residue
                          Origin:
                          activated T-cells, NK-cells
                          Function:
                          species specific
                          – antiviral activity
                          – enhancement of TNF cytotoxicity
                          – increase of cellular cytotoxicity (macrophages, NK-cells)
                          – induction of MHC-class I and class II expression
                          – upregulation of secretory component for IgA and IgM
                          – upregulation of Fc gamma RI on granulocytes
                          – inhibition of osteoclasts, activated by IL-1
                          – inhibition of IL-4 induced isotype switch in B-cells
                          – synergy with TNF in induction of differentiation of human neuroblastoma
                            cells

Trinchieri et al. 1985, Perussia et al. 1980, Ponzoni et al. 1992, Sato et al. 1992, Nakamura et al. 1984, Leibson et al. 1984, Sidman et al. 1984, Petroni et al. 1988, Sollid et al. 1987, Pace et al. 1983, Gerrard et al. 1988, Giacomini et al. 1988, Wong et al. 1983.

IFN gamma Receptor	*Domains:*	IFN gamma rec.	Soluble rec.
	Extracellular	228 aa	228 aa
	Transmbembrane	23 aa	
	Intracellular	221 aa	
	Molecular weight:	90 kDa	
	Distribution:	on nearly all cells except erythrocytes (including B-cells, macrophages, fibroblasts, endothelial cells) species-specific, ≈ 52 % homology to IFN-γ-receptor of other species; homology to IFNα receptor	
	Receptors/cell:	200–10 000	
	Affinity (Kd):	5–0,05 pM	
	Signal transduction:	phosphorylation of serine and threonine after ligand binding, generation of cAMP and hydrolysis of phosphoinositide	
	Regulation:	glycosylation in ER + Golgi (5 glycosylation sites); traffics along the plasma membrane; extracellular exposure of only 20–33 % of total pool: ligand receptor conjugates are internalized, dissociated, dephosphorylated and recycled	
	Sequence homology:	to IFNα receptors, to IFN gamma receptors of other species (strong species specificity)	

Schreiber et al. 1991; Sheehan et al. 1988; van Loon et al. 1991; Hershey et al. 1990; Mao et al. 1990; Finbloom et al. 1985; Aguet et al. 1988; Gray et al. 1989.

1.2.7 IGF, TNF, TGF, PDGF, EGF, FGF

Insulin-like Growth Factor (IGF)

Synonym: somatomedin A/C, SmA/SmC

Size and structure:
- polypeptide, two major forms:
  * IGF-I: 7,65 kDa, 70 aa, single chain
  * IGF-II: 7,47 kDa, 70 aa, single chain sequence homology to IgFI 62%
- IGF (I,II) binding protein (in serum)
  * α-subunit: 80 kDa
  * β-subunit: 53 kDa (BP53) or 28 kDa (BP28) IGF binding subunits
- complexed IGF: 150 kDa or 115 kDa
  * IGF is inactive by complex formation
  * complexes release IGF

Origin:
- IGF-I: liver cells, fibroblasts, other parenchymal cells
- IGF-II: fibroblasts, others (?)

Function:
paracrine and autocrine growth factor for parenchymal cells

Zapf et al. 1986, Froesch et al. 1985, Schwander et al. 1983, Scott et al. 1985, Schimpf et al. 1981, Marquardt et al. 1981, Rechler et al. 1980, Dercole et al. 1984, Sara et al. 1982.

IGF-Receptor

	IGF-Receptor (type I)	IGF-Receptor (type II)
Domains:		
Extracellular	disulfide linked hetero-dimer consisting of	2207 aa
Transmembrane	extracellular α-subunit and transmembrane β-unit	
Intracellular		164 aa
Molecular weight:	130 kDa + 90 kDa	250 kDa
Distribution:	hepatocytes, adipocytes, chondrocytes, fibroblasts, erythrocytes, lymphocytes, pituitary cells, neural cells	
Affinity (Kd):	IGF-I: 1–2 nM	
	IGF-II: 2–4 nM	IGF-II: ?
	Insulin: 100 nM	
Signal transduction:	association of hetero-dimers to tetrameric structures, activation of intrinsic tyrosine phosphokinase	mannosephosphat receptor; cycles among golgi, endo-somal and plasma membrane compart-ments

Baxter et al. 1986, Steele-Perkins et al. 1988, Chou et al. 1987, Roth et al. 1988, Czech et al. 1989.

Tumor Necrosis Factor (TNF)		TNF-α (cachectin)	TNF-β (lymphotoxin)
Size and structure:		polypeptide	glycoprotein
	MW (monomer)	17,4 kDa, 157 aa (formation of multimers of two or three identical subunits)	20–25 kDa, 169 aa (formation of multimers of two or three identical subunits)
	Carbohydrates	Ø	single site
	Cysteins	2 (1 disulphide bond)	Ø
	Homology α/β	56%	56%
Origin:		macrophages NK-cells (free and membrane bound)	T-cells NK-cells
Induced by:		LPS, activation of producing cells	activation of producing cells
Function:			
Induction of			
	– GM-CSF, G-CSF, M-CSF	+++ (endothelial cells)	– (endothelial cells)
	– IL-1	+++	(+)
	– Adhesion molecules (LCAM)	+++	(+)
	– TNF-Rec.	+++ (T-cells)	
	– IL-2-Rec	+++ (T-cells)	
	– MHC-I	++ (T-cells)	
	– MHC-II	++ (T-cells)	
	– IFN gamma	++ (T-cells)	
	– Hypercalcemia	–	+++
	– Shock	+++	–
	– Coagulation	+++	
Suppression of			
	– Coagulation inhibitor	+++	
	– Lipoprotein lipase	+++ (induction of cachexia)	–
Activation of			
	– Neutrophils	+++	+++
	– Endothelium	+++	+++
	– Chondroclasts	+++	–
	– Osteoclasts	+++	+++
Protection against			
	– Parasites (platelets)	–	+++
	– Parasites (eosinophils)	+++	–
	– Bacteria	+++	–
	– HSV, HIV	+++	
Synergism with IL-1		+++	+++
Cytotoxicity		+++	+++

Porter 1991; Beutler 1989; Paul et al. 1988; Porter 1990; Kawahami et al. 1982; Le et al. 1987; Vogel et al. 1987; Munker et al. 1986.

TNF-Receptor

		TNF receptor p55–60	TNF receptor p75–80	Soluble TNF receptor 190/235 aa
Domains:				
Extracellular		190 aa	235 aa	
Transmembrane		21 aa	30 aa	
Intracellular		223 aa	196 aa	
Molecular weight:		60 kDa	80 kDa	
Distribution:		ubiquitous		
Receptors/cell:		1000–15 000	1000–15 000	
Affinity (Kd):	monomer:	1–10 nM	1–10 nM	
	oligomer:	300–500 pM	50–100 pM	
		(both for TNFα and TNFβ)		

Signal transduction: trimeric TNF induces formation of oligomeric high affinity receptor, activation of PLA2 and activation of cellular TPKs TNFα receptor complexes are internalized and degraded via the lysosomal pathway. Manipulations, which block receptor internalization or lysosomal processing inhibit the action of TNFα.

Niitsu et al. 1985, Lautz et al. 1990, Nophar et al. 1990, Heller et al. 1990, Pennica et al. 1992, Goodwin et al. 1991, Tartaglia et al. 1992.

| **Transforming Growth Factor-β (TGFβ)** | Synonym: dicidual suppressor factor, DSF |

Size and structure:
- polypeptide MW 25 kDa, 112-114 aa,
- two polypeptide chains linked by -S-S-bonds
- no glycosylation site

subtypes:

TGF-β_1, -β_2, -$\beta_{1,2}$, -β_3, -β_4, -β_5 (70–79% sequence homology)
- activation of pro TGFβ via:
- cleavage by proteinases (plasmin)   Lyons et al. 1988, 1989
- acid or alkali treatment   Lawrence et al. 1985
- inactivation by:
- binding to α_2-macroglobulin   O'Connor-Mc Court et al.
- trapping to the liver   1987
     Huang et al. 1988
     Coffey et al. 1987

Affinity (Kd):
1–60 pM   Wakefield et al. 1987
Type I-Rec.: 65 pM   Cheifetz et al. 1986, 1988
Type II-Rec.: 85 pM   Segarini et al. 1988
Type III-Rec.: 280 pM

Origin:
- mRNA expressed in nearly all cells   Derynck et al. 1987
- mostly secreted in inactive precursor   Lawrence et al. 1985
  form (unable to bind to receptor)   Wakefield et al. 1987
- main source: platelets and bone
- main source of TGFβ$_3$: mesenchymal cells   Lyons et al. 1990

Function:
- inhibition of epithelial cells and endo-   Boyd et al. 1989
  thelial cells (cell growth, fibronectin
  production) TGFβ$_1$ = TGFβ$_2$
- inhibition of hematopoiesis in general   Okta et al. 1987
  (TGFβ$_1$ > TGFβ$_2$) incl. megakaryocytopoiesis
- growth stimulation of fibroblasts   Assioan et al. 1986
  (in combination with TGF alpha, EGF)   Childs et al. 1982
- growth stimulation of osteoblasts   Centrella et al. 1987
  (depending on density) and osteoclasts   Taskjian et al. 1985
- induction of differentiation of
  * mesenchymal cells into bone cells   Seyedin et al. 1986, 1987
    (secretion of cartilage specific
    proteoglycan and collagen type II)
    and chondrocytes   Assioan et al. 1983
  * bronchial epithelia in squamous cells   Masui et al. 1986
  * fibroblasts (secretion of extra-
    cellular matrix proteins)
- inhibition of differentiation of   Florini et al. 1986
  * myeloblasts
  * adipose cells (by insulin)   Ignotz et al. 1985
- mediator of healing processes
  * induces the formation of granulation   Sporn et al. 1983
    tissue (accumulation of fibroblasts,
    formation of collagen fibrils,   Sporn et al. 1983
    induction of angiogenesis)
  * acceleration of wound repair and   Mustoe et al. 1987
    tensile strength of scar tissue
- stimulation of IgA secretion of B-cells   Weinberg et al. 1992
- enhancement of T-helper cell function

TGF-Receptor	Type I	Type II soluble TNF-R-II	Type III	Type IV	Type V
Domains:					
Extracellular	136 aa	762 aa			
Transmembrane	30 aa	27 aa			
Intracellular	376 aa	41 aa			
Molecular weight:	53–65 kDa	83–110 kDa	250–310 kDa	60 kDa	400 kDa
Distribution:				pituitary cells	

ubiquitous, coexpressed

Affinity (Kd):	1–30 pM	1–30 pM	30–300 pM
	(for all isoforms of TGF)		

Signal transduction: type II receptor: via activation of an intrinsic serine/threonine kinase,
type III receptor: cytoplasmic domain has no signaling motif
(could function as a reservoir for TFGβ)
induction of changes in *junB*, c-*fos*, c-*myc* expression, prevention of
phosphorylation of the retinoblastoma protein, involvement of
guanine-nucleotide binding proteins

O'Grady et al. 1991, Massague 1992, Cheifetz et al. 1988, Lin et al. 1992, Wang et al. 1991, Ohtsku et al. 1992, Diaz-Meco et al. 1992.

Platelet-Derived Growth Factor (PDGF)

Size and structure:
– polypeptide
– homo- or heterodimers of
  PDGF A:
  * 6 kDa
  * sequence homology to B = 60%
  * heparin binding site of 18 aa basic region at the carboxy terminus
  * eight intrachain cysteine residues
  PDGF B:
  * 14 kDa
  * eight intrachain cysteine residues
– three different forms: PDGF-AA, -AB, -BB
Origin:
platelets, many transformed nuclear cells
Function:
– growth and proliferation of mesenchymal cells
  * induction of expression of c-*myc* and c-*fos*
– upregulation of the expression of LDL receptors
– activation of glycogen synthase
– stimulation of vasoconstriction
– induction of chemotaxis

Ross et al. 1973, 1989; Berridge et al. 1984; Cooper et al. 1982; Bochus et al. 1984; Habenicht et al. 1986; Chan et al. 1987; Grotendrost et al. 1982; Seppa et al. 1982.

PDGF-Receptor

Domains:	Subunit α	Subunit β
Extracellular	501 aa	499 aa
Transmembrane	24 aa	25 aa
Intracellular	541 aa	543 aa

Molecular weight: 170–180 kDa   170–180 kDa

Distribution: mesenchymal cells: fibroblasts, smooth muscle cells, osteoblasts, glial cells, myeloblasts

Receptors/cell: 500–300 000

Affinity (Kd): dimers   αα   50–200 pM
(noncovalent   αβ   10–100 pM
association)   ββ   100–500 pM
subunit α binds   subunit β binds
A or B chain of   only B chain
PDGF

Signal transduction: PDGF binding initiates dimerization of receptors, activation of intrinsic TPK, autophosphorylation, phosphorylation of cellular proteins
receptor ligand complexes are internalized and degraded

Glenn et al. 1982; Pike et al. 1983; Frachelton et al. 1984; Heldin et al. 1982, 1983; Yarden et al. 1986; Hart et al. 1988; Nister et al. 1989; Seifert et al. 1989.

Epidermal Growth Factor (EGF)

Synonym: β-urogastrone

Size and structure:
- polypeptide 6 kDa, 53 aa
- three intrachain disulfide bonds
- β-sheet conformation (with C terminal hairpin involved in receptor binding)
- sequence homology with
  * TGFα (40%)   } display
  * vaccinia virus P16 } EGF activity

Origin:
- epithelial cells, neuroectodermal cells, α-granules of platelets
- found in nearly all body fluids (blood, milk, urine, saliva, sweat, others) and in multiple organs and tissues
- growth and differentiation during fetal development
- enhancement of epidermal growth and keratinization
- promotion of angiogenesis and wound healing
- inhibition of gastric acid secretion

Cohen et al. 1963, 1965, 1987; Gregory et al. 1975; Montelione et al. 1987; Makino et al. 1987; Defize et al. 1986; Oka et al. 1983; Fallon et al. 1963.

EGF-Receptor	*Domains:*	Monomer	Dimer	Soluble receptor
	Extracellular	621 aa	noncovalent association, bound to a	621 aa
	Transmembrane	23 aa	single molecule of EGF	
	Intracellular	542 aa		
	Molecular weight:	170 kDa	340 kDa	
	Distribution:	nearly all cell types except those of the hematopoietic lineage		
	Receptors/cell:	20 000–20 0000		
	Affinity (Kd):	1 nM	0,1 nM	

Signal transduction:
- dimerization of receptor by EGF binding; activation of intrinsic TPK, autophos-phorylation (Tyr 1173) via GRB-SOS-RAS
- induction of phosphatidyl inositide hydrolysis and generation of diacyl-glycerol (DAG), activation of PKC, phosphorylation of threonine of the EGF-receptor (position 654), attenuation of intrinsic TPK activity
- increased expression of c-*myc*, c-*fos* and *junB*

Truncated receptor:
- coded by oncogene v-*erbB* (transforming gene of the avian erythroblastosis virus, derivative of chicken EGF-receptor)
- lacks a ligand binding domain as well as a small portion of the C-terminus
- may send a constitutive signal which may induce cellular transformation

Downward et al. 1984, King et al. 1982, Kawamoto et al. 1983, Ullrich et al. 1984, Boni-Schnetzler et al. 1987, Defize et al. 1986, Gamett et al. 1986.

Fibroblast Growth Factor (FGF-1, -2)

Size and structure:
- acidic FGF: 16–17 kDa, 154 aa
  (FGF-1)   140 aa truncated forms
                       134 aa biol. active
  * one N-glycosylation site
  * four intrachain cysteine residues
- basic FGF: 16–17 kDa, 154 aa (55% homology to aFGF)
  (FGF-2)   146 aa truncated forms
                       131 aa biol. active

Origin:
    basic FGF: ubiquitous
    acidic FGF: brain, retina, bone matrix
    FGFs may undergo crinopexy: storage and stabilization of excreted factors in the extracellular matrix

Function:
- proliferative responses in cells/tissues derived from mesoderm and neuro-ectoderm
  * wound healing, angiogenesis
  * nerve regeneration
- release of plasminogen activator by endothelial cells
- increase of hormonal responsiveness in the pituitary
- promotion of chondrossification in cartilagenous tissue
- induce keratinocyte locomotion

Burgess et al. 1986; Gimenez-Gallego et al. 1985; Harper et al. 1986; Gospodarowicz et al. 1986; Baird et al. 1985, 1987; Monkesan et al. 1986; Kato et al. 1985; Sarrett et al. 1992.

FGF-Receptor

	High-affininity receptor I	High-affininty receptor II
Molecular weight:	125 kDa	145 kDa
Distribution:	cell of mesodermal and neuroectodermal origin (including endothelial cells, smooth muscle cells, fibroblasts, chondrocytes, hepatocytes, epithelial cells)	
Receptors/cell:	$\approx$ 10 000	$\approx$ 10 000
Affinity (Kd):	50–500 pM (aFGF > bFGF)	50–500 pM (bFGF > aFGF)
Signal transduction:	via activation of intrinsic tyrosine kinases and activation of MAP kinase. Upon binding to the receptor, aFGF and bFGF are internalized and degraded in the lysosomal compartment. Unlike other peptide growth factors, both FGFs are slowly degraded to low molecular weight fragments which may persist for up to 24 h inside the cell.	

Burgess et al. 1989, Dionne et al. 1990, Neufeld et al. 1986, Sano et al. 1992, Imamura et al. 1992, Sarett et al. 1992.

1.2.8 Oncostatin, CNTF

Oncostatin M

Size and structure:
- native glycoprotein 18–28 kDa, 228 aa
- differences in size due to propeptide, which undergo proteolysis to be converted into mature fully active form (proteolysis is extracellular)
- intramolecular disulfide bonds: 2
- N-glycosylation sites: 2

Origin:
secreted by macrophages and activated T-lymphocytes

Function:
- not species specific
- growth inhibition of selected tumor cell lines
- increase in LDL receptor expression on hepatoma cells, in increase of LDL uptake
- expression of uPA by synovial cells
- increase in IL-6 production by endothelial cells
- activation of endothelial cells

Zarling et al. 1986, Malik et al. 1989, Grove et al. 1991, Hamilton et al. 1991, Brown et al. 1991.

Oncostatin M-Receptors

	High affinity receptor	Low affinity receptor
Molecular weight:	150 kDa	(150 kDa)
		68 kDa
		48 kDa
Distribution:	endothelial cells, T-cells, B-cells, monocytes, granulocytes, megakaryocytes, hepatocytes, fibroblasts, carcinoma cells	
Receptors/cell:	100–200	5000–9000
Affinity (Kd):	3–11 pM	0,4–1 nM
	binding of oncostatin M occurs directly to the gp 130 protein which is part of the Oncostatin receptor	
Sequence homology:	gp 130 subunit is identical to the gp 130 of the IL-6 receptor/LIF receptor. Oncostatin M can bind to LIF receptor like LIF (no direct binding to gp 130)	
Signal transduction:	via phospholipid metabolization and cellular protein tyrosine phosphorylation	

Linsley et al. 1988, Liv et al. 1992, Gearing et al. 1992, Grove et al. 1991.

Ciliary Neurotrophic Factor (CNTF)

Size and structure:
- 20–24 kDa
- homologies: IL-6, LIF, Oncostatin M

Origin:
Schwann cells (peripheral nervous system)
astrocytes (central nervous system)

Function:
- neuronal differentiation
- "survival factor" for neurons (sensory neurons, motor neurons, hippo-campal neurons, preganglionic sympathetic spinal cord neurons)
- promotion of cholinergic differentiation in sympathetic neurons
- additive action with FGF (acidic and basic) on motor neuron survival

Barbin et al. 1984; Blottner et al. 1989; Sendtner et al. 1990, 1991; Rose et al. 1991; Ip et al. 1991, 1992; Skapper et al. 1986; Oppenheim et al. 1991; Ensberger et al. 1989; Saadat et al. 1989; Lillien et al. 1988.

CNTF-Receptor

Domains:
- no transmembrane domain
- extracellular domain is associated with the membrane by a glycosyl-phosphatidylinositol linkage (GPI-linker)
- association with gp 130 subunit

Molecular weight:
72 kDa

Sequence homology:
α-subunit of the IL-6 receptor

Distribution:
cells of nervous system, skeletal muscle cells

Signal transduction:
tyrosine phosphorylation of gp 130

Rose et al. 1991, Ip et al. 1992, Davis et al. 1991, Hibi et al. 1990.

1.2.9 Approaches to Inhibit the Biological Effect of Growth Factors

Target	Inhibition of action	Inhibition of synthesis
Growth factor – – –	– soluble receptors antiidiotype antibodies for antibodies specific for binding site of receptors specific antibodies for growth factors specific immunization	– IL-10 – cytokine suppressive antiinflammatory drugs (CSAIDs) – corticosteroids – antisense oligonucleotides
Receptor – Binding site	– antagonists: * natural inactive analogues(IL-1RA) * synthetic peptide domains of growth factors * MAb anti receptor binding site – growth factor–cytotoxic drug conjugates – growth factor–toxin conjugates/-fusion protein – polyanionic compounds (suramin, dextran)	– antisense oligonucleotides – cross-linking and downregulation * by MAbs * by cytokines – decrease in formation (FK 506)
– Signal transduc- tion	– inhibition of dimerization by peptides – MAbs to nonbinding extracellular domains – inhibition of intrinsic tyrosine phosphokinase (erbstatin, tyrphostins, Flavopiridol) – inhibition of cellular tyrosine phosphokinase Flavopiridol	– mutation of receptors by antisense, oligonucleotides, viruses

2 Cell-Adhesion Molecules

2.1 Overview

2.1.1 Classification

Adhesion molecules enable cell-cell interactions necessary for their communication and cooperation.

Adhesion molecules are either constitutively and constantly expressed or they are formed on the cell membrane in response to a specific stimulation.

Based on differences in the primary sequence, adhesion molecules can be separated into three groups:

– *Immunoglobulin gene super family*

    ICAM-1, -2   (intercellular adhesion molecule)
    LFA-2, -3   (leukocyte function-associated antigen)
    VCAM-1   (vascular cell adhesion molecule)
    N-CAM   (neuronal cell adhesion molecule)

– *Integrins*

    LFA-1   (leukocyte function-associated antigen)
    VLA-1, -2, -3,   (very late activation antigen)
    -4, -5, -6, -7
    VNR   (vitronectin receptor)
    MAC-1   (monocyte adhesion complex)
    p150/95
    GPIIb/IIIa

– *Selectins*

    LECAM-1   (lectin-like cell adhesion molecule)
    GMP 140 (LECAM-3)   (granule membrane protein)
    ELAM-1 (LECAM-2)   (endothelial-leukocyte adhesion molecule)
    PECAM   (platelet endothelial cell adhesion molecule)

Adhesion between molecules of the immunoglobulin gene super family and integrins is mediated by protein-protein interactions, whereas adhesions between selectins and their ligands is realized by lectin–carbohydrate bindings.

Ligands for selectins belong to glycam/SOL (glycosylated cellular adhesion molecules/sialylated oligosaccharide ligands)

– *Ligands for ELAM*
    * Carbohydrates containing sialic acid $\alpha 2$–3 galactose and fucose $\alpha 1$–3/4

3-sialyl Lewis x
3-sialyl Lewis a
VIM-2
3-sialyl di Lewis x
– *Ligands for CMP 140*
  * Carbohydrates containing lacto-*N*-fucopentaose II or sialic acid α2–6 galactose and fucose α1–3
    Lewis x
    3/6 sialyl Lewis x
– *Other carbohydrate ligands*
    SgP 50   (sialylated glycoprotein 50 kDa)
    SgP 100   (sialylated glycoprotein 100 kDa)
    MECA-79

– *CD44* (synonym: hermes antigen) is an 80- to 90-kDa membrane glycoprotein expressed on lymphoid and myeloid cells. Its ligand is hyaluronic acid and CD44 variants. CD44 is expressed on actively trafficking lymphoid cells but is absent on sessile cells residing in germinal centers.

– *Cadherins* are transmembrane proteins which bind to one another and enable cell to cell linkages
    E-cadherins   (epithelial cell adhesion molecule)
    N-cadherins   (neural and muscle cell adhesion molecule)
    P-cadherins   (placenta and epithelial cell adhesion molecule)

2.1.2 Function

For leukocytes
– Adhesion to vascular endothelium
– Transmigration through endothelium
– Adhesion to extracellular matrix (fibronectin, laminin, collagen)
For lymphocytes
– Lymphocyte adhesion and homing
– Adhesion to antigen presenting cell
For platelets
– Leukocyte adhesion
– Endothelial cell adhesion

2.2 Characteristics

Members of: *Common properties:*
Immunoglobulin family
ICAM-1, -2   – structural homology to immunoglobulins
VCAM-1
LFA-2, -3   – act as ligands to integrins
N-CAM

Integrin family

LFA-1	– non covalently linked glycoprotein dimers of
MAC-1	1 heavy (α) and 1 light (β) chain
p150/95	– connecting the intracellular cytoskeleton with
VLA-1, -2, -3	extracellular environment
VLA-4, -5, -6	– cell adhesion, cellular locomotion, binding to
GPIIb/IIIa	extracellular matrix
VNR	– cell aggregation

Selectin family

LECAM	– N-terminal lectin like domain (L)
GMP-140	– epidermal growth factor-like domain (E)
ELAM-1 (E)	– repeated motives similar to those found on
PECAM	complement receptors CR-1 and CR-2 (C)
	– bind specific carbohydrate structures on
	glycoproteins and glycolipids

Cadherin family

Epithelial (E)cadherins	– calcium dependent transmembrane cell-cell
Neural (N)cadherins	adhesion molecules
Placenta (P)cadherins	– bind to one another by means of homophilic
	interactions

CD44

Hermes (H-)cell adhesion	– integral membrane protein
molecules	– different molecular sizes (85–160 kDa), highly
	glycosylated, related to cartilage link proteins

Haskard 1991; Phillips 1988

2.2.1 Immunoglobulin Gene Superfamily Type

Most of the members of the immunoglobulin gene superfamily are adhesion or binding molecules.

Molecules of this family are characterized by 1 or more immunoglobulin domain structures (see chapter on B-cell proliferation).

The main proteins belonging to the immunoglobulin gene superfamily are:
– Immunoglobulins (IgM, IgG, IgE, IgA, IgD)
– T-cell receptor (TCR)
– CD3 (γ, δ, ϵ) chains
– MHC-class I, -class II, CD-1
– CD_4, CD_8
– Fc γ2b/γ1R receptors
– Receptor for PDGF

– Carcinoembryonic antigen group
  * Carcinoembryonic antigen
  * Non-cross-reacting antigen
  * Biliary glycoprotein I
  * Normal fetal antigen
– Adhesion molecules
  * Intercellular adhesion molecules (ICAM-1, -2)
  * Leucocyte function-associated antigen (LFA-2/-3)
  * Vascular cell adhesion molecules (VCAM-1)
  * Neuronal cell adhesion molecules (N-CAM)

Schematic structure of adhesion molecules (immunoglobulin gene superfamily)

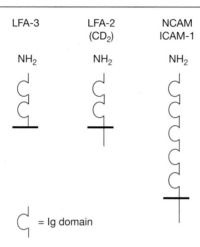

LFA-3

LFA-2 (CD$_2$)

NCAM ICAM-1

NH$_2$ NH$_2$ NH$_2$

= Ig domain

2.2 Integrin Type

– Mediate cell to cell as well as cell to matrix interactions.
– Bind to molecules which expose the RGD-sequence (Arg-Gly-Asp).
– Are heterodimers which consist of two chains (α- and β-chain) which are non covalently associated.
– The β-chain is coded in chromosome 21, the α-chain in chromosome 16.
  The β- and α-chains are formed as precursors, associated non covalently in the ER and either stored in intracellular vesicles or immediately transported to the cell membrane.
– Are transmembrane glycoproteins which mediate the linkage between the ligand and the cytosceleton within the cell.
– Differences in the β-chain define the subfamily:
  β1 – very late activation antigens (VLA 1–7)
  β2 – leucocytes-integrins (LFA1–LeuCAM)
  β3 – glycoprotein IIb/IIIa and vitronectin receptor
– Differences in the α-chain define its ligand specificity.

**Schematic Structure
of Integrins**

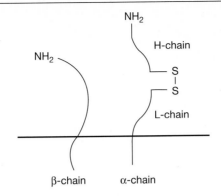

**Integrin Receptor
Family**

Name	α-Chain	(kDa)	β-Chain	(kDa)	Ca⁺⁺ binding repeats	Occurence
GPIIb-IIIa	GPIIb	(125–25)	GPIIIa	(105)		platelets
	VnRα	(125+25)				endothelial cells, many others
VLA-5 (FuR)	FuRα	(140+25)	FuRβ	(140)		fibroblasts, many others
VLA-1	VLA-α₁	(200)				lymphocytes (T-cells), others
VLA-2	VLA-α₂	(165)				lymphocytes, platelets
VLA-3	VLA-α₃	(135)				lymphocytes, platelets
VLA-4	VLA-4α₄	(150)				lymphocytes, monocytes
VLA-6						lymphocytes
Leucocyte Adhesion Proteins	Mac-1	(170)	β-chain	(95)		monocytes, granulocytes
	p150,95	(150)				monocytes, granulocytes
	LFA-1	(180)				lymphocytes

Classification of Inte- | *Integrins for cell to cell contact* | *Ligand:*
grins Based on Binding | $\alpha L/\beta_2$ (LFA-1) | ICAM-1
Characteristics | $\alpha M/\beta_2$ (MAC-1) | ICAM-1, C3bi endotoxin

$\alpha x/\beta_2$ (gp 150/95) — ?
$\alpha 4/\beta_1$ (VLA-4) — VCAM-1

Integrins for binding to basement membrane   *Ligand:*
$\alpha 1/\beta_1$ (VLA-1) — laminin/collagen
$\alpha 2/\beta_1$ (VLA-2) — collagen/laminin
$\alpha 3/\beta_1$ (VLA-3) — laminin/collagen/fibronectin

$\alpha 6/\beta_1$ — laminin
$\alpha 6/\beta_4$ — laminin

Integrins for binding to other proteins   *Ligand:*
$\alpha 4/\beta_1$ (VLA-4) — fibronectin (CSII site)
$\alpha 5/\beta_1$ — fibronectin (RGD = Arg-Gly-Asp site)

$\alpha v/\beta_1$ — fibronectin

$\alpha v/\beta_3$ — vitronectin, fibrinogen, thrombospondin
$\alpha v/\beta_5$ — vWF, vitronectin

Hynes et al. 1987; Albeda et al. 1993.

Function of Leukocyte
Integrins

Synonym: LFA-1 family, leukocyte adhesion proteins, LeuCAM
– Increase of adhesion of activated neutrophils and monocytes to endothelial cells of blood vessels
– Extravasation
– Migration to inflamed regions
– Interaction with target cells
– Adhesion to LPS and to bacteria

Activated leukocytes express
– High levels of integrins (MAC-1, p150,95)
– Activated integrins. Activation stage of integrins is defined by its degree of phosphorylations and cluster formation and by its linkage to actin and talin in the presence of divalent cautions ($Mg2+$, $Ca2+$, $Mn2+$).

Leukocyte integrins deactivate by dephosphorylation and dearrangement of linkages.

Leukocyte Integrins	LFA-1	MAC-1	p150,95
Structure:	α_1 (L)–β_2	α_1 (M)–β_2	α_1 (X)–β_2
MW (kD):	180/95	170/95	150/95
CD terminology:	CD11a/CD18	CD11b/CD18	CD11c/CD18
Ligand:	ICAM-1 ICAM-2	C3b: fibrinogen factor X LPS (binding site different to RGD)	C3bi

Occurrence:	← monocytes, macrophages, granulocytes →
	← NK-cells →
	← Langerhans cells →

	LFA-1	MAC-1	p150,95
	T-, B-lymphocytes thymocytes	B-lymphocytes (CD5+)	
Increased expression after cell activation:	no	yes	yes
Integrin activation:	yes (··-chain)	yes (β-chain)	yes (β-chain)
Co-factor for the function of	TCR-mediated function – T help – CTL NK cytotoxicity Fc-receptor mediated function – ADCC – phagocytosis cell aggregation and extravasation	CR-3-mediated function – binding of C3bi – phagocytosis – cytotoxicity for C3b′ coated bacteria Fc-receptor mediated function – ADCC – phagocytosis adhesion, aggregation, chemotaxis of granulocytes	

Activation of LFA-1

Example: Interaction between cytotoxic T-lymphocytes (CTL) and the specific target cell.

- The first contact is mediated by ICAM-1 (on the target cell) and the "inactivated" LFA-1 (on CTL). This binding is of low affinity.
- Subsequently, the antigen presented by MHC-class I (on the target cells) binds to the T-cell receptor and MHC-class I to CD8.
- Activation of the TCR/CD3 complex on the CTL stimulates phospholipase C (PLP-C), which catalyses the hydrolysis of phosphatidyl-inositol-biphosphate (PIP) into inositol-triphosphate (IP). IP mobilizes intracellular calcium and diacylglycerol (DG) thus, leading to activation of the proteinkinase C. Proteinkinase C phosphorylates the β-chain of LFA-1. Hereby, LFA-1 is "activated" to bind ICAM-1 with high affinity.
- Inactivation of activated LFA-1 is performed by reduction of the proteinkinase level and action of phosphatase (i.e. CD45).

Increased Expression of Mac-1 (p150,95)

Unstimulated cells expose Mac-1 on the cell surface and store Mac-1 in (gelatine containing) organelles.

Chemotactic factors (i.e. C5a, leukotriene B_4) lead to cell membrane expression of stored Mac-1 molecules within 5–10 min. In this way the number of Mac-1 molecules on the cell membrane is increased by a factor of 5–10 (to about 65 000 Mac-1 molecules/cell).

Simultaneously, Mac-1 is activated similar as described for LFA-1 (increase of affinity by a factor of 2–3).

Integrins Belonging to Very Late Activation Antigens

	VLA-1	VLA-2	VLA-3	VLA-4	VLA-5	VLA-6	VLA-7
Structure:	α_1–β_1	α_1–β_1	α_1–β_1	α_1–β_1	α_1–β_1	α_1–β_1	α_1–β_1
CD-terminology:	–/ CD29	CDw49b/ CD29	–/ CD29	CDw49b/ CD29	–/ CD29	CDw49f/ CD29	–
Ligand:	collagen laminin	collagen	laminin fibro-nectin collagen	fibro-nectin VCAM	fibro-nectin	laminin	?
Occurrence:	◄——————— broad distribution on various cell types ———————►						
Function:	◄——————— morphogenesis and wound healing ———————►						

Integrins Belonging to Cytadhesins		gpIIb/IIIa	vitronectin receptor (VNR)
	Structure:	$\alpha_1-\beta_3$	$\alpha_1-\beta_3$
	CD-terminology:	CD41/CD61	CD51/CD61
	Ligand:	fibrinogen	thrombospondin
		fibronectin	fibrinogen
		vitronectin	vitronectin
		von Willebrand factor (F VIII)	von Willebrand factor (F VIII)
		thrombospondin	
	Occurrence:	platelets	various cells
	Function:	morphogenesis and wound healing	

2.2.3 Cell Distribution

Cell	Adhesion molecule	Class	Ligand
Endothelial cells	GMP-140 (CD68)	selectin	Lewis X
	ELAM-1	selectin	S-Lewis X
	ICAM-1	immunoglobulin	LFA-1 Mac-1
	ICAM-2	immunoblobulin	LFA-1
	VCAM-1	immunoblobulin	VLA-4
	PECAM	selectin	PECAM
Neutrophil granulocytes and monocytes	Lewis X, S-Lewis X	carbohydrate	GMP-140, Elam 1
	LECAM-1	selectin	?
	LFA-1 (CD11a/CD18)	integrin	ICAM-1, ICAM-2
	MAC-1 (CD11b/CD18)	integrin	ICAM-1
monocytes	p150/95 (CD11c/CD18)	integrin	?
Monocytes, lymphocytes	VLA-4	integrin	VCAM-1, fibronectin
Lymphocytes	?	?	ELAM-1
	LECAM-1	selectin	?
	LFA-1 (CD11a/CD18)	integrin	ICAM-1, ICAM-2
	VLA-6	integrin	laminin
	VLA-1	integrin	fibronectin, laminin
Platelets, lymphocytes	VLA-2	integrin	fibronectin, laminin
	VLA-3	integrin	fibronectin, laminin
Fibroblasts, lymphocytes, others	VLA-5	integrin	fibronectin
Platelets	GPIIb-IIIa	integrin	fibrinogen, fibronectin, v. W. Factor
Others, endothelial cells	VNR	integrin	vitronectin

Carlos 1990; Pober 1990; Koch 1991; Corkill et al. 1991; Haskard 1991; Hemler 1989; Hogg 1991; Johnston 1989; Simmon 1988, 1990; Bevilacqua 1989; Philipps 1988.

2.2.4 Binding Partners

Partner I				Partner II
Platelets	endothelial cells	GMP-140 (CD68)	←→ Lewis x (CD15)	PMN, monocytes
Platelets	endothelial cells	ELAM-1	←→ S-Lewis X	PMN, monocytes, lymphocytes (?)
Platelets	endothelial cells	ICAM-1	←→ LFA-1 (CD11a/CD18)	PMN, monocytes, lymphocytes
Platelets	endothelial cells	ICAM-1	←→ Mac-1 (CD11b/CD18)	PMN, monocytes
Platelets	endothelial cells	ICAM-2	←→ LFA-1 (CD11a/CD18)	PMN, monocytes, lymphocytes
Platelets	endothelial cells	VCAM-1	←→ VLA-4	lymphocytes
PMN	monocytes	LECAM-1	←→ ? (carbohydrates)	
		p150/95 (CD11c/CD18)	←→ ?	
Monocytes	lymphocytes	VLA-4	←→ fibronectin, VCAM-1	
Others, fibroblasts	lymphocytes	VLA-5	←→ fibronectin	
	lymphocytes	VLA-6	←→ laminin	
	platelets	PECAM	←→ PECAM	endothelial cells
	lymphocytes	VLA-1	←→ fibronectin, laminin	
Platelets	lymphocytes	VLA-2	←→ fibronectin, laminin	
Platelets	lymphocytes	VLA-3	←→ fibronectin, laminin	
	platelets	GP11b/IIIa	←→ fibrinogen, fFibronectin, ←→ v. Willebrand Factor	
Others	endothelial cells	VNR	←→ fibronectin	

GMP = granul membrane protein
ELAM = endothelial leucocyte adhesion molecule
VCAM = vascular cell adhesion molecule
PECAM = platelet endothelial cell adhesion molecule
LECAM = lectin like cell adhesion molecule
VLA = very late activation antigens
MAC = monocyte adhesion complex
LFA = lymphocytes functional association antigen
VNR = Vibronectin receptor

2.2.5 Modulation of Expression and Function

Adhesion molecule	Size (KDa)	Cytokine modulation	Time	Translocation from stores	Alteration of mol. avidity	Synthesis + expression	Shedding
Integrins							
LFA-1	275 (α, β)	–			+		
MAC-1	265 (α, β)	–		+			
GPIIIb/IIIa	255 (α, β)	–		+	+		
VnR	255 (α, β)	–		+	+		
p150/95	245 (α, β)	–		+	+		
VLA-1	340 (α, β)	–		+	+		
VLA-2	305 (α, β)	–		+	+		
VLA-3	400 (α, β)	–		+	+		
VLA-4	290 (α, β)	–		+	+		
VLA-5	305 (α, β)	–		+	+		
VLA-6				+	+		
Immunoglobulins							
ICAM-1	95	+	12–24 hrs.			+	
ICAM-2	46	–					
VCAM-1	110	+	6–10 hrs.			+	
Selectins							
LECAM		–			+		+
GMP-140	140	+	minutes	degranulation			
ELAM-1	115	+	3–4 hrs.			+	
PECAM	130	–					
Ligands							
Lewis X (CD15)	135	–					
S-Lewis X	135	–					

Hemler 1989; Hogg 1991; Johnston 1989; Simmon 1988, 1990; Bevilacqua 1989; Philipps 1988; Haskard 1991.

2.2.6 Structure and function of CD44

Synonyms: hermes antigen, H-CAM, ECM-receptor III
– Transmembrane glycoprotein, highly glycosylated molecular size ranging from 85 to 160 kDa
– Related to cartilage-like proteins and a related proteoglycan core protein
– Ligands for CD44 are glycosaminoglycans, such as hyaluronate (distributed in extracellular matrix and on the luminal cell surface of high endothelial venules)

– Two classes
  * 90 kDa protein
  Occurrence: – lymphoid and myeloid cells
                – only expressed on actively trafficking lymphoid cells,
                  absent on sessile cells residing in germinal centers
  Function: – matrix adhesion, lymph node homing, progenitor homing
                  and lymphopoiesis
  * 150–160 kDa protein
  Occurrence: – epithelial and mesenchymal cells
  Function: – receptor for hyaluronic acid

Albelda 1993, Galandrini et al. 1993.

2.2.7 Structure and Function of Cadherins

– Transmembrane proteins, 723–748 aa, overall homology 50–60%
– Enable cell to cell adhesion, bind to one another by means of homophilic inter-
  actions; binding is selective to identical cadherin types
– Three classes:
  * E-cadherins (uvomorulin, cell CAM 120/80, Arc-1, L-CAM)
  Occurrence: epithelium (all layers)
  * N-cadherins (A-CAM, N-CAL-CAM)
  Occurrence: neural tissues
                lens
                cardiac and skeletal muscle
  * P-cadherins
  Occurrence: placenta, epithelium (basal layer)

Takeichi 1991, Nose et al. 1990, Albelda 1993.

3 Antigen Presentation

3.1 Overview

Antigen presenting cells (APC) participate in the afferent pathway of the immune reaction.
Specialized cells for antigen presentation are
– Dendritic cells
– Macrophages/monocytes
– B-lymphocytes
Antigens are presented by specialized molecules on the cell membrane of APC
– MHC-class I
– MHC-class II
– CD1
– Membrane immunoglobulins

Antigen Presentation

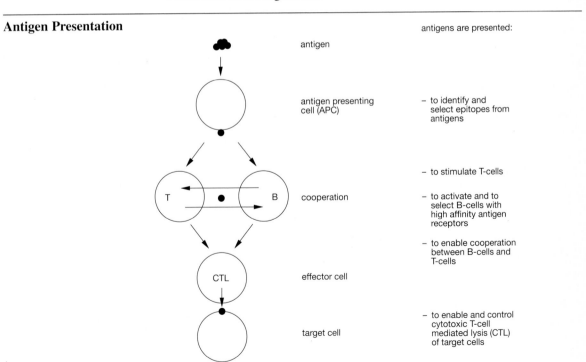

antigens are presented:

antigen

antigen presenting cell (APC)
– to identify and select epitopes from antigens

– to stimulate T-cells

cooperation
– to activate and to select B-cells with high affinity antigen receptors

– to enable cooperation between B-cells and T-cells

effector cell

target cell
– to enable and control cytotoxic T-cell mediated lysis (CTL) of target cells

3.2 Details

3.2.1 Dendritic Cells

Proven Immunocompetent Dendritic Cells and Their Location

Dendritic cell	Organ	Location
Lymphoid	spleen	randomly distributed
Interdigitating	spleen lymphnodes	paracortical T-cell areas
Follicular	spleen lymphnodes tonsils	B-cell rich follicles
Veiled cells	lymphoid	afferent lymph
Langerhans	thymus lymphnodes spleen skin	medulla
Thy-1 positive	skin (mouse)	epidermis
Dermal	skin	collagenous dermis subcutis
Synovial	joints	synovial lining (many) synovial interstitium (few)
Pulmonary	lung	bronchial mucosa and submucosa
Thyroid	thyreoidea	peripheral to follicles
Cardiac	heart	myointerstitium

Headington et al. 1990.

Hypothetical Common Origin of Dendritic Cells and Macrophages

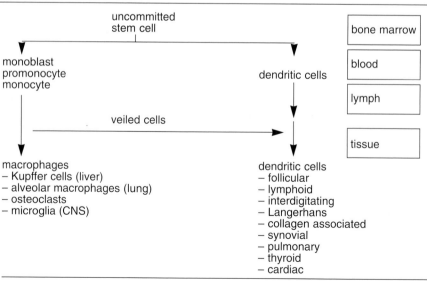

Headington et al. 1990.

**Ontogenesis
of Dendritic Cells**

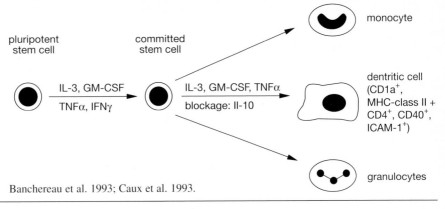

Banchereau et al. 1993; Caux et al. 1993.

**Homing of Dendritic
Cells**

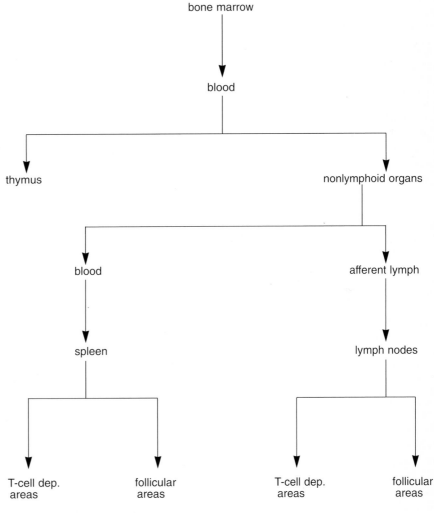

Lanciavecchia 1993.

Function of Dendritic Cells (DC)

Antigen presentation to T-cells
– 100–2000 MHC-class II molecules loaded with peptides are necessary (<0,1% MHC-class II occupancy)
– Long retention of peptide loaded MHC-II enables memory
– One DC can stimulate 80–100 T-cells/day
– Differentiation into DC: stimulated by TNFa + II-3 + GM-CSF inhibited by II-10
– DC can present particular derived proteins (i.e. PPD from mycobacteria)

Stimulation of B-cells
– Mediated by follicular dendritic cells (FDC)
– FDC bind immune complexed antigen via Fc-receptors
– Antigens bound on FDC crosslink membrane Ig of activated B-cells, which leads to antigenic selection
– Co-stimulation with CD40L (or Il-4, Il-2 or MAb anti-CD40) prevents apoptosis of B-cells

Inaba et al. 1993; Caux et al. 1993; Gray et al. 1993; Mac Lennan et al. 1993.

Stimulation of Human Dendritic Cells

Expression of	Stimulated by		
	GM-CSF + Il-4	TNF	CD40L
MHC-I	+	+	+
MHC-II	+	+	+
CD1	+		
CD40	+		
ICAM-1 (CD54)	+	+	+
LFA3 (CD58)	+		
Antigen presentation (MLR)	+ (50–100x)	+	+
FcγR	+	–	–

Sallusto and Lanciavecchia 1993

3.2.2 Antigen Binding Molecules

These belong to the immunoglobulin superfamily and are characterized by
– Constant immunoglobulin domains (loops bridged by disulfide bonds)
– Antigen (peptide) binding variable domains
Antigen binding molecules are TCR and surface immunoglobulins.

Antigen Binding and Presenting Molecules

MHC-class II is a dimer with:
– Two membrane anchoring chains (α, β) each containing one peptide binding and one immunoglobulin domain
– Is involved in antigen presentation by APC (afferent pathway)

CD1 is a monomer which:
- Has one membrane anchoring heavy chain, which contains one immunoglobulin domain (α_3) and two peptide binding domains (α_1 and α_2)
- Is associated with β_2-microglobulin, which provides the second immunoglobulin domain and stabilizes the CD-1 molecule
- Is involved in antigen presentation by APC (afferent pathway)

MHC-class I is a monomer:
- Similar in structure to CD-1
- Associated with β_2 microglobulin
- Involved in antigen presentation by target cells; essential for recognition of target cells by cytotoxic T-lymphocytes (CTL, efferent pathway)

Parkam 1989; Porcelli et al. 1993.

Antigen-Binding Molecules Belong to the Immunoglobulin Superfamily. They are Characterized by the Typical Domain Structure and Variable Regions Binding to Epitopes.

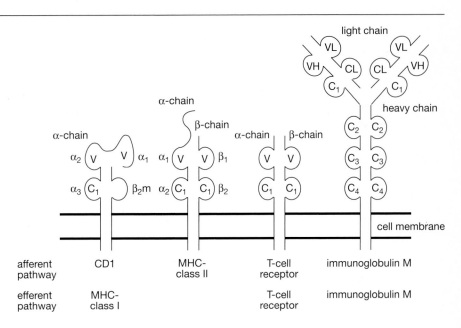

Porcelli et al. 1993

Characterization of CD1

Chromosome: 1q 22–23 (man)
Heterotype: CD1a, -b, -c, -d, -e
Consensus: 26% to MHC-I
              38% to MHC-II-β
Association: β_2-microglobulin, association weaker compared to MHC-I
Occurence: Dendritic cells (Langerhans cells, interfollicular DC)
              monocytes (increase after GM-CSF + Il-4 stimulation)
              T-cells (CD4/CD8 negative)

	Function:	– afferent antigen presentation to T-cells (TCR-$\alpha\beta$ or -$\gamma\delta$ positive, double negative for CD4 and CD8)
		– response to *M. tuberculosis* needs CD1-presentation (inhibited by MAb anti CD1)
		– CD1a and CD1c may be autoantigens
	Loading:	intracellular (also extracellular)

Porcelli et al. 1993

Role of MHC-class II molecules	– Present mostly exogenous antigens	Deverson et al. 1990
		Cerundolo et al. 1991
	– Antigenic peptides are 11–16 aa in size	McMichael et al. 1992
	– Loading takes place in endosomes	Monaco et al. 1990
	– Peptides settle in the groove formed	Parkam 1989
	by peptide binding domains (α_1, β_1)	Garrett 1989
	of the α- and β-chain	Björkman et al. 1988
		Stern et al. 1993
	– The peptide MHC-class II complex is	Brown et al. 1988
	transported to the cell surface	
	– Peptide is recognized by the TCR; in	Rosenthal et al. 1973
	case the CD4 molecule identifies MHC-class II as syngeneic, the TCR is activated by the peptide	Zinkernagel et al. 1974
	– Costimulatory signals are essential; Costimulatory signals are	
	* B7/CD28 for APC/T-cells	Linsley et al. 1991
	B7/CTLA-4 interaction	Schwartz 1992
	* CD40L/CD40 for T-cell/B-cell interaction	Gauchet et al. 1993
	- T-cell and B-cell cooperations with involvement of MHC-class II are similarly restricted to syngeneity	Katz et al. 1972
		Kindred et al. 1973
	– Responses of T-cells to single peptide epitope are polyclonal but not as much heterogenous as responses of B-cells	McMichael 1992

Role of MHC-Class I Molecules	– Present mostly endogenous antigens (including viral antigens).	Sweetser et al. 1989
	– Antigenic peptides are $\approx$ 8–9 aa in size.	Rötzschke et al. 1990
		Schuhmacher et al. 1991
	– Loading takes place in endoplasmatic reticulum.	Nüchtern et al. 1989
		Townsend et al. 1990
	– Peptides settle in the groove of MHC-I formed by the α_1 and α_2 domains.	Björkman 1987 a, b

– Loading stabilizes the MHC-I β_{2m} complex.   Schnabl et al. 1990

      Rock et al. 1991

– Complex is transported through the Golgi   Möller et al. 1992
complex to the cell membrane.

– Peptide is recognized by the TCR   Rosenthal et al. 1973
in case the CD8 molecule identifies   Zinkenagel et al. 1974
MHC-class I as syngeneic.

– No co-stimulatory signal is necessary for   Schwartz et al. 1992
recognition by T-cells and CTL, but LFA-1/
ICAM interaction increases cytotoxic reaction.

– About 200 MHC-class I/β_{2m}/peptide   Christink et al. 1991
complexes per target cell seem to
be sufficient for CTL (TCR) mediated lysis.

– Presentation of tumor antigen by MHC-I only   Lurguin et al. 1989
proven in selected murine models (P815).   van den Eynde et al. 1991

– The α_3 domain of the MHC-class I molecule   Salter et al. 1989
is the site of physical contact with CD8.

3.2.3 MHC genes

The genes for the human MHC are located on the short arm of chromosome 6.
The whole locus comprises class I, II and III genes and spans 4000 kbp.
The locus therefore has a 4% chance for a crossover at any meiosis.
The gene for β_2-microglobulin that associates with MHC-class I molecules is
located on chromosome 15.

**MHC Antigens Are
Coded on Human
Chromosome 6**

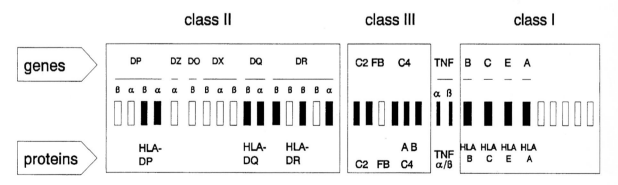

Class I Region

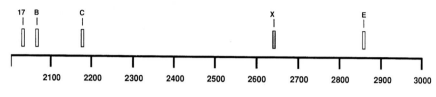

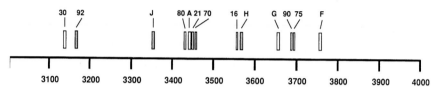

Class II Region

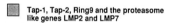

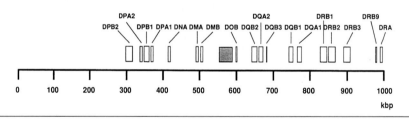

Class III Region

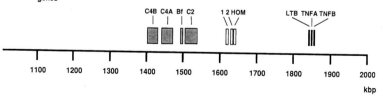

Campbell and Trowsdale 1993.

3.2.4 Regulation of MHC gene expression

MHC class I:
- Mediated through positive regulatory elements in the 5′ region of the genes as the enhancer A and interferon (IFN) responsive elements.
- Three factors are known that bind to enhancer A: RIBP, RIIBP and NF-B.
- Factor ICSBP binds to the IFN responsive element.
- Negative regulatory element (NRE) is located within the IFN responsive element.
- Class II Y box binding proteins bind to NRE (see below).
- The availability of peptides for the loading of MHC class I molecules seems to be crucial for high level expression.
- In general MHC class I molecules are present on almost all nucleated cells.

MHC class II:
- X and Y elements are essential for transcription, but other elements are also found in the 5′ region of class II genes.
- In addition sequences far upstream of the promotor region are also involved in regulation of expression.
- RR-X is a 979 amino acid protein that binds to the X box as monomer and as a dimer.
- RF-X does not share homologies to known DNA binding proteins or transcription factors.
- X-BP1 and X-BP2 are members of the leucine zipper transcription factor family (as the AP1 complex proteins *jun* and *fos*) X-BP1 has been shown to form heterodimers with c-*jun*.
- NF-Ya and NF-Yb are 318 and 207 amino acid proteins respectively that can bind to the Y element probably as heterodimers.
- W element binding factors have been identified but not cloned: H3, H1, H4, Zc, NF-W1, NF-W2.
- The interaction between X and Y element binding proteins may be important for maintaining transcriptional regulation.
- IFN-γ can upregulate MHC class II gene expression, response elements have not yet been defined.

Accolla et al. 1991.

**MHC Class II Gene
Promotor Region**

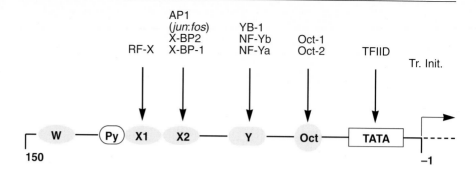

Schematical representation of the 5' region of MHC-class II genes covering 100 bp.

Given are binding sites and the respective cognate transcription factors. Horizontal arrow marks transcription initiation by RNA polymerase II.

3.2.5 Loading of Antigen Presenting Molecules

MHC-class II (for afferent pathway)
– Antigens are phagocytosed and degraded in lysosomes.
– MHC-class II molecules protrude in lysosomes.
– Peptides (6–30 aa) bind into the groove of MHC-class II molecules.
– Loaded MHC-class II are transported to cell membrane.

CD-1 (for afferent pathway)
– May be similar to MHC-class I

MHC-class I (for efferent pathway)
– Endogenous antigens (and presumably endocytosed exogenous antigens) are cleaved by proteasomes into peptides (6–16 aa). Formation of proteasomes is controlled by genes located in the MHC-class II locus of chromosome 6 (Spies et al. 1991).
– Peptides (optimal length 8–11 aa) are transported (transporter for antigen presentation = TAP) into endoplasmatic reticulum.
– Peptides bind into the groove of the MHC-class I molecule.
– By binding of peptides and associated with ·2m the structure of MHC-class I is stabilized.
– Loaded and stabilized MHC-class I is transported via Golgi to the cell membrane.

Loading and Presentation of Antigens by MHC Class II Antigens

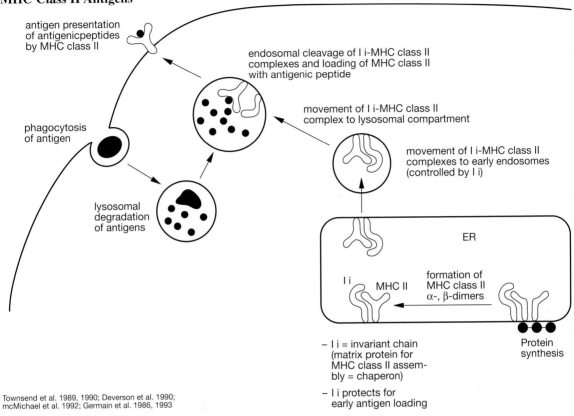

antigen presentation
of antigenicpeptides
by MHC class II

endosomal cleavage of I i-MHC class II
complexes and loading of MHC class II
with antigenic peptide

movement of I i-MHC class II
complex to lysosomal compartment

phagocytosis
of antigen

movement of I i-MHC class II
complexes to early endosomes
(controlled by I i)

lysosomal
degradation
of antigens

ER

I i   MHC II   formation of
MHC class II
α-, β-dimers

Protein
synthesis

– I i = invariant chain
(matrix protein for
MHC class II assem-
bly = chaperon)

– I i protects for
early antigen loading

Townsend et al. 1989, 1990; Deverson et al. 1990;
mcMichael et al. 1992; Germain et al. 1986, 1993

Loading and Presentation of Antigens by MHC Class I Molecules

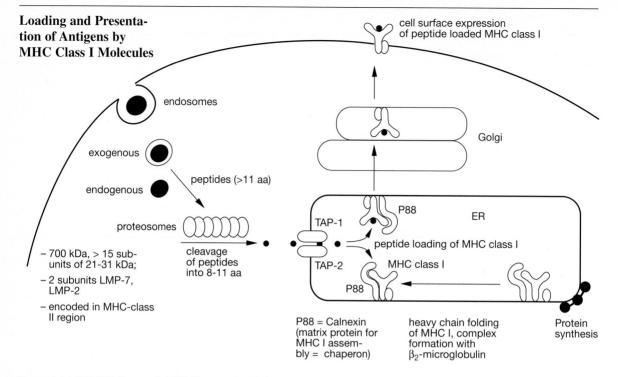

- 700 kDa, > 15 subunits of 21-31 kDa;
- 2 subunits LMP-7, LMP-2
- encoded in MHC-class II region

cleavage of peptides into 8-11 aa

P88 = Calnexin (matrix protein for MHC I assembly = chaperon)

heavy chain folding of MHC I, complex formation with β_2-microglobulin

Protein synthesis

Townsend et al. 1989, 1990; Deverson et al. 1990; Monaco et al. 1990; Cerundolo et al. 1991; mcMichael et al. 1992; Momburg et al. 1993; Peterson 1993

Transporter for Antigen Presentation (TAP) by MHC-Class I Molecules (Encoded in the MHC-Class II Region Between DP and DQ)

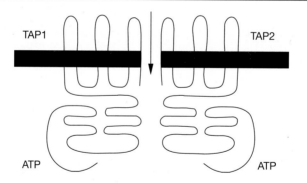

Structure: heterodimer molecule
TAP1: 77 kDa – no polymorphism
TAP2: 71 kDa – moderate polymorphism

Function: ATP-dependent
– peptides of 8–11 aa are transported
– transport variable according to type of aa
– polymorphism of TAP2 influences selection of peptides

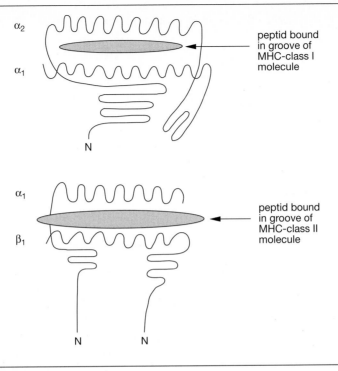

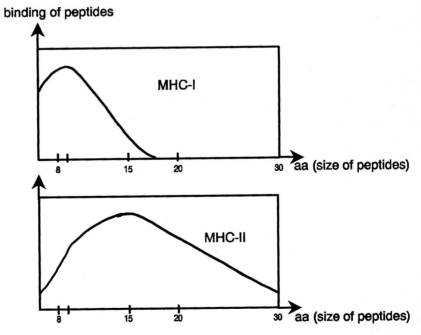

Size of Peptides Binding to MHC-Classes II and I

Stern et al. 1995.

3.2.6 Antigen Presentation by B-Cells

Resting B-cells (Kakuichi et al. 1983, Krieger et al. 1985, Chessnut et al. 1981, Roch et al. 1984)
– Uptake of antigen by endocytosis (precondition: high concentration of antigen)
– Cleave antigen into peptides by lysosomal enzymes
– Load MHC-II with peptides
– Present peptides via MHC-II mainly to T-cells
    * Present to TH0 cells (costimulation: B7-CD28/CTLA-4)
    * Cooperate with TH2 cells (costimulation: CD40-CD40L)

Activated B-cells (Snider et al. 1989, Gosselin et al. 1988, Abbas et al. 1985, Denis et al. 1993)
– Capture antigen by specific membrane immunoglobulin (low concentration of antigen)
– Internalize antigen after cross-linking of membrane immunoglobulins
– Cleave antigen into peptides by lysosomal enzymes
– Load MHC-II with peptides
– Present peptides via MHC-II mainly to T-cells
    * Present to TH0 cells (costimulation: B7-CD28/CTLA-4)
    * Cooperate with TH2 cells (costimulation: CD40-CD40L)

Membrane Ig of all isotypes are similar effective in antigen presentation (Patel et al. 1993).
B-cells seem to present antigen via MHC-II mainly to TH2 cells.
APC present antigen via MHC-II mainly to TH1 cells.
(Gajewski et al. 1991, Snapper et al. 1988, Sornasse et al. 1992)

Additional Structures for Presenting Antigens

Lipase-sensitive membrane structures (Falo et al. 1986, 1987)
Proteins related to heat shock proteins (Smolenski et al. 1990)

Antigen Presentation by B-Cells

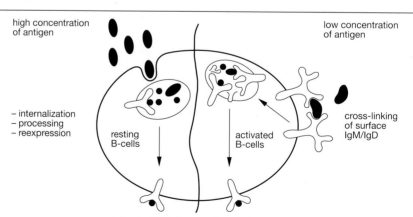

high concentration of antigen

low concentration of antigen

– internalization
– processing
– reexpression

resting B-cells

activated B-cells

cross-linking of surface IgM/IgD

presentation by MHC-II molecules to helper T-cells
– B-cell present mainly to TH$_2$ cells
– dentritic cells and macrophages present mainly to TH$_1$ cells

Chesnut et al. 1981; Kakiuchi et al. 1983; Krieger et al. 1985; Gajewski et al. 1991: Snapper et al. 1988; Sornasse et al. 1992; Denis et al. 1993: Snider et al. 1989; Gosselin et al. 1988; Abbas et al. 1985

Endocytosis of Antigens by B-Cells for Loading of and Presentation by MHC-II

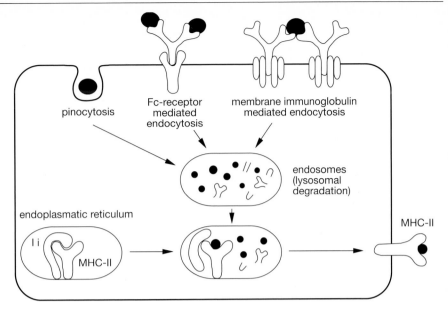

3.2.7 Expression of MHC-Molecules

MHC-I molecules are expressed on nearly all adult tissue cells, whereas MHC-II is expressed mainly on antigen-presenting cells (APC).

Tissue	MHC-I	MHC-II
B-lymphocytes	++	++
T-lymphocytes	++	+
Macrophages/monocytes	++	+++
Dendritic cell family	++	+++
Langerhans cells (epidermis, stomach)		
Interdigitating cells (thymus, lymph nodes)		
Veiled cells (lymph vessels)		
Dendritic cells (spleen, lung, visceral organs)		
Kupffer cells (liver)		
Liver-parenchymal cells	(+)	–
epithelial cells of		
Stomach	+	+
Colon rectum	+	+
Lung	+	+
Kidney	+	+
Skin	+	+
Breast	+	+
Endometrium	+	+
Melanocytes	+	–

Tissue	MHC-I	MHC-II
Endothelial cells (blood vessels)	+	+
Endothelial cells (lymph vessels)	–	
Skeletal muscle cells	(+)	–
Smooth muscle cells	–	
Gia cells	(+)	–
Nerve cells	(+)	–
Embryonic cells	–	–

Steinman et al. 1979; Van Furth 1982; Eliott et al. 1989; Becker 1992.

Congenital Immune Deficiency BARE (CID)

– High infection rate, high mortality
– Lack of MHC-class II expression (HLA-DR, -DQ, -DP)
– Autosomal
– Defect in nucleoprotein RFX or C II TA, which stimulate promotor for MHC-class II

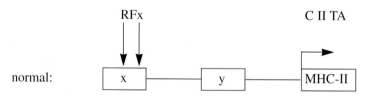

normal:

type 1 CIC:
type 2 CID:

– Gene for RFx has not yet been cloned
– Gene for C II TA codes for a novel 1130 aa protein
  mutations in CID
  * aa 940-963 are deleted
  * no genomic delection (possibly splicing error)
– Transfection or normal C II TA gene in CID lymphocytes repairs MHC-II expression
– Expression of C II TA (and MHC-II) enhanced by IFNγ

Mach et al. 1993; Steimle et al. 1993.

3.2.8 Modulation of Expression of MHC Molecules

	Manipulation	Dendritic cells	Effect	Reference
Compounds Acting on Dendritic Cells	Smoking	cervical mucosa	number ↓	Barton et al. 1988
	Smoking	lung	number ↑	Soler et al. 1989
	UV-B irradiation	skin	function ↓	Baadsgaard 1991 Kripke 1979
	DMBA (7,12-dimethylbenz-anthrazen)	skin	number ↓	Müller et al. 1985 Schwartz et al. 1981
	TPA (12-0-tetradecanoyl-phorbol 13-acetate)	skin	number ↓	Halliday et al. 1988 Baxter et al. 1988
	4-Nitroquinoline N-oxide	oral mucosa	number ↑	Pitigala-Aracheki et al. 1988
	Cyclophosphamide	skin	function ↓	Gruner et al. 1990
	Dexamethasone	skin	function ↓	Gruner et al. 1990
	Aromatic retinoid	skin	number ↑	Shiokara et al. 1987
	Retinoid acid	skin	function ↑	Bedford et al. 1989
	Splenopentin (Args-Lys-Glu-Val-Tyr)	skin	function ↑	Gruner et al. 1990
	Il-1	skin	function ↑	Steinmann 1988
	Il-1	thymus	function ↑	Steinmann 1988
	GM-CSF	blood	function ↑	Markowicz et al. 1990
	IFNγ	lung	function ↑	Kradin et al. 1991
	Il-4	skin	number ↓	Becker 1992
			function ↓	Becker 1992
	TNF	skin	function ↑	Becker 1992

Modulation of MHC-class I expression

	Normal cell	By IFN (α, β, γ)	By TNF	By others	reference
Liver parenchymal cells	(+)	+	+		Barbatis et al. 1981
Endothelial cell (lymph vessels)	(+)	+	+		Koretz et al. 1987
Sceletal muscle cells	(+)	+	+		Emslie-Smith et al. 1989
Smooth muscle cells	0	0	0		Koretz et al. 1987
B-, T-lymphocytes	+	++			Heron et al. 1978
Other tissue cells	+	++	++		Wallach et al. 1982 Hakem et al. 1989
B-lymphocytes	+			++ (EBV)	Jilg et al. 1991
T-leukaemia cells	+			0 (HIV)	Scheppler et al. 1989 Pals et al. 1993 Steinmann et al. 1993
Fibroblasts, keratinocytes	+			++ (UV-light + BPDE)	Lambert et al. 1989
B-, T-lymphocytes	+			0 (cortico-steroids)	Hokland et al. 1981
Keratinocytes	+			0 (cortico-steroids)	von Knebel-Doebe-ritzet al. 1990
Fibroblasts	+	++		(+) (RSV) (+) (AV-12)	Gogusev et al. 1988 Grand et al. 1987

Concept for Vaccines: Search for MHC-1 (vaccine) and MHC-II (Blocking) Peptides

Target	HLA	Library	Reference
Rheumatoid arthritis	DR1, DR4	YXXMXAXXL	Sinigaglia et al. 1993
Type I diabetes	DQW 3,2		
Multiple sclerosis	DR2		
Pemphigus vulgaris	DR4, DR6		
HBV vaccine	HLA 2.1	WLSLCVPFV (IC_{50} 6,9 nmol)	Sette et al. 1993
HCV vaccine		YLVAQATV (IC_{50} 45 nmol)	Sette et al. 1993
HIV vaccine		RMY—	Sette et al. 1993
HPV-16 (E-7) b	D^b	RAHYNIVTF	Melief et al. 1993
Malaria vaccine	B53	YPAEITLTW EPAPFDETL HPSDGKCNL (thrombospondin-related anonymous protein, TRAP)	Hill et al. 1993 Hill et al. 1993

4 Differentiation of T-Cells

4.1 Overview

Differentiation and Action of T-Cells:

The mature immune system is programmed to destroy foreign material entering the body.

Reactions with self antigens have to be excluded.

Deletion or inactivation (induction of anergy) of autoreactive T-cell clones during ontogeny prevents the generation of autoimmune reactions.

The thymus plays a crucial role in this inactivation process as it is the primary site for T-cell differentiation and generation of the T-cell receptor repertoire.

T-cells which leave the thymus can only "see" antigens when they are presented as peptides bound to major histocompatibility complex (MHC) molecules.

Only those T-cells leave the thymus that do not recognize the majority of autologous soluble or cell surface molecules.

T-cells which recognize self antigens presented by MHC-molecules on tissues outside the thymus are kept in an anergic state or are deleted in the periphery.

T-cells develop with the help of Il-7 and other cytokines. TH0 cells differentiate either into TH1 or into TH2 cells. Differentiation is modulated mainly by Il-4, Il-12, IFN gamma and Il-10.

The T-cell receptor CD4 complex identifies antigenic peptides presented by syngeneic MHC-class II molecules.

T-cells are activated if the TCR/CD4 complex and the CD28/ CTLA-4 molecule are stimulated by binding to their respective ligands. CD28 is stimulated by B7/BB1 of the APC.

Without co-stimulatory CD28, TCR/CD4 activation leads to anergy or apoptosis of T-cells.

Memory helper T-cells can be activated by antigens with the help of CD26. CD26 is a dipeptidylpeptidase IV, associated with CD45 (membrane linked protein tyrosine phosphatase).

Pullen et al. 1989; Bjorkman et al. 1988; Brown et al. 1988; Goodnow et al. 1988; Qin et al. 1989; Rammensee et al. 1989; Morahan et al. 1989.

T-cell differentiation

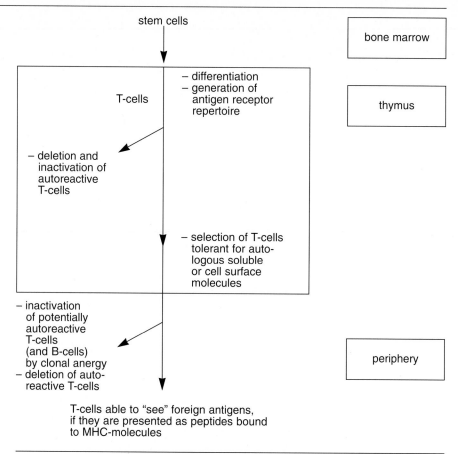

Pullen et al. 1989; Bjorkman et al. 1988; Brown et al. 1988; Goodnow et al. 1988; Quin et al. 1989; Rammensee et al. 1989; Morahan et al. 1989.

4.2 Details

4.2.1 T-Cell Development

Distinct developmental stages are controlled by TCR expression.

The initial TCR $\beta\beta$ homodimer controls expansion of population, regulates allelic exclusion, initiates CD4+, CD8+ positive T-cell expansion, and transscription of TCRα.

TCR $\alpha\beta\cdot$ heterodimer controls whether cells:

– Die by apoptosis when no binding to ligand presented by MHC-class II takes place
– Die when self antigen is recognized
– Are rescued when binding to specific peptide presented by MHC takes place

TCR expression (increase of density of TCR) leads to selective expression of CD4, CD8.

T-cell Development in the Thymus

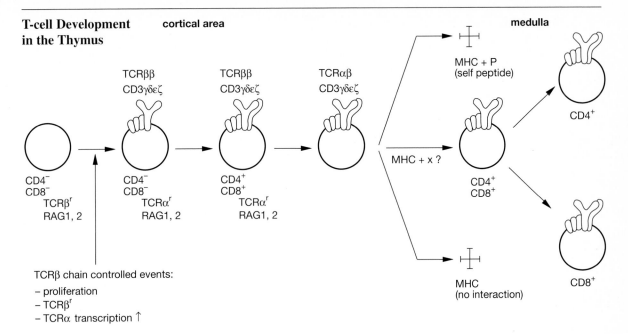

cortical area

TCRββ
CD3γδεζ

TCRββ
CD3γδεζ

TCRαβ
CD3γδεζ

medulla

MHC + P
(self peptide)

CD4⁻
CD8⁻
TCRβ^r
RAG1, 2

CD4⁻
CD8⁻
TCRα^r
RAG1, 2

CD4⁺
CD8⁺
TCRα^r
RAG1, 2

MHC + x ?

CD4⁺
CD8⁺

CD4⁺

CD8⁺

MHC
(no interaction)

TCRβ chain controlled events:

– proliferation
– TCRβ^r
– TCRα transcription ↑

Effect of Il-7 on T-Cell Development

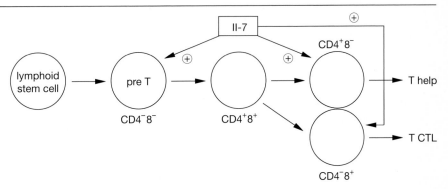

Il-7

lymphoid
stem cell

pre T

CD4⁻8⁻

CD4⁺8⁺

CD4⁺8⁻

CD4⁻8⁺

T help

T CTL

Masuda et al. 1991; Namen et al. 1988; Kishimoto et al. 1992

Development of Helper T-Cells in Mice

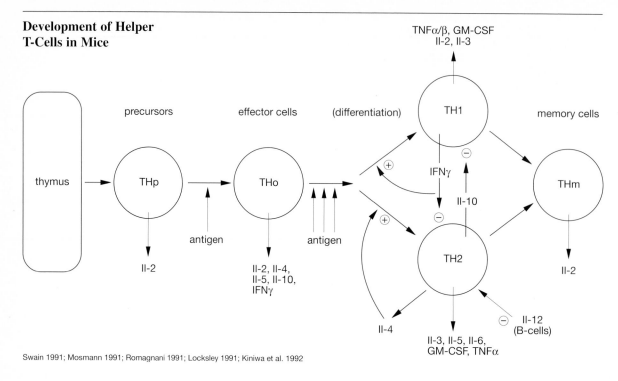

Swain 1991; Mosmann 1991; Romagnani 1991; Locksley 1991; Kiniwa et al. 1992

Arguments for TH₁–TH₂ Differentiation in Man

CD4+ T-cell clones from (biopsies) or specific for	Secreted cytokines			
	Il-4	IFN gamma	Other	Reference
Hashimoto thyreoiditis	–	++	TNFalpha	Del Prete et al. 1989
SCID patients	–	++	Il-2, Il-5, GM-CSF	Bacchetta et al. 1990
Candida albicans/				
Tetanus toxoid	–	++		Goldman et al. 1991
PPD	–/+	++	Il-2 (no Il-5)	Parrouchi et al. 1991
PPD	–	++	Il-2 (no Il-5)	Romagnani 1991 TH1
Contact dermatitis (Nickel)	–/+	++	Il-2, TNFβ, (Il-5 +/–)	Kapsenberg (Romagnani 1991)
TH₁ phenotype cultures	–	++	Il-1, TNFα, β, Il-3, Il-6, GM-CSF (no Il-4, Il-5) no B cell help (IgE) slight B cell help (IgM, IgG, IgA)	Romagnani 1991

CD4+ T-cell clones from (biopsies) or specific for	Secreted cytokines			Reference
	Il-4	IFN gamma	Other	
Vernal conjunctivities	++	–/+		Maggi et al. 1991
Severe atopic disorders	++	–/+		Romagnani 1990
Severe atopic disorders	++	–	Il-5, Il-3, GM-CSF	Kay et al. 19
Toxocariasis *(T. canis)*	++	–/+	Il-5 (no Il-2)	Romagnani 1990, 1991
Filariasis	++	–/+		Romagnani 1990, 1991
Intrinsic asthma		–	Il-5	Hamid et al. 1991
Atopic dermatitis	++	–/+	Il-5	Parrouchi et al. 1991 TH2
(Lolium perenue)	++	–/+	Il-5	
TH₂ phenotype cultures	++	–	Il-5, Il-3, Il-6, TNFα, GM-CSF (no Il-2, TNFβ) no cytolytic activity strong B cell help (IgE, IgM, IgG, IgA)	Romagnani 1991

4.2.2 The T-cell Receptor (TCR)

The TCR is a complex of several polypeptide chains expressed on the T-cell surface. It is consisting of variant and invariant regions, which are functionally closely associated with each other and with CD3 peptides.

Some 95% of human peripheral blood T-cells express the $\alpha\beta$-heterodimer, 3–5% of human peripheral T-cells express the $\gamma\delta$-heterodimer of the TCR. All chains (α, β, γ, δ) comprise constant (C) and variable (V) regions. The TCR-$\gamma\delta$ has a smaller repertoire of V-regions compared with the TCR-$\alpha\beta$.

The V-region is involved in antigen recognition. Each V-region owns three complementarity-determining regions (CDR), which presumably bind to the MHC as well as the antigenic peptide in the groove of the MHC. CDR3 is located in the region of hypervariability and seems to bind to the antigenic peptide.

Associated with the $\alpha\beta$-heterodimer (or the $\gamma\delta$-heterodimer) are the γ, ϵ and δ-chains of the CD3 and the η and ζ-chains. These five invariant chains are responsible for signal transduction and possibly also involved in antigen binding.

The γ-, δ- and ϵ-chains of CD3 are usually expressed as ϵ–γ or ϵ–δ heterodimers and the η- and ζ-chains as η–ζ or ζ–ζ dimers.

According to sequence analysis η- and ζ-chains are differently spliced products of the gene and belong to the ζ-chain family.

It is assumed that by expressing different combinations of these dimers of invariant chains the cell can be responsive to a variety of signals.

Williams et al. 1988; Potocnik et al. 1990; Dustin et al. 1988; Abbas et al. 1991; Fraser et al. 1993; Linsley et al. 1991, 1992; Freemant et al. 1991; Harper et al. 1991; Lenchow et al. 1992; Schwartz et al. 1992; Mustelin et al. 1993.

The T-Cell Receptor

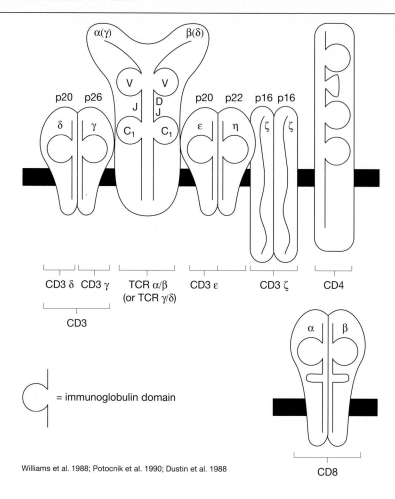

Williams et al. 1988; Potocnik et al. 1990; Dustin et al. 1988

**Comparison Between
TCR-αβ und TCR γ δ
Positive T-Cells**

	TCR-γδ		TCR-αβ	
Structure	heterodimer (associated with CD3) covalent dimerization: only type I, but not type IIabc and type IIbc V-, J- and C-regions, with an additional D-region		heterodimer (associated with CD3) covalent dimerization V-, J- and C-regions, β with an additional D-region	
Ontogeny	thymus: early expression other organs: yes		thymus: late expression (first β, than α) other organs: nearly no	
Variability Gene localisation	low γ: chromosome 7 δ: chromosome 14		high α: chromosome 14 β: chromosome 7	
Molecular weight	γ-type I: 40 kD (protein 32–34 kD) type IIabc: 55–60 kD (protein 40 kD) type IIbc: 40 kD (protein 35 kD) differences caused by different degrees of glycosylation, size of the CII-region, existence of cystein for SS bridges (only type I). δ: 33, 34, 37, 40 kD (dependent on size of V and degree of glycosylation)		α: 39,46 or 50 kD (dependent on degree of glycosylation) β: 50 kD	
CD4/CD8 phonotype an occurrence	CD4$^+$ CD8$^-$: 0 CD4$^-$ CD8$^+$: 20–50% CD4$^-$ CD8$^-$: 50–80% CD3$^+$: ≈8%	0,5–10% of CD3$^+$ lymphocytes in peripheral blood, skin ≈15% in spleen and gastrointestinal tract	CD4$^+$ CD8$^-$: 60% CD4$^-$ CD8$^+$: 35% CD4$^-$ CD8$^-$: < 1% CD3$^+$: >92%	>92% of CD3$^+$ lymphocytes in peripheral blood, >95% of thymocytes, majority in spleen, tonsilla, lamina propria of gut

Variability of the T-Cell Receptor: Number of T-Cell Receptor V, D, J and C Genes

chain	genes			
	V	D	J	C
α	50–100	–	50–100	1 (α)
β	75–100	1 (β₁)	7 (β₁)	1 (β1)
γ	–	–	3 (γ₁)	1 (γ1)
δ	4	2	3	1

Abbas et al. 1991.

4.2.3 The CD4 molecule

It is located on TH-cells, important in APC-T, T-T, T-B and probably T-monocyte cooperation (certain cytolytic T-cells are also CD4+). CD4 is also expressed on monocytes, dendritic cells (Langerhans, microglia) and subsets of B-cells (Bierer et al. 1989, Lifson et al. 1989).

It is a 50 kDa glycoprotein with 4 extracellular domains, the most distal from the membrane having homologies with VL of immunoglobulin.

It is in close physical proximity to the T-cell antigen receptor during T-cell activation (Saizawa et al. 1987).

With its domain similar to VL, it binds to MHC-class II (Krensky et al. 1982, Doyle et al. 1987).

By analogy with the immunoglobulin variable region, complementarity determining regions (CDR) have been defined on the Ig like domains of the CD4 molecules.

Despite their spatial separation, the CDR-like loops from both domain 1 (CD1 and 3) and domain 2 (CDR2) contribute to the binding site for MHC-class II molecules (Fleury et al. 1991).

The binding site for the HIV glycoprotein gp 120 localizes to the CDR2-like loop of the aminoterminal domain.

On the MHC-class II β-chain the binding takes place on a homologous loop (residues 137 to 143 of the class II β-chain) to the CD8 binding site on MHC-class I (Parham 1992).

4.2.4 The CD8 Molecule

It is located on CTLs, important for the recognition of syngeneic target cells and the activation of CTL by the T-cell receptor.

Heterodimer with an α- and a β-chain. The distal extracellular immunoglobulin domain of the α- as well as the β-chain is an immunoglobulin domain.

With its immunoglobulin domain the CD8α-chain binds to the (non-antigenic peptide binding) positions 223, 227, 228 and 245 of the α_3-domain of (preferably syngeneic) MHC-class I molecules (Salter et al. 1990, Newberg et al. 1992).

The cytoplasmic domain of CD8 is associated with the tyrosine kinase p56*lck* of the *src* family. Activation of CD8 by binding to the α_3-domain of the syngeneic MHC-class I molecule leads to activation of p56*lck* (Beyers et al. 1992).

The tyrosine kinase p59*fyn* is associated with the T-cell receptor and activated by binding of the TCR to the antigenic peptide presented by MHC-class I molecules. The CD3 ε, γ and ζ-chain of the TCR are substrates for p56*lck* and p59*lyn* (Beyers et al. 1992).

Costimulation of the TCR and the CD8 molecules induces activation of both the p56*lck* and p59*fyn* and activation of T-cells, i.e. CTL (Newberg et al. 1992).

In addition to syngeneic CTL responses, allogeneic as well as xenogeneic CTL responses can be observed. The interaction between the CD8 molecule and the α_3-domain of MHC-class I seems to be of low significance for xenogeneic and allogeneic CTL responses (Newberg et al. 1992).

The amino acid sequence of the CD8 binding site of the MHC-class I α_3-domain is highly conserved between different MHC-class I molecules (Teitel et al. 1991).

4.2.5 Activation of T-Cells by Antigen-Presenting Cells

T-cell activation in response to antigen displayed by MHC-II or CD1 on the surface of an antigen presenting cell involves the interaction of multiple receptor – co-receptor pairs.

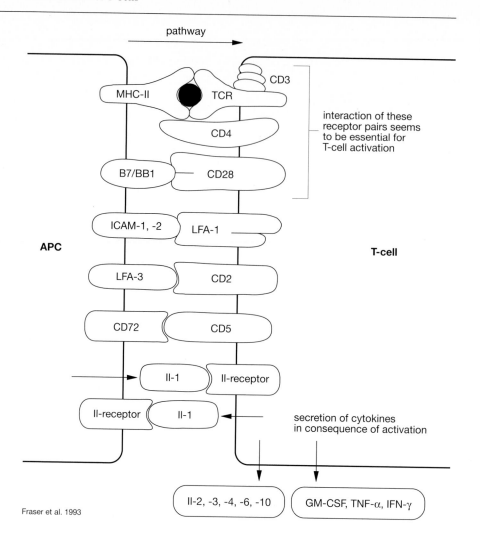

Fraser et al. 1993

**Specific Stimulation
and Co-stimulation of
T-Cells by APC**

	APC	T-cell	
Specific stimulators:	– peptides presented by MHC-II – peptides presented by CD1	– TCR, CD4 dependent – TCR, CD4 independent	

Co-stimulators:	– B7/BB1
	  * 30 kDa, 2 extracellular
	    Ig- domains
	
	  * expressed on APC and B-cells
	    upon activation
	    (i.e. by Il-4, IFN γ gamma, Il-1)
		– CD28
		  * 44 kDa, homodimer
		  * expressed on CD4+
		    T-cells
		  * kDa (B7/BB1) ca. 200 nM
		  * activation leads to aug-
		    mentation of Il-2 production
		  * partner (for B7/BB1) in
		    primary immune response
			– CTL A-4
			  * homologous to CD28
			  * expressed on CD4+ and
			    on CD8+ T-cells
			
			  * appears (max. 24 h)
			    after TCR stimulation
			  * 3% of level of CD28
			  * KD (B7/BB1) ca. 10 nM
			  * additional partner for
			    secondary immune
			    response

	– ICAM-1
	  * 90–120 kDa (peptide: 55 kDa)
	  * 5 extracellular Ig domains
	  * increase in expression by Il-1,
	    IFN gamma, TNF
	  * binding to LFA-1 active energy
	    consuming process
		– LFA-1 (CD11a, CD18)
		  * alpha-chain 180 kDa
		    beta-chain 95 kDa } integrin
		  * phosphorylation of beta-chain
		    increases affinity of binding
		  * linked to G-protein	

	– LFA-3 (CD58)
	  * 60 kDa, transmembrane
	    glycoprotein linked to G-protein
		– CD2 (LFA-2, T11, Leu5, SRBC-rec.)
		  * 49 kDa, membrane glycoprotein
		  * helper function to ICAM-1/LFA-1	

Linsley et al. 1991, 1992; Lindsten et al. 1989; Freeman et al. 1991; Harper et al. 1991; Lenchow et al. 1992; Schwartz 1992.

4.2.6 Signal Transduction After Activation of the TCR-Complex

Stimulation of the TCR-CD3 complex causes tyrosine phosphorylation of CD3δ.

It is unclear, whether phosphorylated CD3δ suppresses phosphotyrosine phosphatase (PTPase) or recruits cellular PT kinases. Probably, cellular PT kinases are activated.

CD3 is associated with the cellular PTK *fyn* (p59); CD4 respectively CD8 is associated with the cellular PTK *lck* (p56). Coaggregation of CD4 and TCR-CD3 enhances phosphorylation of both PTK.

Phosphorylation at Tyr 505 for *lck* and Tyr 528 for *fyn* inhibits the PTK activity of both enzymes, whereas phosphorylation of Tyr 394 *(lck)* and Tyr 417 *(fyn)* activates the respective enzymes.

The activation stage of both *lck* and *fyn* is positively regulated by the phosphotyrosine phosphatase CD45 (leucocyte common antigen; CD45 accounts for more than 90% of the total membrane bound PTPase activity). The PTPase activity of CD45 is counteracted by the kinase activity of the cytosolic PTK CDK (p50).

Dephosphorylation of Tyr 505 and Tyr 528 of *lck* and *fyn* and phosphorylation of Tyr 394 and Tyr 417 leads to activation of both enzymes which may phosphorylate ZAP-70 and by this induce cellular activation.

The Signal-Transduction Complex in T-Cells

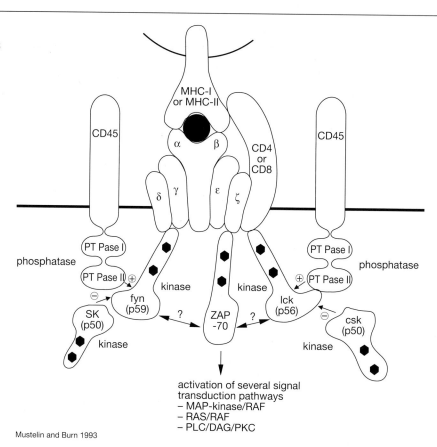

Mustelin and Burn 1993

Expression of *src* Family Kinases in Leukocytes

gene	molecular weight (kDa)	Expression T-cells	B-cells	Other cells
c-*src*	60	–		platelets
c-*yes*	62	+	+	ubiquitous
fyn	59	+	+	ubiquitous
c-*fgr*	55/53**	–	+	natural killer cells, granulocytes
lyn	56/53	–	+	granulocytes
lck	56,58,60,62	+	–	T-cells, natural killer cells
hck	59,56		–	granulocytes, mast cells
blk	55		+	
*csk**	50	+	+	ubiquitous

*)   *csk* resembles *src* family kinases in having *src* homology domains SH3, SH2 and the kinase domains but differs in having an amino-terminal membrane attachment motif, a tyrosine autophosphorylation site and a carboxy-terminal regulatory sequence.

**) Where more than one molecular weight is given, multiple forms exist due to alternative splicing or posttranslational modifications.

Association of cell surface proteins with *src* family tyrosine kinases

Receptor	Cell type	*src* family PTK
TCR-CD3	T-cell	*fyn*
CD2	T-cell	*fyn*
CD4	T-cell	*lck*
CD8	T-cell	*lck*
CD45	T-cell	*fyn, lck*
BCR	B-cells	*blk, fyn, lyn, lck*
FcγRIII (CD16)	natural killer cells	*fyn*
Il-2R	T-cell, natural killer cells	*lck, lyn*
FcεRI	mast cells, basophils	*yes lyn, src*
FcεRIIb (CD23)	mast cells, basophils	*fyn*
CD36	platelets	*lyn, fyn, yes*

4.2.7 Activation of T-Cells

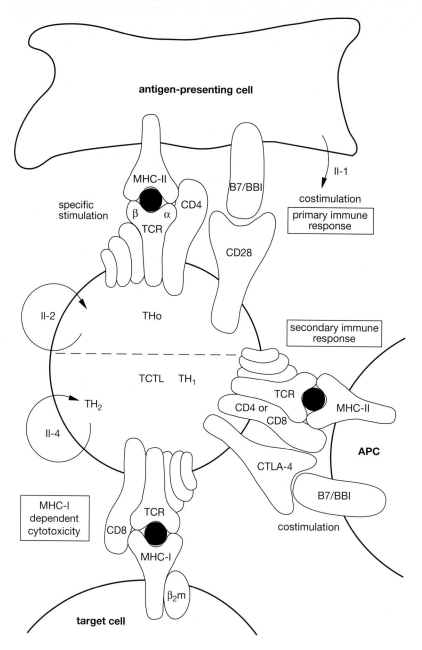

Antigen Presentation by CD$_1$

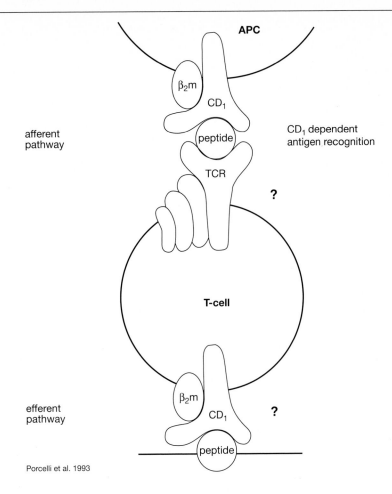

afferent pathway

efferent pathway

Porcelli et al. 1993

Regulation of the Immune Response by T Helper Cells

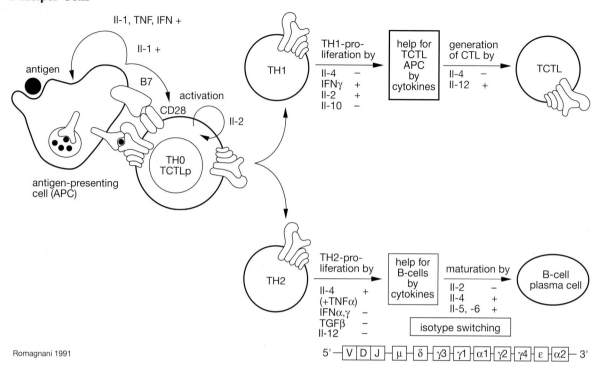

Romagnani 1991

5'—| V | D | J |—| μ |—| δ |—| γ3 |—| γ1 |—| α1 |—| γ2 |—| γ4 |—| ε |—| α2 |— 3'

Cytokine Secretion of T-Cells in Mice

Cytokine secretion	CD8+	CD4+				
		TH prec	TH$_0$	TH$_1$	TH$_2$	TH memory
Il-2	+/–	++	++	++	–	+
IFN γ gamma	++		++	++	–	
TNFβ	+		–	++	–	
GM-CSF	+		+	++	+	
TNFα	+		–	++	+	
Il-3	+		+	++	++	
Il-4	–		++	–	++	
Il-5	–		++	–	++	
Il-6	–		–	++	++	
Il-10	–		++	–	++	

Mosmann et al. 1986, 1989, 1991; Cher et al. 1987; Gajewski et al. 1988; Romagnani 1991.

The balance of stimulating and suppressing factors in the afferent immune response is guaranteed by Il-4, Il-10, Il-12, IFN γ gamma, PGE2 and histamine

	APC/ macro-phages	TH0 cells	TH1 cells	TH2 cells	B-cells	Eosino-phils	Granulo-cytes basophils	Neutro-phils
Il-1	+	+			+	+	+	+
Il-2	+	+	+		+		+	
Il-3	+	+	+	+	+	+	+	+
Il-4	⊖		⊖	+	+	+	+	+
Il-5			+	+	+		+	
Il-6			+		+			
Il-7		+	+		+			
Il-8							+	
Il-10	⊖	+	⊖		+		+	
Il-11	+				+			
Il-12			+		⊖			
Il-13	+				+	+		
IFN γ gamma	+	+	+	⊖	⊖	+		+
TNF α alpha	+	+						+
TNF β beta	+							+
GM-CSF	+					+	+	+
PGE2	⊖	⊖	⊖	⊖	⊖	⊖	⊖	⊖
Histamine	⊖		⊖	⊖	⊖			
TGF β beta		+			+			

+ = stimulation   − = inhibition

di Giovine et al. 1990, Banchereau et al. 1991, Romagnani et al. 1991, Gauchat et al. 1993, Bogen et al. 1993, Armitage et al. 1992, Kiniwa et al. 1992, Naume et al. 1992, Hsieh et al. 1991, Punnonen et al. 1993, Dugas et al. 1993, Emilie et al. 1992, Koch et al. 1992, Uotila 1993.

**The Main Cytokines
Involved in the Afferent
Immune Response**

Main cytokine	main source	Stimulation	Inhibition
Il-1β	macrophages, APC	– TH cells to secrete Il-2, Il-2 + Il-1β stimulate TH cells (proliferation, secretion of IFN γ gamma) – basophils/mast cells to secret Histamine – macrophages to secrete Il-1b, other cytokines (and PGE2)	– Histamine increases cyclic AMP and inhibits APC/macrophages and TH cells – PGE2 increases cyclic AMP and inhibits APC/macrophages and TH cells (expression of cyto-kines and of Il-2 receptors)
IFN γ gamma	TH cells (TH1)	– APC to secrete Il-1β + other cytokines – proliferation of TH1 cells and differentiation into cytotoxic T-cells	– suppression of TH2 cells (helper T-cells)
Il-4	TH-cells (TH2)	– proliferation and differentiation of helper T-cells (TH2), secretion of cytokines – isotype switch in B-cells – proliferation and differentiation of basophils and eosinophils (in cooperation with Il-3 or Il-5)	– suppression of release of Il-1b + other cytokines by APC/macro-phages – induction of apoptosis (dendritic cells) – inhibition of TH1 cells and CTL (in the absence of Il-2)
Il-10	TH cells (TH2)	– isotype switch in B-cells	– inhibition of macrophages/APC (expression of cytokines, MHC-class II) – inhibition of TH1-cells and CTL
Il-12	B-cells	– stimulation of TH1 cells (cytotoxic T-cells)	– inhibition of TH2-cells, decrease of secretion of cytokines (Il-4, others)

**The Main Cytokines
Involved in the Afferent
Immune Response**

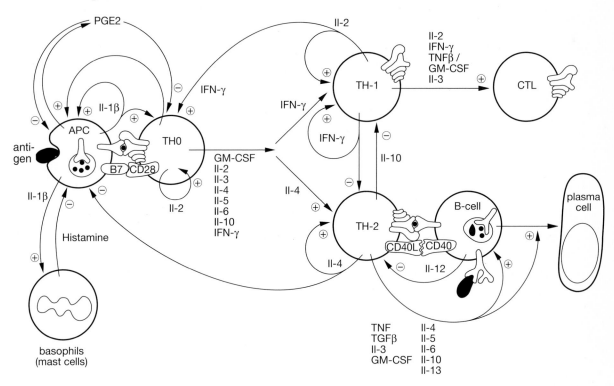

4.2.8 Activation of Memory T-Cells

CD26 (synonym: 1F7) is expressed only on CD4[+] memory/helper T-cells and on CD8[+] T-cells (Geppert et al. 1990, Fox et al. 1984).

   CD4[+]/CD26[+] T-cells are the only cells, which can:
– Respond to (soluble) recall antigens
– Induce B-cell immunoglobulin synthesis
– Activate MHC restricted CTL (Dang et al. 1990, Morimoto et al. 1989).
CD4[+]/CD26[−] T-cells cannot be triggered to elicit helper functions, but they can respond to mitogens and alloantigens.
CD26 is
* A functional collagen receptor of the integrin family (Dang et al. 1990)
* A dipeptidyl peptidase IV ectoenzyme (Ulmer et al. 1990)
* Of 110 kDa in size with
   – extracellular domain: 766 aa
   – cytoplasmic domain: 7 aa (Tanaka et al. 1992)
CD26 is associated with CD45 (membrane linked protein tyrosine phosphatase) for signal transduction (Torimoto et al. 1991).

CD26 can also be associated with the adenosine deaminase protein (ADA, 41 kDa) (Daddona et al. 1984, Aran et al. 1991) for signal transduction. ADA-deficiency causes severe combined immunodeficiency (SCID) (Hirschhorn 1990).

Dipeptidyl peptidase IV activity of CD26 seems to be essential for the costimulatory activity of CD26. Final result of the costimulatory activity of CD26 is the enhancement of the Il-2 production by the stimulated cell.

Via Costimulation of TCR and CD26–CD45 Memory CD4+ T-Cells Can Respond to Soluble Recall Antigens

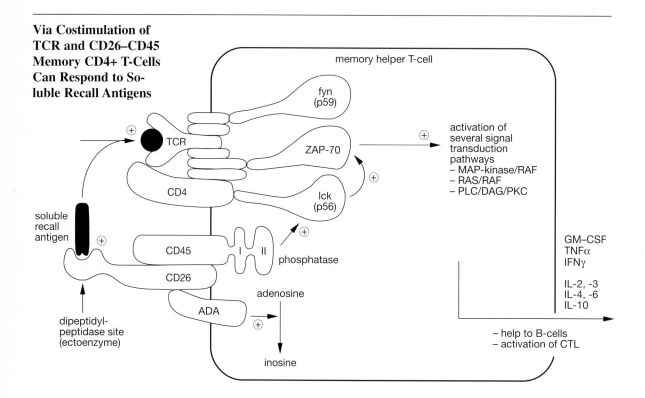

Role of CD26 in HIV Infection

CD4+ T-cells in patients with AIDS have an intrinsic defect in their ability to recognize and to respond to recall antigens.

In HIV infected patients a selective decrease of CD4+ CD26+ T-cells occurs prior to general reduction in CD4+ T-cells.

The HIV Tat-protein binds to and (partially) inhibits dipeptidyl peptidase IV of CD26.

CD26 seems to be a co-receptor with CD4 for entry into the cell.

Blazquez et al. 1992, Subramanyam et al. 1993, Hovanessian et al. 1993.

Pharmacological Inter-   **4.2.9 Pharmacological Intervention of T-Cell Activation**
vention of APC T-cell
Interaction

Target	Compound	Effect	Reference
TCR	– specific peptide	anergy by blockage of * Il-2 gene transcription * responsiveness to Il-4	Lindsten et al. 1989 Schwartz 1990 Kang et al. 1992
	– MAb anti TCR	anergy by blockage of * Il-2 gene transcription * responsiveness to Il-4	
B7/BB1	– Il-4, IFN γ gamma	induction of expression of B7/BB1	Linsley et al. 1991
	– CTLA-4-Fc (IgG)	blockage of T-cell priming * blockage of primary anti-body response even 48 hrs after immunization * blockage of xenograft re-jection * prolongation of allograft survival	Linsley et al. 1992 Lenschow et al. 1992 Turka et al. 1992
	– MAb anti B7	increase of Il-2 production (30 x)	Lindsten et al. 1989
	– transfection of B7/BB1 into tumor cells	strong immune response to original tumor cell (CTL reaction not dependent on tumor cells)	Chen et al. 1992

**Mechanism of Negative
Selection of T-Cells by
Apoptosis**

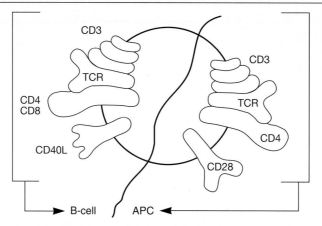

apoptosis may
be induced by:

– MAb anti CD3γ
– MAb anti CD3δ
– MAb anti CD3ε
– antigen without
  activation of CD4/CD8
– no co-stimulatory
  activation via
  B7/CD28 or
  CD40/CD40L

apoptosis: programm of active cell death

– chromatin condensation

– DNA fragmentation
  (oligonucleosomal "ladder")

– membrane blebbing

– fragmentation of cells into
  apoptotic membrane bound bodies

Green et al. 1992   – phagocytosis

5 Superantigens

5.1 Overview

Superantigens stimulate T-cells by crosslinking the MHC-class molecules with the T-cell receptor.

Stimulation of T-cells by superantigens is independent of the
- Antigen processing by APC
- Antigen specificity of the MHC-class molecules and the T-cell receptor (Herman et al. 1991)
- Helper molecules like CD8 and CD4 (for foreign superantigens) or CD8 (for self superantigens)
- MHC-haplotype matched presentation (no MHC-restriction: xenogeneic, allogeneic and autologous MHC-II can present superantigens).

Superantigens stimulate to a primary response by far (10^3–10^4 fold) more T-cells than antigens processed by APC.

Foreign superantigens can stimulate CD4$^+$ (T-help) as well as CD8$^+$ (CTL) T-cells (Fleischer et al. 1988).

Stimulation of T-cells by foreign superantigens needs a cell associated co-stimulatory signal (Miethke et al. 1991).

Self superantigen can only stimulate CD4 positive (T-help) T-cells (Janeaway et al. 1980).

5.1.1 Comparison between conventional antigens and superantigens

Property	Conventional antigen/peptide	Superantigen Self (mouse)	Foreign
Processing by APC	+	B-cells	−
Binding to K_d (M)	MHC-II MHC-I	MHC-II ?	MHC-II 10^{-7}–10^{-11}
Presentation on B-cells, APC by	MHC-II MHC-I	MHC-II	MHC-II
MHC-restriction (MHC-haplotype matched presentation)	+	−	−
Binding site on T-cells	CDR of TCR ($V\alpha$ Jα + $V\beta$ Dβ Jβ)	site of TCR away from CDR ($V\beta$)	site of TCR away from CDR ($V\beta$)
Need of CD4	+	−	−
Need of CD8	+	+	−
Response of CD4+ T-cells	+	+	+
Response of CD8+ T-cells	+	−	+
Frequency of responding T-cells (primary MLC)	10^{-4}–10^{-6}	10^{-1}–10^{-2}	10^{-1}–10^{-2}
Antigen specificity of T-cell response	+	−	−
Cell-associated co-stimulatory signal needed to stimulate T-cells	+	?	+

Janeaway et al. 1980; Pullen et al. 1990; Choi et al. 1990; White et al. 1989; De Kruyff et al. 1986; Zinkernagel et al. 1975; Bjïrkman et al. 1987; STeinman et al. 1983; Larsson Sciad et al. 1990; Herman et al. 1991; Fleischer et al. 1988, 1989; Herrmann et al. 1990; Hedland et al. 1990; Miethke et al. 1991.

Superantigen Cross-links the Vβ-Chain of the T-Cell Receptor with the β-Chain of MHC-Class II Molecule

5.1.2 Function

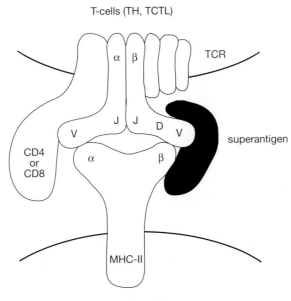

5.2 Details

5.2.1 Foreign Superantigens

Origin	Antigen	MW	Affinity to MHC-II (Kd)	Vb specificity (human)	Disease
Staphylococcus aureus	Enterotoxin A	27 800	$8 \times 10^{-7}\ M$	?	food poisoning
	Enterotoxin B	28 300	$3 \times 10^{-6}\ M$	3,12,14,15,17,20	
	Enterotoxin C1	26 000	$3 \times 10^{-6}\ M$	12	
	Enterotoxin C2	26 000	$3 \times 10^{-6}\ M$	12–15,17,20	
	Enterotoxin C3	28 900	$3 \times 10^{-6}\ M$	5,12	
	Enterotoxin D	27 300	$3 \times 10^{-6}\ M$		
	Enterotoxin E	29 600	$3 \times 10^{-6}\ M$	8	toxic shock syndrome
	toxic shock syndrome toxin 1	22 000	$3 \times 10^{-8}\ M$	2	
	exfoliating toxins A, B			2	scaled skin syndrome (toxic shock)
Streptococcus pyogenes	erythrogenic toxin A	29 200	$\approx 10^{-6}\ M$	12,14	toxic shock syndrome
	toxin B		$\approx 10^{-6}\ M$		
	toxin C	24 200	$\approx 10^{-6}\ M$		rheumatic fever
	toxin D		$\approx 10^{-6}\ M$		
					scarlet fever
Mycoplasma arthritidis	MA supernatant MAS	$\approx 26\ 000$	?	?	arthritis toxic shock

Herman et al. 1991; Fleischer 1991.

**Activation of T-Cells
by Superantigens**

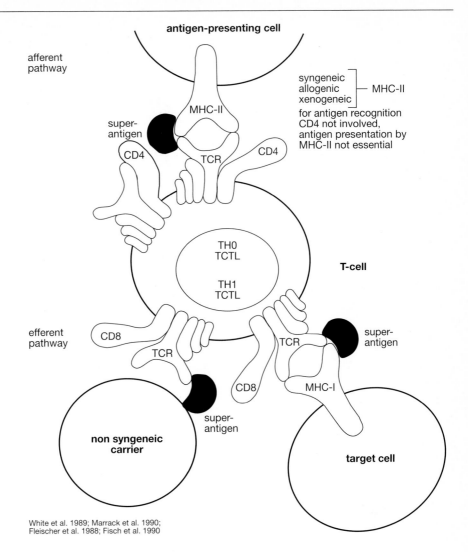

antigen-presenting cell

afferent
pathway

syngeneic
allogenic
xenogeneic } — MHC-II

for antigen recognition
CD4 not involved,
antigen presentation by
MHC-II not essential

MHC-II

super-
antigen

CD4

TCR

CD4

TH0
TCTL

TH1
TCTL

T-cell

efferent
pathway

CD8

TCR

super-
antigen

TCR

CD8

MHC-I

super-
antigen

**non syngeneic
carrier**

target cell

White et al. 1989; Marrack et al. 1990;
Fleischer et al. 1988; Fisch et al. 1990

5.2.2 Self superantigens of mouse mammary tumor virus (MMTV)

MMTV is a type B retrovirus that can exist either in an infectious (milk-trans-mitted) or integrated (in the genome as a provirus) form.

More than 40 endogenous MMTV proviral loci have been identified in mice with 2-8 loci in a given mouse strain.

MMTV possess an open reading frame (ORF) in their 3′LTR that encodes the minor lymphocyte stimulatory (Mls) antigen, which is a self superantigen. Most of the well characterized MMTV proviral integration sites have now been linked to genes encoding functional superantigens.

Mls antigens are nearly exclusively presented by B-cells not by other APC.

Reactivity to Mls antigens is exclusively determined by the variable domain of the β-chain of the T-cell receptor (TCR Vβ).

Mls can stimulate up to 20% of a T-cell population. (The stimulation rate within an antigen-specific conventional MHC-restricted T-cell response to peptide antigens is in the range of 10^{-4}–10^{-6} of the T-cell repertoire).

Mls antigens – despite their potent in vitro activating properties – cannot induce skin graft rejection or lethal graft versus host diseases in vivo.

With the help of Mls antigen definite evidence could be elaborated that autoreactive immature T-cells occuring during thymic development are deleted in the thymus.

Moreover, a clonal non-responsiveness (anergy) can be established following exposure of mature T-cells to neoself antigens in their periphery (Festenstein 1983; Kappler et al. 1988; MacDonald et al. 1998, 1992; Janeway 1991; Corley et al 1992).

6 Differentiation of B-cells

6.1 Overview

B-cell develop their B-cell receptor (BCR) via transient formation of surrogate L-chain/p55 complexes.

Il-7 stimulates pre B-cells to differentiate into B-cells.

The BCR is a complex of membrane bound IgM (or IgD) and heterodimers of nonpolymorphic transmembrane proteins (Igα, Igβ); Igα and Igβ are probably involved in signal transduction.

The BCR is activated by binding of the antigens to the membrane immuno-globulin. Cross-linking of the BCR with the complement receptor-2 (CR-2) through antigen ($\pm$ antibody) C3dg complexes enhances activation of BCR.

Enhancer elements (μ-enhancer, κ-enhancer) assure B-cell specific expression of Ig genes.

6.2 Details

6.2.1 B-cell Development

λ5 and VpreB contain Ig domain.

Both form a surrogate L-chain and associate with p55.

p55 is replaced by VDJCμ in preBII.

Unproductive rearrangement of VDJ and VJ genes leads to null cells or to the initiation of apoptosis at stages preBII and to immature B-cells.

Productive rearrangement leads to synthesis of complete IgM B-cell receptor (μ, δ-double producers exist also).

B-Cell Development

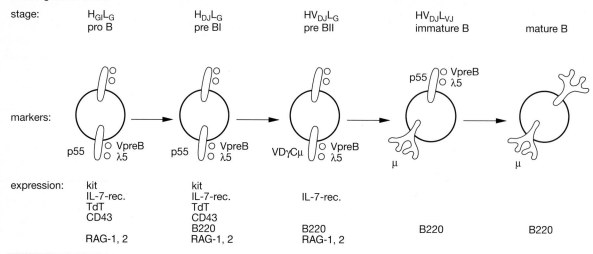

rearrangement event:

stage: $H_{Gl}L_G$ $H_{DJ}L_G$ $HV_{DJ}L_G$ $HV_{DJ}L_{VJ}$
           pro B   pre BI   pre BII   immature B   mature B

markers:

expression:

kit	kit			
IL-7-rec.	IL-7-rec.	IL-7-rec.		
TdT	TdT			
CD43	CD43			
	B220	B220	B220	B220
RAG-1, 2	RAG-1, 2	RAG-1, 2		

Effect of Il-4, -5, -6 and -7 on B-Cell Development

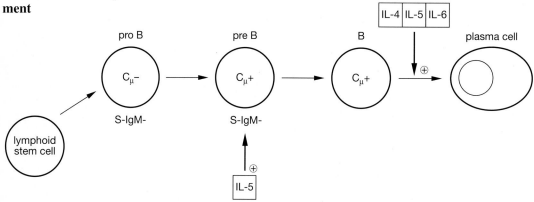

Masuda et al. 1991; Namen et al. 1988; Kishimoto et al. 1992

6.2.2 The B-Cell Receptor

The B-cell antigen receptor complex comprises at least four different molecules: the membrane bound Ig heavy and light chains and a heterodimer of nonpolymorphic transmembrane proteins.

These proteins are called Igα and Igβ and belong to Ig super gene family.

The extracellular domain of Igα and Igβ contains one Ig domain.

Igα and Igβ are about 90% identical between human and mouse.

Both Igα and Igβ can noncovalently associate with the H-chain of all five Ig classes.

The intracellular portion of Igα and Igβ are probably involved in signal transduction.

The Igα/Igβ heterodimer significantly enlarges the potential of the cell membrane immunoglobulin to interact with other molecules, because the cytoplasmic tail of mIgM or mIgD is only three amino acids long.

Igα/Igβ both in human and mouse can serve as substrates for protein tyrosine kinase (protein motifs with two highly conserved tyrosine residues).

Within the B-cell receptor a new protein kinase (PTK72) has been detected, which seems to have structural homology with the CD3-associated protein ZAP. Moreover, several SRC-protein kinases seem to be associated with the B-cell receptor.

The B-Cell Receptor

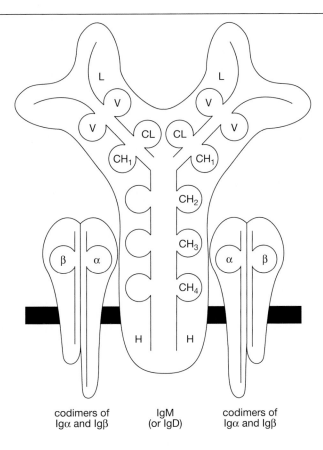

Immunoglobulin domain structure
– Regions of 70–110 amino acids with homology to either Ig variable or constant domains.
– Sandwich-like arrangements of β-pleated sheats.
– cysteine residues form intramolecular disulfide bonds and form a loop of about 55–75 amino acids.

– Ig domains are homology units that are found in many other proteins as for example Thy1 or MHC-class I or class II molecules.
– all proteins that contain one or more Ig homology unit belong to the Ig gene superfamily.

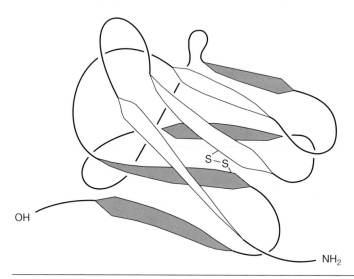

Abbas et al. 1991.

Activation of the B-Cell Receptor (BCR)

The antigen receptors on B-cells (BCR) are coupled via Guanine-binding proteins to the phospholipase C (PLC-C). Moreover, BCR is associated with protein tyrosine kinases (PTK-75, SRC-like PTK).

Upon binding of antigen to the BCR, PLC-C is activated, which mediates hydrolysis of phosphatidylinositol 4,5-biphosphate (PIP_2) to generate intracellular second messangers, namely inositol 1,4,5 triphosphate (IP_3) and diacylglycerol (DAG).

IP_3 mobilizes intracellular stores of calcium (Ca2+) and DAG; it is a physiological activator of protein kinase C (PKC).

Controversy exists concerning the role of G-proteins versus SRC-related PTK in the regulation of PLC activation.

Evidence exists, that G-proteins and PTKs couple to different isoforms of PLC activity (PLC-β, PLC-γ gamma).

Harnett et al. 1992

**BCR-Mediated
Signaling**

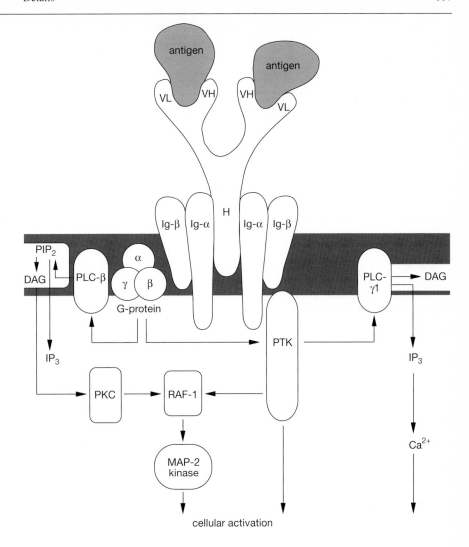

cellular activation

Activation of B-Cell via B-Cell Receptor (BCR) and Complement Receptor-2 (CR2)

Antigen activates directly or indirectly (via bound antibodies) complement. The arising C3-convertase cleaves C3 into C3dg. C3dg binds to antigen or bound antibody.

The complex consisting of antigen (± antibody) and C3dg cross-links the BCR (binding of antigen to specific membrane Ig of the BCR) and the complement receptor 2 (CR-2)/CD-19/TAPA-1 complex.

The CR-2/CD19/TAPA-1 complex consists of
- CR-2: synonym: CD21, transmembrane glycoprotein
  (short cytoplasmic tail)
  140 kDa, member of selectin family, natural ligands: C3dg, EBV, specific MAbs
- CD-19: transmembrane glycoprotein, 95 kDa
  member of the Ig superfamily
  natural ligand: unknown
  specific MAb can block or stimulate (dependent on immobilization of membrane Ig)
- TAPA-1: serpentin-like protein
  20 kDa
- Lyn: SRC-like TPK associated with CD19

CD19/TAPA-1/Lyn seems to function as signal transduction unit for the CR-2.

After cross-linking the CR-2/CD19/TAPA-1 complex is activated whereby clustering of CD19/Lyn may induce its activation through phosphorylation of CD19.

Assembly of Lyn at CD19 may activate the BCR by direct or indirect phosphorylation of Igα and Igβ of the BCR.

Soluble CR2 molecules completely suppress primary B-cell responses in vivo.

van Noesel et al. 1993, Hebell et al. 1991.

**Activation of B-Cells by
Cross-linking of BCR
and CR-2**

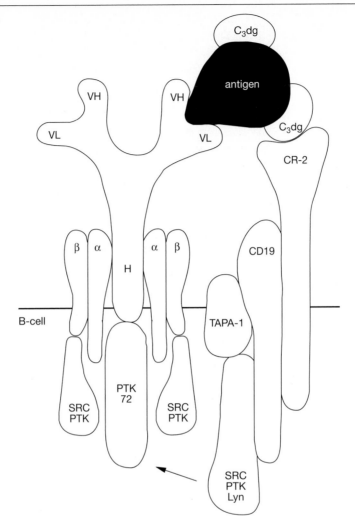

6.2.3 Transcriptional Control of Ig Heavy- and Light-Chain Genes

Enhancer elements (μ enhancer, κ enhancer):
- Assure B-cell specific expression of Ig genes.
- Contain multiple protein binding sites that bind B-cell specific and ubiquitous transcription factors; so called E-boxes (core: CACGTG) and octamer sites (core: ATGCAAAT).
- The POU factors Oct-1 and Oct-2 bind to the octamer sites, the transcription factors NF-Eμ1, -Eμ2, -Eμ3, -Eμ5 to E-boxes.
- E12, E47, E2-2, E2-5, TFE-3, TFE-B, USF are transcription factors from the helix-loop-helix (HLH) type and bind also to E-boxes.
- c-*myc*, N-*myc*, MAX and AP4 are transcription factors from the HLH-leucine zippertype and bind also to E-boxes.

The B-cell specificity of transcriptional regulation for ubiquitous factors as c-*myc*, MAX, USF, TFE-3 is assured through the action of specific inhibitors in other cell types or B-cell precursors.

The k-enhancer contains E-boxes octamer binding sites and a recognition site for NF-kb.

Ig H Enhancer (230 bp)

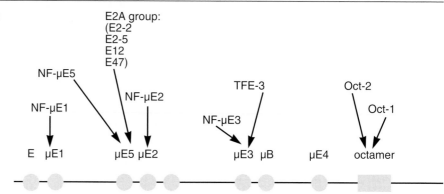

Schematical representation of the 5 region of the Ig heavy- and light-chain genes covering 100 bp.

Given are binding sites and the respective cognate transcription factors.

Ig k Enhancer (300 bp)

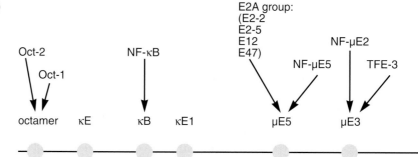

**Transcription
of V genes**

Transcription of the V-regions of rearranged heavy and light chains is enhanced only when V-region promotors are brought to the vicinity of the enhancer elements (E).

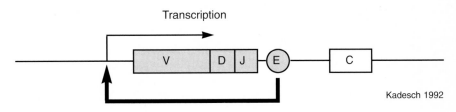

Kadesch 1992

7 Antibody Formation

7.1 Overview

Steps in Antibody Formation

B-cells are stimulated after recognition of antigen by BCR.

Antigen is either recognized directly or indirectly (via bound antibody) complexed with complement protein C3dg.

– Mice depleted of C3 have impaired memory B-cell formation (Matsuda et al. 1978).

– Humans with complement deficiencies are known to suffer from defective humoral immune responses (Jackson et al. 1979).

B-cells are helped by T-cells (TH2-cells) in antibody formation. Interaction between T-cells and B-cells takes place via the TCR on TH2 and antigen loaded MHC-II of B-cells.

Costimulation is essential for B-cell proliferation. Costimulation is mediated via interaction of CD40L on TH2-cells and CD40 on B-cells.

Moreover, TH1-cells help B-cells by secretion of Il-2 and TH2-cells by Il-4, -5, -6, -10. Such cytokines stimulate proliferation and differentiation of B-cells.

During proliferation of B-cells (centroblasts in germinal centers of lymphnodes) somatic hypermutation takes place.

B-cells producing high affinity antibodies are selected by the strengths of cross-linkage to follicular dendritic cells via antigen or antigen-antibody complexes (affinity maturation).

High affinity binding to the BCR and co-stimulation by the CD40/CD40L interaction and by cytokines (Il-2, Il-4) induce proliferation of B-cells (centrocytes) into plasmablasts.

Low affinity binding to the BCR induces apoptosis of B-cells.

Isotype switch of immunoglobulins within the B-cell is mediated by the type and the concentration of cytokines (Il-4, -5, -6, -7, -10, -12, -13, IFNα, γ, TNFα).

Main Steps in Antibody Formation

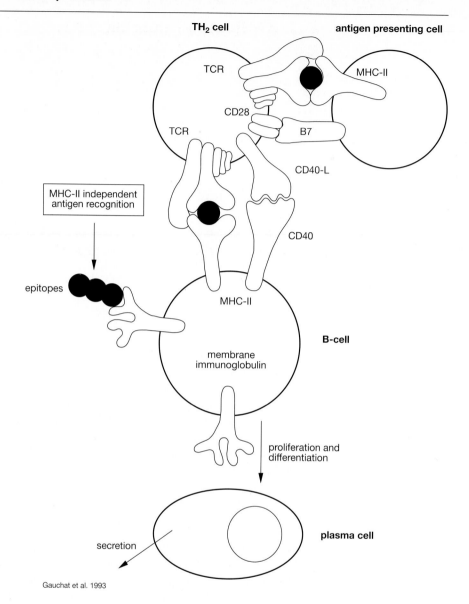

Gauchat et al. 1993

7.2 Details

7.2.1 VDJ Recombination

Requires activity of V(D)J recombination enzymes RAG-1 and RAG-2.

Requires the recognition of RS (recognition signal sequences) elements (heptamer-spacer-nonamer sequences) that flank each of the V, D and J germline genes.

Involves the introduction of double-stranded breaks between elements to be joined.

Involves potential loss or gain of nucleotides at the junctions of VD or DJ joinings (N-segments) as a result of TdT (terminal deoxynucleotidyl transferase) activity.

Is controlled by the developmental stage in B-cell differentiation: heavy chain rearrangement occurs in pre-B-cells before the light chain rearrangement in B-cells.

Is controlled by the lineage, i.e. occurs exclusiveley in B-cells and not in other lineages.

Is controlled by allelic exclusion, i.e. functionally joined VDJ gene segments (coding joins) lead to the inhibition of rearrangements of V, D or J gene segments of the second allele in the same cell.

Is controlled through the accessibility of the V-genes, accessibility correlates with transcriptional activity which itself is controlled by the μ and κ enhancer elements.

Alt et al. 1992

Immunoglobulin V, D, J and C Genes

Chain	Genes			
	V	D	J	C
Human heavy	100	?	6 (3*)	1 (μ)
				1 (δ)
				1 (γ3)
				1 (γ1)
				1 (γ2)
				1 (α1)
				1 (γ2)
				1 (γ4)
				1 (α2)
κ	100	–	5	1
λ	100	–	6	6
Mouse heavy	250–1000	12	4	1 (μ)
				1 (δ)
				1 (γ3)
				1 (γ1)
				1 (γ2b)
				1 (γ2a)
				1 (ε)
				1 (α)
κ	250	–	5 (1*)	1
λ	2	–	3	3

* pseudogenes

**Variable-Region
Heavy-Chain Locus**

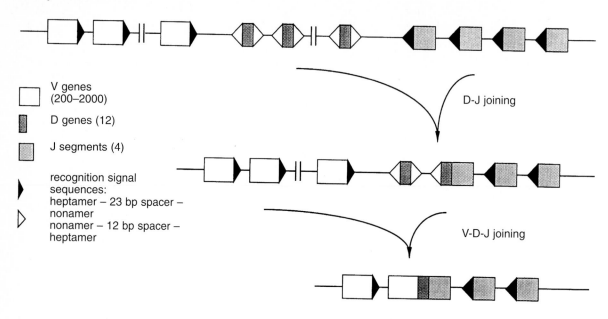

V genes
(200–2000)

D genes (12)

J segments (4)

recognition signal
sequences:
heptamer – 23 bp spacer –
nonamer
nonamer – 12 bp spacer –
heptamer

D-J joining

V-D-J joining

7.2.2 Cooperation of B-Cells with T-Cells

Cooperation between T-cells and B-cells involves the interaction of at least two
stimulatory signals.

One signal is given by antigen loaded MHC-class II molecules (MHC-II) on
B-cells and the T-cell receptor CD4 complex on T-cells. The other signal the
CD40 molecule on B-cells and the CD40 linker on T-cells. In addition, help is
given by the T-cell through expression of cytokines activating B-cells.

Loading of MHC-class II molecules with antigenic peptides is done in early
endosomes (post-Golgi-compartment) (see chapter on antigen presentation).

B-cells endocytose antigens for loading of MHC-II via different mechanisms:
– Constitutive, fluid phase pinocytosis (high concentration of antigen)
– Fc-receptor mediated endocytosis (of antibodies and antibody-antigen com-
   plexes)
– B-cell receptor mediated endocytosis (binding of (and cross-linking by) speci-
   fic antigens, even at low concentration).
B-cells can present their own Ig by two mechanism:
– Endocytosis of membrane Ig (free BCR or BCR complexed with antigen)
– Loading of MHC-II with intracellular Ig in the endoplasmic reticulum or in the
   early endosomes.

Cooperation between T-cells and B-cells involves the interaction of multiple receptor–co-receptor pairs

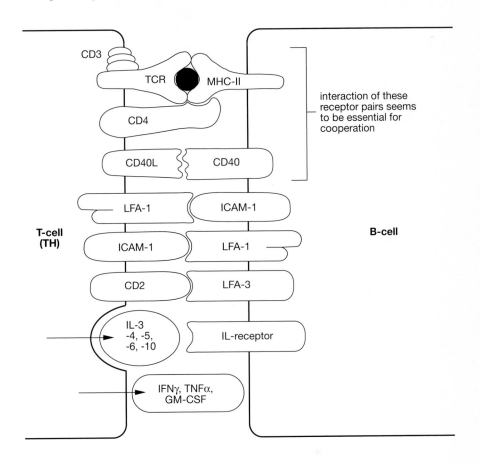

**Two Different Modes of
Cooperation Between
B-Cells and T-Cells**

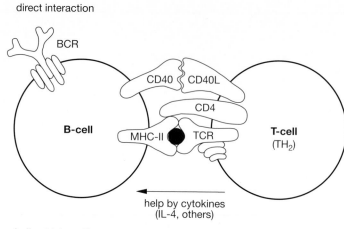

direct interaction

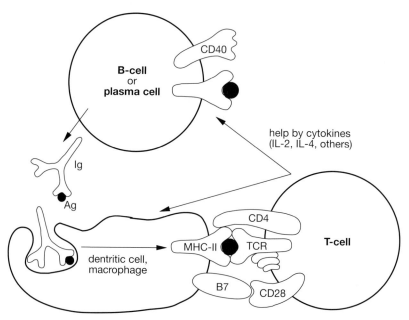

indirect interaction

Bogen et al. 1993

The CD40–CD40-L (Linker) System		CD40	CD40-L

	Structure:	– 277 aa, glycoprotein
		– homology with
		  NGF-receptor
		  TNF-receptor
		– probable dimer
			– 260 aa, glycoprotein MW ≈ 33 kDa
			– no homology with any known protein
			– probable dimer
			– K_a: 2 x 10^9 M^{-1}

	Expression:	– B-cells – epithelial cells (carcinoma cells)	– T-cells (activated)

	Function:	– B-cell activation and
		  function enhancement of
		  proliferation
		  (short -, long term)
		  adhesion, differention
		  prevention of apoptosis in
		  case of simultaneous
		  activation of CD40
		  and antigen receptor
		– CD40-Fc (soluble) is a
		  competitive inhibitor
		– forms heterotypic
		  adhesions between
		  B-cells and T-cells
			– B-cell proliferation in the absence
			  of costimulus
			
			– IgE production in the presence of
			  Il-4
			
			– only membrane bound (unsoluble)
			  seems to be effective
			
			– MAb anti-CD40 can mimic CD40-L
			
			– CD40-Fc (soluble) is a competitive
			  inhibitor
			
			– forms heterotypic adhesions between
			  T-cells and B-cells

Armitage et al. 1992; Liu et al. 1989.

7.2.3 B-Cell Differentiation in Lymph Nodes

Germinal Centers

Follicles consisting of a network of follicular dendritic cells are filled with re-circulating sIgM/sIgD bearing B-cells.

Antigen is taken up by FDCs in form of immune complexes.

B-cell blasts fill the FDC network in the first stage of germinal centers formation. B-cell blasts move to the dark zone and become centroblasts that do not express sIg anymore.

They divide rapidly and produce progeny: the centrocytes; these reexpress sIg and enter the dense follicular network, the basal light zone.

Centrocytes die by apoptosis if they do not recognise antigen presented on FDCs.

Upon interaction with antigen on FCDs cells move to the apical light zone; they survive and give rise to plasma cells and memory B-cells.

Liu et al. 1992; Korsmeyer 1992.

**Schematic Diagram
of Lymph Nodes**

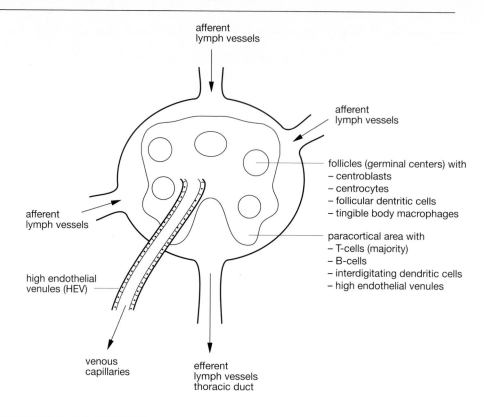

afferent
lymph vessels

afferent
lymph vessels

follicles (germinal centers) with
– centroblasts
– centrocytes
– follicular dentritic cells
– tingible body macrophages

paracortical area with
– T-cells (majority)
– B-cells
– interdigitating dendritic cells
– high endothelial venules

afferent
lymph vessels

high endothelial
venules (HEV)

venous
capillaries

efferent
lymph vessels
thoracic duct

**Functions of Germinal
Centers**

Follicular dendritic cells (FDC)
– Form the framework of the germinal center.

– Bind and present antigen in the form of antigen-
  antibody complexes for long periods of time.
– Essential for proliferation and differentiation
  of B-cells. Germinal B-cells cultured without
  FDC come to apoptosis.
– Release immune complexes in the form of
  immune complex coated bodies (iccosomes).
– Release CD23, which in combination with Il-1α
  prevents apoptosis of B-cells.

B-cells
– Proliferate (via centroblasts) into centrocytes.
– Undergo somatic hypermutation and are selected
  for high affinity.
– Low affinity B-cells are eliminated by apoptosis.

– Undergo immunoglobulin isotype switch.

Nossal et al. 1968
Szakal et al. 1968
Tew et al. 1979
Klaus et al. 1980
Tew et al. 1990
Kosco 1991

Szakal et al. 1988, 1989

Gordon et al. 1989
Liu et al. 1991

Griffiths et al. 1984

Wyllie et al. 1984
Liu et al. 1989, 1991
Kraal et al. 1982
Kocks et al. 1989

– Retire to memory B-cells.   Klaus et al. 1980
                                                                 Gray et al. 1988, 1991
– Bind iccosomes through their surface Ig-Rec.,   Kosco et al. 1988
  endocytose, process and present it via MHC-
  class II to T-cells.
– Activate T-cells.

T-cells (TH$_2$)
– Activate and lead to differentiation of B-cells.   Jacobsen et al. 1974
                                                                 von der Heide et al. 1990

Lymphocyte-Specific Adhesion Molecules on High Endothelial Venule Cells	Rolling	Glycam	– glycosylated cell adhesion molecule; mol. w 55 kDa; (70% sugar) – recognized by L-selectin, exact structure unknown – expressed in peripheral and mesenteric LN, but not in Peyer's patches and spleen
	Adhesion	CD44	– hyaluronate receptor (CM-Rec. III); MW 90–200 kDa (family of molecules with posttranslational modifications, splice variants, widely expressed)
	Adhesion	VAP-1	– vascular adhesion protein-1; mol. w 90 (180) kDa (expressed on FDC and HEV in peripheral lymphatic system on skin, brain, liver, kidney, heart cells, but not in mucosal lymphatic tissue and on leukocytes) – upregulated at inflammatory sites in venules – ligand on lymphocytes not yet known
	Transmigration	Mad CAM-1	– ligands integrin L-PAM-1 and (less) VLA-4

Salmi et al. 1993; Kraal 1993; Strauch et al. 1993.

B-cell Differentiation
in Lymph Nodes

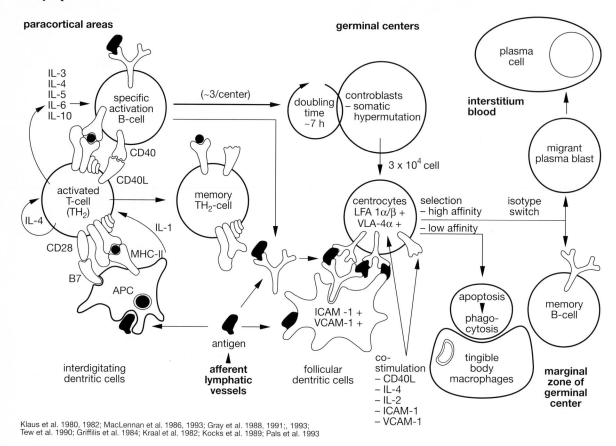

Klaus et al. 1980, 1982; MacLennan et al. 1986, 1993; Gray et al. 1988, 1991;, 1993;
Tew et al. 1990; Griffilis et al. 1984; Kraal et al. 1982; Kocks et al. 1989; Pals et al. 1993

**Effect of Il-4 on
Antibody Production**

Il-4 stimulates IgM, IgG1, IgG4, IgE
(switch to IgE) production.

CD4+ T-cells co-stimulate.
– Co-stimulation is inhibited by MAbs
  specific for TCR, MHC-II, CD2, CD4
  or LFA-1.
– Presence of antigen is not necessary
  (no MHC-II restriction).
– Physical contact between B-cells and
  CD4+ T-cells is essential.
– CD40/CD40L interaction seems to be
  involved.

Coffman et al. 1986,
1988
Finkelman et al. 1990
Gascan et al. 1991
Lundgren et al. 1989
Pene et al. 1988
Vercelli et al. 1989
Parrouchi et al. 1990
Gascan et al. 1991

Nüsslein 1993

No co-stimulation by CD8+ T-cells or   de Vries et al. 1991
CD4-, CD8- T-cells (rather inhibition).   Gascan et al. 1991
Co-stimulation by TNFα in the membrane   de Vries et al. 1991
of T-cells.
CD4+ T-cells can be replaced by MAb   Jabara et al. 1990
anti CD40, EBV or hydrocortisone.   Zhang et al. 1991
                                              Gascan et al. 1991
                                              Thyphronitis et al. 1989
                                              Wu et al. 1991

Il-4 inhibits LPS induced IgG2a,   Coffman et al. 1988
IgG2b, IgG3 production.
Blockage of Il-4 induced IgE synthesis by:
− IFNα, IFN γ gamma   Pene et al. 1988
− TGFβ   de Vries et al. 1991
− Il-10   de Waal et al. 1991
− Il-12   Kiniwa et al. 1992
Enhancement of Il-4 induced IgE synthesis by:
− Il-5 (only at suboptimal concentrations of Il-4)   Pene et al. 1988
− Il-6 (MAb anti Il-6 completely block IgE   Jabara et al. 1990
  production)
− TNFα (switch to IgE in synergy with Il-4)   de Vries et al. 1991
Il-4 inhibits production of:
− Il-6, TNFα, Il-10 (by monocytes)   de Waal et al. 1991
                                              Hart et al. 1989
                                              Te Velde et al. 1990

− Il-1β, PGE2 (by monocytes)   Hart et al. 1989
                                              Te Velde et al. 1990
− IFN γ gamma (by monocytes, NK-cells)   Peleman et al. 1989

B-Cell Stimulation by Il-4

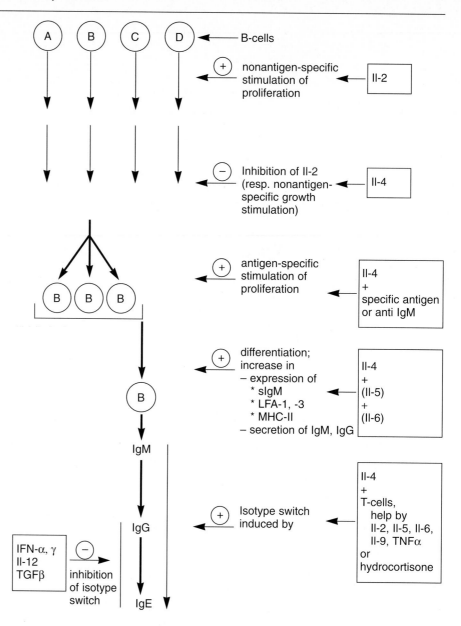

Kiniwa et al. 1992, Finkelmann et al. 1990, Snapper et al. 1987, Pene et al. 1988, Tan et al. 1992, Gauchat et al. 1992, Pukerson et al. 1992.

Ig Isotype Class Switching Control by Cytokines (Mouse)

Cytokine	cellular source	T-cell independent type 1 (LPS)	T-cell independent type 1 (dextran)	T-cell dependent T-cells
Il-4	T-cells, mast cells	IgG1, IgE	IgG1	IgG1, IgE
IFN-γ	T-cells, nat. killer cells	IgG2a	IgG2a, IgG3	IgG2a, IgG3
TGF-β	T-cells, B-cells, macrophages	IgG2b, IgA	IgA	IgG2b, IgA

The B-cell activator is given in parentheses.

Snapper and Mond 1992.

Inhibitory and Stimulatory Effect of Mediators on Isotype Switching

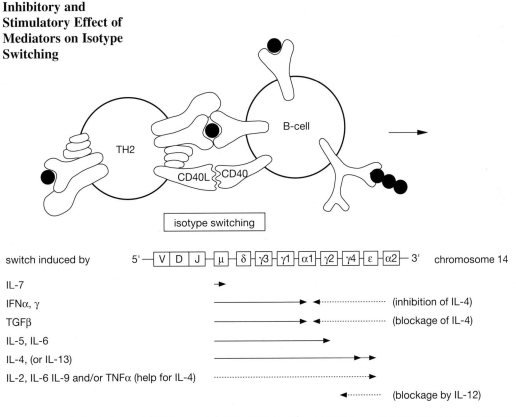

van Vlasselaer et al. 1992; Coffman et al. 1987; Snapper et al. 1987a, 1987b; Lundgren et al. 1989; Gascan et al. 1991; Pene et al. 1988a, 1989b; Del Prete et al.1988, Kehrl et al. 1987, 1989; Corrigan 1992; Gauchat et al. 1992; Kiniwa et al. 1992; Tan et al. 1992; Dugas et al. 1993; Punnonen et al. 1993

7.2.4 Main Cytokines Involved in Differentiation to Plasma Cells

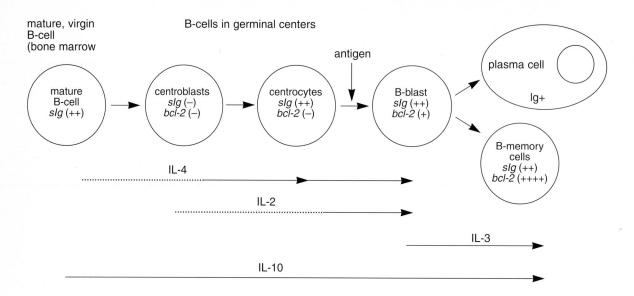

Dechanet et al. 1993; Korsmeyer 1992; Liu et al. 1992

8 Fc-receptor and Antibody Interaction

8.1 Overview

Fc-receptors are defined structures in the cell membrane which bind to the Fc (crystalline fragment) part of IgG, IgE, IgA, IgM or IgD.

Binding of IgG to Fc-recptors is dependent on the concentration of IgG and/or on its conformational change upon binding to antigen or upon chemical or physical influence.

Fc-receptors are involved in:

- Enhancement (opsonisation) of phagocytosis of antibody-coated antigen by macrophages and granulocytes.
- Inflammatory reactions induced by antigen-antibody (immune) complexes (exocytosis of lysosomal enzymes, release of cytokines and mediators).
- Blood clotting by immune complex-mediated aggregation of platelets.
- Allergic reactions by release of mediators through basophils and mast cells after antigen-mediated cross-linking of Fc-receptor bound IgE.
- Control of steady state plasma level of immunoglobulins by Fc-receptor mediated endocytosis and metabolization of immunoglobulins.
- Transcytosis of immunoglobulins (placenta).
- Feedback suppression of B-cells via cross-linking of the Fc-receptor and the B-cell receptor.
- Cytotoxic reactions to target cells via specific antibodies stimulating cytotoxic cells with their Fc part.

8.2 Details

8.2.1 Properties of Murine Fc-Receptors

	Fc γ RIIa	Fc γ RIIb	Fc ε R	Fc α R	Fc µ R	Fc δ R
Lymphocyte distribution	T-cells (/) NK-cells	B-cells T-cells (part)	B-cells (IgD$^+$/IgM$^+$) T-cells, activ. (CD4+/CD8+)	B-cells T-cells, activ. (CD4+/CD8+)	B-cells T-cells, activ. (CD4+/CD8+)	B-cells T-cells, activ. (CD4+)
Specificity	IgG1, -2b, -2a	IgG1, -2b, 2a	IgE	IgA	IgM	IgD
Molecular weight	40 kDa	40 kDa	45 kDa	38 kDa	?	40 kDa
Structure	Ig-like domain	Ig-like domain	lectin-like domain	?	?	?
Soluble form	?	+	+	+	+	+
Affinity	low	low	low	low	low	low
Efect of IFNα/β	+	+	+	–	?	?
Il-4			+			
IFN γ gamma			–			
TGFβ			–			

Friedman et al. 1980; Yodoi et al. 1983; De France et al. 1987; Conrad et al. 1987; Berg et al. 1990, Lynch et al. 1990.

8.2.2 Human Fc-Receptors

Type		Syno-nym	CD, Ly	Affinity (K_a M^{-1})	Specificity	Structure	Glycol. site	Number (aa)	Molecular weight (kDa)
Fcγ	RI		CD64	10^8–10^9 (IgG)	1=3>4≫2	1 chain	6	374	72
	RII - A	- a	CDw32	<10^7 (IgG)	1=3≫2,4	1 chain	2	325	40
	- B	- b, - C	CDw32	<10^7 (IgG)	1=3≫2,4	1 chain	3	310	40
	- C	- a', -B	CDw32	<10^7 (IgG)	1=3≫2,4	1 chain	3	321	40
	RIII - A α	- 2	CD-16	<10^7 (IgG)	1,3≫2,4	α+γ+γ; α+γ+ζ; α+ζ+ζ	5	254	50–80
	- A γ				association subunit	–	1 chain	0	86	7–9
	- A ζ	TCR/CD3ζ			association subunit	–	1 chain	0	163	16
	- B	- 1	CD-16	<10^7	1,3≫2,4	GPI anchoring	6	233	50–80
Fc ε	RI - α			10^{10} (IgE)	IgE	α+β+γ+γ	6	260	45–65
	- β			association subunit	–	1 chain			
	- γ			association subunit	–	1 chain	0	86	7–9
	RII - A		CD23	<10^7 (IgE)	IgE		1	321	ca. 40
	- B		CD23	<10^7 (IgE)	IgE		1	321	ca. 40

A, B, C = structurally related but distinct genes; α, β, γ, ζ = protein subunits; GPI = glycosyl-phosphatidyl inositol anchoring

Burton 1985; von de Winkel 1991; Ravetch et al. 1991; Yokota et al. 1988, 1992; Kikutani et al. 1986.

Expression and Function of Human Fc Receptors

		Mon./ M0	Eosin.	Neutro.	Baso.	Mast. c.	NK	B	T	plate-lets	Function (+ expression on other cells)
Fc γ	RI	+	+	(+)	−	−	−	−	−	−	internalization, delivery to lysosomes
	RII - A	+	+	+	?	?	−	−	−	+	phagocytosis, ADCC, IC, (Langerhans cells, endothelium)
	- B	+	−	−	?	?	−	+	−	−	internalization, delivery to lysosomes, ADCC, inhibition of Ig synthesis (feedback suppression)
	- C	+	+	+	?	?	−	−	−	−	phagocytosis, ADCC
	RIII - Aα	+	−	−	?	?	+	−	+	−	ADCC, phagocytosis, IC (mesangium, trophoblast)
	- B	−	+	+	?	?	−	−	−	−	Synergism with RII A, binding of IC (without activation)
Fc ε	RI - α	−		−	+	+	−	−	−	−	degranulation (allerg. mediators), secretion of cytokines
	- γ	+		−	+	+	+	−	+	−	(functional subunit)
	RII - A	−	−	−	−	−	−	+	+	−	endocytosis (antigen presentation)
	- B	(+)	+	−	−	−	−	(+)	−	−	phagocytosis (antigen presentation) (only on μ+, δ+ positive B-cells)

Burton 1985; van de Winkel 1991; Ravetch et al. 1991; Yokota et al. 1992; Bieber et al. 1989, 1992; Valent et al. 1990; Lin et al. 1990.

Structure of Fc Receptors

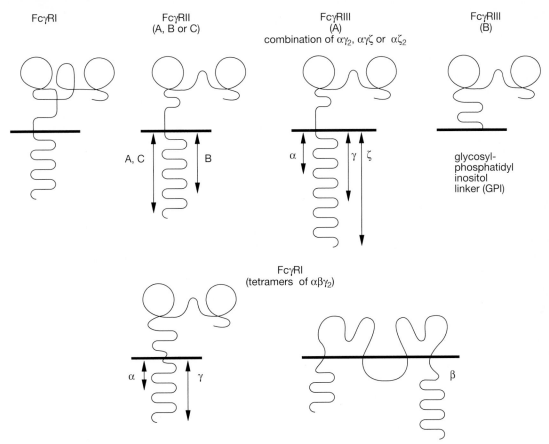

FcγRI

FcγRII
(A, B or C)

FcγRIII
(A)
combination of $\alpha\gamma_2$, $\alpha\gamma\zeta$ or $\alpha\zeta_2$

FcγRIII
(B)

A, C   B

α γ ζ

glycosyl-
phosphatidyl
inositol
linker (GPI)

FcγRI
(tetramers of $\alpha\beta\gamma_2$)

α γ

β

based on review of Ravetch and Kinet 1991

Fc ε Receptors Bind
IgE at Its CH3 Domain

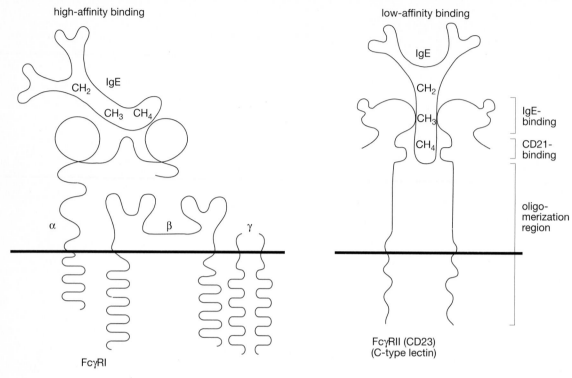

high-affinity binding

low-affinity binding

Gould et al. 1991; Stadler et al. 1993

Organ Distribution and Function of Fc γ Receptors	Cells	Fc γ RI (72KdA, CD64)	Fc γ RII (40KDa, CD32)	Fc γ RIII A, B (50-80KDa, CD16)
	Monocytes	+	+	+ (subpopulation)
	Macrophages	+	+	+
	Neutrophils	–	+	+
	Eosinophils		+	+
	Basophils		+	
	B-cells		+	
	LGL/NK-cells			+
	T-cells			+ (subpopulation)
	Platelets		+	
	Langerhans cells		+	
	Endothelial cells (placenta)		+	
	Mesangial cells (kidney)			+
	Trophoblast cells			+
	Function			
	Recycling		+	
	Phagocytosis	+	+	+ (A)
	O_2-generation (granulocytes)	+	+	+ (A)
	Exocytosis		+	+ (B)
	ADCC by monocytes	+	+	+ (A, B)
	by neutrophils		+(+GM-CSF)	
	by NK-cells		+	+
	by eosinophils		+(+GM-CSF)	
	TNFα release	+	+	+ (A)
	Il-6 release	+		
	Ig production		+	
	Transport of IgG			+

Burton 1985; van de Winkel 1991; Fanger 1989.

Structures Interacting with IgG Constant Regions

	C1q binding Ka (1/M)	C' activation	Binding to human Fc receptors (K_a; 1/M)		Binding to mouse Fc receptors		
			Fcγgamma RI	Fcγgamma RII	Fcγgamma RIII A,B	Trypsin sensitive	Trypsin resistant
Human							
Monomeric							
IgG1	1×10^4	+	$\sim5 \times 10^8$	$\sim5 \times 10^6$	$\sim4 \times 10^7$		++
IgG2	6×10^3	(+)	$<10^6$	$\sim5 \times 10^6$	(< IgG4)		–
IgG3	3×10^4	+	5×10^8– 1×10^9	$\sim10^7$	$\sim4 \times 10^7$		+++
IgG4	4×10^3	–	$\sim10^7$	$<10^6$	(<IgG3)		+
Aggregated							
IgG	5×10^3– 2×10^4	+	5×10^8– 3×10^9	$\sim2 \times 10^7$	$\sim4 \times 10^7$		
Fc (IgG1/4)	1×10^4	–	50^5–10^6				
Mouse							
Monomeric							
IgG1		+	$\sim10^6$	$\sim10^6$	(<IgG2b)		5×10^5
IgG2a		+	5×10^8	(<Ig2b)	$\sim10^6$	2×10^7	5×10^5
IgG2b			$\sim10^6$	$<10^6$	$<10^6$		5×10^5
IgG3		+	5×10^8	(<IgG2b)	$\sim10^7$		
Aggregated							
IgG		+	10^7–10^8				$\sim1 \times 10^6$
Fc		–			5×10^6		

Burton 1985; van de Winkel 1991

Signal Transduction via Fc-Receptors

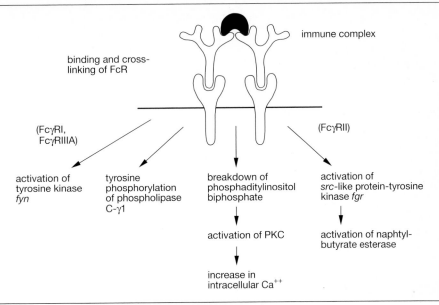

immune complex

binding and cross-linking of FcR

(FcγRI, FcγRIIIA)

(FcγRII)

activation of tyrosine kinase *fyn*

tyrosine phosphorylation of phospholipase C-γ1

breakdown of phosphaditylinositol biphosphate

↓

activation of PKC

↓

increase in intracellular Ca^{++}

activation of *src*-like protein-tyrosine kinase *fgr*

↓

activation of naphtyl-butyrate esterase

Function of the Fc ε RII (CD23)

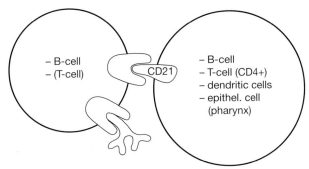

– B-cell
– (T-cell)

CD21

– B-cell
– T-cell (CD4+)
– dendritic cells
– epithel. cell (pharynx)

Fc ε RII
receptor for:
– IgE (low affinity)
– CD21

Function
stimulation of
– growth (myeloid precursors, B-cells)
– survival (B-cells in germinal centers)
– maturation (prothymocytes)
– antigen presentation (MHC-II)
MAb anti-CD23
– stimulate B-cell proliferation
– block differentiation into IgE secreting B-cells in response to IgE

CD21 (MW 135-170 K)
receptor for:
– C3d (C3dg, iC3b)
– EBV (gp 350/220 env. GP)
– Interferon α alpha
Function
stimulation of
– proliferation by ligands (MAb anti CD21) or soluble CD23
– IgE synthesis in response to Il-4

Aubry et al. 1992

8.2.3 Modulation by Cytokines

**Cytokines Affecting Fcγ
Receptor Expression
and Function**

Density of receptors (x 10^3 / cell)

Cells and cytokines	FcγRI	FcγRII	FcγRIII A, B	FcγRI	FcγRII A,B
– Monocytes	15–40	30–60	1–5	–	–
– Macrophages	50–100	30–80	40–100	–	–
+ IFN γ gamma	▲ (100–300)	▼ (ADCC▲)	–		▲ (B)
TGFβ	–	–	▲ (A)		
TNFα	–	–	▼ (B)		
Il-4	–	–	▼	–	▲ (B)
G-CSF, M-CSF					
Il-1, Il-2	–	–	–		
Il-2, Il-6					
– Neutrophils	<2	30–60	100–200	–	–
+ IFN γ gamma	▲ (5–20)	– (ADCC▲)	–		
G-CSF	▲	–	–		
TNFα	–	–	▼ (50–100)		
GM-CSF	–	– (ADCC▲)	–		
Il-3	–	–	–		
– Eosinophils	<3	25–35	5–15	–	5 (B)
+ IFN γ gamma	–	–	–		
GM-CSF	–	– (ADCC▲)	– (ADCC▲)		
TNF, Il-5					
– Basophils/ mast cells-	?	?	?	+	–
+ Il-4	–	–	–	▲	–
Il-3	–	–	–	▲	–
– Lymphocytes (B-/T-cells)	–	10 (B-Ly)	5 (T-Ly)	–	+ (B-Ly,A)
+ Il-2		▲			
Il-4	–	▼			▲ (B-Ly,B)
IFN γ gamma	–	▲			
– Platelets	–	<2	–	–	–

Daeron et al. 1990; Yokota et al. 1988; Lazlo et al. 1988; Fanger 1989; van de Winkel 1991; Ravetch et al. 1991; Yokota et al. 1992; Kay 1992; Bieber et al. 1989, 1992; Valent et al. 1990; Lin et al. 1990.

▲ = increase   ▼ = decrease

8.2.4 Release of Immunoglobulin Binding Proteins (IBFs) and Its Modulation

Cell	Caused by	Secretion of soluble form	Reference
T-cells	–	FcγRI	Friedman et al. 1974
T-cells	Il-2, Il-4	FcδRI	Amin et al. 1988
T-cells	IgG	FcγRII	Daeron et al. 1988
B-cells	Il-4, IFN gamma	FcεRII	Bonnefoy et al. 1988

Selective Release of Il-1 Receptor Antagonists (Il-1 RA) by Polyclonal Antibodies

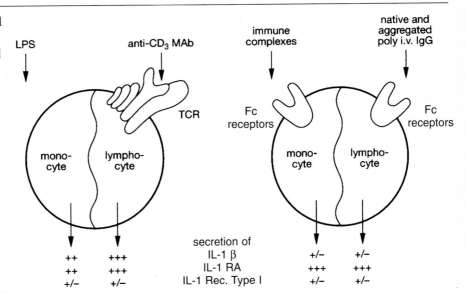

Arend et al. 1985, 1991; Kurrle et al. 1992

8.2.5 Blockage of Antibody Production

Mechanism	Responsible structure	Author
Blockage of idiotypes (Fab, haptens)	V region of antibody	Möller 1985 Zalcberg et al. 1987
Feedback suppression – by IgG (all subclasses)	Fc part of IgG carbohydrates on Fc Fc receptors on B-cells	Voisin 1980 Morgan et al. 1987 Heyman et al. 1985 Uhr et al. 1968
– by anti Fc γ gamma rec. antibodies (MAb)	V region of MAb	Gergely et al. 1992
– by immunoglobulin binding substance (IBFs)	soluble Fc γ gamma rec. (presumably Fc γ gamma RII)	Fridman et al. 1974 Thi Bick Thui et al. 1980 Khagat et al. 1987 Santes et al. 1990
– cross-linking of Fc γ gamma RII and mIg	idiotype and Fc part (IgG) of immune complexes	Abrahams et al. 1973 Kölsch et al. 1980 Rigley et al. 1989
– cross-linking of complement receptors (CRH2) and mIg	idiotype of antibodies in immune complexes and C3b bound to Fc part of immune complexes	Tsohos et al. 1990 Carter et al. 1988
– blockage of CR2 receptors without cross-linking	monomeric C3b, C3d or monovalent antibodies to CR2 receptors	Howard et al. 1983

Feedback Suppression of B-Cells by Cross-linking of Fc γ gamma RII Receptor and Membrane IG (m Ig)

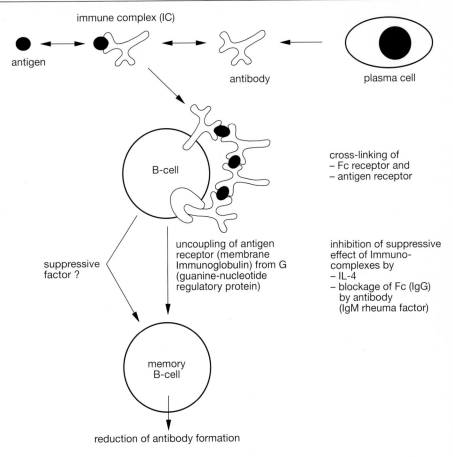

immune complex (IC)

antigen

antibody

plasma cell

B-cell

cross-linking of
– Fc receptor and
– antigen receptor

suppressive factor ?

uncoupling of antigen receptor (membrane Immunoglobulin) from G (guanine-nucleotide regulatory protein)

inhibition of suppressive effect of Immuno-complexes by
– IL-4
– blockage of Fc (IgG) by antibody (IgM rheuma factor)

memory B-cell

reduction of antibody formation

Kohler et al. 1977; Uhr et al. 1961; Sinclair et al. 1969; Hoffmann et al. 1978; Unkeless et al. 1988; Kölsch et al. 1980; Sinclair et al. 1971; Cambier et al. 1987; Klaus et al. 1989; Kinashi et al. 1986; Sinclair et al. 1987; Kalsi 1991; Rigley et al. 1989; Bijsterbosch et al. 1985

Feedback Suppression of B-Cells by Antiidiotype Antibodies

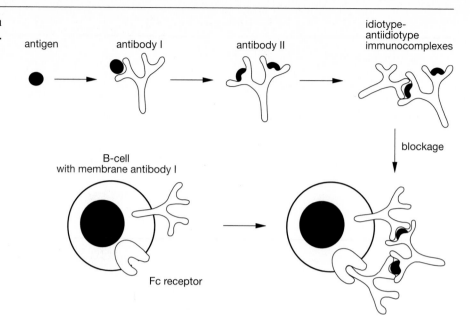

antigen   antibody I   antibody II   idiotype-antiidiotype immunocomplexes

B-cell with membrane antibody I

blockage

Fc receptor

9 Generation of the IgA response

9.1 Overview

Secretory immunoglobulin A (sIgA) protects mucosal epithelial cells by:
- Inhibition of adhesion, colonization and function of bacteria (Dhar et al. 1985; Abraham et al. 1985)
- Prevention of attachment and internalization of viruses (Taylor et al. 1985)
- Reduction of potential infestation of parasites (Kaplan et al. 1985)
- Neutralization of toxins and suppression of toxin induced damage (Tamaru et al. 1985)

Generation of the IgA Response

About 30% of total IgA ($\approx$85% IgA1, 90% monomeric IgA) is produced by B-cells (plasma cells) in the bone marrow. IgA in lymphatics and blood vessels is bound to the asialoglycoprotein receptor (hepatic binding protein) on liver (Kupffer) cells, internalized and metabolized.

Less than 0,01% of total IgA is secreted via bile and bile duct into the gut.

More than 65% of total IgA ($\approx$60% IgA1, $\approx$90% polymeric IgA) is produced by B-cells (plasma cells) in the villi of the gut. Transport of IgA through the epithelium of the gut is performed with the help of the secretory piece protein of the polymeric immunoglobulin receptor.

Generation of enteral IgA starts by microfold cells, which take up antigen from the gut lumen, transport it to the dome of Peyer's patches and deliver it there to APC.

Via APC, T-cell and B-cell interaction B-cells, which secrete specific IgA, are generated.

Such B-cells migrate from Peyer's patches to mesenteric lymphnodes, where they differentiate to plasmablasts. Plasmablasts leave the lymphnodes.

Differentiation of IgA producing plasma cells takes place in the lamina propria of the epithelium of the gut.

Plasma cells in the lamina propria of the epithelium secrete polymeric (mainly dimeric IgA). IgA is complexed by the 15 kDa polypeptide called J (joining) chain.

9.2 Details

9.2.1 Properties of secretory and serum IgA

	Serum	Secretory
Form	monomeric (M-IgA)	polymeric (P-IgA)
Sedimentation	7 S (90% of total)	11 S (90% of total)
Molecular weight	165 kDa	390 kDa
J(oining) chain	–	+ (produced in plasma cells, 15 kDa, one N-glycosylation site, has Ig domain structure, complexes M-IgA by binding to the penultimate cysteine in the C-terminal region)
Secretory piece (polymeric Ig receptor)	–	+ (produced in epithelial cells, 80 kDa, part of the Ig-super-family, serves as a receptor for P-IgA, binds to the CH2 domain of one monomer in the P-IgA)
IgA1 (carries a 13 aa proline rich peptide, site of cleavage by IgA proteases)	80–90%	50–75%
IgA2 (has no cleavage site and is resistent to bacterial IgA proteases)	10–20%	25–50%

Tomasi 1989; Mostov et al. 1984; Krajci et al. 1989.

9.2.2 Circulation and Metabolization of IgA

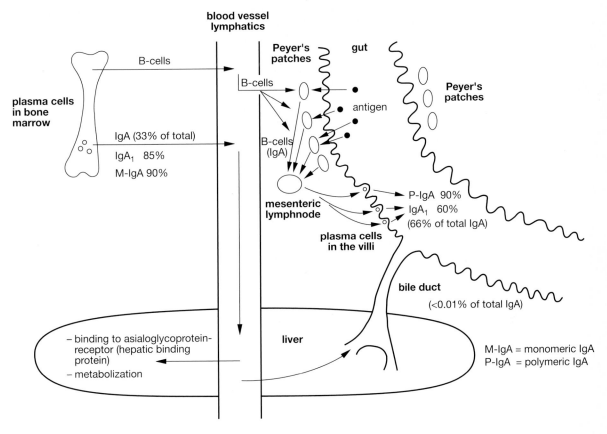

Tomasi 1989; Mestecky et al. 1987; Biewenga et al. 1993

9.2.3 Enteral IgA Response

Immunogenicity of antigens:

– live microorganisms (can selectively attach to mucosa and enter the Peyer's patches via microfold cells)	+++	Tse et al. 1991 Pappo et al. 1989
– Dead microorganisms/particular antigens (are taken up by microfold cells)	+/++	Sminia et al. 1990 London et al. 1987
– soluble antigens (anergy due to limited digestion, less efficient uptake or phagocytosis by macrophages not involved in the immune response)	+/–	Paoli et al. 1990 Michael 1989 van den Dobbelsteen et al. 1992

Functional properties of IgA:
– Produced by plasma cells residing in bone   Mestecky et al. 1987
  marrow (monomeric serum IgA) or in the lamina   Conley et al. 1987
  propria of epithelia (dimeric secretory IgA)

– Actively transported by epithelial cells into   Brandtzaeg et al. 1981
  lumen (glands, gut)

– Specific secretory IgA can agglutinate micro-   Conley et al. 1987
  organisms and neutralize toxins without
  activating complement system
  (protection of mucosal surfaces)

Gastrointestinal Generation of IgA Response	Particulate antigen is taken up from the (gut) lumen by microfold (M) cells in the epithelium overlying Peyer's patches.	Mestecky et al. 1987
	M-cells transport antigens to the dome of Peyer's patches (M-cells do not degrade the antigen and are not antigen presenting cells).	Trier 1991 van Rooijen 1990
	In the dome of Peyer's patches APC (macrophages, less dendritic cells) process and present the antigen.	Sminia et al. 1991 Ermak et al. 1990 Kraal et al. 1983 Pavli et al. 1990
	On antigen contact, dome macrophages produce cytokines to activate TH2 cells, which subsequently secrete cytokines (Il-4, Il-5, Il-6); Il-4, Il-5 and Il-6 cooperate with TGF· and induce switch to IgA in antigen specific activated B-cells.	Kawanishi et al. 1983 Dunkley et al. 1986 Spalding et al. 1986 Sonoda et al. 1989 Coffman et al. 1989 Picker et al. 1992 Harriman et al. 1990
	Probably, the follicular dendritic cells of Peyer's patches play a decisive role in directing virgin B-cells to switch to IgA expression.	Schrader et al. 1990
	IgA$^+$ B-cells migrate from Peyer's patches to mesenteric lymph nodes or parathymic lymph nodes (draining the peritoneal cavity); there they differentiate to IgA producing plasmablasts under the influence of cytokines (Il-5, Il-6) secreted by TH2 cells.	Mega et al. 1991 Biewenga et al. 1993 Becky Kelly et al. 1991
	Plasmablast leave the lymphnode via HEV and settle in the villi of the gut.	Biewenga et al. 1993

Differentiation of plasmablast to IgA   Mosmann et al. 1989
secreting plasma cells takes place in the villi
(lamina propria of epithelium) under the
influence of cytokines secreted by TH2 cells

Transport of polymeric IgA from the lamina propria   Tomasi 1989
through mucosal epithelium into the lumen of the gut
is mediated by the secretory component.

**Generation of IgA
Response in the Gut**

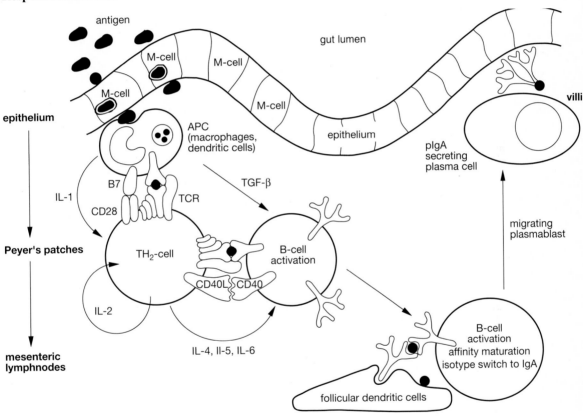

Synthesis of Secretory Component (SC), Linkage to and Transcytosis of Polymeric IgA or IgM

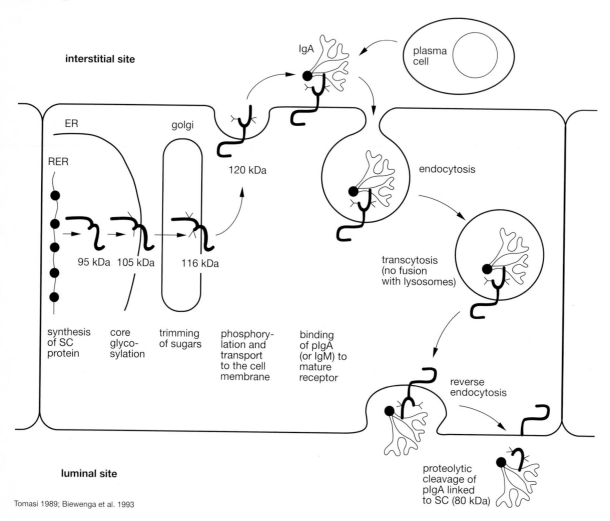

interstitial site

IgA

plasma cell

ER   golgi

RER

120 kDa

endocytosis

95 kDa   105 kDa   116 kDa

transcytosis (no fusion with lysosomes)

synthesis of SC protein

core glycosylation

trimming of sugars

phosphorylation and transport to the cell membrane

binding of pIgA (or IgM) to mature receptor

reverse endocytosis

luminal site

proteolytic cleavage of pIgA linked to SC (80 kDa)

Tomasi 1989; Biewenga et al. 1993

**The Polymeric
Immunoglobulin
Receptor**

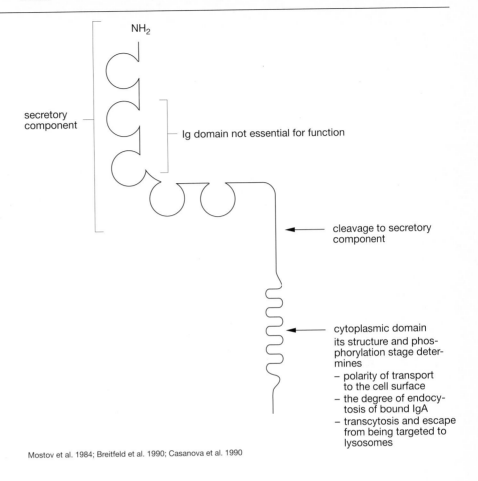

NH$_2$

secretory
component

Ig domain not essential for function

cleavage to secretory
component

cytoplasmic domain
its structure and phos-
phorylation stage deter-
mines
– polarity of transport
  to the cell surface
– the degree of endocy-
  tosis of bound IgA
– transcytosis and escape
  from being targeted to
  lysosomes

Mostov et al. 1984; Breitfeld et al. 1990; Casanova et al. 1990

9.2.4 Secretory Immunoglobulin A (sIgA) in Tears

The principal tissue involved in ocular mucosal immunity is the lacrimal gland (Sullivan et al. 1989).

Lacrimal gland tissue contains a very high density of IgA-containing cells and produces the secretory component (SC) in both acinar and ductal cells (Allansmith et al. 1980; Hann et al. 1989).

The SC appears to control the binding and transcytosis of polymeric IgA into tears against an apparent gradient (Brandtzaeg 1983; Sullivan et al. 1988).

The resulting tear IgA concentrations are among the highest of all mucosal secretions and are accompanied by substantial levels of free SC (Delacroix et al. 1983; Sullivan et al. 1988).

The number of IgA containing lymphocytes in the lacrimal gland, the production of IgA and SC by lacrimal tissue and the levels of IgA and SC in tears are significantly greater in males as compared to females (Sullivan et al. 1986, 1984, 1985; Hann et al. 1988).

Hormonal Influence on the Secretory Immune System of the Eye

Androgens:
– Stimulate the synthesis of secretory component (SC) by acinar cells
– Augment the secretion of SC from the lacrimal gland
– Considerably increase the tear levels of IgA and SC

This effect of androgens:
– Is not duplicated by the administration of other steroid hormones
– Requires an intact hypothalamic pituitary axis
– Is unique to the eye
– Is caused by an enhanced production of IgA by plasma cells (rather than increased recruitment of IgA positive cells) and an enhanced transfer of IgA from lacrimal tissue to tears
– Is supported by the hypothalamic pituitary gonadal axis. Orchidectomy reduces the effect of androgens.
– Is supported by (but not dependent on) insulin.

Androgens have no influence on IgG level in tears.

Sullivan et al. 1984, 1985, 1987, 1988, 1989.

10 Complement Activation and Inhibition

10.1 Overview

Complement may be activated via the classical and the alternative pathway.

Antibodies bound to the corresponding antigen activate complement via the classical pathway (C1q-C1r-C1s).

Activation of the complement cascade via the classical or alternative way leads to the generation of the anaphylatoxins C3a, C4a, C5a. Anaphylatoxins induce chemotaxis, degranulation of basophils and mast cells, activation of neutrophil granulocytes, hypotension and the capillary leak syndrome (see chapter systemic inflammatory reaction syndrome).

Final end point of the complement activation is the generation of the membrane attack complex (MAC). This membrane attack complex can either lead to leakage of the cell membrane and cell death or to stimulation of the target cell. Stimulation of granulocytes, macrophages, synovial cells, osteoclasts, glomerular epithelial cells and other cell by the MAC seems to be an essential pathway of acute and chronic inflammation.

Activation of the complement cascade is inhibited and thereby controlled by various inhibitors present in blood plasma and other extracellular fluids and/or on the cell membrane. Due to the presence of such inhibitors on the cell membrane, nucleated cells are largely resistant to complement mediated lysis. Elimination of MAC from the cell membrane by endocytosis, exocytosis or transcytosis significantly contributes to resistance of nucleated cell to complement mediated lysis.

MAC's themselves may stimulate cells, including endothelial and synovial cells and may participate in chronic Rhematoid arthritis.

Complement receptors (esp. CR1 and C1qR) significantly participate in the elimination of immune complexes.

10.1.1 Classification

Proteins	Activation sequence	Inhibitors/regulators	Receptors
Plasma proteins	C1q, C1r, C1s, C4, C2 B, D, C3 C5, C6, C7, C8, C9	C1 inhibitor (C1-INH) C4b binding protein (C4b-BP) factor I, factor H, factor J protein S, SP40/40 carboxypeptidase N	
Cell membrane proteins		decay-accelerating factor (DAF) membrane cofactor protein (MCP) homologous restriction factor/ C8 binding protein (HRF) MAC inhibitory protein (MIP) membrane inhibitor of reactive lysis (MIRL)	complement receptor 1 (CR1) complement receptor 2 (CR2) complement receptor 3 (CR3) complement receptor 4 (CR4) complement receptor 5 (CR5) C3e receptor C3a receptor C5a receptor C1q receptor factor H receptor (HR)

Porcel et al. 1992

10.1.2 Activation

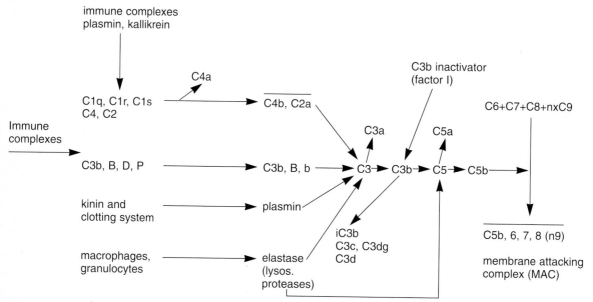

Müller-Berhaus 1977; Müller-Eberhard 1975, 1977; Dierich et al. 1988; Goldstein et al. 1993.

10.1.3 Blockage of Complement-Mediated Lysis by Nucleated Cells

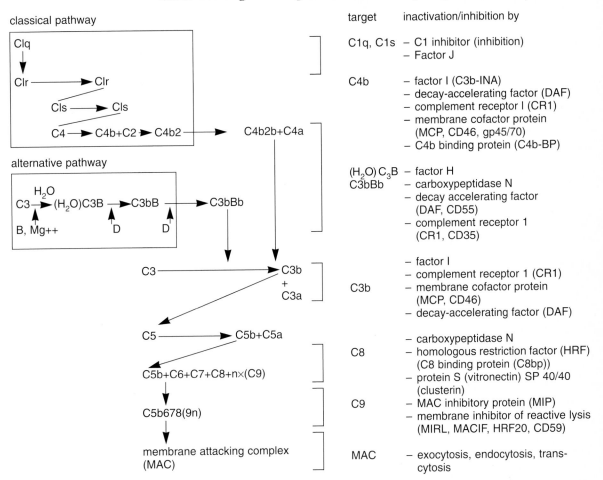

classical pathway

C1q

C1r ──────► C1r

C1s ──────► C1s

C4 ──► C4b+C2 ──► C4b2 ──────► C4b2b+C4a

alternative pathway

H_2O

C3 ──► $(H_2O)C3B$ ──► C3bB ──────► C3bBb

B, Mg^{++} D   D

C3 ──────────────► C3b + C3a

C5 ──────► C5b+C5a

C5b+C6+C7+C8+n×(C9)

C5b678(9n)

membrane attacking complex (MAC)

target	inactivation/inhibition by
C1q, C1s	– C1 inhibitor (inhibition) – Factor J
C4b	– factor I (C3b-INA) – decay-accelerating factor (DAF) – complement receptor I (CR1) – membrane cofactor protein (MCP, CD46, gp45/70) – C4b binding protein (C4b-BP)
$(H_2O)\,C_3B$ C3bBb	– factor H – carboxypeptidase N – decay accelerating factor (DAF, CD55) – complement receptor 1 (CR1, CD35)
C3b	– factor I – complement receptor 1 (CR1) – membrane cofactor protein (MCP, CD46) – decay-accelerating factor (DAF)
C8	– carboxypeptidase N – homologous restriction factor (HRF) (C8 binding protein (C8bp)) – protein S (vitronectin) SP 40/40 (clusterin)
C9	– MAC inhibitory protein (MIP) – membrane inhibitor of reactive lysis (MIRL, MACIF, HRF20, CD59)
MAC	– exocytosis, endocytosis, transcytosis

Parker 1992; Davitz et al. 1986; Fearon 1979; Medof et al. 1984, 1986; Müller-Eberhard 1988; Ross et al. 1985; Weisman et al. 1990; Morgan 1992; Porcel 1992.

10.2 Details

10.2.1 Function of Complement Inhibitors

Target	Location of inhibitor		Function of inhibitor
	Blood	Cell membrane	
C1q, C1r, C1s	C1-INH		– inhibition of activation (C1q), dissociation of C1q from C1r2 C1s2, formation of complexes C1r C1s-CI-INH
C4b2b (C3-convertase)	factor J		– inhibition of binding of C1q with C1r2 C1s2
	C4b-BP		– inhibition of C4b-C2 interaction, inactivation of C4b2b
	factor I		– enzymatic cleavage of C4b
		DAF	– accelerates inactivation of C4b2b
		CR1	– accelerates inactivation of C4b2b (cofactor for degradation of C4b), transport of IC by erythrocytes
		MCP	– cofactor for degradation of C4b
C3bBb (C3 convertase)	factor H		– accelerates inactivation of C3bBb
	factor I		– enzymatic cleavage of C3b
		CR1	– accelerates inactivation of C3bBb (cofactor for degradation of C3b), transport of IC by erythrocytes
		DAF	– accelerates inactivation of C4b2b
		MCP	– cofactor for degradation of C3b
C3a, C4a, C5a	carboxy-peptidase N		– inactivation of anaphylatoxins by cleavage of arginin in the carboxy terminal position
C5b67	protein S	–	– inhibition of association of C5b67 with the cell membrane, binds the complex SC5b-9
	SP40/40		– inhibition of association of C5b67 with the cell membrane, formation of inactive SC5b6789 complexes
C8 (C5b678n9)		HRF	– binding to C8, inhibition of C8 to complex with C5b67 (acts on homologous MAC)
		MIP	– inhibition of polymerization of C9 (acts on homologous MAC)
		MIRL	– inhibition of polymerization of C9 (acts on homologous MAC)

Parker 1992; Morgan et al. 1992; Porcel 1992; Agostoni et al. 1992.

Enzymes Inhibited by
C1 Inhibitor
(C1 Inactivator C1-IA)

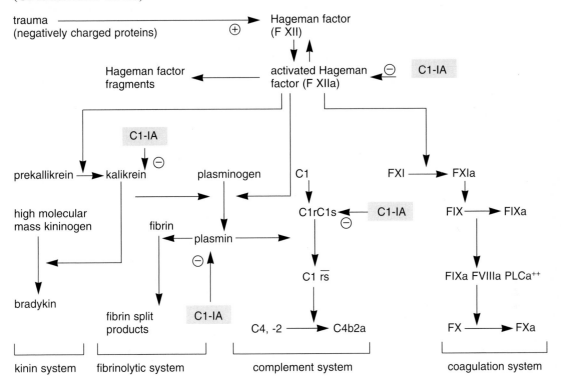

Lepow et al. 1954, 1956; Ratnoff et al. 1957; Forbes et al. 1970; Ratnoff et al. 1969; Gigli et al. 1970; Carreer 1992.

10.2.2 Activity of Complement Split Products on Cells

Binding to cells	C1q	C4b	C4a	C3a	C3b	iC3b	C3d/dg	C5a	C5b67
T-lymphocytes							+		
B-lymphocytes	+	+			+	+	+		
mast cells/basophils			+	+				+	
Eosinophils				+				+	(+)
Neutrophils	+	+		+	+	+		+	(+)
Monocytes/macrophages	+	+		+	+	+		(+)	
Platelets	+					+		(+)	
Erythrocytes		+							
follicular dendritic cells					+	+	+		
Natural killer cells						+			
Function on cells									
Clearance of immune complex	+	+			+	+	+		
(B) cell activation							+		
Cellular adhesion				+		+			
Chemotaxis						(+)		+	(+)
Mediator release			+	+				+	

Sorkin et al. 1970; Spilberg et al. 1978, Dierich et al. 1993, Porcel et al. 1992.

10.2.3 Complement Receptors

Receptor	Ligand-Main	Ligand-Low affinity	Ery.	Mo/M	B-Ly	T-Ly	PMN	Eos	Bas./mast	Dentr. cells	NK cells	Plate-lets	Other cells
CR1 (CD35)	C3b	C4b, C3b, C3c	+	+	+	+	+	+		+			Schwann's
CR2 (CD21)	C3dg, C3d, EBVgp350/220	iC3b, C3b			+	+				+			epithelial
CR3 (CD11b/18, Mac-1)	iC3b	C3d		+		+	+	+		+	+		mesangial
CR4 (CD11c/18, p150/95)	iC3b			+		+	+	+			+		
CR5	C3dg, C3d						+					+	
C3aR	C3a, C4a			+		+	+		+				smooth muscle
C5aR	C5a, C5a des-Arg			+			+		+			+	smooth muscle
C3eR	C3e, C3dk			+			+						
C1qR	C1q	collagen		+	+		+					+	fibroblasts
HR	factor H			+	+		+						
DAF	C4b2a, C3bBb		+	+	+	+	+	+	+	+	+	+	epithelial
MCP	C3b, C4b			+	+	+						+	epithelial fibroblasts
HRF/C8bp	C8, C9		+	+	+	+	+	+	+	+	+	+	epithelial
MIRL	C8, C9		+	+	+	+	+	+	+	+	+	+	epithelial mesenchymal

Becherer et al. 1989; Ross 1989; Herbert et al. 1991; Tausk et al. 1990; Chevalier et al. 1989; Schifferli et al. 1986; Cooper et al. 1990; Kuypers et al. 1989; Roberts et al. 1989; Soulder et al. 1989; Vogt et al. 1986; Porcel et al. 1992.

Specific Biological Functions of Complement Receptors	Receptor	C′-regulator protein	Other biological function
	CR1 (CD35)	+	adherence and phagocytosis of C3b carrying cells or immune complexes (IC)
	CR2 (CD21)	–	B-cell activation by cross--linking BCR and CR2; binding of IC, infection by EBV, HIV-1, HTLV-1
	CR3 (CD11b/18, Mac-1)	–	cellular adhesion (Ca++, Mg++), phagocytosis, infection by HIV (monocytes, macrophages)
	CR4 (CD11c/18)	–	cellular adhesion (Ca++, Mg++), phagocytosis
	C3eR	–	chemotaxis (PMN, monocytes), leucocytosis
	C3aR	–	chemotaxis, mediator release
	C5aR	–	stimulation of cytokine (Il-6, others) synthesis, oxydative metabolism, release of eicosanoids and lysosomal enzymes (neutrophils, macrophages) degranulation (mast cells, basophils) chemotaxis (leukocytes)
	C1qR	–	clearance of IC, glycolipides, mannose coated cells infection by HIV
	HR/FH	+	⎫
	DAF	+	⎬ resistance to lysis by complement (inhibition of formation of membrane attacking complex)
	MCP	+	⎬
	HRF/C8bp	+	⎬
	MIRL	+	⎭

Dierich et al. 1993; Porcel et al. 1992; Frank et al. 1991; Tomlinson 1993.

Complement Receptor Type 1 (CR1)	Synonyms:	C3b-receptor, C3b/C4b-receptor, immune adherence receptor CD35
	Structure:	single glycoprotein chain with one of four allotypic molecular weights A: 250 kDA, frequency 82 % B: 290 kDA, frequency 18 % C: 330 kDA, (rare) D: 210 kDA, (very rare) encoded on chromosome 1 (region of regulator of complement activation)
	Specificity:	for C3b (i.e. C3c region, binding is bivalent) displaces Bb and prevents more factor B from binding to C3b C4b (binding is bivalent) dissociates C2 and prevents more C2 from binding to the C4b iC3b
	Occurrence:	in erythrocytes, granulocytes (neutrophil, eosinophil) monocytes, macrophages B-cells, subset of T-cells Langerhans cells, follicular dendritic cells Kupffer cells, glomerular podocytes, peripheral neurons

Function:	inhibits classical and alternative pathway C3 and C4 convertases	

Function: inhibits classical and alternative pathway C3 and C4
convertases
is a co-factor for factor I cleavage of C3b or C4b
is a co-factor for factor I cleavage of iC3b (into C3c, C3dy)
on erythrocytes CR1 transport immune complexes and bacteria
to macrophages for clearance (inhibition of immune complex
diseases)
on phagocytes CR1 promote adherence and phagocytosis of
immune complexes (particles)
on lymphocytes CR1 enhance antigen recognition with low
antigen dose

Medof et al. 1982, 1984; Fearon 1979; Dykman et al. 1983, 1984, 1985; Weisman et al. 1990, Bescherer et al. 1988, Ross 1992.

C1q-Receptor

Structure: – single chain glycoprotein (20% carbohydrate) — Peerschke et al. 1983 / Malhotra et al. 1989
– MW 56 kDa
– high cysteine content
– aspartic acid, asparagine, gluta-mine, and glycine account for 45% of total aa — Malhotra et al. 1989

Occurence: – leucocytes (B-cells, T-cells, monocytes, neutrophils, eosinophils) (10^4–3 x 10^5/cell) — Tenner et al. 1981
– platelets (distinctive from collagen receptor) (4 x 10^3/cell) — Peerschke et al. 1987/1988
– fibroblasts (collagen site receptor and binding site receptor) (8 x 10^6/cell) — Bordin et al. 1983, 1988
– endothelial cells (5 x 10^5/cell) — Peerschke et al. 1983
– epithelial cells (1 x 10^6/cell) — Bordin et al. 1982
– smooth muscle cells (2 x 10^6/cell) — Bordin et al. 1982

Specificity: – collagen tail of C1q (region which is occupied by C1r2 C1s2) — Malhotra et al. 1990
– collagen like sequence of — Malhotra et al. 1990
  * mannan binding protein
  * lung surfactant protein A
  * lung surfactant protein D
  * conglutinin

	Signal transduction			
		–	mediated by Ca++ influx, causing increase in cytosolic free Ca++ activated K$^+$ channels	Oiki et al. 1988
		–	in platelets inositol phosphate pathway	Peerschke et al. 1993
		–	maybe additional pathways involved (including tyrosine phosphokinase)	Tenner et al. 1993

Function of C1q-Receptor I	Cells	Biological effect of ligand binding	Reference
	B-cells	– enhancement of Ig synthesis (by polymeric, less by monomeric C1q)	Daha et al. 1990 Young et al. 1991
		– down regulation of Il-1 expression by enhanced secretion of Il-1 RA	Habicht et al. 1987
		– inhibition of proliferation (mainly by monomeric C1q)	Ghebrehiwet et al. 1990
	T-cells	– subpopulation (~8%) which binds C1q	Tenner et al. 1981
		– inhibition of mitogen induced proliferation	Ghebrehiwet et al. 1993
	Neutrophil granulocytes	– phagocytosis of species bearing C1q	
		– stimulation of oxydative burst (by polymeric, not by monomeric C1q, SPA or MBP)	Tenner et al. 1982 Goodman et al. 1992
	Monocytes/ macrophages	– synthesize and secrete C1q, its degree correlates with capacity for Fc-receptor mediated phagocytosis and ADCC	Müller et al. 1978 Len et al. 1989
		– enhancement of phagocytosis via Fc-receptors and CR1 (by polymeric C1q) via opsonisation by C1q and activation via C1q-receptor	Sorvillo et al. 1986 Bobak et al. 1988
		– surfactant protein (SPA), mannose binding protein (MBP) can enhance Fc-receptor and C1 receptor mediated phagocytosis via C1q-receptor	Kuhlman et al. 1981 Tenner et al. 1989 Jiang et al. 1992
	Fibroblasts	– high affine receptor for binding site of C1q mediates complement activation, MAC generation and cell activation for connective tissue regeneration	Andrews et al. 1981 Bordin et al. 1988
		– low affine receptor for collagen tail of C1q induces chemotactic response towards the C1q-concentration gradient	Oiki et al. 1988
		– phagocytosis/uptake of parasites (*Trypanosoma cruzi*)	Rimoldi et al. 1989
	Eosinophil granulocytes	– cytolysis of species bearing C1q	Hamada et al. 1987

Cells	Biological effect of ligand binding	Reference
Endothelial cells	– adherence of immune complexes induction of inflammation and vasculitis	Daha et al. 1988
	– stimulation of oxydative burst, superoxide anion release and phagocytosis (i.e. of bacteria)	Ryan et al. 1989
Smooth muscle cells (vascular)	– involvement in inflammatory reaction in consequence of damage (i.e. by infarction)	Rossen et al. 1988
platelets	– phagocytosis of detritus bearing C1q	Shingu et al. 1989
	– inhibition of collagen-mediated aggregation (by monomeric C1q)	Peerschke et al. 1987 Suba et al. 1976
	– no inhibition of collagen induced platelet adhesion	Chiang et al. 1985 Peerschke et al. 1990

Receptors with Functional/Structural Similarity to C1q-Receptor

	Macrophage scavenger receptor	Ro SSA (calreticulin)	Onchocerca volvulus antigen (RAL-1)	B50 melanoma antigen
Structure	helical and collagen-like coiled coils	low cysteine content, high protein sequence homology to C1q-rec.	63% protein sequence homology to Ro SSA	high protein sequence homology to C1q-rec.
Occurrence	cell membrane of macrophages	intracellular	outer membrane of microfilaria	cell membrane of melanoma cells, non-melanoma cell lines
Function	ingestion of lipoprotein cholesterol similarities to C1q, competes with C1q		immobilization of C1q in an orientation (tail of C1q binds to parasite), which prevents C1q mediated interaction of microfilariae with phagocytic cells	immobilization of C1q in an orientation, which might prevent C1q mediated interaction of tumor cells with phagocytic cells
Reference	Kodama et al. 1990 Acton et al. 1993	McCauliffe et al. 1990 Rokeach et al. 1991	Unnasch et al. 1988	Gersten et al. 1991

10.2.4 Interaction Between Complement Components and Platelets

Complement component	Involvement of platelets	References
C1q	– ~4000 C1q-receptors on platelets (≙ collagen receptor gpIa/IIa)	
	– binding of C1q-mediated via collagen part of C1q, C1q inhibits binding of and activation by collagen	Peerschke et al. 1987
	– monomeric C1q inhibits binding and activation of platelets by collagen	
	– aggregated C1q activates platelets and induces platelet aggregation	Cazenawe et al. 1976
	– by binding of monomeric C1q platelets may inhibit complement activation via the classical pathway	Devine 1992
C1-INH	– stored in α-granules of platelets and release upon stimulation by thrombin and collagen	Schmaier et al. 1985
Factor D	– inhibits platelet aggregation in response to thrombin, but does not affect response to arachidonic acid or collagen	Davis et al. 1979
C3a	– may induce aggregation of human platelets, but results are contradictory	Polley et al. 1983
	– may inhibit platelet aggregation in response to collagen or arachidonic acid	Gyongyossy-Issa et al. 1989
C3dg	– platelet responses to C3b/C3dg are varied	Devine 1992
DAF	– expressed on membrane surface of platelets, platelets of patients with paroxysmal nocturnal hemoglobinuria are deficient in DAF	Nicholson-Weller et al. 1982 Devine et al. 1987
MCP	– expressed on platelets	Sega et al. 1989
CR1, CR2, CR3, p150/95	– complement receptors are not present on human platelets but on nonprimate platelets (clearance of IC)	Devine 1992
C3dg-receptor	– present on platelets, functional role unclear	Vik et al. 1987 Devine et al. 1989
Factor H	– stored in α-granulocytes of platelets and released upon activation or exposure to C3bBb	Kenny et al. 1981 Devine et al. 1987
C-8, C-9	– platelet secrete the terminal proteins of complement (esp. C8, C9) in response to stimulation by collagen	Houle et al. 1989

Complement component	Involvement of platelets	References
MAC	– platelet can initiate assembly of MAC in the absence of known complement activators, by shedding of C5b678(9n) depositions – platelets exposed to C5b678(9n) do not activate, but release α-granule content including FV	Zimmermann et al. 1976 Sims et al. 1986 Ando et al. 1988, 1989 Wiedmer et al. 1986
Protein S (vitronectin)	– platelets bear the protein S receptor, mediates binding of platelets to damaged vessels and modulates MAC activity on the platelet surface – platelets contain an internal pool of vitronectin that is released in response to stimulation by thrombin	Suzuki et al. 1987 Ginsberg et al. 1987
MIRL HRF (C8bp)	– present on the surface of platelets – present on the surface of platelets, binds free C8	Sims et al. 1989 Blaas et al. 1988

Endocytosis/Exocytosis Induced Resistance of Nucleated Cells (NC) to Lysis by the Membrane Attack Complex (MAC) of Complement

Resistance to MAC caused by:

– endocytosis and enzymatic degradation of MAC
  (neutrophils, Ehrlich ascites cells)

Campbell et al. 1985
Morgan et al. 1987
Carney et al. 1985, 1986

– Exocytosis of MAC
  (glomerular epithelial cells, oligodendrocytes,
  rheumatoid synovial cells, platelets)

Cammussi et al. 1987
Scolding et al. 1989
Morgan 1992
Sims et al. 1986

– Endocytosis and exocytosis of MAC
  (neutrophils, more than 25 000 MAC/cell)

Campbell et al. 1985
Morgan et al. 1987

– Transcytosis of MAC into the urinary space
  (glomerular epithelial cells)

Kerjaschki et al. 1989
Morgan 1992

Half-life of MAC on the cell membrane (neutrophils)
is about 3 min at 37 °C.

Morgan et al. 1984
Morgan et al. 1985

Endocytosis (followed by lysosomal degradation) and
transcytosis utilizes clathrin coated pits and the
intracellular vesicle transport system.

Carney et al. 1986
Kerjaschki et al. 1989

Biochemical pathways for MAC elimination:

– Increase in intracellular Ca^{++} (from 0,2 M to
  5 M within 1 min after MAC formation) by
  release from intracellular stores (and influx)

Campbell et al. 1981
Morgan et al. 1985

– Level of intracellular Ca^{++} is regulated by MAC
  induced protein kinase activation and calmodulin
  modulation

Campbell et al. 1982
Cox 1988
Colbran et al. 1989

– Increase of intracellular Ca^{++} is followed by
  increase of cAMP

Cox 1988

– Interaction of MAC with G-protein, release of
  inositolphospholipids leads to increase of
  cAMP and Ca^{++}

Carney et al. 1990
Daniels et al. 1990

10.2.5 Resistance of Nucleated Cells (NC) to Lysis
by Membrane Attack Complex (MAC) of Complement

– No consistent relationship between degree of lysis and	Cikes 1970
	Ferrone et al. 1973
* antigen density	Pellegrino et al. 1974
* amount of early or late complement components	Ohanian et al. 1975
	Cooper et al. 1974

– NC have an active resistance mechanism	Goldberg et al. 1959
	Green et al. 1960

– increase of resistance by treatment with	
* Anabolic hormones (insulin, hydrocortisone)	Segerling et al. 1975
	Schlager et al. 1976
* cAMP	Kaliner et al. 1974
* Cholesterol (increase in concentration)	Boyle et al. 1976
by condensing membrane phospholipids	Cheetham et al. 1990
* MAB for aggregation of MACs to patches	Morgan et al. 1987

– Decrease of resistance by treatment with	
* Cytostatics (puromycin, doxorubicin, actinomycin D)	Segerling et al. 1975
	Schlager et al. 1976
* Enzymes (neuraminidase, trypsin, pepsin, pronase)	Boyle et al. 1978
	Morgan et al. 1985
* EDTA to chelate Ca^{++}	Morgan 1992
* Inhibitors for PKC or calmodulin	Roberts et al. 1985
* 2-Chloroadenosine to reduce cAMP	Carney et al. 1990
* Inhibitors for G-protein	

– NC tolerate some degree of membrane leakiness	Boyle et al. 1976
	Hallett et al. 1981

10.2.6 Activation of Nucleated Cells by Membrane Attacking Complex

Cell	Parameter	Reference
Neutrophil granulocytes macrophages	generation of radical oxygen (O_2; OH; H_2O_2)	Hallet et al. 1981 Campbell et al. 1985 Roberts et al. 1985
Glomerular mesangial cells		Hansch et al. 1984, 1987 Adler et al. 1986 Lovett et al. 1987
Rheumatoid synovial cells		Morgan et al. 1988
Cartilage cells rheumatoid synovial cells	release of lysosomal enzymes (including collagenases)	Lachmann et al. 1969 Jahn et al. 1990
Osteoclasts macrophages	synthesis of PGE2	Raisz et al. 1974 Hansch et al. 1984, 1987
Glomerular mesangial cells glomerular epithelial cells rheumatoid synovial cells pulmonary endothelial cells amniotic epithelial cells		Lovett et al. 1987 Hansch et al. 1988 Daniels et al. 1990 Suttorp et al. 1987 Rooney et al. 1990
Neutrophil granulocytes rheumatoid synovial cells oligodendrocytes	synthesis of leukotrienes	Seeger et al. 1986 Daniels et al. 1990 Shiraziet al. 1987
Neutrophil granulocytes	synthesis of thromboxanes	Seeger et al. 1986
Glomerular mesangial cells macrophages	release of Il-1	Lovett et al. 1987 Hansch et al. 1987
Rheumatoid synovial cells	release of Il-6	von Kempis et al. 1989 Daniels et al. 1990
Glomerular epithelial cells	synthesis of type IV collagen	Hansch et al. 1989 Torbohm et al. 1990

The Membrane Attack Complex (MAC) of Complement Activates Nucelated Cells for Their Recovery and to Their Function

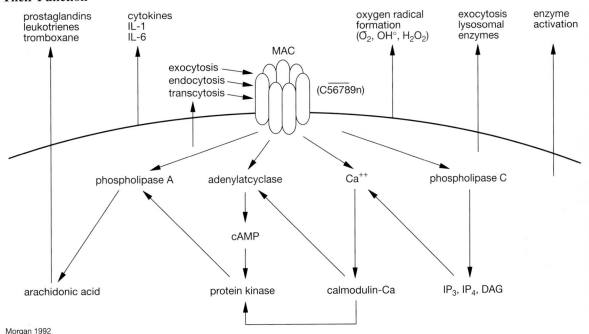

prostaglandins
leukotrienes
tromboxane

cytokines
IL-1
IL-6

oxygen radical
formation
(O_2, $OH°$, H_2O_2)

exocytosis
lysosomal
enzymes

enzyme
activation

MAC

exocytosis
endocytosis
transcytosis

($\overline{C56789n}$)

phospholipase A   adenylatcyclase Ca^{++} phospholipase C

cAMP

arachidonic acid   protein kinase   calmodulin-Ca IP_3, IP_4, DAG

Morgan 1992

The Membrane Attack Complex (MAC) May Have a Role in Auto-immune Diseases

Rheumatoid arthritis:
– MAC can be found in synovial fluids (free or in membrane fragments) or deposited in the synovial membrane.
– MAC activated synovial cells secrete mediators and interleukins.
– Synovial fluid contains cytokines, prostaglandins, leukotriens, radical oxygen species, exocytosed enzymes.
– In spite of MAC presence, cell infiltration and proliferation is a major histological feature of Rheumatoid arthritis rather than cell death.
Conclusion: MAC may be an essential factor for chronic rheumatoid arthritis

Other autoimmune diseases:
– MAC can be found in lesions of autoimmune disease
Nephritis   lupus erythematodes membranous nephropathy
Arthritis   PCP, psoriasis, Sjögren syndrome, Behcet disease
Dermatitis   pemphigus vulgaris, bullous pemphigoid
Neurological   multiple sclerosis, myasthenia gravis,
inflammations   cerebral lupus

Sanders et al. 1986; Morgan et al. 1988, 1992.

10.2.7 Diseases Associated with (Inherited or Acquired) Deficiency of Complement Components

CR1	systemic lupus erythematodes, lepra immune complex disease	⎤
C1q	immune complex disease, infections	
C1r	systemic lupus erythematodes, infections	
C1s	dermatomyositis, infections	
C2	glomerulonephritis, infections, SLE	auto
C4	vasculitis, infections	immune
C4b-BP	atypic Behcet disease	and immune
C3	immune complex disease, infections	complex diseases
Factor I	infections, immune complex diseases	
Factor H	glomerulonephritis, *Neisseria* meningitis infections, immune complex diseases	infections with bacteria (preference for
Factor D	immune complex diseases	encapsulated bacteria:
CR4, CR3	infections	– *pneumococci*
Properdin	*Neisseria* meningitis infections	– *N. meningococci*
C5	*Neisseria* meningitis infections	– *Hemophilus influenza*
C6	*Neisseria* meningitis infections	
C7	*Neisseria* meningitis infections	
C8	bacterial infections	
C9	*Neisseria* meningitis infections	⎦
CI-INH	hereditary angioedema	⎤
DAF,		
HRF,		damage of cell
MIRF	hemoglobinuria paroxistica nocturna	membranes
C3Nef	glomerulonephritis membrane proliferation	⎦

Agostoni et al. 1992; Schifferli et al. 1988; Ross et al. 1984; Nagata et al. 1989; Orren et al. 1987; Tedesco 1986; Hauptmann 1986; Sjoholm et al. 1982; Zimran et al. 1987; Schlesinger et al. 1990; Passwell et al. 1992; Porcel et al. 1992.

10.2.8 Approaches for Immunotherapy with Regulators
of Complement Activation

Compound	Source	Pharmacological effect	Species	Reference
C1-INH	blood	– inhibition of capillary leak syndrome – reversal of shock symptoms in sepsis	human human	Hack et al. 1991
CR1	recomb.	– reduction of infarct size after induced myocardial ischemia	rat	Weisman et al. 1990
		– reducing tissue injury after intradermal IC injection	rat	Yeh et al. 1991
		– protection against complement dependent lung and dermal injury by IC deposition, cobra venom factor and thermal trauma	rat	Mulligan et al. 1992
		– reduction of organ injury after intestinal ischemia reperfusion	rat	Hill et al. 1992
		– prolongation of xenograft survival by inhibition of natural antibodies	rat	Xia et al. 1992 Pruitt et al. 1992
DAF	recomb.	– reduction of reversed Arthus reaction induced by immune complexes	guinea pig	Moran et al. 1992
C1q	blood	– reduction of glomerular deposition of immune complexes and reduction of shock reaction by IC	mouse	Sedlacek et al. 1979
		– inhibition of immune complex mediated platelet aggregation and complement activation (in vitro)	human	Sedlacek et al. 1979
		enhancement of phagocytosis (in vitro)	human	Bobak et al. 1988
		– stimulation of oxidative metabolism (in vitro)	human	Tenner et al. 1982
		– enhanced binding to endothelial cells of immune complexes (in vitro)	human	Daha et al. 1988
		– enhanced secretion of immunoglobulin by B-cells (in vitro)		Tenner et al. 1987 Tenner et al. 1987
		– enhanced secretion of Il-1R antagonist (in vitro)	human	Habicht et al. 1987

11 Cell-Mediated Cytotoxicity

11.1 Overview

The final step in the immune reaction is the cytotoxic reaction to the target cell. This cytotoxic reaction can be antigen specific:
- Antibody mediated by activation of complement and generation of the membrane attack complex (MAC) (see chapter on complement activation and inhibition)
- Cell mediated by cytotoxic T-cells (CTL)
- Antibody and cell mediated by activation of killer cells through the bifunctional activity of antibodies (antibody dependent cellular cytotoxicity)

The cytotoxic reaction can also be non-antigen-specific:
- Induced by activation of the apoptosis receptor or by incomplete (monovalent) activation of the target cell
- By phagocytosis (macrophages, granulocytes)
- By so-called natural killer cells
- By release of cytotoxic mediators (IFN, TNF, IL-1)
- By superantigens

11.2 Details

11.2.1 Cytotoxicity by T-Lymphocytes

Cytotoxic T-lymphocytes (TCTL) interact with the specific target cell in the following way:
- The first contact is mediated by ICAM-1 (on the target cell) and the "inactivated" LFA-1 (on TCTL). This binding is of low affinity.
- Subsequently the antigen presented by MHC-class I (on the target cells) binds to the T-cell receptor and MHC-class I to CD 8.
- Activation of the TCR/CD3 complex on the TCTL stimulates phospholipase C (PLP-C) which catalyses the hydrolysis of phosphatidyl-inositol biphosphate (PIP) into inositol triphosphate (IP). IP mobilizes intracellular calcium and diacylglycerol (DG), thus leading to activation of the proteinkinase C. Proteinkinase C phophorylates the β-chain of LFA-1. Hereby, LFA-1 is "activated" to bind ICAM-1 with high affinity.

– Inactivation of activated LFA-1 is performed by reduction of the proteinkinase level and action of phosphatase (i.e. CD45).

Activation of Cytotoxic T-Cells by Antigen-Presenting Target Cells

Activation of cytotoxic T-cells in response to antigen displayed by MHC-I on the surface of an antigen-presenting target cell involves the interaction of multiple receptor-coreceptor pairs.

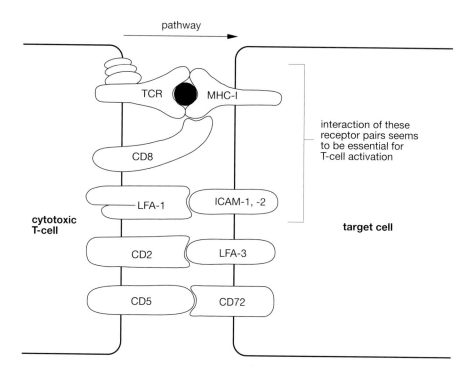

Fraser et al. 1993

Regulation of LFA-1 Dependent Cell Adhesion

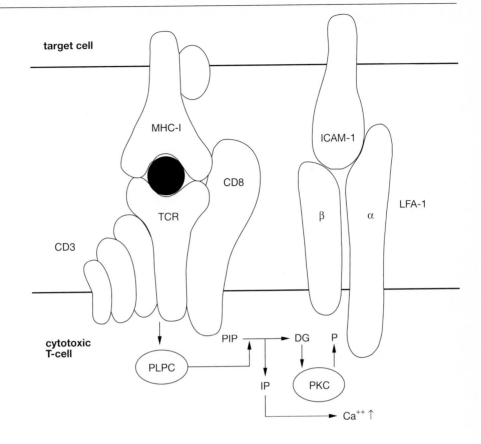

Cell Death Mediated by CTL

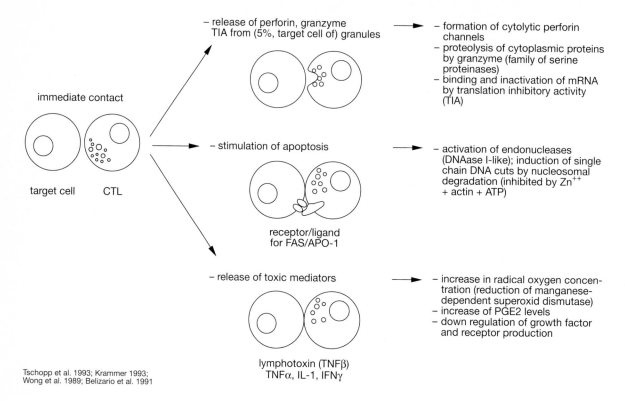

- release of perforin, granzyme TIA from (5%, target cell of) granules

→ - formation of cytolytic perforin channels
- proteolysis of cytoplasmic proteins by granzyme (family of serine proteinases)
- binding and inactivation of mRNA by translation inhibitory activity (TIA)

immediate contact

target cell　　　CTL

- stimulation of apoptosis

→ - activation of endonucleases (DNAase I-like); induction of single chain DNA cuts by nucleosomal degradation (inhibited by Zn^{++} + actin + ATP)

receptor/ligand for FAS/APO-1

- release of toxic mediators

→ - increase in radical oxygen concentration (reduction of manganese-dependent superoxid dismutase)
- increase of PGE2 levels
- down regulation of growth factor and receptor production

lymphotoxin (TNFβ)
TNFα, IL-1, IFNγ

Tschopp et al. 1993; Krammer 1993; Wong et al. 1989; Belizario et al. 1991

Formation of Cytolytic Perforin Channels

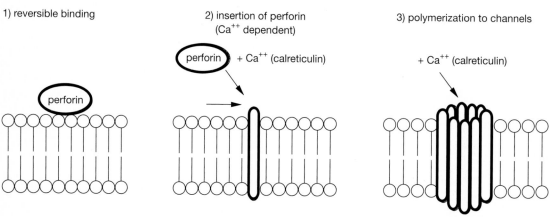

1) reversible binding

perforin

2) insertion of perforin (Ca^{++} dependent)

perforin + Ca^{++} (calreticulin)

3) polymerization to channels

+ Ca^{++} (calreticulin)

Tschopp et al. 1993

The Level of CTL Response is Dependent on the Nature of the Antigen	Nature of antigen	Degree of CTL response	References
	Soluble protein	(+)	Wraith et al. 1985
	Immunocomplexed proteins	++	Randall et al. 1987
	Soluble proteins within cells	++	Moore et al. 1988 Carbone et al. 1989
	Foreign cells	++	McMichael 1992
	Proteins in bacteria	+	Aggarwal et al. 1990
	Proteins in protozoa	+	Romero et al. 1989
	Proteins of viruses Influenza	+++ +++	McMichael et al. 1983 Yap et al. 1978 McMichael et al. 1983
	RSV	+++	Cannon et al. 1988 Isaacs et al. 1990
	HIV	+++	Walker et al. 1986
	EBV	+++	Moss et al. 1978 Crawford et al. 1980
	CMV	+++	Quinnan et al. 1982

Escape from CTL Control	Antigen	Mechanism	References
	Virus		
	LCM	mutation of epitope sequence	Pircher et al. 1990
	HIV	mutation of epitope sequence quicker than switching of CTL-response from one epitope to another	McMichael 1993 Philipps et al. 1992
	Adenovirus 12	downregulation of MHC-I expression	Schrier et al. 1983 Anderson et al. 1985
	EBV	downregulation of adhesion molecules expression (LFA-3, ICAM-1)	Gregory et al. 1988
	Tumor cells		
	Melanoma	change of epitope	Ernst et al. 1986 Frankel et al. 1985 Knuth et al. 1989
	Various tumors (colorectal, others)	abnormal expression of MHC-I	Gopas et al. 1989 Momberg et al. 1989 Smith et al. 1989
	Various tumors	abnormal expression of MHC-I molecules	Vanky et al. 1990

11.2.2 Cellular Cytotoxicity via Mechanisms not Involving Recognition of Antigen Presented by MHC-I

T-cells activated by Il-2 secrete mediators (IFN γ gamma, TNFα, TNFβ, Il-1):
- Directly cytotoxic for the target cell
- Induce local or systemic inflammatory reactions, which kill the bystander target cell

Interaction between T-cells or killer cells and target cells can be mediated by:
- Cross-linking of TCR and MHC-I by superantigens
- Binding of killer cells to the target cell by cell adhesion molecules (LFA-1/ICAM-1 and/or CD2/LFA-3); interaction of CD2/LFA-3 is competitively inhibited by LFA-3 on red blood cells
- Cross-linking of Fcγ receptors on killer cells and antigens on the cell membrane of target cells by antibodies (antibody dependent cellular cytotoxicity)
- Activation of apoptosis

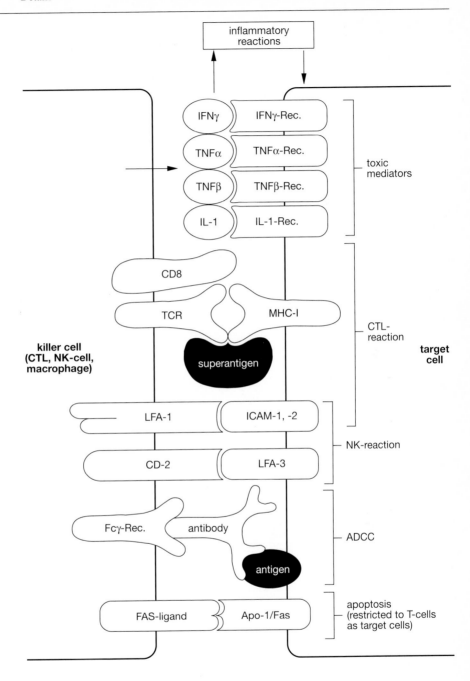

Cytotoxicity by Natural Killer Cells Mediated via Cell Adhesion Molecules

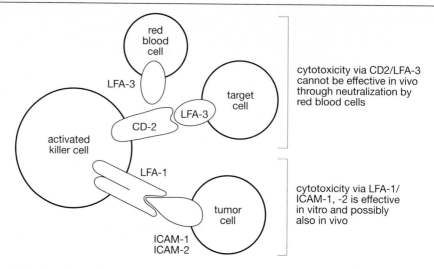

cytotoxicity via CD2/LFA-3 cannot be effective in vivo through neutralization by red blood cells

cytotoxicity via LFA-1/ ICAM-1, -2 is effective in vitro and possibly also in vivo

LFA = lymphocyte function antigen (LFA-1 = CD11/18; LFA-3 = CD58)
ICAM = intercellular adhesion molecule (ICAM-1 = CD54)

Oblakowski et al. 1991; Selvaraj et al. 1987: Davignon et al. 1981; Martin et al. 1987; Staunton et al. 1989; Imamura et al. 1988; Brenner et al. 1991

Interaction Between T-Cells and Killer Cells

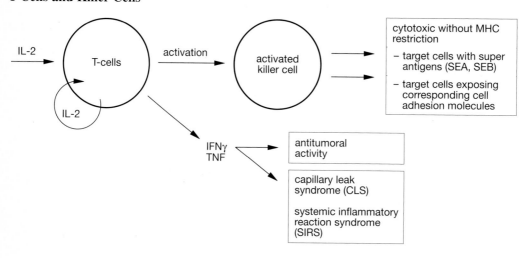

Lotzova et al. 1987; Broxmeyer et al. 1986; Price et al. 1987; Gottleib et al. 1989; Rosenberg et al. 1988; Smith et al. 1988; Fisch et al. 1990; Delvaraj et al. 1987; Oblakowski et al. 1991; Davignon et al. 1981; Martin et al. 1987; Staunton et al. 1989;

12 Immune-Mediated Inflammatory Reaction

12.1 Overview

Immune mediated inflammation is induced through a cascade of events. The steps in this cascade are:

– Activation of
  * Leukocytes
  * Endothelial cells
  * Platelets
  * Mesenchymal cells

– Release of
  * Cytokines
  * Mediators of inflammation

– Afferent antigen-specific immune response

– Autocrine and parakrine activation of cells

– Activation of the
  * Clotting system
  * Complement system
  * Kallikrein system

– Generation of
  * Anaphylatoxins
  * Kinins
  * Fibrin

– Release of
  * Lysosomal enzymes
  * Prostaglandins
  * Histamine/serotonin
  * Leukotriens
  * Oxygen radicals

– Efferent antigen specific immune response
  * CTL
  * Antibodies (immune complexes, ADCC)

– Inflammation with
  * Vasodilatation/extravasation
  * Invasion of leukocytes
  * Destruction of extracellular matrix
  * Cell death
  * Angiogenesis/proliferation of mesenchymal cells

12.1.1 Cascades of the Inflammatory Response

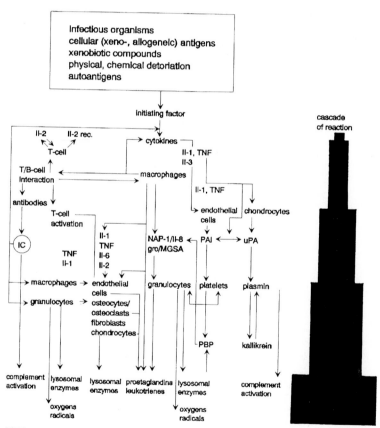

TNF = tumor necrosis factor, UPA = urokinase-like plasminogen activator, PAI = plasminogen activator inhibitor, NAP = neutrophil-activating protein, Gro/MGSA = melanoma growth stimulating activity, IC = Immune complexes, IL-1 rec. = interleukin 2 receptor, PBP = platelet basic protein.

Sedlacek et al. 1992.

12.1.2 Central Role of the Hageman Factor

Activation of the Hageman factor (F XII F XII a) plays a central role for activation ot the:
– Clotting system
– Fibrinolytic system
– Complement system
– Kinin system

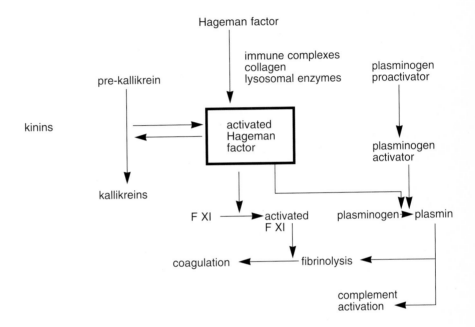

12.1.3 Complexity of Interactions (Cells, Cytokines, Mediators)

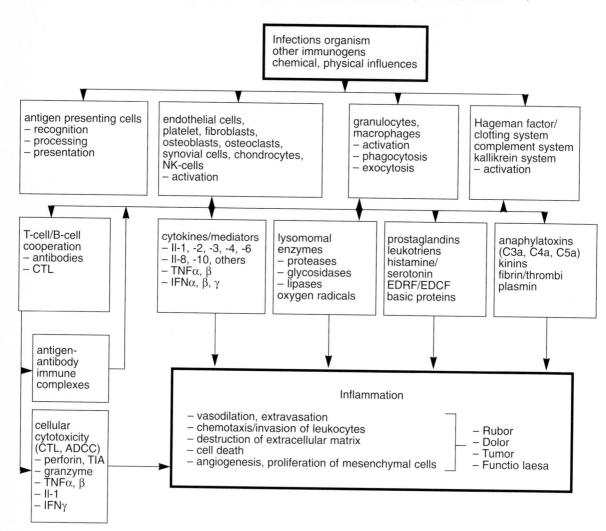

12.2 Details

12.2.1 Activation and Action of Kinins

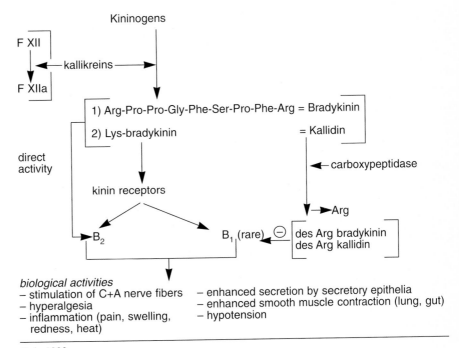

Kyle 1992.

12.2.2 Biological Action of Mediators of the Arachidonic Acid Pathway

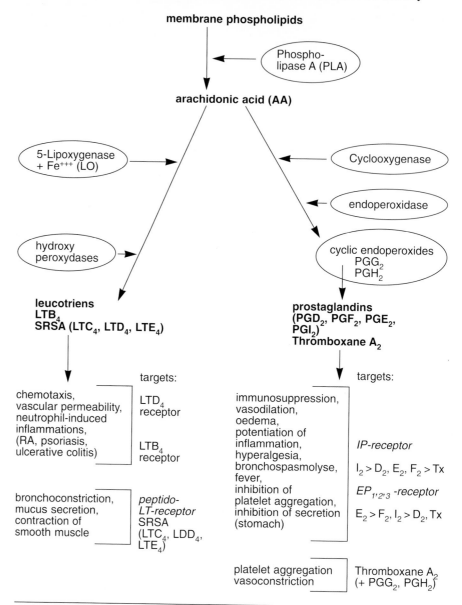

MacMillan 1991; Kirwan 1991; Forth et al. 1980; Claesson 1992.

**Synthetic Pathway
of Prostaglandins and
Leukotriens**

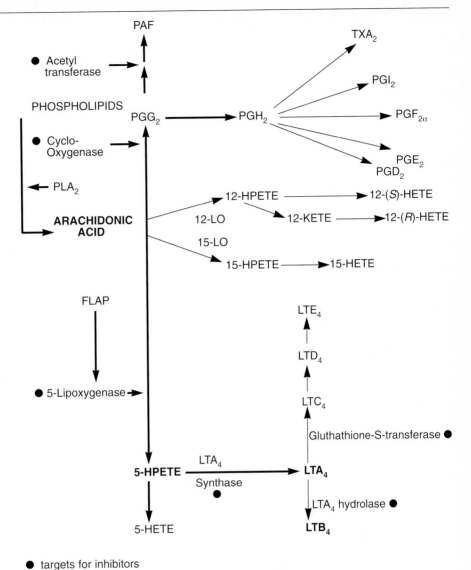

● targets for inhibitors

Djurie et al. 1992.

Synthesis of Leuko-
triens by Lymphocytes,
Monocytes and Granu-
locytes

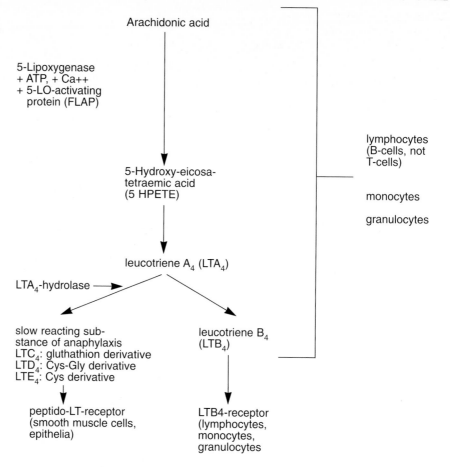

Arachidonic acid

5-Lipoxygenase
+ ATP, + Ca++
+ 5-LO-activating
 protein (FLAP)

5-Hydroxy-eicosa-
tetraemic acid
(5 HPETE)

leucotriene A_4 (LTA_4)

LTA_4-hydrolase ⟶

slow reacting sub-
stance of anaphylaxis
LTC_4: gluthathion derivative
LTD_4: Cys-Gly derivative
LTE_4: Cys derivative

leucotriene B_4
(LTB_4)

peptido-LT-receptor
(smooth muscle cells,
epithelia)

LTB4-receptor
(lymphocytes,
monocytes,
granulocytes

lymphocytes
(B-cells, not
T-cells)

monocytes

granulocytes

Macmillan 1991; Claesson et al. 1992.

**Cooperation of Mono-
cytes and Lymphocytes
in Formation of
Mediators of the
Arachidonic Acid
Pathway**

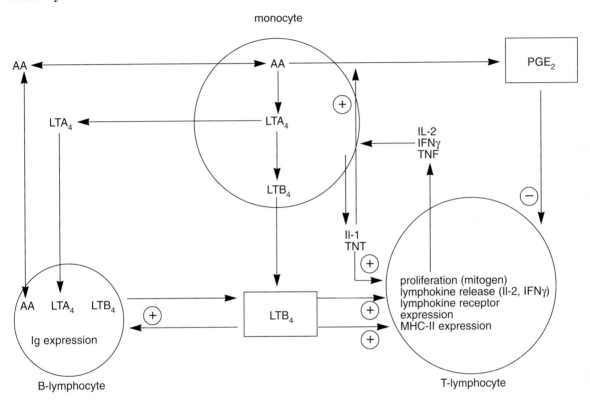

Biological Action of Leukotriene B_4 on Neutrophil Granulocytes	Cell	Effect	Test system	References
	Neutrophil granulocytes	chemotaxis	in vitro	Smith et al. 1980
		degranulation	in vitro	Rae et al. 1981
		aggregation	in vitro	Rae et al. 1981
		accumulation	in vivo	Camp et al. 1985
		activation	in vivo	Brag et al. 1981
		endothelial cell adhesion	in vivo	Björk et al. 1982 Lindstrom et al. 1990
		increase of vascular permeability	in vivo	Björk et al. 1981
		synergy with C5a	in vivo	McMillan et al. 1988
	Eosinophil granulocytes	chemotaxis	in vitro	Goetze et al. 1980

12.2.3 Diseases Associated with Prominent Neutrophil Infiltrates

Rheumatoid arthritis
Ankylosing spondylitis
Asthma
Gout
Hemodialysis associated neutropenia
Allergic contact dermatitis

Dishydrotic eczema
Bullous pemphigoid
Psoriasis
Inflammatory bowel disease
Acquired respiratory distress syndrome

Ahmadzaden et al. 1991
Klickstein et al. 1980
Shindo et al. 1990
Rae et al. 1982
Strasser et al. 1990
Barr et al. 1984
Thorsen et al. 1990
Rosenbach et al. 1985
Rosenbach et al. 1985
Barr et al. 1990
Sharon 1984
Davies et al. 1990

12.2.4 Metabolic Changes Induced by Cytokines

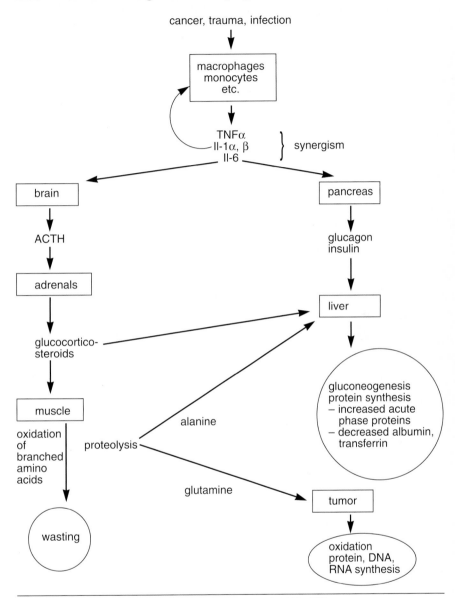

Hall-Angeras et al. 1990; Mealy et al. 1990; Argiles et al. 1989, 1992.

12.2.5 Putative Mechanism of the Delayed-Type Hypersensitivity Reaction

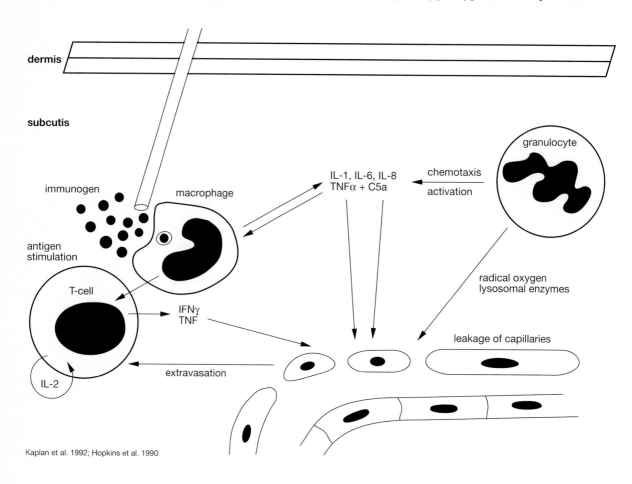

Kaplan et al. 1992; Hopkins et al. 1990

12.2.6 Approaches for the Therapy of Inflammatory Reactions

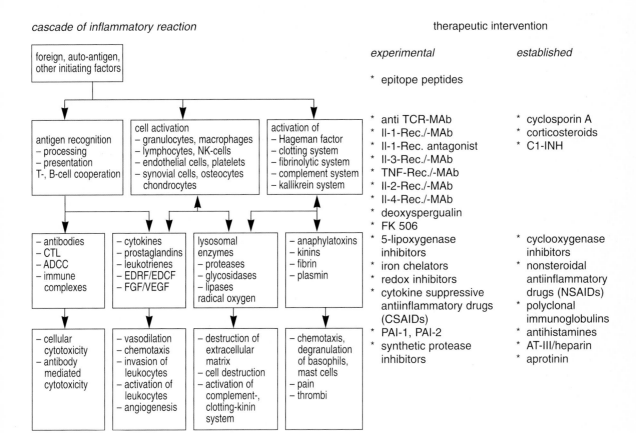

cascade of inflammatory reaction

foreign, auto-antigen, other initiating factors

antigen recognition
– processing
– presentation
T-, B-cell cooperation

cell activation
– granulocytes, macrophages
– lymphocytes, NK-cells
– endothelial cells, platelets
– synovial cells, osteocytes
  chondrocytes

activation of
– Hageman factor
– clotting system
– fibrinolytic system
– complement system
– kallikrein system

– antibodies
– CTL
– ADCC
– immune
  complexes

– cytokines
– prostaglandins
– leukotrienes
– EDRF/EDCF
– FGF/VEGF

lysosomal
enzymes
– proteases
– glycosidases
– lipases
radical oxygen

– anaphylatoxins
– kinins
– fibrin
– plasmin

– cellular
  cytotoxicity
– antibody
  mediated
  cytotoxicity

– vasodilation
– chemotaxis
– invasion of
  leukocytes
– activation of
  leukocytes
– angiogenesis

– destruction of
  extracellular
  matrix
– cell destruction
– activation of
  complement-,
  clotting-kinin
  system

– chemotaxis,
  degranulation
  of basophils,
  mast cells
– pain
– thrombi

therapeutic intervention

experimental

* epitope peptides

* anti TCR-MAb
* Il-1-Rec./-MAb
* Il-1-Rec. antagonist
* Il-3-Rec./-MAb
* TNF-Rec./-MAb
* Il-2-Rec./-MAb
* Il-4-Rec./-MAb
* deoxyspergualin
* FK 506
* 5-lipoxygenase
  inhibitors
* iron chelators
* redox inhibitors
* cytokine suppressive
  antiinflammatory drugs
  (CSAIDs)
* PAI-1, PAI-2
* synthetic protease
  inhibitors

established

* cyclosporin A
* corticosteroids
* C1-INH

* cyclooxygenase
  inhibitors
* nonsteroidal
  antiinflammatory
  drugs (NSAIDs)
* polyclonal
  immunoglobulins
* antihistamines
* AT-III/heparin
* aprotinin

Biological Action of Antiinflammatoric Inhibitors of the Arachidonic Acid Pathway

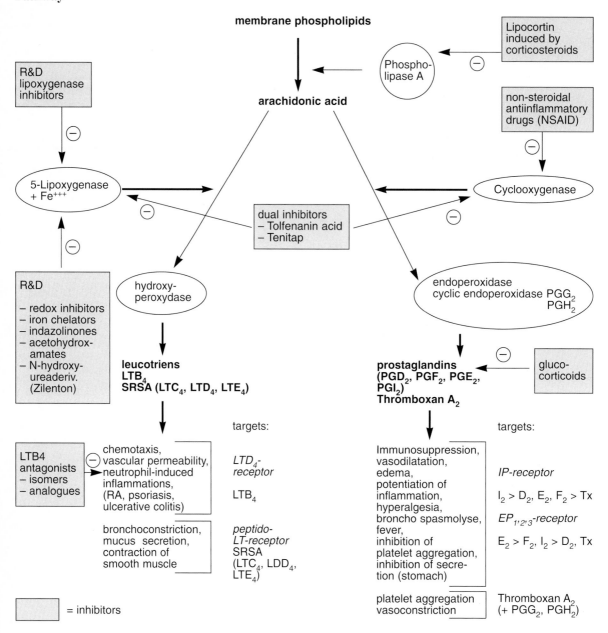

MacMillan 1991; Kirwan 1991; Forth et al. 1980; Claesson 1992; Djuric et al. 1992.

Cytokine Suppressive Antiinflammatory Drugs (CSAIDs)	Pharmacological class	Name of compound	Cytokine suppressed	Reference
	Antiarthritic	auranofin	Il-1β, Il-1RA	Chang et al. 1990
		penicillamine	I-1β	Rordorf-Adam et al. 1989
		tenidap	Il-1β	Otterness et al. 1991
	Corticosteroids	dexamethasone	Il-1β	Lee et al. 1988
		mometasone furoate	Il-1β	Barton et al. 1991
	Antioxidant	probucol	Il-1β	Ku et al. 1988
		tetrahydropapa-veroline	Il-1β, TNF, Il-6	Engui et al. 1993
		probucol	Il-8	De Forge et al. 1992
		butylated hydroxyanisol	Il-1β via Il-1RA	Waters et al. 1993
	Lipoxygenase inhibitors	BW 775C	Il-1	Dinarrello et al. 1984
		SK 86002	Il-1β, TNF, Il-8	Lee et al. 1993
	Phosphodiesterase inhibitors	pentoxifylline	TNF	Chao et al. 1992
		rolipram	TNF, Il-β	Endres et al. 1991
	Alkaloids	tetrandine	TNF	Ferrante et al. 1990
	Antibiotics	chlarithromycin	Il-1β	Takeshita et al. 1989
	Cytokines	Il-10	Il-1β, TNF	Malefyt et al. 1991
	Imidazoline derivative	TA-383	Il-6	Sugita et al. 1993

Macrophage-associated Activation of Il-1β by Converting Enzyme May Be a Target for Antiinflammatory Drugs

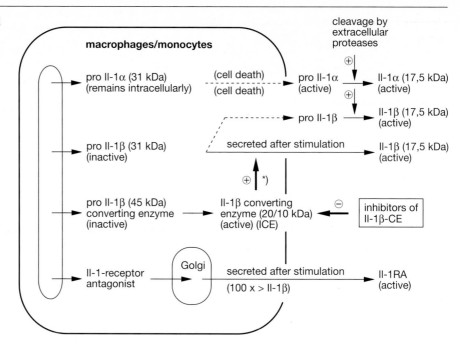

*) Il-1β converting enzyme is a Thiol (cysteine) protease specific for cleavage of pro Il-1β at the Asp (116) - Ala (117) bond.

Miller et al. 1993

**Inhibition of Il-1
Synthesis by Enzyme
Inhibitors**

Mechanism – target   Theoretical approach

Il-1 precursor (31,5 kDa)

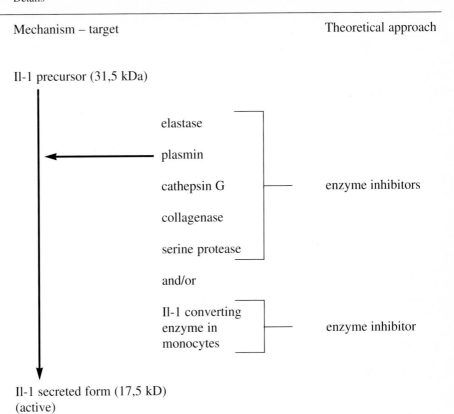

elastase

plasmin

cathepsin G   enzyme inhibitors

collagenase

serine protease

and/or

Il-1 converting
enzyme in   enzyme inhibitor
monocytes

Il-1 secreted form (17,5 kD)
(active)

Lewis et al. 1992

13 Interaction with Endothelial Cells

13.1 Overview

13.1.1 Granulocytes and Endothelial Cells

Steps of inflammatory reactions:
- Histamine and/or thrombin preactivates endothelial cells. These express selectins (GP-140, ELAM-1), low concentrations of ICAM-1, -2 and GlyCAM.
- Nonactivated polymorphic neutrophil granulocytes (PMN) attach to preactivated endothelial cells with low strength (rolling). Attachment of PMN is mediated via their LECAM-1 to GLyCAM (sialylated oligosaccharide ligands) and with their ligands SLex and LeCAM-1/Lewis X to ELAM-1 and GMP-140.
- Attached PMN are activated by factors (C4a, LTB4, cytokines), released from fully activated endothelial cells. Activated PMN shed LECAM-1, which neutralizes free GlyCAM and GMP-140 and thus limits the number of attaching PMN.
- Activated PMN express LFA-1, MAC-1 and VLA-4, which mediate strong attachment to ICAM-1, -2 and VCAM-1, produced by fully activated endothelial cells. This attachment remains for about 1 h and can be followed by transmigratory extravasation of PMN.
- A long lasting ($\geq$ 24 h) attachment and subsequent transmigration of PMN can be induced by activation of endothelial cells with cytokines (IL-1, TNFα) and LPS. Such activated endothelial cells secrete IL-8, which activates PMN to express high amount of VLA-4, which binds to extracellular matrix. Transmigration of PMN is the consequence.

Hallmann et al. 1991, Parekh 1991, Zimmerman et al. 1992.

Steps of Interaction Between Neutrophil Granulocytes and Endothelial Cells

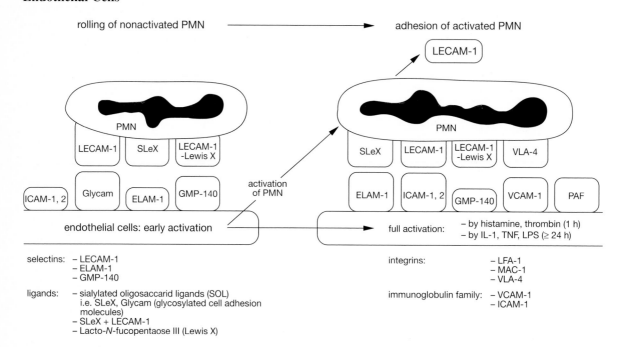

selectins: – LECAM-1
            – ELAM-1
            – GMP-140

ligands: – sialylated oligosaccarid ligands (SOL)
             i.e. SLeX, Glycam (glycosylated cell adhesion
             molecules)
           – SLeX + LECAM-1
           – Lacto-*N*-fucopentaose III (Lewis X)

integrins: – LFA-1
                            – MAC-1
                            – VLA-4

immunoglobulin family: – VCAM-1
                            – ICAM-1

13.1.2 Lymphocytes and Endothelial Cells

Steps of inflammatory reactions:
– Extravasation of lymphocytes is possible
  * In normal spleen (from arteriols into pulpa)
  * Through the endothelial lining of "high endothelial venules" (HEV) in spleen, lymphnodes and Peyer's patches.
– Number and size of HEV in lymphoid organs is increased by local immune reactions. Stimulation of lymphnodes by antigens leads to change of normal capillaries into HEV by proliferation and differentiation of endothelial cells.
– Adhesion to HEV cells and transmigration of lymphocytes takes place via adhesion molecules (CD44 on lymphocytes). Nonorganspecific adhesion takes place mainly via LFA-1/ICAM-1.
– T-cells transmigrate mainly peripheral lymphnodes, B-cells mainly lymphoid tissues associated with mucous epithelia.
– Adhesion to HEV cells in peripheral lymphnodes (but not in gut or tonsil associated lymphoid tissues) of T-cells is specifically mediated by LECAM-1/sialylated fucosylated glycoproteins (sLex, Sgp50, Sgp100, MeCa-79).

- Memory T-cells mainly accumulate in the afferent lymph (ductus thoracicus) after leaving lymphnodes. They express only low amounts of LECAM-1.
- Naive T-cells mainly accumulate in the efferent lymph and recirculate between blood and peripheral lymphnodes. Naive T-cells express high amounts of LECAM-1.

Anderson et al. 1991, Brandley et al. 1990, Hamann et al. 1988, Imai et al. 1991, Mackay et al. 1990, Pals et al. 1988, Shimizu et al. 1992.

Main Adhesion Molecules on Lymphocytes and Monocytes

Endothelial cell

  VCAM-1 (vascular adhesion molecule)

  ICAM(-1), -2, -3, -R (intercellular adhesion molecules)

  Glycam (SOL) (glycosylated cellular adhesion molecule, sialylated oligo-saccharide ligands, Lex, Sgp 50, Sgp 100, MECA-79)

  Sialyl Lewis X

  Sialyl Lewis X

  Lacto-*N*-fucopentaose III

  Hyaluronic acid

Lymphocyte

  VLA (very late activation antigens: $\alpha4\beta1$ (VLA-4), $\alpha4\beta7$)

  LFA-1 (CD11a/CD18) (leukocyte function associated antigen)

  MAC-1 (CD11b) (monocyte adhesion complex)

  gp 95/150 (CDIIc)

  LECAM-1 (lectin-like cellular adhesion molecules)

  ELAM-1 (endothelial cell adhesion molecules)

  PECAM-1 (platelet endothelial cell adhesion molecules)

  GMP-140 (granule membrane protein)

  CD44 (hermes antigen)

**Tissue-Specific
Enhanced Expression
of Adhesion Molecules
by Endothelial Cells**

Tissue	Vessels	Causing agent/disease	Increase of	Decrease of
Lymphoid tissue	HEV	antigen stimulation	ICAM-1 GMP-140	
Normal tissue	post capillary venules	histamine, thrombin	GMP-140 ICAM-1 ELAM-1	
		IL-1, TNF-α, LPS	ICAM-1 ELAM-1 VCAM-1	GMP-140
Kidney	glomeruli	acute inflammation	ICAM-1 ELAM-1	
		chronic, progressive disease		ICAM-1
	tubuli (epithelial cells)	glomerulonephritis	ICAM-1	
		rejection after transplantation	ICAM-1	
Liver	interlobular bile vessels, endothelial cells	chronic hepatitis	ICAM-1 ELAM-1	
	hepatocytes	rejection after transplantation	ICAM-1	
Heart	capillaries	rejection after transplantation	ICAM-1	
Lung	serum	cold infection	s-ICAM-1	
Joints	synovium	rheumatoid arthritis	s-ICAM-1	
	serum	osteoarthritis	s-ICAM-1	
		rheumatoid arthritis	s-ICAM-1	

Briscoe et al. 1991, Faull et al. 1989, Lhotta et al. 1991, Suzuki et al. 1991, Popp et al. 1992, Herold et al. 1992.

13.2 Details

13.2.1 Activation of Endothelial Cells by Cytokines and Growth Factors

Parameter (synthesis or formation)	Endothelial cells		Mediators that induce activation
	Resting	Activated	
General			
increase in thickness	–	2–3x	IL-1α/β, TNF, IFN-γ, LT
loss in contact inhibition	–	+	IL-1α/β, TNF, IFN-γ, LT
permeability	–	+	IL-1α/β, TNF, IFN-γ, LT
proliferation rate	47–23 000 days	2,4–13 days	FGF, PDGF, TNF, LT
(doubling time)			IL-1, GM-CSF, G-CSF
generation of NO (EDRF =	–/+	++	IL-1β, TNF
endothelial derived relaxing factor)	–	– –	TGF-β
generation of endothelin	–/+	++	IL-1β, TNF
Coagulation			
tissue factor	–/+	+	IL-1α/β, TNF, LT
thrombomodulin	+	–	IL-1α/β, TNF, LT
plasminogen activator			IL-1α/β, TNF, LT
inhibitor (PAI)	–/+	–	TGF-β, TGF-α
plasminogen activator	+	–	TGF-β
(uPA, tPA)	+	+++	bFGF, TNF-α
Acute inflammatory			
endothelial leucocyte			
adhesion molecule (ELAM)	–	++	IL-1α/β, TNF, LT, TGF
intercellular adhesion			
molecule (ICAM 1, 2)	+	++	IL-1α/β, TNF, LT, IFN
vascular cell adhesion			
molecule (VCAM)	(+)	+	IL-1α/β, TNF, LT, IFN
platelet activating			
factor (PAF)	–/+	+	IL-1α/β, TNF, LT, IFN
IL-1α, IL-6, G-CSF,	–/+	+	IL-1α/β, TNF, LT
GM-CSF, M-CSF, IL-8,	–/+	+	IFN-γ
MCAF	–	+	IL-1, TNF-α
Chronic inflammatory			
FGF, PDGF	–/+	+	IL-1α/β, TNF, LT, IFN
angiogenesis	–	++	TNF, FGF, PDGF
PGE$_2$, PGI$_2$, LTB$_4$, TBXA$_2$	+/–	++	IL-1α/β, TNF, LT, IFN
Immune reaction			
MHC-class I	+	++	TNF, IL-1α/β, LT, IFN
MHC-class II	–	+	IFN-γ
interstitial cell adhesion molecule			
(ICAM-1)	+	++	IL-1α/β, TNF, LT, IFN
membrane IL-1α			IL-1α/β, TNF, LT

Rubanyi 1992; Bone 1992; Bevilacqua et al. 1985, 1987, 1989; Bussolino et al. 1989; Cotran et al. 1988; Furchgott et al. 1989; Hobson et al. 1984; Laiho et al. 1989; Meinardus-Hager et al. 1991; Osborn et al. 1989; Pfeilschifter et al. 1991; Pober et al. 1982, 1983, 1986, 1988; Herlyn et al. 1991; Sica et al. 1990.

Endothelial Reactions
Induced by Cytokines
(General Reactions,
Inflammation,
Coagulation,
Immune Reaction)

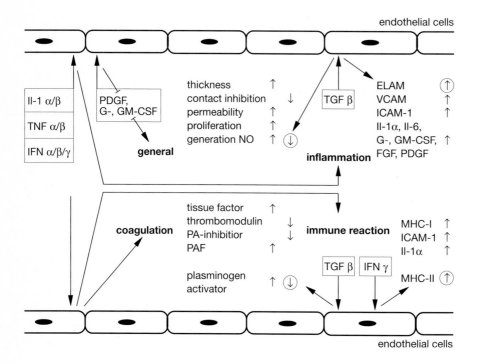

Endothelial Injury
Induced by Leukocytes

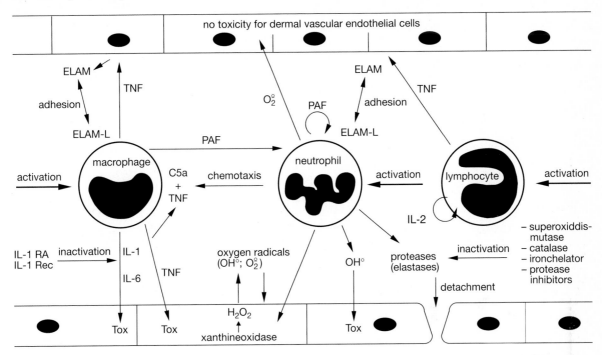

Word et al. 1991; Johnson et al. 1974, 1981; Lee et al. 1987; Phan et al. 1989; Prober et al.1986; Sachs et al. 1978; Smedly et al. 1986; Spragg et al. 1985; Varani et al. 1985; Warren et al. 1989a, b

Generation of Oxygen Radicals

Haber-Weis Reaction

$$H_2O_2 \xrightarrow{\;O_2^{\circ}\;} O_2 + OH^{\circ} + OH^{\ominus}$$

$$(H - \overline{\underline{O}} - \overline{\underline{O}} - H + \langle \overset{\circ}{O} \overset{\circ}{=} O\rangle \longrightarrow O_2 + |\overline{\underset{\circ}{O}} - H + |\overline{\underline{O}} - H^{\ominus})$$

Fenton reaction

$$H_2O_2 + Fe^{\text{②+}} \longrightarrow Fe^{\text{③+}} + OH^{\circ} + OH^{\ominus}$$

$$(H - \overline{\underline{O}} - \overline{\underline{O}} - H + Fe^{\text{②+}} \longrightarrow Fe^{\text{③+}} + \overline{\underset{\circ}{O}} - H + |\overline{\underline{O}} - H^{\ominus})$$

Reaction catalyzed by xanthine oxidase

$$H_2O + O_2 \xrightarrow[\text{substrate}]{\text{xanthine oxidase}} H_2O_2 + \text{oxidized substrate}$$

13.2.2 Endothelium-Derived Relaxing Factors (EDRF)

Cells of the vascular endothelium produce and release autocrine and paracrine substances which can:
- Relax the tonus of the surrounding smooth muscle
- Inhibit the aggregation of platelets

They can also contribute to the "thromboresistant" and "vasodilator" function of the endothelium.

Prostaglandin PGI_2 (Moncada et al. 1976)
- acts by increasing of cAMP levels in smooth muscle cells and platelets

EDRF (Furchgott et al. 1980, 1987)
- Has been shown to be nitric oxide (NO) or a labile nitroso compound formed from L-arginine in the endothelial cells (Furchgott et al. 1987; Ignarro et al. 1988; Palmer et al. 1987)
- Acts by increasing cGMP levels in smooth muscle cells and platelets (Rubanyi 1992)

EDHF (endothelium derived hyperpolarizing factor; Feleton et al. 1988; Kauser et al. 1989)
- Still unidentified; diffusible endothelium derived factor
- Acts by membrane hyperpolarization presumably via activating K^+ channels

**Action of Endothelium-
Derived Relaxing
Factors**

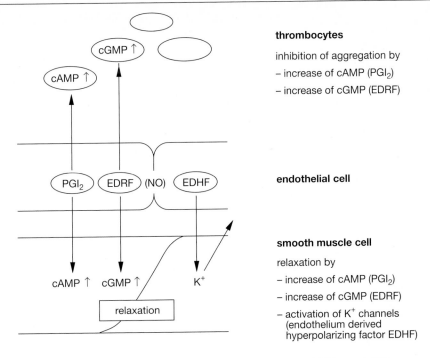

thrombocytes

inhibition of aggregation by
– increase of cAMP (PGI$_2$)
– increase of cGMP (EDRF)

endothelial cell

smooth muscle cell

relaxation by
– increase of cAMP (PGI$_2$)
– increase of cGMP (EDRF)
– activation of K$^+$ channels
  (endothelium derived
  hyperpolarizing factor EDHF)

Moncada et al. 1976; Furchgott et al. 1980, 1987; Ignarro et al. 1988; Palmer et al. 1987; Feleton et al. 1988;
Kauser 1989; Rubanyi 1992

13.2.3 Endothelium-Derived Contracting Factors (EDCF)

Cells of the vascular endothelium produce and release substances, which provoke contraction of the surrounding smooth muscle cells and lead to vasoconstriction:

Thromboxane A_2; Prostaglandin H_2
– Inhibits cyclooxygenase, prevents thereby endothelium dependent vascular contractions evoked by stretch and various agonists. The mediator is probably TXA_2/PGH_2 (Rubanyi et al. 1992).

Angiotensin II
– The renin-angiotensin system has been localized in endothelial cells (Rubanyi et al. 1992).

Endothelin
– Endothelins are peptides of 21 aa. At least 3 isoforms exist (-1, -2, -3). The stimuli, which trigger its synthesis/release, are unknown (Rubanyi 1992). ET-1 is about 20-fold more potent than ET-3 in vasoconstriction (Warner et al. 1989).
– Endothelins (mainly ET-1) may also induce:
  * Bronchoconstriction (Advenier et al. 1990)
  * Uterine contraction (Bousso-Mittler et al. 1989)
  * Cardiac effects (Galron et al. 1989) and
  * Aldosterone secretion (Gomez-Sanchez et al. 1990)
– All endothelins
  * Induce initial vasodilatation (Warner et al. 1989; Inoue et al. 1989)
  * Induce stomach ulcers (Wallace et al. 1989)
  * Inhibite platelet aggregation (Lidburg et al. 1990)
– Receptors for endothelins belong to the G-proteincoupled receptors of the rhodopsin receptor super family (Rubanyi 1992).
– Two structurally different receptors exist:
  * the ETB receptor on endothelial cells (Sakurai et al. 1990; Rubanyi 1992)
  * the ETA receptor on vascular smooth muscle cells (Rubanyi 1992)
– Endothelin is produced following proteolytic cleavage in two steps (Yanagisawa et al. 1988; Rubanyi 1992):

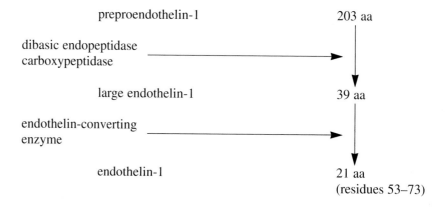

preproendothelin-1   203 aa

dibasic endopeptidase
carboxypeptidase

large endothelin-1   39 aa

endothelin-converting
enzyme

endothelin-1   21 aa
                                                               (residues 53–73)

**Endothelium-Derived
Contracting Factors**

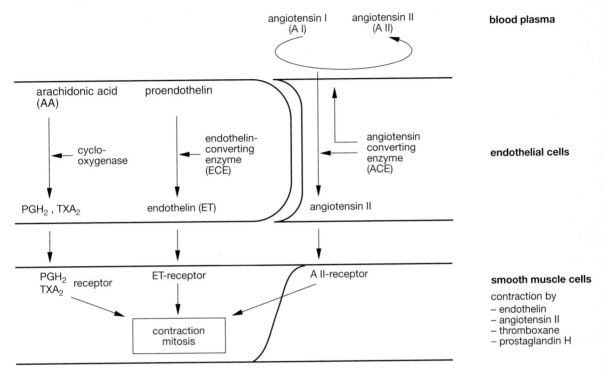

Rubanyl et al. 1985, 1988, 1992; Hickey et al. 1985; Yanagisawa et al. 1988

13.2.4 Immunological Aspects of Arteriosclerosis

Arteriosclerosis is a common histopathological feature of chronic rejection in all organ transplants.

Pathophysiological changes of allograft arteriosclerosis include
– Inflammation of the tunica adventitia
– Necrosis of the tunica media
– Thickening of the intima

Disease can develop by the following pathway:
– Damage of the vascular endothelium by:
  – Cytokines or toxic compounds released from leukocytes
  – Lipid abnormalities, hypertension, diabetes
– Activation of endothelial cells with
  – Adhesion of native (and oxidized) LDLs (fatty streak)
– Release of cytokines (IL-1, others) and growth factors (bFGF, PDGF, IGF)

– Attachment and activation of T-cells and macrophages (foam cell through pha-
  gocytosis) and platelets; release of growth factors (bFGF, PDGF, IGF)
– Diapedesis of macrophages into the intima with:
  – Edema of intima
  – Eelease of growth factors
– Proliferation of smooth muscle cells and fibroblasts; invasion of smooth
  muscle cells from media into intima; thickening of intima; formation of fibro-
  tic cap; deposition of LDLs
– Expression of tissue factor (thromboplastin) by smooth muscle cells; activation
  of F VIII by tissue factor (TF)/F VIII complexes, fibrin and platelet clots
– Necrosis of smooth muscle cells; calcification
– Rupture of arteriotic plaque; thrombus formation infarction

The disease can experimentally be prevented by:
– ±15-Deoxyspergualin (see chapter on immune suppression)
– Mycophenolic mophetil (see chapter on immune suppression)

Hävry 1994, Raisänen-Sokolowski et al. 1994.

Immunological Aspect
for Artheriosclerosis

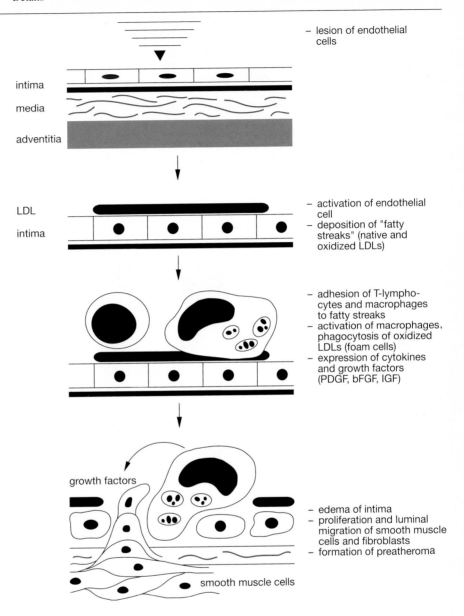

– lesion of endothelial
  cells

intima

media

adventitia

LDL

intima

– activation of endothelial
  cell
– deposition of "fatty
  streaks" (native and
  oxidized LDLs)

– adhesion of T-lympho-
  cytes and macrophages
  to fatty streaks
– activation of macrophages,
  phagocytosis of oxidized
  LDLs (foam cells)
– expression of cytokines
  and growth factors
  (PDGF, bFGF, IGF)

growth factors

– edema of intima
– proliferation and luminal
  migration of smooth muscle
  cells and fibroblasts
– formation of preatheroma

smooth muscle cells

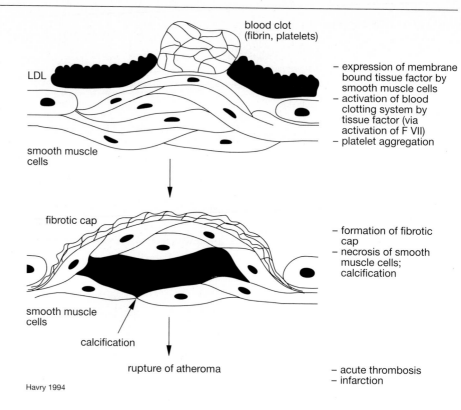

blood clot
(fibrin, platelets)

LDL

smooth muscle
cells

– expression of membrane
  bound tissue factor by
  smooth muscle cells
– activation of blood
  clotting system by
  tissue factor (via
  activation of F VII)
– platelet aggregation

fibrotic cap

smooth muscle
cells

calcification

– formation of fibrotic
  cap
– necrosis of smooth
  muscle cells;
  calcification

rupture of atheroma

– acute thrombosis
– infarction

Havry 1994

14 Involvement of the Clotting System and Platelets

14.1 Overview

The clotting system and platelets are involved in the immune reaction via various mechanisms:
- Direct activation of the intrinsic and extrinsic pathway
- Activation of monocytes, macrophages, granulocytes, lymphocytes and release of mediators and cytokines
- Activation of the complement system
- Activation of endothelial cells
- Activation of platelets

Activation and Inhibition of the Clotting System

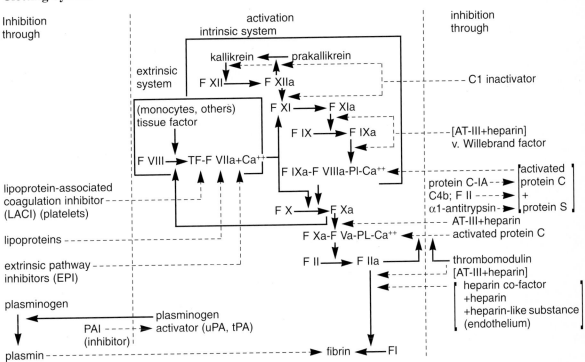

Patterson et al. 1990; Langley et al. 1992; Kyle et al. 1988.

14.2 Details

14.2.1 Inhibition of Coagulation in Normal Epithelium

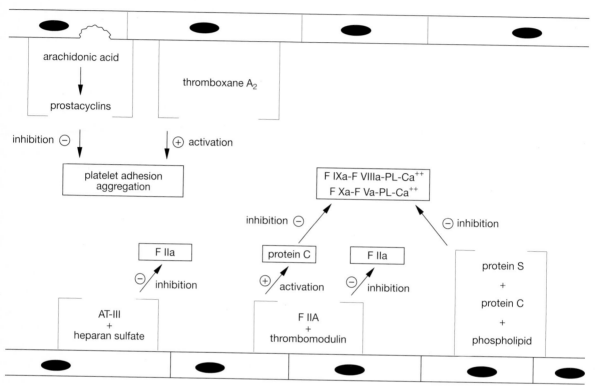

Patterson et al. 1990

14.2.2 Effect of Growth Factors and Cytokines on Plasminogen Activator Secretion

| Growth factors | Cell type | Effect on production of | | Other effects | References |
		PA	PAI		
EGF	fibroblasts	+ (uPA, tPA)	+ (PAI 0 (PAI-1)		Eaton 1983 Laiko 1986
	carcinoma cells kidney cells	− (uPA, tPA) +		growth stimulation anchorage-independent growth (?)	Stoppelli 1986 Jetten 1983
TFG-α	fibroblasts	+ (uPA, tPA)			Laiko 1986
bFGF	endothelial cells	+ (uPA, tPA)	+ (PAI-1		Montesano 1986
TGFβ	fibroblasts	+ (uPA	+ (PAI-1)	activation of TGFβ by plasmin inhibition of TGFβ by macroglobulin	Laiko 1986
	endothelial cells carcinoma cells sarcoma cells	− (uPA, tPA) + (uPA) − (uPA)	+ (PAI-1) + (PAI-1)		Sakzela 1987 Keski-Oja 1988 Laiko 1987
CSF	monocytes	+	+ (PAI-2)		Lin 1979
IL-1	endothelial cells fibroblasts	0 (tPA)	+ (PAI-1)	increase of TIMP increase of proteins	Nachman 1986 Postlethwaite 1988
TNF-α	endothelial cells	0 (tPA	+ (PAI-1)		Schleef 1988
IFN α	macrophages	+			Hovi 1981
Thrombin	endothelial cells fibroblasts	+ (tPA) +	+ (PAI-1) + (PAI-1)		Gelehrter 1986 Eaton 1987

14.2.3 Activation and Aggregation of Platelets

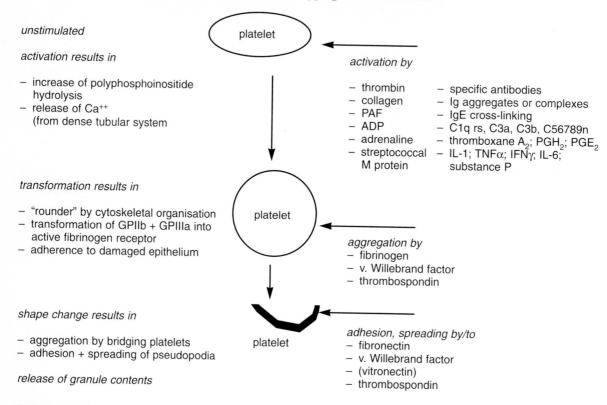

unstimulated

activation results in

- increase of polyphosphoinositide hydrolysis
- release of Ca^{++} (from dense tubular system

activation by

- thrombin
- collagen
- PAF
- ADP
- adrenaline
- streptococcal M protein

- specific antibodies
- Ig aggregates or complexes
- IgE cross-linking
- C1q rs, C3a, C3b, C56789n
- thromboxane A$_2$; PGH$_2$; PGE$_2$
- IL-1; TNFα; IFNγ; IL-6; substance P

transformation results in

- "rounder" by cytoskeletal organisation
- transformation of GPIIb + GPIIIa into active fibrinogen receptor
- adherence to damaged epithelium

aggregation by

- fibrinogen
- v. Willebrand factor
- thrombospondin

shape change results in

- aggregation by bridging platelets
- adhesion + spreading of pseudopodia

release of granule contents

adhesion, spreading by/to

- fibronectin
- v. Willebrand factor
- (vitronectin)
- thrombospondin

Philipps et al. 1988; Devine et al. 1992; Henson et al. 1977, 1981; Cheng et al. 1979; Amelsen et al. 1985; Rolley et al. 1981, 1983, 1979; Gresele 1992; Joseph 1992; Martin 1992.

Main Physiological Role of Platelets	Physiological role	mechanism
	Inhibition of bleeding	– platelet aggregation (fibrinogen) – stabilization of platelet aggregates (thrombomodulin) – bridging of platelets to damaged endothelial cells (vWF)
	Vascular repair	– spreading of platelets
	Vasodilatation and disaggregation of platelets	– release of NO (EDRF)
	Allergic reaction	– release of PF4, PF, BHRS to activate mast cells, basophils – release of stored Histamin and Serotonin – increase of eosinophil activity by PF4
	Inflammation	– release of β-thromboglobulin, PDGF, catalase, TGFβ, chemotactic factor, 12-HETE for tissue degradation, attraction and activation of leukocytes
	Vascular permeability	– filling of intercellular gaps by adhering to exposed extracellular matrix via the GpIIb/IIIa receptor – release of adenosine which increases cAMP levels in endothelial cells and reduces transendothelial permeability

Joseph et al. 1992; McGregor 1992; Martin 1992; Tuffin 1992; Malik 1992.

Human Platelet Surface Glycoproteins

Glycoprotein	Classification	Ligand	Function
GpIIb-IIIa (GpIIb + GpIIIa)	integrin IIbβ3	fibrinogen, fibronectin, vWF, vitronectin	– platelet aggregation (fibrinogen) and adhesion – uptake of fibrinogen, fibronectin and vWF; storage in the granule; release after activation for platelet aggregation – binding of thrombospondin via fibrinogen
GpIb-IX (GpIb (GpIbα + GpIbβ) + GpIX)	CD42b	vWF	– bridging between platelets and damaged endothelium in arterial vessels at higher shearing forces
GpIc-IIa	integrin 5β1, VLA-6 integrin bβ1	fibronectin, collagen	– platelet adhesion
GpIa-IIa	integrin 2β1, VLA-2	laminin, thrombo-spondin collagen	– platelet adhesion – stabilization of platelet aggregates
GpIIIb	GpIV, CD36	thrombospondin, collagen	– stabilization of platelet aggregates
GMP-140	P-selectin, PADGEM, CD62 (expressed following degranulation)	Lewis-X	– expressed following degranulation of platelets – stabilization of platelet aggregates
PECAM-1	CD31, Ig super family	?	– platelet adhesion (?)
GpIc'IIa	CD49f, CD29	laminin	– platelet adhesion

Fox et al. 1988; Ikeda et al. 1991; Tuffin 1992; McGregor 1992; Roth 1992.

Function of a Human Platelet Surface Glycoprotein

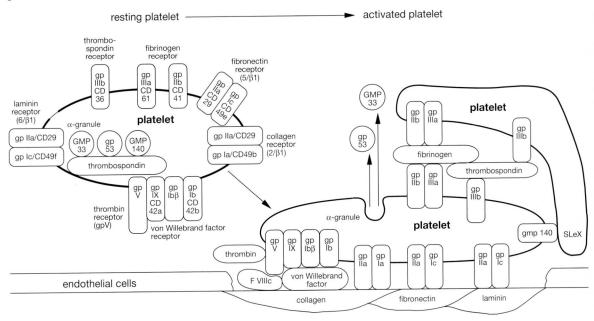

The Fibrinogen Receptor on Platelets Synonym: GPIIb–IIIa complex

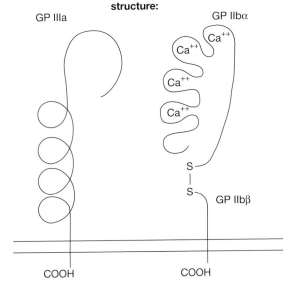

structure:

GP IIIa

GP IIbα

GP IIbβ

COOH   COOH

size (KDa):

GP IIIa   105
GP IIbα   125
GP IIbβ   25

density:

50 000/platelet
70%   exposed
30%   cryptic
(canalicular system,
α-granules)

1-2% of the total
platelet protein

inactivation:

by chelating agents
by monoclonal antibodies

Ligands:
- Fibrinogen   Kd: 10^{-7} M
                      (aggregation by bridging platelets)
- Fibronectin   (adhesion, spreading; each receptor binds 2
                      fibronectin molecules)
- von Willebrand factor   (aggregation, adhesion, spreading)

Binding to each partner is exclusive:
- Thrombospondin (aggregation, adhesion, binding only related to GPIIb–IIIa, distinct site)

Philipps et al. 1988, Tuffin 1992.

Platelet Aggregation

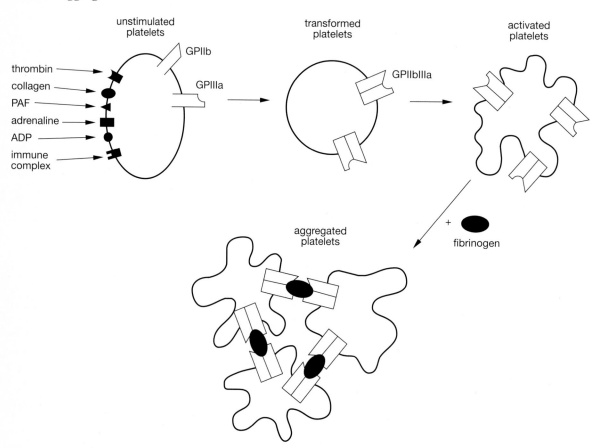

Compounds Released
by Platelets

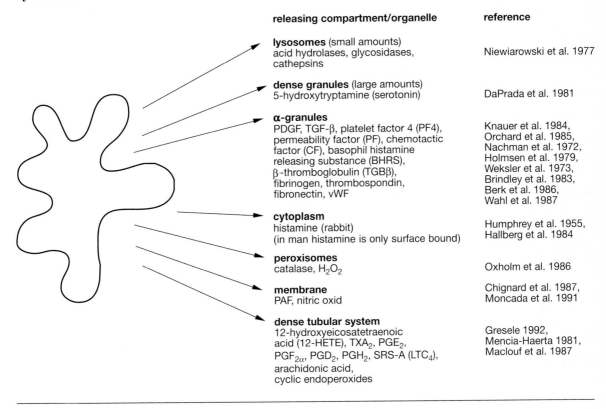

	releasing compartment/organelle	reference
	lysosomes (small amounts) acid hydrolases, glycosidases, cathepsins	Niewiarowski et al. 1977
	dense granules (large amounts) 5-hydroxytryptamine (serotonin)	DaPrada et al. 1981
	α-granules PDGF, TGF-β, platelet factor 4 (PF4), permeability factor (PF), chemotactic factor (CF), basophil histamine releasing substance (BHRS), β-thromboglobulin (TGBβ), fibrinogen, thrombospondin, fibronectin, vWF	Knauer et al. 1984, Orchard et al. 1985, Nachman et al. 1972, Holmsen et al. 1979, Weksler et al. 1973, Brindley et al. 1983, Berk et al. 1986, Wahl et al. 1987
	cytoplasm histamine (rabbit) (in man histamine is only surface bound)	Humphrey et al. 1955, Hallberg et al. 1984
	peroxisomes catalase, H_2O_2	Oxholm et al. 1986
	membrane PAF, nitric oxid	Chignard et al. 1987, Moncada et al. 1991
	dense tubular system 12-hydroxyeicosatetraenoic acid (12-HETE), TXA_2, PGE_2, $PGF_{2\alpha}$, PGD_2, PGH_2, SRS-A (LTC_4), arachidonic acid, cyclic endoperoxides	Gresele 1992, Mencia-Haerta 1981, Maclouf et al. 1987

Biological Activity
of Compounds Relea-
sed by Platelets

Compound	Biological activity	References
Lysosomal enzymes	tissue degradation and cytotoxicity	Niewiarowski et al. 1977 Vlodavsky et al. 1992
5-HT (serotonin)	vasoconstriction, increase of vascular permeability, stimulation of fibroblast growth	Majno et al. 1961 Boncek et al. 1970
PDGF	chemotactic locomotion towards monocytes, neutrophils, fibroblasts; activation of mono- cytes, proliferation of mesenchymal cells	Denel et al. 1982, Page 1988 Grotendorst et al. 1981, Tzeng et al. 1985
TGF-b	chemotactic locomotion towards and activation of monocytes; stimulation of proliferation of mesenchymal cells	Wahl et al. 1987 Laiho et al. 1989

Compound	Biological activity	References
Platelet factor 4 (PF4)	stimulation of basophils to release histamine; chemotactic locomotion for neutrophil granulocytes and monocytes; inhibition of collagenase, stimulation of elastase activity; activation of eosinophils for chemotaxis, exposure of Fcγ and Fcϵ receptors)	Brindley et al. 1983 Denel et al. 1981 Hiti-Harper et al. 1978 Lonky et al. 1981 Chihara et al. 1988
Permeability factor (PF)	degranulation of mast cells	Nachman et al. 1972
Basophil histamine releasing substance (BHRS)	histamine release by degranulation of mast cells and basophils	Holmsen et al. 1979 Knauer et al. 1984
Chemotactic factor (CF)	cleavage of C5, generation of C5a, induces chemotactic locomotion of PMN	Weksler et al. 1973
Histamine	mainly released by platelets from rabbits, only trace amounts in human platelets	Humphrey et al. 1975 Da Prada et al. 1981
Catalase	toxic necrosis of cells and tissues by radical oxygen	Oxholm et al. 1986
Thromboxane B$_2$ (TBXB$_2$)	vasoconstriction and bronchial smooth muscle; contraction enhancement of cholinergic transmission	Samuelson et al. 1978 Chung et al. 1985
Prostaglandin E$_2$	vasodilation, suppression of T-cells	Gresele et al. 1992
12-Hydroxyeicosatetra-enoic acid (5-hete)	chemotactic agent for eosinophil granulocytes stimulation of 5-lipoxygenase activity in leukocytes	Goetzl et al. 1977 Maclouf et al. 1982
Slow-reacting substance of anaphylaxis (SRSA) (LTC$_4$, LTD$_4$, LTE$_4$)	interaction with peptide leukotriene receptor on smooth muscle cells and epithelia	Mencia-Huerta et al. 1981 Claesson et al. 1992
Platelet activating factor (PAF)	platelet activation, activation of LB$_4$ synthesis by leukocytes	Page 1988 Mencia-Huerta et al. 1989 Pretolani et al. 1989 Lin et al. 1982
Arachidonic acid	taken up by leukocytes for their synthesis of 5-hete and LTB$_4$	Marcus et al. 1980, 1986
Cyclic endoperoxides	taken up by leukocytes for their synthesis of prostaglandins	Marcus et al. 1980, 1986
Nitric oxide (EDRF)	dilatation of blood vessels	Moncada et al. 1991
Fibrinogen	platelet aggregation	Tuffin 1992
Thrombomodulin, vWF, fibronectin	stabilization of platelet aggregates bridging of platelets to damaged endothelial cells	Mc Gregor 1992
Adenosine	enhancement of endothelial barrier function by increase of endothelial cAMP levels	Malik 1992

14.2.4 Role of Transforming Growth Factor β (TGFβ)

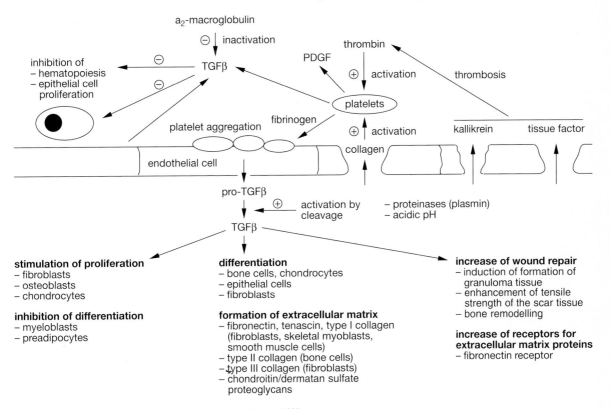

stimulation of proliferation
– fibroblasts
– osteoblasts
– chondrocytes

inhibition of differentiation
– myeloblasts
– preadipocytes

differentiation
– bone cells, chondrocytes
– epithelial cells
– fibroblasts

formation of extracellular matrix
– fibronectin, tenascin, type I collagen
  (fibroblasts, skeletal myoblasts,
  smooth muscle cells)
– type II collagen (bone cells)
– type III collagen (fibroblasts)
– chondroitin/dermatan sulfate
  proteoglycans

increase of wound repair
– induction of formation of
  granuloma tissue
– enhancement of tensile
  strength of the scar tissue
– bone remodelling

**increase of receptors for
extracellular matrix proteins**
– fibronectin receptor

Laiko et al. 1989; Mustoe 1987; Tashijian et al. 1985; Spona 1986; Massaque 1986

14.2.5 Arachidonic Acid Metabolism in Platelets

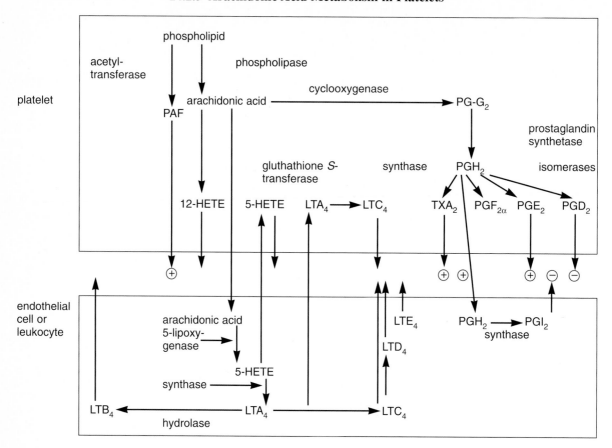

$\oplus$ stimulation $\ominus$ inhibition of platelet activation and aggregation

Marous et al. 1982, 1986; Maolouf et al. 1987; Defreyn et al. 1982; Mehta et al. 1985; Gresele et al. 1992.

14.2.6 Inhibitors of Platelet Aggregation

Target: Fibrinogen Receptor (GpIIb–IIIa) on Platelets

Compounds	References
MAb [F(ab)$_2$, Fab, chimeric]	Coller et al. 1989
Leech proteins (Ornatin, Decorsin)	Mazur et al. 1991
Snake venoms (Echistatin, Bitistatin, Rhodostomin, Barbourin)	Gould et al. 1990 Scarborough et al. 1991
Peptide antagonists	Bunting et al. 1991 Davidson et al. 1991 Roux et al. 1991 Feigen et al. 1991 Scarborough et al. 1991
Nonpeptide antagonists amino alkyloxyphenylpropionic acid others	Nicholson et al. 1991 Gould et al. 1992

Inhibition of Platelet Aggregation

Target	Compound	References
vWF-receptor (GpIbIX)	Mab anti GpI	Nicholas et al. 1991
vWF-receptor	vWF peptides 474–708 RG 12986 (Rhône-Poulenc)	Kasiewski et al. 1991
vWF	aurintricarboxylic acid	Strong et al. 1990
TBS-receptor (GpIa/IIa)	thrombospondin peptides Mab anti GpIa	Catimel et al. 1992 McGregor et al. 1992
TBS-receptor (GpIIIb)	thrombospondin peptides Mab anti GpIIIb	Catimel et al. 1992 McGregor et al. 1992
cAMP phospho-diesterase	inhibition by methyl-xanthines or cilostamide	Haslam et al. 1992
Guanylyl cyclase	activation by compounds releasing NO (e.g. Nitroprusside)	Haslam et al. 1992
Cyclooxygenase	inhibitors (aspirin)	Gresele et al. 1991
Thromboxan synthase	inhibitors (OKY 046, picot amide)	Gresele et al. 1991
TXA$_2$ receptor	antagonists (daltobran, picot amide)	Gresele et al. 1991

14.2.7 Modulation of Platelet Aggregation In Vivo

Accumulation/ aggregation induced by	Effect on aggregation in Modulation by	Rat	Guinea pig	Rabbit	References
ADP	PGI$_2$		–		Page et al. 1982
			–		Humphries et al. 1989
	heparin (high dose)		–		Barrett et al. 1984
	(low dose)		Ø		
	TXA$_2$ antagonist		Ø		Chan et al. 1984
	adrenaline	–			Oyekan & Botting 1986
	EDRF	–			Bhardwaj et al. 1988
	endothelin-1			–	Humphries et al. 1990
	PAF antagonists		Ø	Ø	Thiemermann et al. 1990 Smith et al. 1989
	inhibitor of NO synthesis			+	Herd 1991 May et al. 1991
Collagen	Heparin (high dose)		–		Barrett et al. 1984
	(low dose)		Ø		
	Indomethacin		Ø		Butler et al. 1984
	Acetylsalicylic acid		Ø		
			–		Smith et al. 1989
				–	Herd 1991
	EDRF		–		Humphries et al. 1990
	endothelin-1			–	Thiemermann et al. 1990
	PAF antagonists		Ø		Smith et al. 1989
				Ø	Herd 1991
PAF	heparin (low dose)		Ø		Barrett et al. 1984
	(high dose)		–		
	heparin (high dose)			–	Herd 1991
	acetylsalicylic acid		Ø		Smith et al. 1989
	acetylsalicylic acid			+	Herd 1991
	indomethacin			+	
	endothelin-1			–	Thiemermann et al. 1990
	PAF antagonists	–		–	Smith et al. 1989 Herd 1991
	inhibitor of NO synthesis			+	May et al. 1991
Thrombin (in the lung)	heparin (low dose)		–		Barrett et al. 1984
	endothelin-1			Ø	Thiemermann et al. 1990
	inhibitor of NO synthesis			+	May et al. 1991

Accumulation/ aggregation induced by	Effect on aggregation in Modulation by	Rat	Guinea pig	Rabbit	References
Thrombin (in the brain)	desulfatohirudin			–	May et al. 1992
	PAF antagonist		Ø		
	inhibitor of NO synthesis		Ø		
Arachidonic acid	indomethacin		–		Barrett et al. 1986
	acetylsalicylic acid		–		
Endotoxin	PAF antagonists		–		Beijer et al. 1987
	indomethacin	Ø			
	heparin		–		
	PGI$_2$ analogue		–		

–, inhibition; +, potentiation; Ø, no effect.

14.2.8 Cytokines that Stimulate Megakaryocytopoiesis

Cytokine	Secretion	References
IL-3	paracrine	Teramura et al. 1988 Ganser et al. 1990
IL-6	paracrine + autocrine	Ishibashi et al. 1989 Fuse et al. 1991 Brack et al. 1990
GM-CSF	paracrine	Mazur et al. 1987 Vannuchi et al. 1990
LIF (leukemia inhibition factor)	paracrine	Burstein et al. 1990 Metcalf et al. 1990
IL-11	paracrine + autocrine	Burstein et al. 1990 Teramura et al. 1992 Kobayashi et al. 1993
SCF	autocrine	Avraham et al. 1992

15 Enzymatic Degradation of Extracellular Matrix

15.1 Overview

15.1.1 Destruction of Extracellular Matrix

This is an important process and a consequence of inflammation.
The extracellular matrix (ECM) consists of:
- Basement membranes surrounding all epithelia, endothelia, muscles, adipose cells and nerves
- Interstitial stroma (in which all blood vessels are found)

The ECM is composed of:
- Collagens
- Proteoglycans (heparin sulfate, others)
- Glycoproteins (laminin, elastin, fibronectin)

Cells expose receptors for matrix proteins; such receptors belong to
- Integrins
- Selectins
- Cartilage link proteins

Cells can detach from the ECM by proteolysis. They express proteases such as:
- Matrix metalloproteinases (collagenases, gelatinases, matrilysins/stromelysins)
- Serine proteases (uPA, tPA, elastase)
- Cysteine proteases (cathepsin B and cathepsin L)
- Aspartic acid proteases (cathepsin D)

Several proteases can cleave plasminogen into plasmin. To these belong:
- uPA, tPA
- Cathepsin B, L via activation of pro-uPA
- Cathepsin D via activation of pro-cathepsin L

Secretion and function of such enzymes are regulated by the balance between inhibitors and stimulators or activators.
Certain protease may attach to the membrane on cells. With that bound enzymes cells are able to path their migration through the extracellular matrix.

Monsky et al. 1993, Schmitt et al. 1992.

15.1.2 Interaction of Proteases

**Proteases Destroy ECM
Directly or Bound to
Specific Receptors on
Cells**

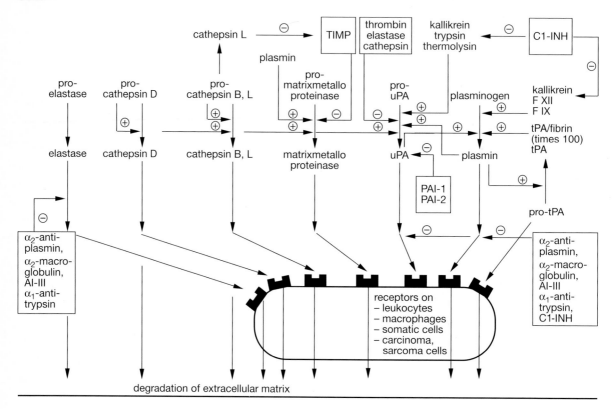

Monsky et al. 1993; Schmitt et al. 1992; Kwaan 1992

15.2 Details

15.2.1 Matrix Metalloproteinases (MMP)

Inhibitors	MMP	Stimulators
inhibitors of expression	secretion: connective tissue cells (fibroblasts, chondrocytes, osteoblasts, endothelial cells, macrophages, neutrophils, synovial cells)	for increased expression
– retinoids		– IL-1α, β
		– TNF-α
– glucocorticoids		– bFGF
	MMP-1 = interstitial collagenases	– stimulants for exocytosis (neutrophils, macrophages)
– TGFβ		
	substrates: collagen type	
inhibitors of activity	I, II, III, VII, X	for activation
	tissue collagenase: proenzyme 55 kDa	
– tissue inhibitors of	enzyme 45 kDa	– proteinases
MMP (TIMP)	neutrophil collagenase: proenzyme 75 kDa	(plasmin?)
	enzyme 58 kDa	– organomercurials
* TIMP-1 (for MMP-1,-3)		– MMP-3 (stromelysins) for
(28,5 kDa)	MMP-2 = gelatinases	collagenases (MMP-1)
* TIMP-2 (for MMR-2)		
(20 kDa)	substrates: dematured collagens (gelatins)	
* large TIMP	collagen type IV, V, VIII, X, XI	
(CIMP, 76 kDa)	type I: proenzyme 72 kDa	
	enzyme 62 kDa	
– α_2-macroglobulin	type II: proenzyme 92 kDa	
	enzyme 84 kDa	
– synthetic inhibitors		
	MMP-3 = stromelysins	
	substrates: proteoglycan core and link proteins collagen type IV, IX procollagen I, II, III fibronectin, elastin, laminin	
	types I, II, III: proenzyme 57 kDa	
	enzyme 45 kDa	

Suzuki et al. 1990; Nagase et al. 1990; Docherty et al. 1985; Stelter-Stevenson et al. 1989; Lewis et al. 1992; Galloway 1991; Gravellese et al. 1991; Lawston et al. 1981; Russel et al. 1991; Goldberg et al. 1986; Hasty et al. 1990; Müller et al. 1988; Quantin et al. 1989; van Wart et al. 1990.

15.2.2 Cellular Proteases

Matrix Metallo-proteases

Expression:
- proenzyme, activation by enzymes in the cell membrane to give 59 kDa MMP, 72 kDa MMP, 92 kDa MMP
- stimulation of expression by TGFβ, IL-1, cell activation

Source:
leukocytes, fibroblasts, tumor cells (over-expression)

Cell membrane binding:
- attachment of proenzyme to cell membrane, binding of 72 kDa MMP to high affinity receptor
- receptors concentrated on the invadopodia of invasive cells
- activated enzymes remain attached at the cell membrane

Function:
- destruction of extracellular matrix by invasive cells

Zucker et al. 1990, Moll et al. 1990, Emonard et al. 1992, Brown et al. 1990.

Serine Proteases (uPA, tPA, Elastase)

Expression:

B,

uPA:	– secreted as an enzymatically inactive
tPA:	proenzyme; activated by plasmin, cathepsin L, kallikrein, trypsin or thermolysin; inactivated by elastase, cathepsin G, thrombin
elastase:	– secreted by leukocytes (exocytosis of lysosomal enzymes)

Source:

uPA:	– epithelial cells, endothelial cells, fibroblasts, leukocytes
	– carcinoma cells, sarcoma cells (over-expression)
tPA:	– endothelial cells
	– carcinoma cells, sarcoma cells
elastase:	– leukocytes, platelets, carcinoma cells (prostate, breast, pancreas)

Cell membrane binding:

uPA:	– pro uPA or uPA binds to high affinity uPA-receptor (GPI-lipid anchor) on leukocytes, stromal cells, tumor cells
	– after binding of PAI-1, trimeric complex (PAI-1/uPA/uPA-rec.) is internalized
tPA:	– pro-tPA or -tPA binds to high affinity tPA-receptor (mannose receptor) on endothelial cells
elastase:	– associates with membrane receptor (fibroblasts)

Function: uPA, tPA: – cleavage of plasminogen to plasmin,
                              plasmin degrades * fibrin
                                                * ECM
                                     activates * proteases
                                                  (metalloproteinases,
                                                  uPA, tPA)
                                                * hormones
              elastase: – degradation of ECM
                          – degradation of uPA, tPA

Schmitt et al. 1992, Blasi et al. 1988, Hajjar et al. 1990, Ottter et al. 1992, Campbell et al. 1987, Kao et al. 1986, Monsky et al. 1993.

Serine Protease Plasmin   Expression: proenzyme: – plasminogen (92 kDa)
                                                     – activated by extracellular cleavage (uPA, tPA,
                                                       tPA/fibrin complex, factor XI, factor XII,
                                                       kallikrein, streptokinase/plasmin complex) at the
                                                       Arg-560 and Val-561 peptide bonds into plasmin
                                          plasmin: – heterodimer (L-chain, H-chain, 1-disulfide bond)
                                                     – L-chain (25 kDa) contains the active site; trypsin-
                                                       like specificity; hydrolyses proteins and peptides
                                                       at lysyl and arginyl bonds
                                                     – inhibited directly by   * α_2-antiplasmin
                                                                               * α_2-macroglobulin
                                                                               * C1-inhibitor
                                                     – inhibited indirectly by * C1 inhibitor (kallikrein,
                                                                                 factor XII)
                                                                               * PAI-1, PAI-2 (uPA, tPA)

Source: liver cells (secretion of plasminogen)

Cell membrane
binding: attachment of plasminogen as well as plasmin to binding
              proteins

Function: – reproduction (ovulation, fertilization)
             – tissue modulation (embryogenesis, adaptation)
             – activation of hormones and enzymes by cleavage of pro-
               hormones and proenzymes
             – fibrinolysis
             – inflammation and wound healing
             – tumor growth and metastasation

Kwaan 1992, Monsky et al. 1993, Schmitt et al. 1992.

Activation and Degradation of Urokinase – Type Plasminogen Activator

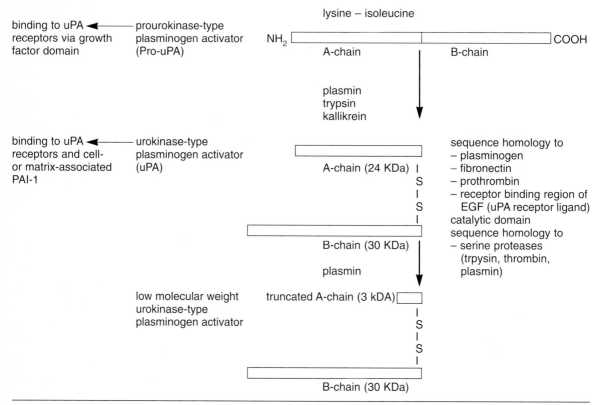

binding to uPA ◄——— prourokinase-type plasminogen activator (Pro-uPA)

lysine – isoleucine

binding to uPA ◄——— receptors via growth factor domain

NH$_2$ | A-chain | B-chain | COOH

plasmin
trypsin
kallikrein

binding to uPA ◄——— receptors and cell- or matrix-associated PAI-1

urokinase-type plasminogen activator (uPA)

A-chain (24 KDa)

B-chain (30 KDa)

plasmin

sequence homology to
– plasminogen
– fibronectin
– prothrombin
– receptor binding region of
  EGF (uPA receptor ligand)
catalytic domain
sequence homology to
– serine proteases
  (trpysin, thrombin,
  plasmin)

low molecular weight urokinase-type plasminogen activator

truncated A-chain (3 kDA)

B-chain (30 KDa)

Laiko et al. 1989; Barnathan 1992.

Plasminogen Activator
Inhibitors

	Endothelial type plasminogen activator inhibitor (PAI-1)	Placental type plasminogen activator inhibitor (PAI-2)	Protease nexins (PN)
Produced by	endothelial cells smooth muscle cells (vascular) granulosa cells platelets tumor cells	placenta, epidermis, monocyte/macrophages, lymphoma cells	fibroblasts, platelets
MW	43 KD	47 KD	45–100 KD
Activation	by conformational change half-life of activated form: 2h resistant to reducing agents/SDS conformational change is induced by: phospholipids phosphatidyl inositol phosphatidyl serine inhibited by: excessive Ca^{++} uPA, tPA (not Pro uPA)	storage in unglycosylated form secretion in glycosylated form	PNI sensitive to reducing agents and SDS PNII resistant to reducing agents complex formation with EGF binding protein, trypsin, NGF and PNII or (NGF) PNIII
Production	stimulated by: thrombin, LPS, dexamethasone inhibited by: gonadotropin	stimulated by: phorbols, choleratoxin MDP, LPS inhibited by: dexamethasone	
Specificity	uPA, tPA, irreversible complex formation (suicide substrates)	uPA, tPA, plasmin	uPA, thrombin

Laiko et al. 1989; Barnathan 1992.

Role of Plasminogen Activators and Plasmin in Normal and Pathological Processes

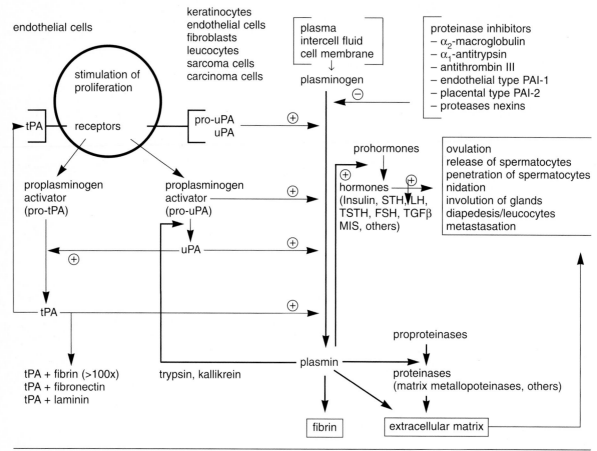

Lalko et al. 1989; Barnathan 1992.

Binding to and Function of Plasminogen Activator (uPA, tPA) on Endothelial Cells

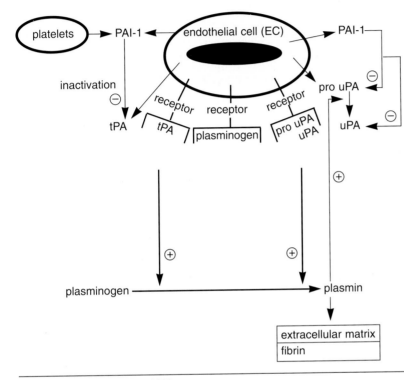

activation of endothelial cells

– shift to and increase of uPA production (bFGF)
– increase of uPA receptor expression (IFNγ, TNFα, thrombin, bFGF)
– increased PAI-1 secretion (LPS, IL-1β, TNFα)
– suppression of PAI-1 secretion (heparin + endothelial growth factor)

receptor for plasminogen activators

– uPA receptor MW 55–60 kD
– increased expression by bFGF
– not internalized after binding uPA or tPA
– internalized after complex-formation of bound tPA or uPA with PAI-1 or PAI-2

plasminogen activator inhibitor (PAI-1)

– present in excess amounts (intra-extravascularly)
– inactivates tPA/uPA irreversibly
– no or only slight inactivation of receptor bound tPA or uPA

Lalko et al. 1989; Bamathan 1992.

Cathepsins: Cellular Proteases

Expression:
– lysosomal enzymes
  * cysteine proteases (cathepsin B, L)
  * aspartic acid proteases (cathepsin D)
– correlated with extent of *ras* H expression and metastatic potential

Source:
– leukocytes
– stromal cells
– sarcoma and carcinoma cells (over-expressed)

Cell membrane binding:
– attachment to cell membrane
– binding to mannose receptor on macrophages (cathepsin D)

Function: – degradation of ECM, cleavage by
                     cathepsin L: – elastin, proteoglycans
                     cathepsin B: – laminin, proteoglycans, fibronectin, collagens
                                I, II, IV, V, IX, XI
                     cathepsin D: – laminin, fibronectin, proteoglycans
        – activation of uPA, matrix metalloproteinases
          (cathepsin B, L)
        – activation of cathepsin B, L (cathepsin D)
        – tumor growth and metastasation

Monsky et al. 1993, Kane et al. 1990, Denhardt et al. 1987, Young et al. 1991, Schmitt et al. 1992.

15.2.3 Modulation of Secretion of Cellular Proteases

Factor	Cell treated	Enzyme secreted Proteases	Inhibitors
IL-1	fibroblasts granulocytes macrophages tumor cells endothelial cells	tPA uPA stromelysin collagenase	
IL-4	endothelial cells	tPA	
IL-6	fibroblasts	stromelysin	
IFNγ	macrophages	uPA	
TGFβ	fibroblasts	cathepsins	TIMP PAI-1
	melanoma cells fibrosarcoma carcinoma cells (various)	collagenases gelatinases cells stromelysin	
TNFα	endothelial cells osteosarcoma cells fibrosarcoma cells	uPA collagenase	
bFGF	endothelial cells fibroblasts	tPA collagenase	
EGF	colon carcinoma cells fibroblasts	uPA stromelysin	PAI-1
PDGF	normal cells carcinoma cell	cathepsin	

Herlyn et al. 1991, Brown et al. 1990, Collart et al. 1986, Emeis et al. 1966, Van Hinsberg 1990, Kwaan 1992, Prence et al. 1990.

16 Angiogenesis

16.1 Overview

The starting point in the regeneration of vascularization by angiogenesis is pre-existent intact capillaries around damaged tissue. The sequence of reaction is:

- Engorgement, increase in permeability of vessels; loosening of cell junctions; disruption of basal membrane of intact capillaries.
- Movement of endothelial cells through their own basal membrane towards source of angiogenic stimulus and via secretion of degradative proteinases.
- Formation of cords of endothelial cells and sprouts.
- Proliferation of endothelial cells within the sprout but not usually in its tip.
- Simultaneous proliferation of pericytes and fibroblasts of perivascular tissue.
- Average capillary growth rates between 1,2 and 3 mm/day.
- Growth of capillary sprouts appear to follow the path of least resistance.
- The tip of one sprout joins with another to form a capillary loop.
- The lumen of new vessels develops between overlapping cells within the sprouts by the accumulation of blood and tissue secretions in the intercellular space.
- New basal membrane is laid down around the new vessels with the participation of pericytes.
- Fibroblasts migrate towards the new vessel, surround it and subsequently develop into the cellular and adventitial layer.
- Reticular and collagen fibrils are first seen four to 7 days after the initiation of fibroblast migration.

Mignatti et al. 1989; Moses et al. 1990; Auerbach et al. 1976; Cogan 1949; Folkman et al. 1971, 1974, 1983, 1986, 1987; Engerman et al. 1967; Cavallo et al. 1972; Hobson et al. 1984; Tannock et al. 1972; Schor et al. 1983; BŇr et al. 1972.

Angiogenesis

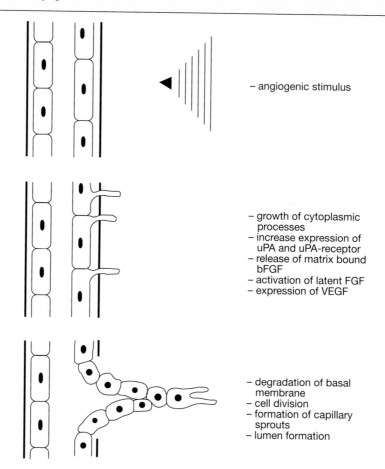

– angiogenic stimulus

– growth of cytoplasmic
  processes
– increase expression of
  uPA and uPA-receptor
– release of matrix bound
  bFGF
– activation of latent FGF
– expression of VEGF

– degradation of basal
  membrane
– cell division
– formation of capillary
  sprouts
– lumen formation

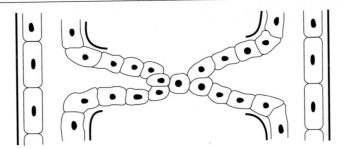

– confluence of capillary sprouts
– cessation of migration
– inhibition of cell devision
– basal membrane reconstitution
– junctional complex formation

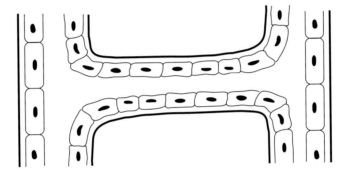

16.2 Details

16.2.1 Angiogenic or Mitogenic Peptides

	Can act as angiogenic factor	Is a mitogen for endothelial cell
Fibroblast growth factor (FGF)	+	+
Epidermal growth factor (EGF, transforming growth factor (TGFα)	+	+
Vascular endothelial growth factor (VEGF), vascular permeability factor (VPF)	+	+
Substance P	+	+
Platelet derived endothelial cell growth factor (PD-ECGF)	+	+
Angiogenin	+	
Angiotensin II	+	
G-CSF		+
GM-CSF		+
IL-4		+
Erythropoietin		+
Endothelin		+
Hepatocyte growth factor		+
Human growth hormone		+
Calcitonin-related peptide		+
Platelet-derived growth factor (PDGF)	+	
Angiotropin	+	

Bichnell et al. 1992, Klagsbrunn et al. 1991.

The Main Angiogenic
Factors in Detail

Fibroblast growth factor family (FGF)

Basic FGF (bFGF)	MW: 18 kDa, pI: 9.6	Eschetal 1985
	MW: 21–26 kDa (n-terminal extens.)	Florkiewicz et al. 1989
	affinity to haparan sulfate proteoglycans	
	$Kd = 2 \times 10^9$	Moscatelli 1987
Acidic FGF (aFGF)	MW: 18 kDa, pI: 5	Gimenez-Gallego et al. 1985
(endothelial cell	affinity to heparan sulfate proteoglycans	
growth factor ECGF)	$Kd = 2 \times 10^9$	
	sequence homology bFGF/aFGF = 50%	Esch et al. 1985
Oncogenes		
int-2 (MTV)	MW: 27 kDa, 40% homology	Dickson et al. 1990
hst (stomach carcinoma)	MW: 23 kDa, 50% homology to bFGF	Yoshida et al. 1988
K-*fgf* (Kaposi)	MW: 23 kDa, 50% homology	Delli-Bovi et al. 1987
FGF-5 (bladder ca)	MW: 29 kDa, 40% homology	Zhan et al. 1988
Keratinocyte growth		
factor (KGF)	MW: 28 kDa	Finck et al. 1989
Properties of bFGF/aFGF	cellular rather than secreted protein	Schweigerer et al. 1987
	(no signal peptide)	
	synthesis: endothelial cells	
	association with extra cellular matrix	Jage et al. 1986
Activity	mitogenic for endothelial cells	Baird et al. 1987
	chemotactic for endothelial cells,	Gospodarowicz et al. 1987
	production of collagenase and plasminogen	Mignatti et al. 1989
	activators	
Vascular endothelial growth	MW: 34–42 kDa	Conn et al. 1990
factor (VEGF),	resistant to acid pH and heating	Connolly et al. 1989
vascular permeability factor	affinity to heparin	
(VPF)	24% homology to PDGF	
	secreted protein, synthesis by follicular	Ferrara et al. 1989
	cells and tumor cells	Levy et al. 1983, 1989
Activity	mitogenic/1 ng/ml) for human endothelial	
	cells (not for fibroblast or other cells)	
	increase in fluid leakage	Connolly et al. 1989

Platelet-derived endothelial cell growth factor (PD-ECGF)	MW: 46 kDa, cationic sensitive to heat and acid does not bind to heparin not secreted, synthesis by platelets, fibroblast and tumor cells	Miyazono et al. 1987 Usuki et al. 1989
Activity	mitogenic (20 ng/ml) for human endothelial cells (not for fibroblasts) chemotactic only for endothelial cells	
Epidermal growth factor (EGF)	MW: 6 kDa secreted into biological fluids	Carpenter et al. 1979
Transforming growth factor-α (TGF-α)	MW: 5,5 kDa, 40% homology to EGF bind to the EGF receptor	Marquadt et al. 1984
	secreted to fibroblast, macrophages and tumor cells	Todaro et al. 1980
Activity	mitogenic for endothelial cells but not specific	Schreiber et al. 1986
Angiogenin	MW: 14,1 kDa	Fett et al. 1985
	68% homology to pancreatic RNAse A secreted by fibroblasts, lymphocytes and tumor cells, liver	Fox et al. 1990
Activity	RNAse activity weak not mitogenic in vitro high angiogenic activity in vivo inhibited by RNAse A inhibitor (placenta)	Shapiro et al. 1986
Angiotropin	MW: 4,5 kDa cooper containing polyribonucleopoly- peptide secreted by monocytes	Hockel et al. 1988
Activity	not mitogenic in vitro specific chemotactic for endothelial cells (4–400 pg/ml) to form tubular structures	
Transforming growth factor-β (TGFβ)	MW: 25 kDa (as homodimer) family of highly homologous peptides (TFGβ 1, 2, 3, 4, 5)	Sporn et al. 1988
	secreted in biologically inactive latent form, activation by proteases	Lawrence et al. 1985

Activity	in vitro: inhibition of endothelial cell proliferation	Roberts et al. 1986
	in vivo: angiogenic, possibly via activation of macrophages	Wahl et al. 1987
Tumor necrosis factor α (TNFα)	MW: 17 kDa	Beutler et al. 1986
	secreted by macrophages and tumor cells 28% sequence homology to TNFβ (lymphotoxin)	Gray et al. 1984
Activity	pleiotropic mediator of inflammation, induction of cachexia	Munker et al. 1986
	activation of macrophages, endothelial cells, induction of GM-CSF, IL-1, ICAM-1 synthesis in vitro: inhibition of endothelial cells proliferation in vivo: strongly angiogenic	Leibovich et al. 1987
Low molecular weight non-peptide angiogenetic factors	1-butyryl-glycerol (monobutyrin) produced by adipocytes	Dobson et al. 1990
	heparin	Roche et al. 1985
	prostaglandins, nicotinamide	Klagsbrun et al. 1991

Activity of Angiogenic Factors

	Heparin binding	Migration (target cells)	Proliferation (target cells)	Specificity (endothelial cells)	Angiogenesis in vivo
FGF	+	+	+	0	+
VEGF/VPF	+	+	+	+	+
PD-ECGF	0	+	+	+	+
TGFα	0	+	+	0	+
Angiogenin	0	0	0	n.e.	+
Angiotropin	n.e.	+	0	+	+
TGFb	0	–	–	0	+
TNFa	0	+	–	0	+

–, inhibition; +, stimulation; 0, no effect; n.e., not evaluated.

Klagsbrun et al. 1991, Bichnell et al. 1992.

16.2.2 Vascular Endothelial Growth Factor (VEGF)

– Synonym: vascular permeability factor (VPF)

Size and structure:
– 34–42 kDa, polypeptides of 186 (165) and 121 aa
– dimeric disulfide-bonded protein with a single amino terminus, 8 cysteines
– 1 N-linked glycosylation site (not required for function)
– sequence homology with both A and B chains of PDGF

Origin:
– pituitary follicular cells
– high levels: lung, kidney, heart, adrenal glands
  low levels: liver, spleen, gastric mucosa, breast, ovary, keratinocytes, macrophages (not in inactivated endothelial cells)
– expression is upregulated by hypoxia (fibroblasts, smooth muscle cells, endothelial cells, other cells)
– tumor cells (express several fold more VPF than the corresponding normal cells)

Function:
– stimulation of growth of endothelial cells from a variety of sources (brain, fetal and adult aortas, umbilical veins) at picomolar concentration
  * less potent at promoting endothelial cell growth than bFGF but synergy with FGF
  * more restricted target cell population than a FGF or bFGF
– transient increase in microvascular permeability without causing endothelial cell damage or mast cell degranulation (not blocked by antihistamins), subsequent infiltration of ECM with plasma proteins and fibrin deposition
  * activity at equieffective dosis of VPF and histamine:
    VPF: $\approx 2 \times 10^{-13}$ mol, histamine: $\approx 1 \times 10^{-8}$ mol
– stimulation of von Willebrand factor release, promotion of platelet binding to ECM, induction of tissue factor (pro coagulant) activity and promotion of hypercoagulable state
– regulation of fibrinolysis by modulating expression of plasminogen activator, plasminogen activator inhibitor and collagenase
– migration and activation of macrophages
– binding to heparin and heparin-like proteoglycans (VPF consisting of 189 aa polypeptides has a greater affinity for heparin containing proteoglycans than other VPFs)

Inhibition:
– no inhibition by hirudin or antihistamins (both compounds inhibit thrombin or histamine induced activation of endothelial cells)
– no competitive inhibition by thrombin and histamine

Receptor: – two types of high affinity (kDa ≈ p moles)
                * FLt-1 with intrinsic *fms*-like tyrosine kinase
                * KDR with intrinsic tyrosine kinase
            – only on endothelial cells (in contrast to FGF-receptors)
                (not on smooth muscle cells, fibroblasts, neutrophils),
                expression is upregulated by hypoxia
            – heparin binding of VPF enhances binding of VPF to receptor

Signal
transduction: increase of intracellular Ca++ through activation of
                phosphoinositide-specific phospholipase C, generation of IP3 and
                1,2-diacylglycerol

Senger et al. 1993, Conn et al.1990, Myoken et al.1991, Keck et al.1989.

16.2.3 Balance Between uPA/PAI-1 and FGF/TGF-β

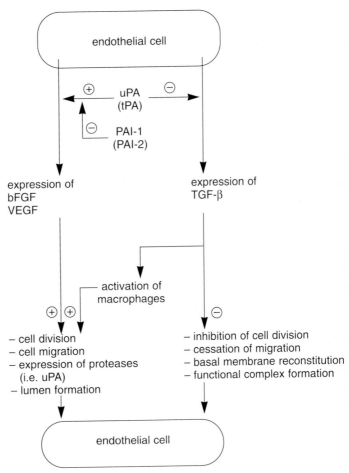

Pepper 1994

16.2.4 Inhibitors of Angiogenesis

	Heparin binding	Endothelial cells		Angiogenesis
		Migration	Proliferation	
Corticosteroids/ angiostatic steroids	0	n.e.	–	–
Heparin fragments	0	–	–	–
Thrombospondin	+	–	–	n.e.
Platelet factor IV	+	–	n.e.	–
TGFβ	0	–	–	+
Interferon-α/β	0	–	–	–
TNFα	0	+	+	–
Protamine	+	–	n.e.	–

–, inhibition; +, stimulation; 0, no effect; n.e. = not evaluated

Klagsbrun et al. 1991, Bichnell et al. 1992.

Inhibitors of Angio-genesis

Corticosteroids	Folkman et al. 1983
Steroid analogues	Crum et al. 1985
Heparin fragments (6 sugar units)	Folkman et al. 1983
Hexauronyl hexosaminoglycan sulfate	Rong et al. 1986
Thrombospondin from platelets (160 kd)	Phillips et al. 1980
	Good et al. 1990
Platelet factor IV (28 kd)	Taylor et al. 1982
Transforming growth factor β (25 kd)	Jennings et al. 1988
Interferon gamma (50 kd)	Friesel et al. 1987
Interferon β	Bichnell et al. 1991
Tumor necrosis factor α (17 kd)	Frater-Schröder et al. 1987
Protamine (43 kd)	Taylor et al. 1982
Tissue inhibitor of metalloproteases (TIMP-1, -4)	Bichnell et al. 1991
Penicillamine	Bichnell et al. 1991
Vitamin D3 and analogues	Bichnell et al. 1991
Herbimycin A	Bichnell et al. 1991
15-Deoxyspergualin	Oikawa et al. 1991
Somatostatin and analogues	Wolterin et al. 1991
Gly-Arg-Gly-Asp-Ser	Nicosia et al. 1991
Sulfated chitin derivatives	Murata et al. 1991

17 Systemic Inflammatory Reaction Syndrome

17.1 Overview

The systemic inflammatory reaction syndrome (SIRS) is a multifactorial systemic disease. The initial local diseases causing SIRS might be:
− Trauma, haemorrhage, burns (Redl 1992, Faist 1992)
− Infections (gramnegative or grampositive bacteria) alone or in consequence of trauma, haemorrhage, burns (Bone 1992)
− Pancreatitis (Bone 1992)

The main steps are:
− Activation of macrophages, granulocytes (via LPS, cytokines, others) and release of mediators, cytokines, lysosomal enzymes, radical oxygen, leukotriens (Wright et al. 1990, von der Poll 1992)
− Aactivation of endothelial cells (via LPS, TNF, cytokines, others) expression of thromboplastin (tissue factor) (Conway et al. 1989)
− Activation of extrinsic way of blood clotting by the initial complexformation of thromboplastin with F VIIIa, which activates F X to form F Xa
− Activation of complement by LPS and bacterial toxins, generation of anaphylatoxins (C3a, C4a, C5a). Anaphylatoxins induce activation of neutrophil granulocytes, hypotension and the "Capillary leak syndrome" (Morrison et al. 1977, Grossman et al. 1984, Lundberg et al. 1987, de Boer et al. 1992, Hack et al. 1989)
− Activation of F XII (Hageman factor) by LPS with generation of F XIIa, activation of the intrinsic blood clotting system, and activation of the kallikrein-kinin system (Kaplan et al. 1987)
− Activation of lymphocytes (T-cells, B-cells), secretion of cytokines
− Failure of the main organs (multiorgan failure, Bone et al. 1992)

17.2 Details

17.2.1 Pathophysiological Pathways

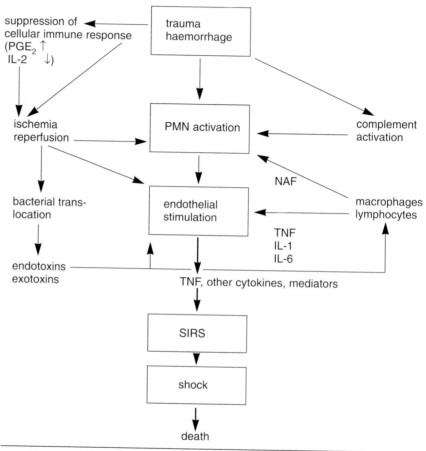

Bone 1992; Redl 1992; Faist 1992.

Incidence rate:	increasing
	1979: 73,6 cases per 100 000 persons
	1987: 175,9 cases per 100 000 persons
Initiating events:	endotoxin and other products from gramnegative bacteria
	toxins and other products from grampositive bacteria
	viral and fungal antigens
	noninfectious stimuli
development of shock:	≈ in 40 % of the cases
Mortality:	≈ 35–45%
Causes of death:	≈ 50% of patients suffer from gramnegative sepsis

Wenzel 1992; Bone 1991, 1992.

induced by:

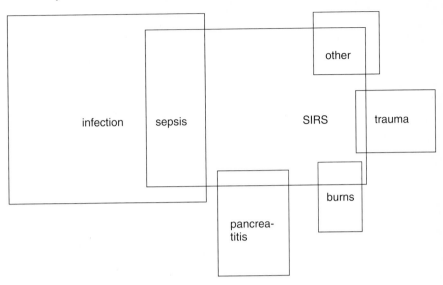

clinical parameters:

- tachypnoe (respiration >20 breaths/min)
- tachycardia (heart rate >90 breaths/min)
- hyperthermia (>38,4 °C) or hypothermia (<35,6 °C)
- lactate level above normal range
- oliguria (urine output <0,5 ml/kg body weight and 1 h)
- hypotension (systolic <90 mmHg)
  early shock: responsive to i.v. fluid administration
  refractory shock: unresponsive to i.v. fluid administration
                      requires vasopressors or higher doses of dopamine

Bone et al. 1991, 1992.

Activation, Stimulation and Damage of Endothelial Cells Provoke the Initiation of an Autocatalytic System Leading to the Development of SIRS

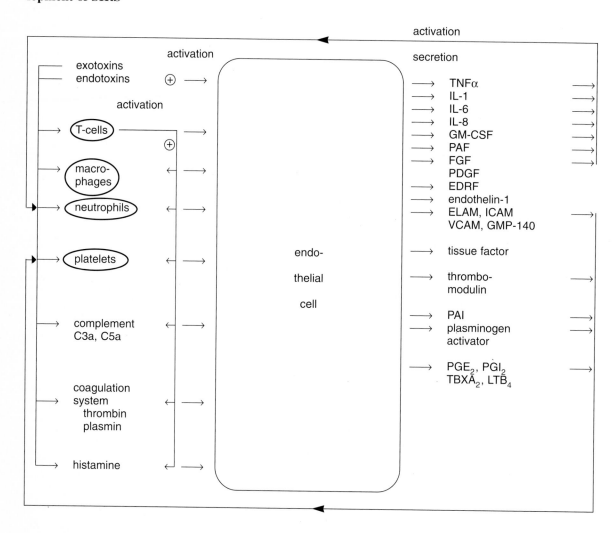

Michalek et al. 1980; Wolff 1973; Jonston 1988; Tracey et al. 1989; Dineman et al. 1990; Vane et al. 1990; Miyanchi et al. 1990; Bone 1991, 1992; Reidl 1992.

Systemic Inflammatory Reaction Syndrome Induced via Macrophages or via T-Cells and Superantigens

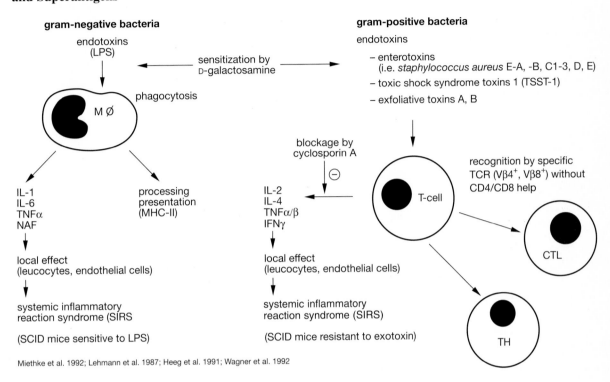

gram-negative bacteria

endotoxins
(LPS)

← sensitization by D-galactosamine →

phagocytosis

M Ø

IL-1
IL-6
TNFα
NAF

processing
presentation
(MHC-II)

local effect
(leucocytes, endothelial cells)

systemic inflammatory
reaction syndrome (SIRS

(SCID mice sensitive to LPS)

gram-positive bacteria

endotoxins

– enterotoxins
(i.e. *staphylococcus aureus* E-A, -B, C1-3, D, E)
– toxic shock syndrome toxins 1 (TSST-1)
– exfoliative toxins A, B

blockage by
cyclosporin A

⊖

IL-2
IL-4
TNFα/β
IFNγ

T-cell

recognition by specific
TCR (Vβ4$^+$, Vβ8$^+$) without
CD4/CD8 help

CTL

TH

local effect
(leucocytes, endothelial cells)

systemic inflammatory
reaction syndrome (SIRS)

(SCID mice resistant to exotoxin)

Miethke et al. 1992; Lehmann et al. 1987; Heeg et al. 1991; Wagner et al. 1992

Pathophysiological Pathways in SIRS Induced by Gram-Negative Bacteria

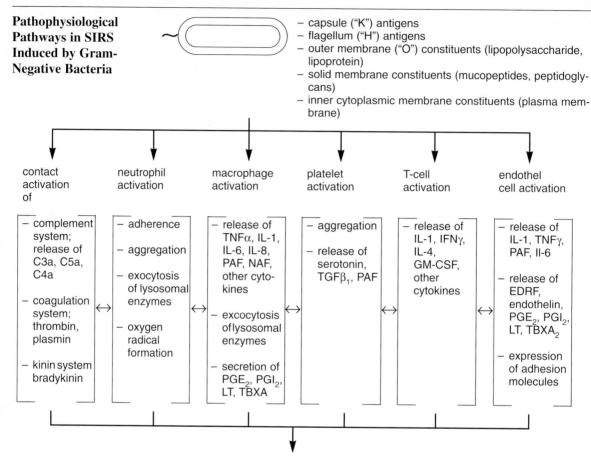

- capsule ("K") antigens
- flagellum ("H") antigens
- outer membrane ("O") constituents (lipopolysaccharide, lipoprotein)
- solid membrane constituents (mucopeptides, peptidoglycans)
- inner cytoplasmic membrane constituents (plasma membrane)

contact activation of

- complement system; release of C3a, C5a, C4a
- coagulation system; thrombin, plasmin
- kinin system bradykinin

neutrophil activation

- adherence
- aggregation
- exocytosis of lysosomal enzymes
- oxygen radical formation

macrophage activation

- release of TNFα, IL-1, IL-6, IL-8, PAF, NAF, other cytokines
- excocytosis of lysosomal enzymes
- secretion of PGE₂, PGI₂, LT, TBXA

platelet activation

- aggregation
- release of serotonin, TGFβ₁, PAF

T-cell activation

- release of IL-1, IFNγ, IL-4, GM-CSF, other cytokines

endothel cell activation

- release of IL-1, TNFγ, PAF, II-6
- release of EDRF, endothelin, PGE₂, PGI₂, LT, TBXA₂
- expression of adhesion molecules

generalized inflammatory response
generalized endothel cell damage

Lipopolysaccharides released by disruptered gram negative bacteria can induce SIRS by the following pathway:

– LPS bind to LPS-binding protein (LPB) secreted from the liver into blood.

– LPS/LPB complex formation enables high affinity binding to CD14, which is either membrane bound on macrophages (mCD14) or shedded to soluble form (sCD14) by the action of proteases and phospholipases.

– LPS alone can bind to CD14 also but with low affinity.

– mCD14 is anchored to the cell membrane by glysosylphosphatidylinositol linker (GPI).
– Binding of LPS/LPB (or LPS) to mCD14 leads to activation of macrophages.

– Binding of LPS/LPB (or LPS) to soluble CD14 (sCD14) enables the complex to bind to and to activate mCD14 negative macrophages and endothelial cells (which are per se CD14 negative). Mechanisms of binding and activation of CD14 negative cells is unknown.

– Activation of macrophages and endothelial cells leads to secretion of mediators (TNF, IL-1, IL-2, IL-6, IL-8, PAF, leukotrienes), radical oxygens and additional factors involved in SIRS.

17.2.2 Role of LPS Binding Protein

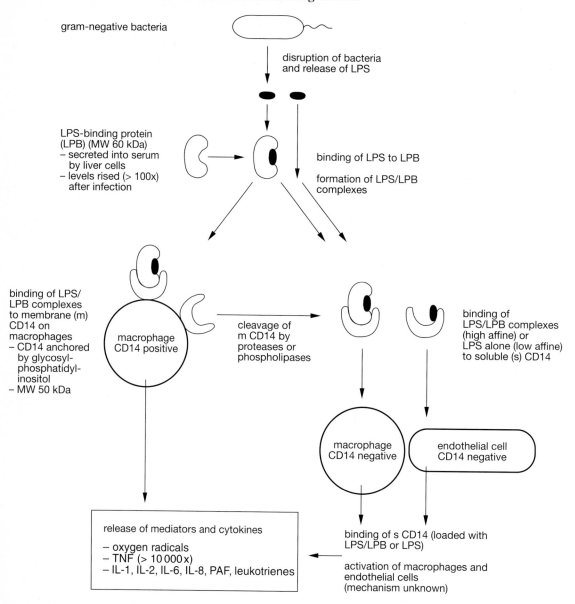

gram-negative bacteria

disruption of bacteria
and release of LPS

LPS-binding protein
(LPB) (MW 60 kDa)
– secreted into serum
  by liver cells
– levels rised (> 100x)
  after infection

binding of LPS to LPB

formation of LPS/LPB
complexes

binding of LPS/
LPB complexes
to membrane (m)
CD14 on
macrophages
– CD14 anchored
  by glycosyl-
  phosphatidyl-
  inositol
– MW 50 kDa

macrophage
CD14 positive

cleavage of
m CD14 by
proteases or
phospholipases

binding of
LPS/LPB complexes
(high affine) or
LPS alone (low affine)
to soluble (s) CD14

macrophage
CD14 negative

endothelial cell
CD14 negative

release of mediators and cytokines

– oxygen radicals
– TNF (> 10 000 x)
– IL-1, IL-2, IL-6, IL-8, PAF, leukotrienes

binding of s CD14 (loaded with
LPS/LPB or LPS)

activation of macrophages and
endothelial cells
(mechanism unknown)

Tobias et al. 1988; Wright et al. 1989, 1990; Sariban et al. 1988; Huber et al. 1988; Akira et al. 1990; van der Poll 1992; Bufler et al. 1993; Stelter et al. 1993;
Loppnow et al. 1993; Schilling et al. 1993

17.2.3 Role of Complement and Neutrophils

Complement activation:
- Caused by LPS and/or TNFα   Berger et al. 1988
- Mediates mast cell degranulation   Frank et al. 1987
- Mediates LPS induced release of   Fink et al. 1989
  thromboxane A_2 and Prostaglandin I_2
- C5a induces capillary leakage   Parrillo et al. 1989
- C5a activates PMN   Frank et al. 1987
  (migration, adherence, aggregation)   Gallin et al. 1980

Polymorphic neutrophil cell activation:
- Respiratory burst   Maleck et al. 1987
  (generation of oxygen radicals O_2°; OH°)   Clark et al. 1990
- Release of lactoferrin   Tate et al. 1983
- Release of lysosomal enzymes (lysozyme,   Zheutlin et al. 1986
  myeloperoxidase, elastase, collagenase etc.)
- Myeloperoxidase may induce formation   Tate et al. 1983
  of hypochloric acid and free chlor   Petrak et al. 1989
  (damage of endothelium, mitochondria, collagen)   Jacobs et al. 1989

17.2.4 Approaches to Influencing SIRS

Influence LPS Toxicity	Enhancement	Neutralisation	
		Direct	Indirect
	LPS binding protein (LPB)	antibodies to LPS antibodies to CD14 bactericidal/permeability increasing protein (BPI)	
	Soluble CD14	soluble CD14	

	Activation of macrophages, endothelial cells, granulocytes, lymphocytes	phagocytosis	protease inhibitors
			   C1 inhibitor
			   antithrombin III/heparin
			   hirudin
			   α_1-antitrypsin

			inhibition of PGE synthesis by cyclooxygenase inhibitors (at early stages of infection)
			immune stimulation by low doses of IL-2 (at early stages of infection)
			inhibition of secretion/function of TNF by xanthine derivatives, antibodies, TNF-receptors
			inhibition of function of IL-1 by antagonists (IL-1-RA, antibodies)

Tobias et al. 1988; Wright et al. 1989; Bahrami et al. 1993; Girior 1993; Graaf et al. 1983; Guerrero et al. 1993; Hach et al. 1992; Jochum et al. 1981, 1993; Dickneite 1990; Dickneite et al. 1993; Faist et al. 1993; Schînhartig et al. 1989; Zabel 1992; Alexander et al. 1991; Langner et al. 1992; Peppel et al. 1991; Mac Vittie et al. 1992.

Inhibition of SIRS

Test compound	SIRS induction	Species	SIRS inhibition	References
MAb against TNF	LPS	mice	+ + – + +	Beutler et al. 1985 Freudenberg et al. 1986 Eskandari et al. 1992 Bagby et al. 1991 Evans et al. 1989
MAb against TNF	*S. aureus* exotoxin B	mice	+	Wagner et al. 1992
MAb against TNF	CLP	mice	– – –	Bagby et al. 1991 Eskandari et al. 1992 Evans et al. 1989
MAb against TNF	*Pseudomonas*	mice	–	Silva et al. 1990
MAb against TNF	*Klebsiella*	mice	–	Silva et al. 1990
MAb against IL-2	*S. aureus* exotoxin B	mice	–	Wagner et al. 1992
MAb against IL-6	LPS	mice	+	Starnes et al. 1990
S. aureus Exotoxin B	*S. aureus* exotoxin B	mice	+	Wagner et al. 1992
Cyclosporin A	*S. aureus* exotoxin B	mice	+	Wagner et al. 1992
MAb against TNF	*E. coli* infection	mice	+ + +	Tracey et al. 1987 Silva et al. 1990 Hishaw et al. 1990
TNF pretreatment	CLP	mice	+ + + +	Alexander et al. 1991 Sheppard et al. 1989 Havell 1987 Echtenacher et al. 1990
	MAb for TNF + *Listeria*	mice	–	Havell 1987 Nahane et al. 1988
Mab against C5a	*E. coli* infection	monkey	+	Stevens et al. 1986

Test compound	SIRS induction	Species	SIRS inhibition	References
C1 inhibitor	sepsis	man	+/– (shock)	Hach et al. 1991
Pentoxyfylline	*E. coli* infection	guinea pig	+	shizaka et al. 1988
Pentoxyfylline	LPS	dogs	+	Welsh et al. 1988
Pentoxyfylline	LPS	mice	+	Schade 1990
MAb against LPS (*E. coli* J5) E5	LPS	sheep	(+)	Wheeler et al. 1990
MAb against LPS (*E. coli* J5) E5	mice		(+)	Young et al. 1989
MAb against LPS (*E. coli* J5) E5	sepsis	man	(+)	Greenman et al. 1991
	sepsis	man	–	Wenzel et al. 1991
MAb against LPS (lipid A) HA-IA	LPS	man	(+)	Ziegler et al. 1991
	E. coli	mice	+	Teng et al. 1985
	local Schwartz-man	rabbit	+	Teng et la. 1985
	Pseudomonas	rabbit	+	Ziegler et al. 1987
	LPS	rat	(+)	Feely et al. 1987
	LPS	rabbit	–	Tune et al. 1989
	LPS	mice	–	Baumgartner et al. 1990
	local Schwartzman	rabbit	–	Baumgartner et al. 1990
IL-1-RA	*E. coli*	mice	(+)	Thompson et al. 1992
IL-1-RA	sepsis	man	(+)	Synergen press release 1993
IL-1-RA	sepsis	man	–	Synergen press release 1993
Superoxide dismutase	sepsis	man	(+)	Marzi et al. 1991

Enzymes Inhibited
by C1 Inhibitor
(C1 Inactivator C1-IA)

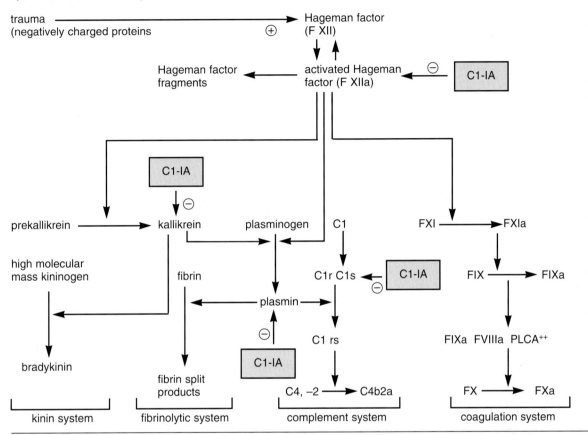

Lepow et al. 1954, 1956; Ratnoff et al. 1957; Forbes et al. 1970; Ratnoff et al. 1969; Gigll et al. 1970; Carreer 1992.

Activation and Action
of Kinins

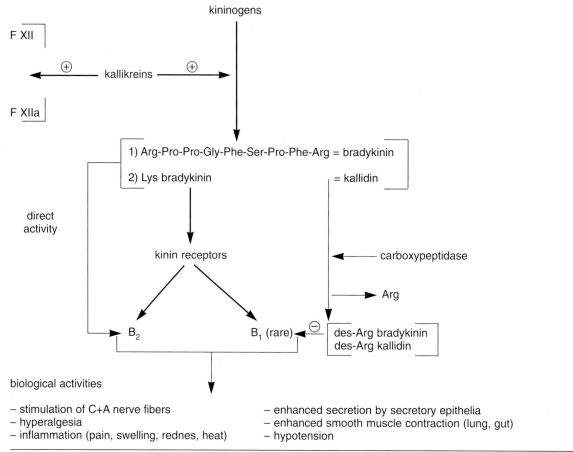

biological activities

– stimulation of C+A nerve fibers
– hyperalgesia
– inflammation (pain, swelling, rednes, heat)

– enhanced secretion by secretory epithelia
– enhanced smooth muscle contraction (lung, gut)
– hypotension

Kyle 1992.

Inhibitors of Tumor Necrosis Factor	Compound	Mechanism	Indications/comments
	MAb to TNFα alpha	neutralization	prevention of LPS shock local treatment of arthritis protection of cerebral malaria
	Glucocorticoids	inhibition of synthesis and release of TNFα alpha	treatment of sepsis (moderate activity)
	Xanthine derivatives (pentoxifylline)	inhibition of synthesis and release of TNFα alpha	prevention of LPS shock (ID_{50} = 100 mg/kg)
	Cyclosporin A	inhibition of synthesis of TNFα alpha and TNFβ (in addition to IL-2, IL-4, IFN-γ, IL-5)	treatment of chronic arthritis
	Cytokine suppressive antiinflammatory drugs (i.e. SKF 105809)	suppression of synthesis and release of IL-1, TNFα alpha, TNFβ	prevention of LPS shock (ID_{50} = 10 mg/kg p.o.) treatment of arthritis
	TNF-Rec. antagonists		
	Rec. TNFα alpha mutants	inhibition of TNFα alpha/β receptors	
	Rec. TNFα alpha/β receptors	neutralization of TNFα alpha/β	prevention of LPS shock (efficacy impaired by free soluble TNF-Rec)
	Synthetic TNFα alpha/β "receptors"	neutralization of TNFα alpha	application of high doses should be possible
	Dibutyryl-AMP	inhibition of TNFα alpha	protection of endothelial cells from TNFα alpha damage

Mackenzie 1991; Greig 1991; Pooter 1991; Beutler 1985; Tracey 1987; Schall et al. 1990; Smith et al. 1990; Oliff et al. 1987; Grau et al. 1987; Brennan et al. 1989; Zengh et al. 1990; Noel et al. 1989.

Inhibitors of Neutrophil Granulocytes	Compound	Activity	References
	Pentoxyphyllin	decrease of exycytosis decrease of oxygen radical formation inhibition of activation by LPS, TNFα alpha, IL-1 increase in cAMP	Bessler et al. 1986 Till et al. 1988 Sullivan et al. 1984 Sullivan et al. 1988
	Adenosine	decrease of respiratory burst decrease of oxygen radical formation	Engler 1987 Thiel et al. 1991
	MAb anti-Mac-1	inhibition of adhesion and trans-endothelial migration	Anderson et al. 1990
	MAb anti-ELAM-1	inhibition of TNFα alpha induced damage in rat lungs	Ward 1991
	Dapsone	inhibition of oxygen radical formation	Martin et al. 1985 von Ritter et al. 1989
	Superoxide dismutase	scavenging of superoxide radicals	Allison et al. 1988 Katz et al. 1988
	Alloparinol	inhibition of xanthine oxidase	Warren et al. 1990
	Deferoxamine	chelation of iron, which is catalytic for oxygen radical formation	Haynes et al. 1990
	Apolactoferrin	chelation of iron, which is catalytic for oxygen radical formation	Ward et al. 1983
	N-Acetylcysteine	scavenging oxygen radicals	Bernard et al. 1984 Lucht et al. 1987
	Ascorbic acid	scavenging oxygen radicals	Kuzuya et al. 1989
	2-Octadelyl-ascorbic acid	scavenging oxygen radicals	Kuzuya et al. 1989
	Eglin	inhibition of elastase	Siebach et al. 1989
	FUT-175	inhibition of proteases	Okuda et al. 1989

18 Immune Complex Mediated Diseases

18.1 Overview

Antigen-antibody immune complexes play an essential role in the immune response by:
- Binding to and neutralization of antigen and infectious organisms
- Activation of the complement system
- Activation of the Hageman factor and thereby activation of the clotting system, fibrinolytic system and kallikrein system
- Activation of granulocytes, macrophages, killer cells
- Activation and aggregation of platelets
- Antigen-specific inhibition of lymphocytes (via the BCR)

Immune complex mediated diseases occur in the course of the elimination of antigens by antibodies

Chronic immune complex diseases are caused by:
- Continuing exposure to relative high amounts of antigen (compared to the amount of antibody)
- Insufficient production of antibodies (quantity, quality)
- Overloading of the system eliminating immune complexes (phagocytosis, solubilization)
- Local immune complex formation inflammation and local damage of tissues

Sedlacek et al. 1983.

Possible human IC diseases
- Glomerulonephritis
- Vasculitis (various forms)
- Endocarditis
- Dermatomyositis and polymyositis
- Anaphylactoid purpura
- Hypersensitivity pneumonitis
- Panencephalitis
- Synovitis
- SC-mediated shock reaction

Examples of antigens detected in established human IC diseases

Administered antigens	*Parasitic antigens*
– Heterologous proteins	– *Toxoplasma* – *Plasmodium malariae* – *Schistosoma mansoni*
Viral antigens	*Autologous antigens*
– Hepatitis B – Rubella – Influenza A	– DNA, nucleoprotein – IgG – Renal tubulus antigen
Bacterial antigens	*Tumor antigens*
– β-Hemolytic streptococci – *Staphylococcus epidermidis* – *Treponema pallidum* – *Salmonella* Vi antigens	– Colon carcinoma – Bronchogenic carcinoma

Haakenstad and Mannik 1976, Niederhoff et al. 1979, Pernice et al. 1979.

18.2 Details

18.2.1 Conformational Change of Antibody

Models

– *Allosteric model:* antigen induces conformational changes within the variable region of the antibody, leading to the expression of secondary binding sites.

– *Distortive model:* antigen binding induces distortion of the relative domain position, leading to the expression of secondary binding sites.

– *Associative model:* multideterminant antigen induces via formation of immune complexes "polymerisation" of the antibody molecules as a necessary step for antibody mediated functions.

Upon Binding to the Antigen

– The three-dimensional structure of antibody molecules is modular with multiple domains (about 110 amino acids long and folded into an antiparallel β-sheet bilayer with two respectively three strands connected by loops) connected into two types of polypeptide chains (light, MW 25 kDa and heavy, MW 50 kDa).

Homologous domains from the light (L) and heavy (H) chains associate via their β-sheet surfaces to form dimeric structures. The complete molecule is a tetramer with the general formula H2L2.

– The two N-terminal domains of each chain contain hypervariable polypeptide segments, whose length and amino acid sequence varies from one molecule to another. This variability allows construction of antigen combining sites fitting a great many antigenic structures with diverse chemical compositions and molecular shapes. Each antibody molecule carries two identical antigen combining sites.

– Binding to the epitope of the antigen is mediated by the hypervariable complementarity determining regions (CDR-1, -2, -3) in the variable domain of the H-chain (VH) and the L-chain (VL) of the antibody. Such CDR form loops connecting two β-strands. All six loops from the two domains (VL, VH) come to close proximity in the immunoglobulin fold, forming the binding site for the epitope.

– Aromatic residues (His, Phe, Tyr, Trp) in the CDR regions favour van der Waals-London and hydrophobic forces for binding. Other amino acids favour hydrogen bonding with the epitope. Transition from the free to the antigen bound stage decreases the entropy and drives the reaction to the formation of antigen-antibody complexes.

– Binding drastically decreases at distances greater than 2–4 Å. Affinity of antigen-antibody binding depends on the steric complementarity between the interacting molecules. The binding site residues need to be positioned precisely in order to take full advantage of van der Waals and hydrophobic interactions and hydrogen bonding.

– Binding of CDR to the epitope induces a relative displacement of the VH and VL domains, which can be followed by Fab arm movement at the hinge region, Fab axial rotation and switch region bending.

– This segmental flexibility of the antibody allows its bivalent attachment to identical epitopes on rigid surfaces. Bivalent binding enhances the effective affinity of binding by orders of magnitude.

– Complement activation is affected by segmental flexibility of the antibody. An IgM molecule, after bivalent binding, disstorts from a star to a staple conformation, which seems to be the essential conformational change required for the exposure of complement binding sites in the CH2 domain. Binding of C1q to the CH2 domain of IgG molecules is apparently inversely correlated with hinge length and thus with segmental flexibility.

Poljak 1991, Bhat et al. 1990, Schumaker et al. 1991, Borsos et al. 1981, Dangle et al. 1988, Tan et al. 1990, Novotny et al. 1992, Mian et al. 1991.

18.2.2 Effector Function of Immunoglobulins

IgG Domain Structure

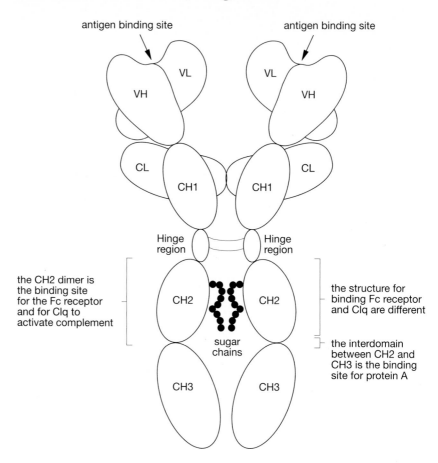

antigen binding site

antigen binding site

VL

VL

VH

VH

CL

CL

CH1

CH1

Hinge region

Hinge region

the CH2 dimer is the binding site for the Fc receptor and for Clq to activate complement

CH2

CH2

the structure for binding Fc receptor and Clq are different

sugar chains

the interdomain between CH2 and CH3 is the binding site for protein A

CH3

CH3

Deisenhofer 1981; Sutton et al. 1983; Parekh et al. 1985; Rudd et al. 1991

The branched sugar chains between the two CH2 domains prevent direct contact between the two CH2 domains. On the other hand, they are bridging these two domains through interaction of the terminal *N*-acetylglucosamine residue with the mannose sugar of the opposing carbohydrate chains. One branch of each sugar chain interacts with hydrophobic (lectin-like) residues of its CH2 domain.

Chemical and Biological Characteristics of Human Immunoglobulins

Immunoglobulins	IgG1	IgG2	IgG3	IgG4	IgA1	IgA2	sIgA	IgM	IgD	IgE
H-chain type	γ_1	γ_2	γ_3	γ_4	α_1	α_2	α_1/α_2	μ	δ	ε
H-chain MW (kDa)	51	51	60	51	56	52	52,56	65	70	72,5
Number of CH domains	4	4	4	4	4	4	4	5	4	5
MW (kDa)	146	146	170	146	160	160	385	970	184	188
Content of carbohydrates (%)	2–3	2–3	2–3	2–3	7–11	7–11	7–11	12	9–14	12
Mean serum concentration (mg/ml)	9(5–12)	3(2–6)	1(0,5–1)	0,5(0,2–1)	3	0,5	0,05	1,5	0,03	0,0005-05
Passage through placenta	++	+	++	++	0	0	0	0	0	0
Half-life time in blood circulation (days)	21–23	20–23	7–8	21–2	6	6	–	5	3	3
Catabolism rate (% per day)	7	7	1	7	25		–	9	37	89
Synthesis rate (mg/kg per day)	~33	~33	~33	~33	~24	~24	–	~3,3	~0,4	~0,02
Percentage in blood circulation (%)	45	45	45	45	42	42	–	80	75	50
Complement activation										
C1q binding	+++	+	+++	0	0	0	0	+++	?	0
Alternate pathway	+	+	+	+	+	+	+	++		(+)
Fc receptor binding										
Human monocytes (Fc γ RI-III)	++	+/–	++	+/–	0	0	0	0	0	0
(Fc μ R)	0	0	0	0	0	0	0	+++	0	0
Human neutrophils (Fc γ RII)	++	+/–	++	+	0	0	0			
Human platelets (Fc γ RII)	++	+	+	+						
Human lymphocytes (Fc γ RII)	++	+/–	++	+						
(Fc ε RII)									+	
Human basophils/mast cells (Fc ε RI)										+++
Binding to protein A *(S. aureus)*	+	+	0	+						
rheumatoid factors	+	+	0	0						

Hamilton 1987, French 1986, Anderson et al. 1986.

The Sugar Chains Between the CH2 Domains are Decisively Involved in Effector Functions of IgG

Treatment   Effect in IgG function

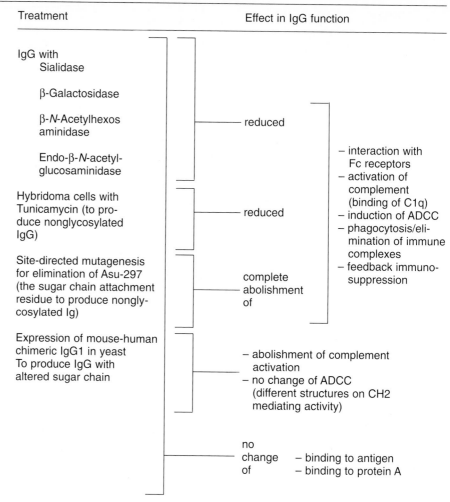

IgG with
   Sialidase

   β-Galactosidase

   β-*N*-Acetylhexos
   aminidase

   Endo-β-*N*-acetyl-
   glucosaminidase   reduced

Hybridoma cells with
Tunicamycin (to pro-   reduced
duce nonglycosylated
IgG)

Site-directed mutagenesis
for elimination of Asu-297   complete
(the sugar chain attachment   abolishment
residue to produce nongly-   of
cosylated Ig)

  – interaction with
    Fc receptors
  – activation of
    complement
    (binding of C1q)
  – induction of ADCC
  – phagocytosis/eli-
    mination of immune
    complexes
  – feedback immuno-
    suppression

Expression of mouse-human
chimeric IgG1 in yeast
To produce IgG with
altered sugar chain

  – abolishment of complement
    activation
  – no change of ADCC
    (different structures on CH2
    mediating activity)

no
change   – binding to antigen
of   – binding to protein A

Furukawa et al. 1991, Leatherbarrow et al. 1985, Heyman et al. 1985, Tsuchiya et al. 1989, Tao et al. 1989, Horwitz et al. 1988.

**Changes in Glycosyla-
tion of IgG in
Rheumatoid Arthritis
May be Associated with
Rheumatoid Factors**

Disease	Galactosylation of IgG	Rheumatoid factors	References
Rheumatoid arthritis	decreased (serum IgG synovial IgG)	+ +	Parekh et al. 1985, 1989
Pregnancy in RA patients	normal/upper level	−	Pekelharing et al. 1988
Osteoarthritis	normal/lower level	−	Parekh et al.
Crohn's disease	normal/lower level	−	Parekh et al.
Sjögren's disease	normal	−	Nagano et al. 1986
Systemic lupus erythematodes	normal	−	Endo et al. 1989

**Bivalent Effector
Functions Induced
by Immune Complexes**

Elimination of IC	◄ Effector function of IC ►	Inflammation induced by IC
Maintaining solubility and inhibition of precipitation of IC through binding of complement factor to antibody Attachment to CR1 on erythro-cytes mediated by C4b/C3b on IC; transport to liver (and spleen) for eliminiation (immune response)	◄ Complement activation (classical pathway and alternative pathway) ►	Via complement activation and release of anaphylatoxins C3a, C5a, C4a; – Chemotaxis: activation of PMN; release of lysosomal enzymes, radical oxygen – Degranulation of basophils/mast cells; release of histamine, serotonin, leukotriens
Endocytosis and phagocytosis – Degradation and elimination of IC – Loading MHC class II molecules and antigen presentation to stimulate immune response Cleavage of native IgG into F(ab')2 and Fab fragments, reduc-tion of Fc γ R mediated reactions through antigen F(ab')2/Fab IC	◄ Attachment to Fc γ gamma and complement receptors (CR1, CR2, CR3, C1g-R) on granulocytes and macrophages ►	Activation of leukocytes: – Generation of oxygen radicals Release of – Cytokines (IL-1, IL-3, IL-8, IFN, TNF, others) – Leukotrienes – Prostaglandins Exocytosis of lysosomal enzymes (degradation of extracellular matrix, activation of clotting system, kinin system, complement system)
Release of C1-INH, factor H, protein S, expression of MCP, MIRL, HRF Attachment to CR1 on (nonprimate) platelet and transport to liver	◄ Attachment to, activation and aggregation of platelets ►	Intravascular coagulation Release of vasoactive amines Release of C-8, C-9
Stimulation of immune response by cross-linking BCR-CR-2 on B-cells Inhibition of B-cells by cross-linking BCR and Fc γ gamma receptors	◄ Attachment to, activation and differentiation of B-cells (and T-cells) ►	Release of cytokines (Il-1, Il-2, Il-3, IL-4, IL-6, IL-8, IFNgamma, TNFalpha, TNFβ)

18.2.3 Size of Immune Complexes

**Antigens and
Antibodies Can Form
Immune Complexes
of Different Sizes**

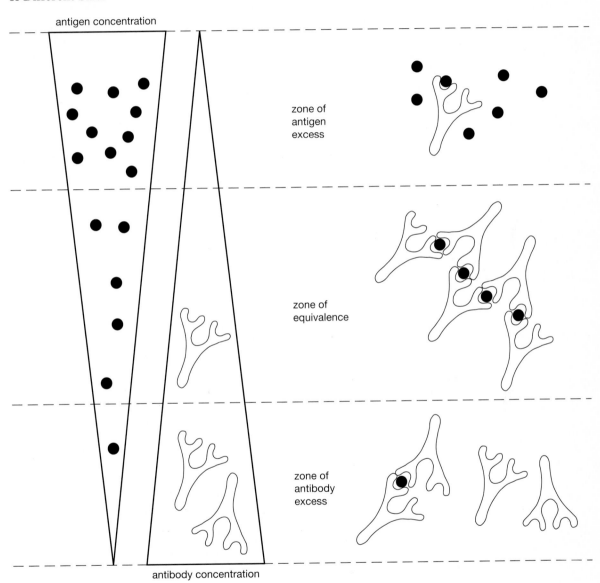

The size of immune complexes (IC) depends on:
– Relative concentration of antigen and antibody
– Mean affinity of (polyclonal) antibodies
– Physical and chemical characteristics of the antigen
    * Molecular weight/structure
    * Number of epitopes
    * Density of epitopes

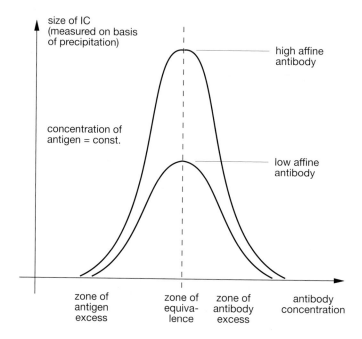

**The Effector Functions
Induced by Immune
Complexes Depend on
the Isotype of the Anti-
body, the Size and the
Composition of Anti-
gens and Antibodies**

| | Reaction of IC of different composition | | | | |
| | Antigen excess | | Zone of equivalent | Antibody excess | |
	Extreme	Slight		Slight	Extreme
Turbidity	–	+	+++	++	–
Binding to rheumatoid factors	(+)	+	+++	++	+
Lymphocytes, binding to					
Fc-receptors	–	+	++	+++	++
C′-receptors	(+)	+	++	+++	++
Platelets					
Release of serotonin	+	++	+++	+++	++
Release of β-thromboglobulin	–	+	++	+	–
Aggregation	–	+	+++	+++	+
Granulocytes					
Phagocytosis/exocytosis	(+)	++	+	+	–
Macrophages					
Phagocytosis/exocytosis	–	(+)	++	+++	+
Shock reaction after i.v. injection of IC	–	++	+++	++	–
Inflammation after local injection	–	+	++	+	–
Complement activation	+	++	+++	+++	+
Stimulation of B-cells (BCR-CR2)	+	+++	+++	+	–
Inhibiton of B-cells (BCR-FcR)	+	++	+++	+++	(+)

Sedlacek et al. 1983.

18.2.4 Inhibition/Solubilization of IC by Complement

Complement-mediated inhibition of immune complex precipitation and solubilization of precipitates is an essential mechanism to prevent IC diseases.

Complement factor	Mechanism of action	References
C1q binding to Fc part	inhibition of Fc-Fc interactions and high lattice formation	Schifferli 1986, 1987
Covalent binding of numerous C3b and C4b molecules to antigen and antibody	inhibition of Fc-Fc interaction and high lattice formation; weakening the bond between antigen and antibody and disrupture of immune complexes	Schifferli et al. 1985
Increase of C4A allotype in relation to C4B allotype	C4B generated from C4A forms with its thioester group amide bonds with the amino acids of the antibody and thereby inhibits high lattice formation (C4B from C4B bind preferably to hydroxyl groups)	Gatenby et al. 1990 Paul et al. 1988
Increase of C2C allotype in relation to C2B allotype	similar as with C4A, but more efficient than C4A	Varga et al. 1991
Increase of IgG4 antibodies after prolonged immunization	IgG4 does not activate complement and thus prevents complement-mediated solubilization of IC	van der Zee et al. 1986
Increase of gp60	interference with the binding of C1q to the Fc part of antibodies	Ahmed et al. 1960
Classical pathway	inhibits by C1q, C4b immune complex precipitation	Schifferli 1986
Alternative pathway	solubilizes by factor D, C3b IC precipitates	Takahashi et al. 1978

18.2.5 Elimination of IC

Involvement of C4 in the elimination process of immune complexes (IC)

– IC activate complement via the classical and/or alternative pathway.

– C4b generated by activation of the classical pathway is bound to the Fc part of the antibody forming the IC.

– C4b (in addition to C3b) is the ligand mediating binding of IC to the complement receptor 1 (CR1) on:

* erythrocytes to transport IC out of the circulation to Kupffer cells of the liver
* granulocytes, monocytes and macrophages to induce endocytosis and/or phagocytosis of IC.

– Two isotypes of C4, namely C4A and C4B exist. They are encoded by two almost identical (99%) genes. Both C4 (after activation) differ in their reactivity due to differences in amino acids.
* C4A reacts with its thioester bond more avidly with amino groups and therefore is more efficient in processing IC bearing amino-rich antigens.
* C4B is more reactive with hydroxyl groups as substrates (it is more hemolytic than C4A).

– Many IC-associated autoimmune diseases are associated with a silent C4A gene.

Moulds et al. 1992, Schneider et al. 1986, Isenman et al. 1984, Law et al. 1984, Paul et al. 1988.

IC Diseases Associated with Genetic Changes in Expression of the Complement Factor C4 Isotypes (C4A, C4B)		Expression of C4 isotypes		References
		C4A	C4B	
	Subacute sclerosing panencephalitis	0	+	Rittner et al. 1984
	Juvenile dermatomyositis	0	+	Reed et al. 1991
	Graves' disease	0	+	Ratanachaiyavong et al. 1989
	Systemic lupus erythematodes	0	+	Goldstein et al. 1988
	Sjögren' syndrome	0	+	Moriuchi et al. 1991
	Rheumatoid vasculitis	0	+	Hillarby et al. 1991
	Scleroderma	0	0	Briggs et al. 1987
		0	+	Mollenhauer et al. 1984
	IgA nephropathy	0	0	McLean et al. 1984
	Rheumatoid arthritis	0	+	O'Neill et al. 1982 van Zeben et al. 1992
	Felty's syndrome	+	0	Thomson et al. 1988
	Glomerulonephritis	+	0	Wank et al. 1984

Involvement of C2 and Factor B in the Elimination Process of IC	Genetic change	IC-associated disease	References
	C2 deficiency	systemic lupus erythematodes, dermatomyositis, vasculitis	Borradori et al. 1991 Agnello et al. 1986 Osterland et al. 1975
	Deficiency of factor B-F	diabetes type 1	Budowle et al. 1982 Mimura et al. 1990
	Expression of factor B-F1	diabetes type 1	

Characteristics of complement receptor type 1 (CR1) and its involvement in the elimination process of IC:

– Expressed on:
  * blood cells
    erythrocytes: 500 CR1 molecules/cell
    leukocytes: 10 000–30 000 CR1 molecules/cell
  * renal podocytes, follicular-dendritic cells

– Four subtypes:
  * CR1-A MW: 220 kDa binding sites of C3b: 2 (81%)
  * CR1-B MW: 250 kDa binding sites of C3b: 3 (18%)
  * CR1-C MW: 190 kDa binding sites of C3b: 1 (1%)
  * CR1-D MW: 280 kDa binding sites of C3b: 4 (<1%)

– Tandemly arranged repeating modules [short consensus repeats (SCR) or complement control protein repeats (CCP)]:
  No. of SCR for CR1-A = 30 SCR
  * SCR-1 + SCR-2:   binding site for C4b
  * SCR-8 + SCR-9:   binding site for C3b
  * SCR-15 + SCR-16: binding site for C3b

– IC bind with attached C4b and C3b to clusters of Cr1 on:
  * Erythrocytes: transport IC to liver and spleen, where fixed macrophages, bearing other complement receptors and Fc receptors strip IC with their proteinases from erythrocytes. In the liver, the IC are degraded in the spleen, the IC serve as immunogen.
  * Granulocytes, monocytes, macrophages: endocytose or phagocytose IC. For phagocytosis binding of IC to CR1, CR2 and Fcγ gamma R takes place.

– The higher the number of CR1 and the bigger the CR1 clusters, the better the elimination of IC.

Moulds et al. 1992, Ahearn et al. 1989, Hourcade et al. 1989, Kalli et al. 1991, Klickstein et al. 1988, Krych et al. 1992, Hebert et al. 1991, Brown et al. 1991, Porcel et al. 1992.

Transport of immune complexes to the macrophage phagocytic system

– Erythrocytes use CR1 to absorb soluble and particulate immune complexes.

– Erythrocytes express only small numbers of CR1 molecules per cell. Formation of large clusters on the cell surface helps to bind immune complexes efficiently (Chevalier et al. 1989; Paccaud et al. 1990).

– Excess of erythrocytes ensures that immune complexes entering the blood bind primarily to erythrocytes and not to leukocytes (Medof et al. 1982).

- – Absorption to erythrocytes prevents deposition of immune complexes in blood vessels and mediation of inflammation and tissue damage.

- – Erythrocytes carry C3b coated immune complexes on their membrane CR1 to the liver where macrophages strip the complexes from the red cell surface (Cornacoff et al. 1983; Schifferli et al. 1986, 1988)

- – Erythrocytes cleared from immune complexes return to peripheral circulation.

- – The process is rapid and effective even in patients with systemic lupus erythematodes where both plasma complement and erythrocyte CR1 have been depleted by chronic exposure to immune complexes (Schifferli et al. 1989).

Clearance from Peripheral Blood of Soluble or Particulate Immune Complexes by CR1 on Erythrocytes

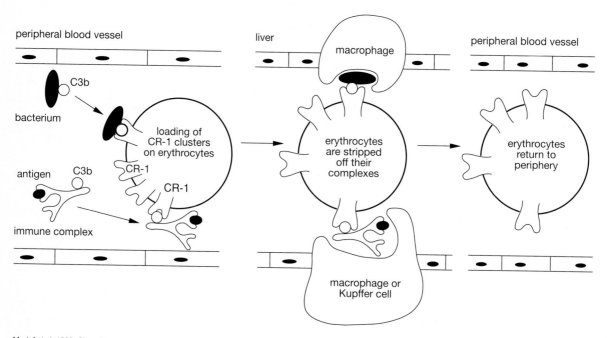

Medof et al. 1982; Chevalier et al. 1989; Paccaud et al. 1990; Cornacoff et al. 1983; Schifferli et al. 1986, 1988, 1989

Characteristics of complement receptor type 2 (CR2) and its involvement in the pathophysiology of IC diseases:

– Expressed on:
  * 145 kDa-protein
    – B-lymphocytes (mature, circulating or in lymphnodes)
    – follicular dendritic cells
    – T-lymphocytes (subpopulation: thymocytes 10–40% of CD4+ CD8+ cells, increase after stimulation)
  * 200 kDa protein
    – Epithelial cells

– Linear arranged repeating modules (short consensus repeats).

– Binds C3b, C3bi, C3dg, EBV.

– Plays a role in B-cell activation and differentiation (cross-linking of BCR and CR2 by immune complexes, see chapter on B-cell activation and differentiation).

– CR2 is also associated with CR1.

– Role of CR2 on T-cells unclear. Possibly adhesion of T-cells to targets bound with C3bi and C3dg (i.e. HIV-1 coated with complement factors may infect T-cells via CR2).

Fujisaku et al. 1989, Moore et al. 1987, Weis et al. 1988, Fischer et al. 1991, Reynes et al. 1985, Tedder et al. 1984, Tsoukas et al. 1988, Young et al. 1989, Carter et al. 1988, Matsumoto et al. 1991, Boger et al. 1991.

Molecules Containing Glycin-Proline-Lysine Repeats Contribute to the Elimination of Degradation Products and Immune Complexes via the C1q Receptor

Collagen (> 15 types)	– extracellular matrix protein	Ramirez et al. 1990 Van der Rest et al. 1991
Macrophage scavenger receptor	– receptor for low density lipoproteins – binding of polyribonucleotides, polysaccharides, phospholipids	Kodama et al. 1990 Rohrer et al. 1990 Krieger 1992
Complement C1q	– secreted protein (18 poly peptide chains: 6xA, 6xB, 6xC) – recognition and binding of activators of the classical pathway of complement binds with collagen part to C1q receptors involved in clearance of immune complexes, glycolipides, mannose-coated cells	Reid 1983, Burton 1985 Thiel et al. 1989 Erdei et al. 1988 Thiel et al. 1988
Pulmonary surfactant apoprotein (SP-A)	– secreted protein – binding of surfactant phospholipids and carbohydrates – lowers surface tension in the alveoli – binds with collagen part to C1q receptors involved in clearance of immune complexes, glycolipids, mannose coated cells	Floros et al. 1986 Hawgood et al. 1987
Mannose binding protein (MBP)	– secreted protein – binding to oligomannose of surface oligo-saccharides of bacteria, fungi – activation of complement and (antibody independent) lysis of microbes or opsonisation – binds with collagen part to C1q receptor involved in clearance of immune complexes, glycolipids, mannose coated cells	Drickamer et al. 1986 Ikeda et al. 1987 Kuhlman et al. 1989
Conglutinin	– secreted protein – binds to degradation product of C3 via polymeric structures – binds with collagen part to C1q receptors involved in clearance of immune complexes, glycolipids, mannose coated cells	Davis et al. 1984 Lee et al. 1990 Linacott et al. 1978
Ficoline α, β	– membrane and secreted protein – binds with collagen part to C1q receptor – possibly involved in TGFβ clearance	Ichijo et al. 1991, 1993

18.2.6 IC Diseases Associated with Changes in the Expression of CR-1, CR-2, CR-3, C1-IA (-INH)

	Change in Expression	IC-associated disease	References
IC Diseases Associated with Changes in the Expression of CR1	High expression of CR1-C (smallest subtype), low expression of CR1-A, -B	systemic lupus erythematodes	Van Dyne et al. 1987
	Low number of CR1 on erythrocytes (genetic or acquired)	systemic lupus erythematodes	Walport et al. 1988 Klopstock et al. 1965
	Low number of CR1 on erythrocytes and auto-antibodies to CR1	systemic lupus erythematodes	Moulds et al. 1991
IC Diseases Associated with Changes in the Expression of CR2, CR3 and C1-INH	Decrease of CR2 on B-cells	systemic lupus erythematodes	Wilson et al. 1986
		rheumatoid arthritis	Kahan et al. 1986
	Increase ($\approx 90\%$) of CR2 on T-cells	systemic lupus erythematodes	Moulds et al. 1992
	Increased expression of CR3	systemic lupus erythematodes	Buyon et al. 1988
	Deficiency of C1-INH	systemic lupus erythematodes (in addition to angioedema)	Liszeski et al. 1991

Therapy of immune complex diseases should eliminate IC, which are able to induce effector functions.

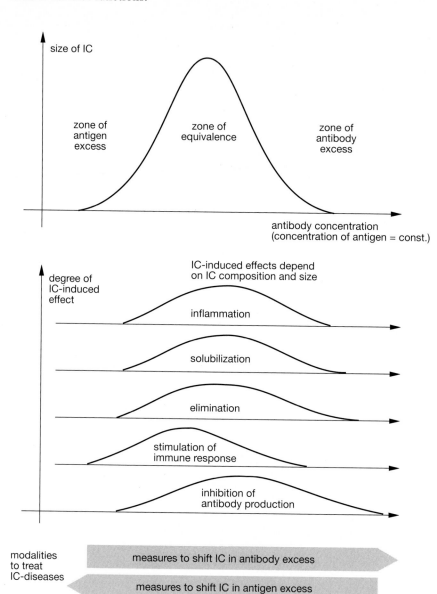

18.2.7 Approaches for Therapy of IC Diseases

Symptomatic	Causative

Plasmapheresis
Plasma exchange transfusion
 	
Antiinflammatory drugs
 	
Histamine and serotonin
antagonist
 	
Inhibitors of complement
activation (C1-INH)
 	
Inhibition of Fc receptor
mediated activation
of leukocytes and platelets
(Fc fragments; anti-Fc Fab/
F(ab′)2-antibodies)
	Suppression of antibody response by
	– Immune suppressives
	  (Cytostatics)
	– Corticosteroids
	  (Induction of tolerance)
	
	Increase of antibody response by
	– Polyvalent antibodies
	  (high dose)
	– Immune stimulation
	  (cytokines, others)
	
	Increase of phagocytosis rate
	– increase in number and activation of
	  granulocytes, macrophages by
	  cytokines
	– Solubilization and opsonization of
	  immune complexes (monomeric C1q)
	Elimination of antigen
	– antibiotics
	– prevention of exposure

Sedlacek et al. 1979, 1981, 1983, 1987; Debre et al. 1993.

For treating acute immune complex diseases, F(ab′)2 antibodies should induce fewer side effects than native IgG. Native IgG is the preparation of choice for suppression of antibody response.

	Comparison on therapeutic properties of different antibody preparations		
	IgG	F(ab′)2	Fab
Natural occurrence	++	+	+
Increase of catabolic rate of endogenous IgG	++	–	–
Half-life time (blood)	18 days	2 days	< 1 day
Suppression of antibody response	++	–	–
Neutralization and elimination of			
Toxins	++	++ (partly via kidney)	++ (partly via kidney)
Viruses	++	++	(+)
Bacteria	++	++	(+)
Complement activation			
Classical pathway	++	–	–
Alternative pathway	++	++	–
Transport of IC by erythrocytes (CR1) to liver and spleen	++	++	–
Phagocytosis of IC via			
Fcγ gamma receptors	++	–	–
C3b receptors	++	++	–
Exocytosis via			
Fc receptors	++	–	–
C3b receptors	++	++	–
Platelet activation and aggregation	++	–	–

Sedlacek et al. 1983.

Digestion of Human Immunoglobulin G (Monomer or Immune Complexes)	IgG1	IgG2	IgG3	IgG4
Hinge amino acid no.	15	12	62	12
Interchain disulfide bond no.	2	4	11	2
Isoelectric point (pH)	8,6 ± 0,4	7,4 ± 0,6	8,3 ± 0,7	7,2 ± 0,8

Digestion by	Efficiency of cleavage			
Papain	+	±	+	+
Plasmin	+++	+	+++	+
Trypsin	+++	+	+++	+++
Pepsin	+	+	+++	+++
Cathepsin D (like Pepsin)	+	+	+++	+++
Elastase (like Plasmin)	+++	+	+++	+

Hamilton 1987, Shakib et al. 1980, Spiegelberg 1974.

19 Allergic diseases

19.1 Overview

Allergic diseases are caused by adverse immune responses (so-called hypersensitivity reactions) to harmless environmental components (so-called allergens).

Type 1 hypersensitivity is mediated by IgE (Ishizaka et al. 1989) and is primarily responsible for allergic diseases such as:
– Allergic rhinitis
– Extrinsic asthma (early asthmatic reaction, EAR; late asthmatic reaction, LAR)
– Food allergies
– Skin allergies (i.e. to cosmetics)
– Allergies to drugs, insect stings, others

Allergic patients sensitized to an allergen produce IgE antibodies specific to that allergen. The IgE molecules circulate in the blood and bind tightly to the high affinity IgE Fc receptors (Fc ε RI) on the surface of basophils in the circulation, and mast cells in various tissues (Metzger et al. 1986).

In an allergic response allergens enter the body via inhalation, ingestion, injection or through the skin. These allergens bind with their epitopes to the antigen-binding sites of IgE on the surface of mast cells and basophils, cross-link the IgE molecules and their (Fc ε RI) receptors and thereby trigger the release of histamine, leukotrienes, prostaglandins, platelet activating factor and other pharmacological mediators.

These mediators cause vasodilatation, increased vascular permeability, edema, smooth muscle contraction and mucus secretion resulting in various allergic symptoms (Ishizaka et al. 1984).

Basophils and Mast Cells Play the Central Role in the Immediate-Type Hypersensitivity Reaction

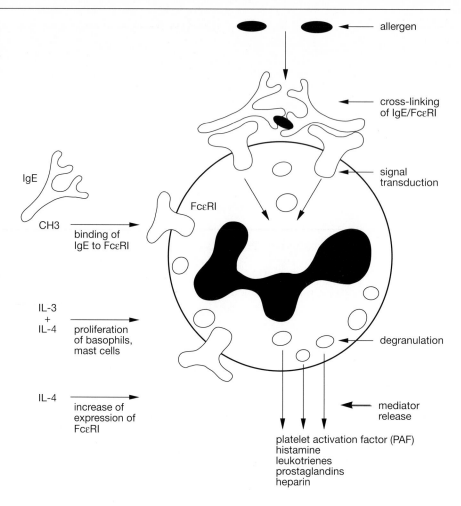

Biological Activity of Histamines	Via H$_1$ receptor	Via H$_2$ receptor
	Contraction of smooth muscle [gut, uterus, bronchi, arterioles arteries (lung), veins (liver)]	Dilatation of smooth muscles [bronchi, arteries (lung), uterus]
	Contraction of endothelial cells (increase of permeability)	Tachycardia
	Secretion of adrenalin	Increase of secretion (stomach)
	↓	↓
	Vasoconstriction and increase of blood pressure	Vasodilatation and decrease of blood pressure
	Increase of capillary permeability	Increase of heart frequence
	Dilatation of coronary arteries	
	Hemoconcentration	
	Increase in lymph flow	

Forth et al. 1980.

The immune protective role of IgE is unclear, but it is a mediator of the immediate-type hypersensitivity reaction.

IgE does not seem to be involved in protective immune responses:
- Individuals who have no detectable or very low IgE in their blood have no impaired immunological functions (Levy et al. 1970).
- Mice rendered IgE deficient by immunological or genetic treatments have also no impaired immunological functions (Haba et al. 1990, Marshall et al. 1985, Kuhn et al. 1991).
- Increase of serum IgE in response to parasitic infections in high responder (BALB/c) mice seems to be associated with mortality, whereas low IgE responder (C57Bl/6) mice show only a mild disease with no mortality (Mogbel et al. 1990, Sadick et al. 1990). Treatment of high IgE responder mice with anti IL-4 MAb results in conversion of the lethal into a non-lethal course of the parasitic infection (Finkelman et al. 1990).

All immediate type hypersensitivity reactions to allergens are strictly dependent on IgE.

- The levels of total IgE in serum are often higher in allergic patients than in nonallergic patients and tend to correlate with disease severity, especially in respiratory allergies (Burrows et al. 1989, Sears et al. 1991).
- The serum concentration of allergen-specific IgE is a measure of the extent of the allergic immune response against the particular allergen in a patient (Burrows et al. 1989).

Atopic dermatitis seems to be an IgE mediated disease:
- Atopic dermatitis is mostly associated with one disease of the allergic triad (atopic dermatitis, asthma, allergic rhinitis; Rajka 1989, Pasternak 1965, Stifler 1965).
- Eczema can be transferred to bone marrow recipients from atopic transplant donors (Agosti et al. 1988).
- Serum IgE is elevated and immediate skin tests and specificity analysis of serum IgE are positive for various dietary and environmental allergens in about 80% of patients (Johnson et al. 1974, Rajka et al. 1975).
- The family history of atopy is positive in 70% to 90% of patients (Sampson et al. 1985).
- The histological appearance of the eczematous lesions suggest a classical (type IV) cell mediated hypersensitivity reaction in the pathogenesis of atopic dermatitis (Mihm et al. 1976).
- However, infiltration of lymphocytes and monocytes can also be the terminal stage of the "late phase" IgE mediated response following allergen-induced mast cell activation (Solley et al. 1976).

19.2 Details

19.2.1 Modulation of IgE Secretion by Cytokines

IL-4
- Induces B-cells to switch to IgE production
- IL-4 alone is unable to induce IgE synthesis
  A prior membrane contact between activated T-cells and B-cells is necessary

IL-1, -5, -6, -7, -9, -10, TNFα
- Have an auxiliary role in and modulate IL-4 dependent IgE production

IL-13
- Induces IL-4 independent IgE synthesis by B-cell switching
- Has no additive or synergistic effect with IL-4 (common signaling pathway?)

IFNα, γ
- Inhibit IL-4 induced switch of B-cells to IgE

TGFβ
– Inhibits IL-2 induced switch of B-cells to IgE

IL-12
– Inhibits IL-4 induced switch of B-cells to IgE

(see chapter on antibody formation)

Cytokines Involved in Switch to IgE: Signal I and Signal II Are Required

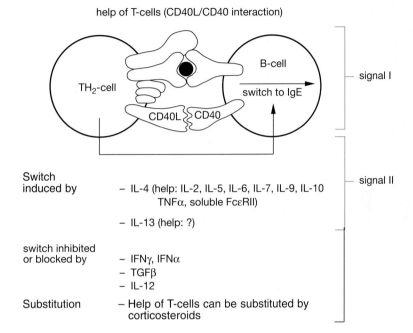

Switch
induced by
– IL-4 (help: IL-2, IL-5, IL-6, IL-7, IL-9, IL-10
    TNFα, soluble FcεRII)

– IL-13 (help: ?)

switch inhibited
or blocked by
– IFNγ, IFNα
– TGFβ
– IL-12

Substitution
– Help of T-cells can be substituted by
    corticosteroids

Regulation of Human
IgE Synthesis In Vivo/
Ex Vivo

	Normal	Atopic patients
Serum IL-4 level	–	–
Cytokine production by PBL/T-cells (in vitro)		
IL-4 (spontaneous)	–	++
IL-4 (after activation)	+	+++
IFN γ gamma (after activation)	+++	+
IL-5 (after activation)	+	+++
IL-2 (after activation)	++	+
Serum IgE level	+	++/+++
IgE production by PBL (in vitro)		
after IL-4 treatment	++	++/+++
after IFNα	–/+	–/+
IgE level after treatment (in vivo) with		
IFNα		+ (50 %)
IFN γ gamma		+

Rousset et al. 1991; King et al. 1990; Wierenga, et al. 1990; Parrouchi et al. 1991; de Vries et al. 1991; Souillet et al. 1989.

19.2.2 Allergic Inflammation

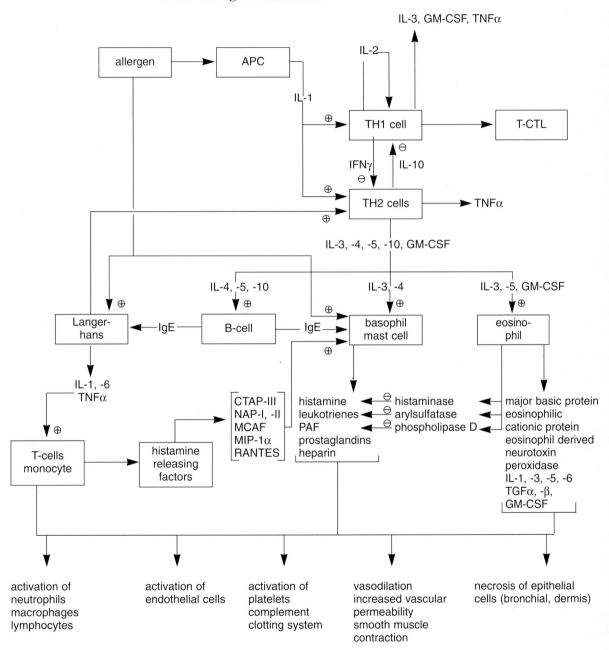

Mast Cells and Eosinophils

Fc ε RI-IgE complexes on the cell membrane of mast cells and basophils are cross-linked by allergen. Cross-linking leads to degranulation and exocytosis of mediators.

During this immediate phase of mast cell activation chemo-tactic factors (LTB4, IL-3, IL-5, GM-CSF, eosinophil chemo-tactic factor A) are generated, which attract neutrophils and eosinophils to the area.

Approximately 4–8 h later neutrophils and eosinophils infiltrate the atopic area (dermis, lung).

Biopsies contain ≈50% lymphocytes, 25–30% eosinophils, 10% neutrophils, 5–10% monocytes (Solley et al. 1976).

Eosinophils release (Slifman et al. 1988, Leiferman et al. 1985):
– Major basic protein (MBP) (cytolytic protein, capable of damaging epithelial cells and promoting further mast cell histamine release)
– Eosinophil cationic protein (ECP)
– Eosinophil derived neurotoxin
– Eosinophil peroxidase
– Histaminase (for degradation of histamine)
– Arylsulfatase [for degradation of SRSA (LTC4)]
– Phospholipase D (for degradation of PAF)

After 24–48 h later lymphocytes and monocytes become the predominant cells.

Allergic Reaction

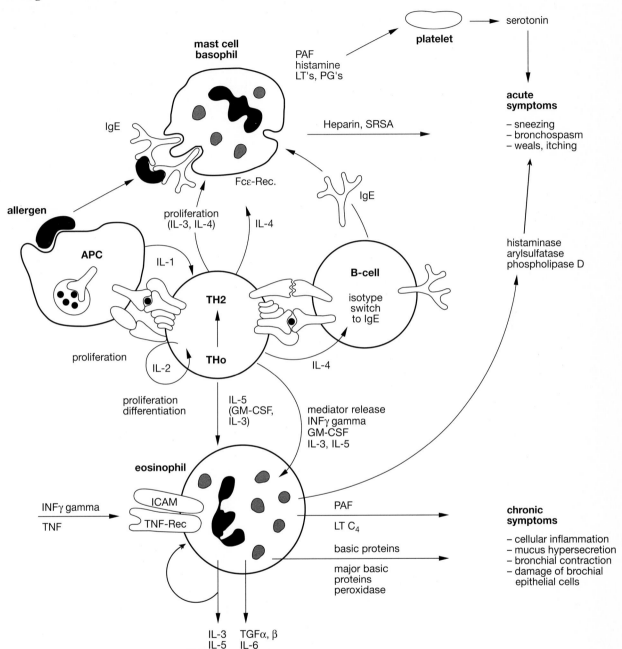

Kay 1992; Mogbel 1992; Czech et al. 1992; Kapp et al. 1992

Influence of Cytokines on Eosinophils

	Maturation/ differen- tiation	Priming/ activation	Cyto- toxicity	Mediator release	Release of cytokines by eosinophils
IL-1	–	–	–	+	–
IL-2	–	–	–	?	–
IL-3	+	+	+	+	+
IL-4	–	–	–	–	–
IL-5	+	+	+	+	+
IL-6	–	–	–	?	+
IL-7	–	–	–	?	–
IL-8	–	–	–	–	–
GM-CSF	+	+	+	+	+
G-CSF	–	–	–	–	–
TNFα	–	+	+	–	–
IFN γ gamma	–	–	+	+	–
TFGα, β	–	–	–	–	–

19.2.3 Role of Langerhans Cells

Langerhans cells contain high affinity Fc ε RI receptors (Beiber et al. 1992, Wang et al. 1992).

Increased numbers are found in skin lesions of atopic dermatitis patients (Kuo et al. 1980).

In mice Langerhans cells can be activated by allergens through cross-linking of Fc ε RI bound IgE.

Activated cells release a variety of cytokines including IL-1, IL-6 and TNFα (Matsue et al. 1992), which in turn attract and activate infiltrating TH2 lymphocytes, which help through their cytokines B-cells to proliferate and switch to IgE.

19.2.4 Role of Fc ε RII (CD23)

Membrane bound Fc ε RII (a, b) is cleaved to produce soluble forms with molecular weights of 25, 33 and 37 kDa (Delespesse et al. 1989).

Soluble Fc ε RII binds competitively IgE and prevents binding of IgE to membrane bound Fc ε RII (Uchibayashi et al. 1989).

Level of soluble Fc ε RII is directly correlated with the expression of membrane bound Fc ε RII (Langerhans cells, T-cells, B-cells) and production of IgE (Cairns et al. 1988, Pene et al. 1989).

IL-4 stimulates expression of Fc ε RII mRNA and production of membrane bound and soluble Fc ε RII (Denoroy et al. 1990, te Velde et al. 1990, Sarfati et al. 1988).

Soluble Fc ε RII functions synergistically with IL-4 in stimulation of IgE production (Pene et al. 1989).

IFNγ gamma also stimulates production of membrane bound and predominantly soluble Fc ε RII, but suppresses IL-4 mediated expression of bound or soluble Fc ε RII (Mayumi et al. 1989; Delespesse et al. 1989; Denoroy et al. 1990, te Velde et al. 1990, Sarfati et al. 1988).

IFNα (and PGE2) also suppress IL-4 induced enhancement of Fc ε RII expression. In addition, IFNα inhibits IFNγ gamma to stimulate on its own production of membrane bound or soluble Fc ε RII (Delespesse et al. 1989, Galizzi et al. 1988).

IL-2 stimulates Fc ε RII production and soluble Fc ε RII stimulates T-cells to produce IL-2. Production of IL-2 is inhibited by IL-4 (Kawabe et al. 1990).

High levels of soluble Fc ε RII can be observed in diseases with high IgE levels such as parasitic and allergic diseases (Yanagihara et al. 1990, Neuber et al. 1991).

stimulation of FcεRII expression: – IL-4 (help by soluble FcεRII, inhibition by IFNγ, IFNα, PGE₂)
                                     – IFNγ (inhibition by IFNα)
                                     – IL-2 (IL-4 inhibits production of IL-2)

19.2.5 Histamine-Releasing Factors (HRF)

– Connective tissue activating peptide (CTAP III):
  * Member of the chemokine family; MW 10–12 kDa (Baeza et al. 1990)
  * Produced by a monocyte dependent T-cell (Sedgwick et al. 1981, Kaplan et al. 1985)
  * Chemotactic for basophils, leads to release of Histamine from basophils; Release dependent on Ca++ and Mg++ (Lett-Brown et al. 1984)

– Neutrophil-activating peptide (NAP II)
  * Cleavage product of CTAP III
  * Has direct HRF activity
  * Chemotactic for neutrophils

– Monocyte chemotactic and activating factor (MCAF; MCP-1):
  * Member of the chemokine family (Kuna et al. 1992)
  * Chemotactic for basophils and most potent HRF (Kuna et al. 1992, Alam et al. 1992)

– Macrophage inflammatory factor (MIP-1α, Alam et al. 1992):
  * Member of the chemokine family
  * Direct agonist causing release of histamine from basophils from allergic and nonallergic patients
  * Chemotactic for monocytes

– Regulated upon activation, normal T-cell expressed and secreted (RANTES; MCP-2):
  * Sequence homology to MIP-1α and Il-8
  * Chemotactic for T-cells, eosinophils and basophils
  * Inhibits histamine release by basophils induced by MCAF (Alam et al. 1992)
  * Directly induces basophils Histamine release. May function through the same or closely related receptor as MCAF or MIP-1α.

– IL-8 (neutrophil activation protein 1, NAP-1):
  * Sequence homology to MIP-1α and RANTES
  * Chemotactic for neutrophils
  * Inhibits histamine release by basophils induced by MCAF (Alam et al. 1991, 1992), IL-2 and CTAP-III (Kuna et al. 1991).
  * May directly induce basophil histamine release (contradicting results) (White et al. 1989, Alam et al. 1991)

– IgE-dependent HRF, Il-3:
  * Produced by macrophages (Schulman et al. 1985)
  * Histamine release is mediated through Fc ε RII bound IgE (Liu et al. 1986)
  * IgE seems to be heterogenous in mediating HRF. Nearly 50% of patients do not respond (MacDonald et al. 1987, 1989).

– Spontaneous basophil histamine release (SBHR)
  * Significantly elevated in atopic patients compared to normal controls (May et al. 1982, Sampson et al. 1993)
  * Reduced by appropriate diet eliminating specific allergen
  * Induced by HRF, produced by macrophages (Sampson et al. 1993)

Histamine-Releasing Factors in Allergic Inflammations

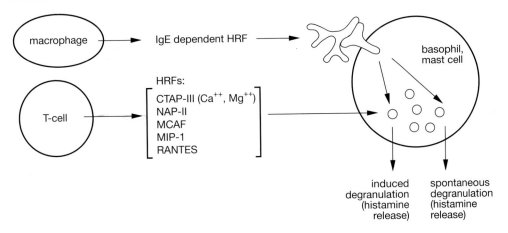

19.2.6 Treatment of Allergic Diseases (Rochlin et al. 1991)

- Avoidance of allergens
  * Food and contact allergens

- Pharmacotherapy with antagonists of vasoactive mediators
  * antihistamines (block H_1 or H_2 histamine receptors on target cells)

- Allergen desensitization
  * Numerous repeated injection of low doses of allergen (induction of IgG4, which blocks allergic reaction, whereas IgG1, -2, -3 has no blocking activity; Aalberse et al. 1983)

- Immune suppression
  * Corticosteroids
    (induction of apoptosis of T-cells and inhibition of inflammation but help of IL-4 to induce switch to IgE)

- Immune modulation
  * IFNγ gamma, IFNα (clinical trials)
    (increase of cellular immune response by stimulation of TH1; Coffmann et al. 1986, Souillet et al. 1989)
  * IL-4 receptor (experimental)
    (blockage of IL-4, which stimulates in B-cells switch to IgE (Finkelman et al. 1986, Paul et al. 1987, Vallenga et al. 1993)
  * MAb anti-IL-4 (experimental)
    (inhibition of IgE response, Davies et al. 1993)
  * IgE receptors (Fc ε RII, CD23, experimental)
    (suppression of IgE synthesis, Delespesse et al. 1989, Ishizaka et al. 1988)

Treatment of Allergic Diseases with Mono-clonal Antibodies Specific for IgE (Experimental)	In vitro prerequisites for anti IgE to be effective: – Specific for the CH3 domain of all human IgE, no cross-reaction with other isotypes – Inhibition of binding of IgE to Fc ε RI and Fc ε RII – No binding to receptor (Fc ε RI, Fcε RII) bound IgE, no induction of histamine release – No complement activation by MAb-IgE complexes – Specific binding to IgE-secreting cells – May mediate low level cytolysis in complement-mediated and antibody-dependent cell mediated cytolysis Indications for in vivo efficacy: – Complete inhibition of IgE synthesis in vitro. – Inhibition of IgE synthesis in vivo by induction of autoanti-IgE response

Davis et al. 1993; Stadler et al. 1993; Marshall et al. 1985, 1989; Haba et al. 1990.

Inhibition of IL-4 Mediated IgE Synthesis (Experimental)	Monoclonal antibodies to Fc ε RII (CD23)	Bonnefoy et al. 1990
	Monoclonal antibodies to IL-4	De Kruyff et al. 1989 Pene et al. 1988 Del Prete et al. 1988 Sato et al. 1993
	Soluble IL-4 receptors	Sato et al. 1993 Renz et al. 1993
	IFNα	de Vries et al. 1991
	IFNγ gamma	Souillet et al. 1989
	TFGβ	de Vries et al. 1991
	IL-10	de Waal et al. 1991
	IL-12	Kiniwa et al. 1992

Interferons and Allergic Diseases	Biological effect	Test system	Interferons α	γ	References
	Suppression of IL-4 induced IgE production	in vitro	+	+	Pene et al. 1988
		in vitro		+	Snapper et al. 1987
		in vitro		+	Coffman et al. 1986
	Inhibition of spontaneous IgE secretion	in vitro		+	Rousset et al. 1988, 1990
	Defect in IFN γ gamma production by lymphocytes of atopic dermatitis or hyper-IgE patients	in vitro		+	Reinhold et al. 1988, 1990
		in vitro		+	Del Prete et al. 1989
	Suppression of IgE production	in vivo		+	Finkelmann et al. 1988
	Improvement of atopic dermatitis	in vivo		+	Reinhold et al. 1990
		in vivo		+	Boguniewicz et al. 1990
		in vivo	−		Mackie et al. 1990
		in vivo	+	+	Pung et al. 1993
	Improvement of hyper-IgE syndrome	in vivo		+	Souillet et al. 1989
		in vivo		+	King et al. 1989

20 Autoimmune Diseases

20.1 Overview

20.1.1 Reasons for Autoimmune Reactions

- Altered self (change of antigen structure) by:
    * Physical influences (change of protein structure by irradiation)
    * Infection (exposure of virus-associated antigens, change of structure by microbiological enzymes)
    * Binding of xenobiotic compounds (pharmaceuticals, chemicals)
    * Dedifferentiation (failure in glycosylation of proteins, mutations)

- Disrupture of anatomical barriers for the immune system:
    * Blood brain barrier, testis and ductus deferens, ocular lenses

- Cross-reaction of antibodies:
    * Immune reaction against streptococci and (self) cardiolipin

- Failure in induction and maintance of tolerance of the immune system against self

20.1.2 Autoantibodies in Normal Persons

Low concentration of nearly all autoantibodies in normal human sera: binding of autoantibodies to:
- Actin
- Tubulin
- Thyroglobulin
- Myoglobulin
- Cytochrome *C*
- Basic myelin
- DNA
- Immunoglobulin G

Normal "autoantibodies" have a considerable polyreactivity:

Specifity	Cross-reaction
Anti-DNA	Cytoskeleton Phospholipids Bacterial cell surfaces
Anti-IgG	DNP-DNA Nucleosomes Bromelain-modified erythrocytes

Normal "autoantibodies" are mainly IgM antibodies with low affinity. Disease-related autoantibodies are IgG, not highly cross-reactive and of high affinity.

Gilbert et al. 1982; Dighiero et al. 1982; Martin 1975; Andrzejewski et al. 1981; Shoenfeld et al. 1983; Carroll et al. 1985; Ternguk 1986; Souroujou et al. 1988; Poncet et al. 1988; Hannestad et al. 1969, 1979; Cunliffe et al. 1980.

20.1.3 Role of B-Cells and T-Helper Cells in Autoimmune Diseases

Macrophages, dendritic cells or B-cells can present autologous molecules with their MHC-class II proteins.

Autoreactive B-cells capture the autologous molecules by their specific membrane immunoglobulin. The resulting antigen-antibody immune complex is internalized and processed into peptides. Such autologous peptides may be loaded on MHC-class II molecules and presented by the B-cell to T-cells reactive for the autologous peptide (Nepom et al. 1991).

In some cases, peptides derived from the B-cell surface antibody molecules bind to the MHC class II molecules and may be presented to so-called anti-idiotypic helper T-cells (Bogen 1993).

T-cells reactive for the autologous peptide help autoreactive B-cells to proliferate. Antiidiotypic helper T-cells sustain this help. How autoreactive T-cells can evade thymic education and selection and peripheral tolerance is yet unclear.

In a conventional protective immune response against exogenous antigens, the autoreactive and anti-idiotypic T-cells will cease generating helper signals, once the foreign antigen is eliminated and cannot be presented any more by APC. In autoimmune diseases the autologous antigens such as immunoglobulin, cardiolipins, DNA or others are constantly present self components, continuously presented by antigen-presenting cells, especially B-cells, to the specific auto-reactive T-cell, thus perpetuating the autologous immune response (Celis 1993, King et al. 1993).

20.2 Details

20.2.1 Specificity of Human Autoantibodies

**Reactions of Human
Autoantibodies with
Autoantigens**

Disease/source of autoantibody	Autoantigen	Cross-reacting species	References
Systemic lupus erythematodes (SLE)	DNA	bacteria, viruses, plants	Stollar et al. 1972
	RNA	bacteria, viruses	Eilat et al. 1978
	histone	ox, chicken	Hardin et al. 1983
	Sm	frog, *Drosophila*	Wooley et al. 1982, Lerner et al. 1980
	U$_1$ ribonucleoprotein (RNP)	ox, *Drosophila*	Reichlin et al. 1969, Monat et al. 1981
	Sjögren's syndrome B-LA	bovine, rat	Chan et al. 1987
	topoisomerase	chicken	Hoffmann et al. 1989
	protein kinase	rat	Stetler et al. 1984
	ribosomal protein	rat, yeast	Francoeur et al. 1986
	fibrillarin (RNP)	frog	Lapegre et al. 1990
	cyclin (prolif. cell nucl. Ag)	mouse, hamster, bird	Bravo 1986
	neurofilaments	rat, ox	Kurki et al. 1986
	RNA polymerase I		Reimer et al. 1987
Myositis	Ki-Ku antigen	ox, guinea pig, rabbit	Francoeur et al. 1986
	tRNA synthetase	ox, rabbit, rat	Yoshida et al. 1983, Yang et al. 1984
Scleroderma	centromere	rat, hamster, mouse	Brenner et al. 1981
	nucleoli	rat	Mole Bayer et al. 1990
	topoisomerase	ox, mouse	Maul et al. 1986, Shero et al. 1986 Alderuccio et al. 1986
	mitochondrial 72 kDa protein	ox, pig, rat, rabbit, yeast	
Sjögren's syndrome	SS-B/LA	ox, mouse, rat, rabbit	Chan et al. 1987
Mixed connective tissue disease	U$_1$ RNP	ox, *Drosophila*	Reichlin et al. 1989, Monat et al. 1981,
	protein kinase	rat	Stetler et al. 1984
Pemphigus	epidermal protein	all mammals, birds	Anhalt et al. 1982

Disease/source of autoantibody	Autoantigen	Cross-reacting species	References
Primary biliary cirrhosis	nucleoli mitochondria pyruvate dehydrogenase E_2 pyruvate dehydrogenase X	rat mouse, rat, yeast, *E. coli* bacteria ox, pig	Bravo 1986 Frazer et al. 1985 Fussey et al. 1990 Surk et al. 1989
Thrombocytopenia	laminin B	rat, hamster, mouse	Guilly et al. 1987
Diabetes	pancreatic islets	rat	Lernmark et al. 1978
Myasthenia	acetylcholin receptor	rat, electric eal	Drachman et al. 1982, Akaronow 1975
Hyperthyroidism	TSH-receptor	rat	Valente et al. 1983
Asthma, rhinitis	β-adrenergic receptor	ox, dog	Venter et al. 1980
Rheumatoid arthritis	histones immunoglobulins IgG	ox, chicken rabbit, ox, pig, horse	Homan et al. 1959 Waaler 1940, Rose et al. 1948, Butler et al. 1964
Anemia	microsomes polysaccharid epitope on cell surface GP	dog, rat, mouse ox, rabbit, pig	Dow et al. 1985 Pirofsky 1969, Childs 1980

Autoantigens in Insulin-Dependent Diabetes

Autoantigen	Characteristics		Immune response		Specificity/function
	Structure	DMA*)	Anti-bodies	Cellular	
Sialoglycoprotein	GM2-1		+		not β-cell specific
Glutamate decarboxy-lase	GAD65 (64 kDa)	+	+	+	cross-reaction with P-2 protein of coxsacky B-virus
	GAD67	+	+	+	
Insulin		+	+	+	
Insulin receptor			+		
Islet cell protein	38 kDa		+	+	induced (cross-reactivity with) CMV
Bovine serum albumin antigen	ABBOS peptides	+	+		cross-reaction with β-cell beta cell p69 protein (PM-1)
Glucose transporter	Glut-2		+		inhibits glucose stimulation
HSP-65	p277	+	+	+	
Carboxypeptidase H			+		Insulin secretory granule protein
Islet cell protein	52 kDa		+		cross-reaction with Rubella virus
Islet cell protein	ICA12/ ICA512		+ +		homology to CD45
Membrane antigen	150 kDa		+		β-cell specific
RIN polar			+		present on insulinoma cells

*) disease modifying antigen

MacCaren et al. 1993; Kaufman et al. 1992; Karjalainen et al. 1992; Atkinson et al. 1990, 1993.

**Autoantibodies
to Immunoglobulins**

Specificity, directed against	Occurrence/isotype	References
Fc part (polyspecific) cross-reaction to DNA, histones, myosin, actin, vimentine	10–15% (spontaneously) mainly IgG enhancement by B-cell activation (LPS, Staph. Tox. A; others)	van Snick et al. 1983 Hartman et al. 1989 Lydyard et al. 1990 Gergely et al. 1992
Isotype specific	induced by immune complexes or in rheumatoid arthritis mainly IgM, IgG, IgA	Coulie et al. 1983, 1985 Stanley et al. 1987 Nemazee et al. 1985 Tarkowski et al. 1984
CH_2–CH_3 interdomain region (IgG1, -2, -4)	rheumatoid arthritis mainly IgM	Nardella et al. 1985, 1987 Sasso et al. 1988
Carbohydrate binding region of IgG3	rheumatoid arthritis	Artandi et al. 1991
CH_3 domain of IgG3 (His-435; Tyr-436)	rheumatoid arthritis	Huck et al .1986
CH_3 domain of IgG1; IgG2a, IgG3	rheumatoid arthritis	Stassin et al. 1983
CH2 domain of IgG1; IgG2a	rheumatoid arthritis, viral infections	Stassin et al. 1983 Coutelier et al. 1987

Association with MHC-II Antigens

	MHC-II association	MHC-II mutation β-1 domain	Epitope (aa)	Susceptibility
Rheumatoid arthritis (man)	DRw10 DR4-Dw10	70, 71 67, 70, 71		increased decreased/normal
Diabetes mellitus (man)	DR5/DQw3.1 DR2/DQw1.12	57 53, 55, 57		increased increased
Myasthenia gravis (man)	DR3/DQw2 DR5	57	257–269 195–212	increased
Pemphigus vulgaris (man)	DRw6/DQB1.9	57		absolute
Exp. autoallergic encephalomyelitis (mouse)	IAα Aβ 1Eα Eβ		1– 20, 89–101 35– 47	high

Steinmann 1990; Brocke et al. 1988; Zamvil et al. 1986, 1988; Sahai et al. 1988; Urban et al. 1989; Todd et al. 1988; Sinha et al. 1988; Scharf et al. 1988.

Allotypic and Isoallotypic Markers of Immunoglobulin G

	IgG1	IgG2	IgG3	IgG4
Allotypic markers (H-chain)	Gm1 a x f z	Gm2 n C3, -5 g-1, -5	Gm3 b1, -3, -4, -5 s t u v	Gm4
Isoallotypic markers				4a, -b

Hamilton 1987, van Loghem 1986.

Autoimmune Responses are Generated Through the Cooperation of Auto-active B-Cells and T-Cells. Antiidiopeptide Reactive Helper T-Cells Amplify the Help

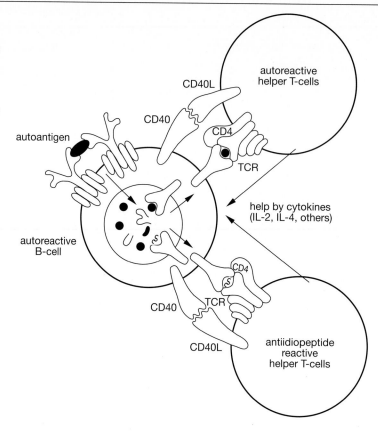

20.2.2 Relationship to Exposure to Xenobiotics

Disease	Heavy metals	Pharma-ceuticals	Organic solvents industrial chemicals	Food additives chemicals in food
Annual incidence 6–35 per 100 000				
– Systemic lupus erythematodes	–	–	hydrazine	tartrazine alfalfa sprouts
– Autoimmune haemolytic anemia	–	penicillin penicillamin α-methyl-dopa nomifensin	–	–
Annual incidence 4,5–12 per 1 000 000				
– Scleroderma	–	–	vinylchloride silica dust	adulterated rapeseed oil
Annual incidence 2–5 per 1 000 000				
– Myasthenia gravis	–	penicillamine	–	–
– Pemphigus		penicillamine pyrithioxine α-mercaptopropio-nylglycine captopril		
– Immune complex nephritis	gold cadmium mercury	various	–	–
– Autoimmune thyroid disease	–	lithium penicillamine amiodarone	polybrominated and polychlorinated biphenyl	–
– Autoimmune hepatitis		α-methyldopa oxyphenisatin halothane		
– Eosinophilic myalyic syndrome	–	impure L-tryptophan	–	–

Talal 1993.

20.2.3 Approaches To Treat Autoimmune Diseases

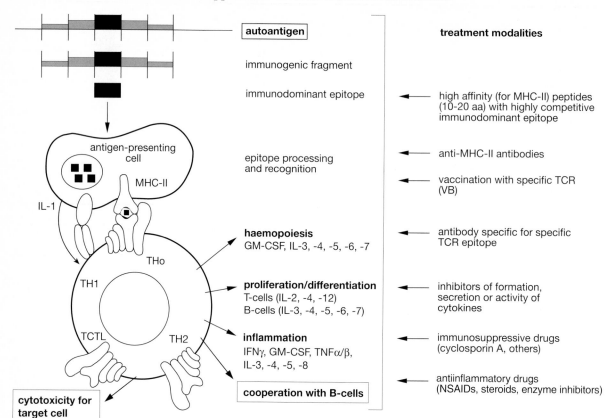

Steinman 1990; Corrigan 1992

**Prevention of
Experimental
Autoimmune Diseases**

	Blocking peptide	MAb anti-MHC-II	TCR vaccination	MAb anti-TCR	
Encephalomyelitis					
Mouse (H-2u)	+	+	0	+	Sakai et al. 1989 Acha-Orbea et al. 1988 Steinman et al. 1981
(H-2s)	0	+	–	0	Sakai et al. 1988 Sriram et al. 1987
Lewis rat	0	0	+	+	Lider et al. 1988, Owhashi et al. 1988
Monkey	0	+	0	0	Steinman 1990
Myasthenia gravis (mouse)	0	+	0	0	Waldor et al. 1983
Diabetes (mouse)	0	+	0	0	Boitard et al. 1988
Collagen-induced arthritis (mouse)	0	+	0	0	Wooley et al. 1985
Thyreoditis (mouse)	0	+	+	0	Maron et al. 1983, Vladutia et al. 1987

Approaches for Therapy of Rheumatoid Arthritis

Drug families	Way of action	Efficacy	
Nonsteroidal anti-inflammatory drugs (NSAIDs) (indomethacin or analogues, azapropazones, salicylates)	– inhibition of prostaglandin synthesis (cyclooxygenase)	short term: long term:	reduction of signs and symptoms of inflammation in 30-50% of patients no significant effect
Disease modifying antirheumatic drugs (DMARDs) Corticosteroids	– promotion of formation of lipocortin (inhibitor of phospholipase A_2) – reduced production of cytokines and inflammatory enzymes (incl. metalloproteinases) – reduction in T-, B-cells, PMN and macrophages number and function	short term: long term:	immediate but transient reduction of inflammation reduction in progression of RA erosions (from 60% to about 20% after 2 years of treatment)
Methotrexate	– antimetabolite	long term:	improvement of symptoms in about 30% of patients
Azathioprine Cyclophosphamide Cyclosporin A	– antimetabolite, cytostatics reduction in IL-1 – inhibition of bone resorbing activity of IL-1; PGE – inhibition of PGE_2 production – inhibition of T-cell cytokine production (TNFα alpha, -β, others)	long term: long term: however:	no significant effect reduction in progression of RA erosions in 25-50% of cases synergistic with NSAIDs in kidney toxicity
Gold preparations (thiomalate) Penicillamin Hydroychloroquine Sulfasalasine	not well defined common mode of action	long term:	reduction in progression of RA erosions in 60-70% of patients (side effects: thrombocytopenia, leucopenia, anaemia in about 30%)

Kirwan 1991; Russel 1991; Mac Kenzie 1991; Bayliss et al. 1991; Lewis et al. 1992; von Rijthove et al. 1991.

Approaches for Selective Immune Suppression in Rheumatoid Arthritis and Associated Diseases

Compound	Mode of action	Efficacy	References

MAb anti-CD4	depletion of TH cells	therapeutic effect in murine
		   collagen arthritis
		   SLE
		   myasthenia gravis
		   EAE
		   diabetes mellitus
		   thyroiditis
		   uveitis
			Ranges et al. 1985
			Wofsy et al. 1987
			Christadoss et al. 1986
			Waldor et al. 1985
			Koike et al. 1987
			Nabozny et al. 1991
			Atalla et al. 1990

MAb anti-CD$_4$	depletion of TH cells depletion of TH cells	clinical trial ongoing effective in out-treated RA patients, suppression of TH cells (pilot studies)	Lewis et al. 1992 Herzog et al.1987 Wendling et al. 1991 Reiter et al. 1991 Horneff et al. 1991 Herzog et al. 1989
		generation of human anti mouse Ig antibodies	Horneff et al. 1991 Goldberg et al. 1991
MAb anti-CD4 (chimaeric)	depletion of TH cells	suppression of TH cells and clinical signs of therapeutic activity in out-treated RA patients (pilot study)	Moreland et al. 1993
Diphtheria toxin IL-2	toxicity on T-, B-cells	25% improvement (12 of 13 RA patients) (numerous side effects)	Lewis et al. 1992
MAb anti-IL-2-Rec.	toxicity on T-, B-cells	trial ongoing	Lewis et al. 1992
Antigenic peptides binding to MHC-II DR1 groove	specific blockage of antigen recognition	trial ongoing	Lamont et al. 1990
Collagen type II (oral)	specific blockage of afferent and efferent immune response	in mice delay of onset and decreased incidence phase I started	Thompson et al. 1990

**Inhibition of IL-1
Secretion and/or
Function**

Compound	Mechanism	Comments	References
Prostaglandins	suppression of IL-1 synthesis		Hoffmann et al. 1991
5-Lipoxygenase inhibitors	suppression of IL-1 synthesis	controversial (zilentone not effective)	Hoffmann et al. 1991 Lewis et al. 1992
Cytokine suppressive anti-inflammatory drugs (CSAIDs) 5-LO-cyclooxygenase inhibitors			
Tenidap	inhibition of IL-1 synthesis	effective in vitro, reduces IL-1 activity in synovial fluid of RA patients	Blackburn et al. 1991 Robinson et al. 1990
SKB 105809	inhibition of IL-1, TNF, IL-6 synthesis and release	effective in vitro, in vivo prevention of LPS shock (10 mg/kg) treatment of arthritis (rat)	Greig 1991
Glucocorticoids, probucol, ciprofloxacin, 5-A-salicylic acid, 3-deazadenosine, pentamidine	inhibition of IL-1 synthesis		Lewis 1992
IL-1 type I-Receptor	competitive inhibition of IL-1	inhibition of allograft rejection (heart, cells)	Dower et al. 1989 Fanslow et al. 1990
IL-1 receptor antagonist	blockage of IL-1-Rec	inhibits acute IL-1 effects in vivo if in 100–1000 fold excess	Hannum et al. 1990 McIntyre et al. 1991

Selective Immune Suppression in Rheumatoid Arthritis and associated Diseases

Compound	Mode of action	Efficacy	References
MAb antiautoantigen MHC complex	specific blockage of antigen recognition	in mice (EAE) effective	Aharoni et al. 1991
Immunization with TCR (Vα, Vβ)	immune response against antigen specific T-cell receptors	in mice (EAE) effective	Howell et al. 1989
MAb anti-β_2-subunit of integrins (LFA-1, Mac-1, p150/95) (CD 18)	inhibition of interaction between leukocytes and partner cells	reduction of acute and chronic arthritis in rabbits	Jasin et al. 1990

Indications for Use of Intravenous Polyclonal Immunoglobulins (ivIg) (consensus statement of the Australasian Society)

Application is indicated in:
– Primary immunoglobulin deficiency
– Autoimmune thrombocytopenia (children, adults)
– Posttransfusion pupura
– Allogeneic bone marrow transplantation (up to day 90)
– Prophylaxis for recurrent bacterial infections in children with AIDS related diseases
– Chronic lymphocytic leukaemia with hypogammaglobulinaemia and repeated bacterial infections (>2/year)
– Kawasaki disease
– Chronic inflammatory demyelinating polyneuropathy (CIDP) in children too small for plasma exchange

Application may be indicated in:
– Recurrent infection in patients with lymphoid malignancy other than chronic lymphocytic leukemia
– Autoantibodies to F VIII
– IgG subclass deficiency and evidence of infection
– Patients with selected neurological diseases where other therapy has failed and plasmapheresis is difficult
  * chronic inflammatory demyelinating polyneuropathy
  * Guillain-Barré syndrome
  * Intractable seizures of childhood
  * Myasthenia gravis
– Autoimmune haemolytic anaemia, resistant to conventional forms of therapy
– Autoimmune neutropenia with recurrent bacterial infection and failure of prophylactic antibodies

– Pregnancy complicated by neonatal alloimmune thrombocytopenia (NAIT) (contradictory: evidence of an effect of ivIg in elevating fetal platelet counts)
– Protection of the fetus in autoimmune thrombocytopenia in pregnancy

The administration of i.v. Ig in indications not cited cannot be justified at present.

Keller et al. 1993.

Improvement of Chronic Autoimmune Diseases After i.v. Injection of Polyclonal Immunoglobulins (Summary of Case Reports, If Not Stated Otherwise*)	Disease	Therapeutic effect	References
	Rheumatoid arthritis	+	Mitroupoulon et al. 1987
	Juvenile rheumatoid arthritis	+	Combe et al. 1985
		+	Groothoff et al. 1988
		+	Silverman et al. 1990
	Crohn's disease, colitis ulcerosa	+	Rohr et al. 1987
		+	Koflach et al. 1990
	Systemic lupus erythematodes	+	Gaedicke et al. 1984
		+	Jordan et al. 1989
		+	Corvetta et al. 1989
		+	Maier et al. 1990
		+	Lin et al. 1989
		+	Ahashi et al. 1990
		+/–	Ballow et al. 1989
		+	Gonzalez et al. 1989
		+/–	Barron et al. 1992
		–	Jordan et a. 1991
		+	Oliet et al. 1992
		+	Saida et al. 1988
		+	Sugisahi et al. 1982
		+	Ben Chetrit et al. 1991
		+/–	Winder et al. 1993
	Juvenile dermatomyositis	+	Roifman et al. 1987
		+	Barron et al. 1992
	Dermatomyositis	+	Cherin et al. 1991
		+	Lang et al. 1991
	Chronic polymyositis	+	Roifman et al. 1987

*) Placebo-controlled study.

Disease	Therapeutic effect	References
Membraneous glomerulonephritis, chronic active hepatitis haemolytic anaemia (autoimmune)	+ + + + + +	Palla et al. 1991 Carmassi et al. 1992 Hillgartner et al. 1987 Salama et al. 1984 Blanchette et al. 1992 Clauvel et al. 1983
Thrombocytopenic (idiopathic), purpura	+ + + + + + + + + + + +	Imbach et al. 1981 Fehr et al. 1982 Bussel et al. 1983 Schmidt et al. 1981 Burdach et al. 1986 Mori et al. 1983 Castaman et al. 1991 Newland et al. 1983 Rodeghiero et al. 1992 Faradji et al. 1982 Bierling et al. 1987 Berchtold et al. 1989
Virus-related thrombocytopenia, pure red cell aplasia	+ + + + + +	Ravich et al. 1991 Clauvel et al. 1983 Etzioni et al. 1986 Kurtzman et al. 1989 McGuire et al. 1987 Ballester et al. 1992
Neutropenia (autoimmune)	+	Pollack et al. 1982
Evans's syndrome (autoimmune haemolytic anaemia + idiopathic thrombocytopenia)	+	Petrides et al. 1992
Severe rhesus alloimmunization, Kawasaki syndrome	+ + + + + + + + +	Margulies et al. 1991 Furusho et al. 1984 Leung et al. 1987 Newburger et al. 1986, 1991 Engle et al. 1989 Barron et al. 1990 Schulman et al. 1992 Saulsburry 1992

Disease	Therapeutic effect	References
Fetal loss by antiphospholipid antibodies, autoantibodies to F VIII	+	Carreras et al. 1988
	0	Parke et al. 1992
	+	Müller-Eckhardt et al. 1983
	+	Sultan et al. 1984, 1991
	+	Green et al. 1987
Acquired von Willebrand disease	+	Delannoy et al. 1988
	+	Castaman et al. 1992
	+	Macik et al. 1988
Myasthenia gravis	+	Balzereit et al. 1986
	+	Sopo et al. 1992
	+/0	Arsura et al. 1989
	+	Gadjos et al. 1984
Epilepsia (Lennox syndrome, Gastaut syndrome, West syndrome)	+	Van Rijchevorsel-Harmant et al. 1986
	+	Echenne et al. 1991
	+	Illum et al. 1990
	+	Pechadre et al. 1977
	+	Laffont et al. 1979
	+	Ariizumi et al. 1983
	+	Standstedt et al. 1984
	+	Bedini et al. 1985
	+*)	Illum et al. 1990
	0	Hara et al. 1985
Multiple sclerosis	+	Rothfelder et al. 1982
	+	Sonko et al. 1986
	+	van Engelen et al. 1992
	+(−)	Schüler et al. 1983
	0	Cook et al. 1992
Chronic inflammatory demyelinating polyneuropathy (CIDP)	+	Vermeulen et al. 1985
	+	Albama et al. 1987
	+	Cook et al. 1987
	+	Curro et al. 1987
	+	Faed et al. 1989
	+	Cornblath et al. 1992
	+*)	Van Doorn et al. 1990
	0*)	Vermeulen et al. 1993

Disease	Therapeutic effect	References
Guillain-Barré syndrome	+*)	van der Meche et al. 1992
	+	Jackson et al. 1993
	+	Rajah et al. 1992
	+	Hidon et al. 1992
	+	Kleyweg et al. 1988
	+	Shahar et al. 1990
	+	Mauro et al. 1989
	+	Heaton et al. 1992
Multifocal motor neuropathy	+	Nobile-Orazio et al. 1993
Lamberg-Eaton syndrome	+	Bird et al. 1992
Infantile opsoclonus poly-myoclonia syndrome	+	Sugie et al. 1992
Graves' ophthalmopathy	+	Antonelli et al. 1992
	+	Dweyer et al. 1991

*) Placebo-controlled study.

Dose Regimen in the Therapy of Auto-immune Diseases with Polyclonal Immuno-globulins

Disease	Total dose of Ig	No. of patients treated	No. of patients responding	References
Rhesus allo-immunization	949 mg/kg per day times 4–5 day (20–28 weeks of gestation)	7	7 (bilirubin low)	Margulies et al. 1991
Graves' ophthal-mopathy	400 mg/kg per day times 5 days 9 cycles every 21 days	7	4	Antonelli et al. 1992
Spontaneous F VIII:C inhibitors	400 mg/kg per day times 5 days	6	5	Sultan et al. 1991
Bleeding due to virus-related thrombocytopenia	1 g/kg per day times 2 days 3 courses every week	14	14	Rarick et al. 1991
Epilepsia	400 mg/kg per day times 5 days every 6 weeks	23	8	Echenne et al. 1991
Red cell aplasia	400 mg/kg per day times 5 days	3	3	Ballester et al. 1992
Idiopathic thrombocytopenic purpura	400 mg/kg per day times 5 days	45	35	Rodeghiero et al. 1992
von Willebrand syndrome	1 g/kg/per day times 2 days	1	1	Rastaman et al. 1992
AIDS	200 mg/kg permonth times 12 months	24	24	Saint-Marc et al. 1992
Juvenile dermatomyositis	1 g/kg per day times 2 days/month for 6 months	5	5	Roifman et al. 1987
	400 mg/kg per day times 4 days followed by 400 mg/kg/month	6	5	Barron et al. 1992

Disease	Total dose of Ig	No. of patients treated	No. of patients responding	References
SLE	2 g/kg per day times 5 days + 400 mg/kg/month for 5 months	7	3	Barron et al. 1992
Demyelinating optic neuritis (multiple sclerosis)	400 mg/kg per day times 5 days	5	5	Baziel et al. 1992
Guillain-Barré syndrome	400 mg/kg per day times 5 days	7	6	Jackson et al. 1993
Progressive MS (multiple sclerosis)	500–200 mg/kg per day times monthly	14	0	Cook et al. 1992
Kawasaki syndrome	400 mg/kg per day times 4 days	15	15	Saulsburg 1992
Chronic inflamma-tory demyelinating polyneurophathy (CIDP)	400 mg/kg/ per day times 5 days	15 13	4 3	Vermeulen et al. 1993
Multifocal motor neuropathy	400 mg/kg per day times 5 days every 2nd month	5	4	Nobile-Orazio et al. 1993
Kawasaki disease	1 g/kg single dose	44	43	Barron et al. 1990
Juvenile arthritis	400 mg/kg per day times 4 days	11	10	Silverman et al. 1990

21 Immune Suppression

21.1 Overview

21.1.1 Therapeutic Activity and Toxicity of Immune Suppressives

Therapeutic Activity	Indication	Most effective compounds
	Rejection of transplanted organs	
	Prevention	cyclosporin A, FK 506, corticosteroids
	Treatment	corticosteroids, azathioprine, 15-deoxyspergualin (experim.)
	Graft versus host disease	cyclosporin A, azathioprine, corticosteroids, FK 506
	Autoimmune reactions	corticosteroids, azathioprine, cyclosporin A, methotrexate, 15-deoxyspergualin (experim.) (cyclophosphamide, chlorambucil)

Toxicity	Dose limiting toxicity	Compound
	Myelosuppression	G-mercaptopurin, azathioprine, cyclophosphamide, chlorambucil
	Nephrotoxicity	cyclosporin A
	Cushing-syndrome	corticosteroids
	Diabetes	corticosteroids
	Neoplasia (lymphoma)	cyclosporin A
	Haemorrhagic cystitis	cyclophosphamide
	Emesis	cyclophosphamide, chlorambucil

21.1.2 Mode of Action of Immune Suppressive Drugs

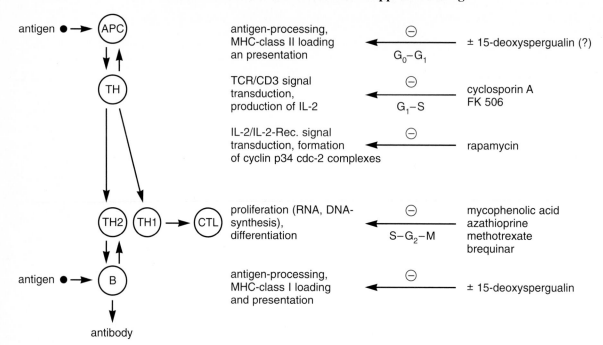

21.2 Details

21.2.1 Mode of Action of Specific Agents

**Cyclosporin A, FK 506,
Rapamycin**

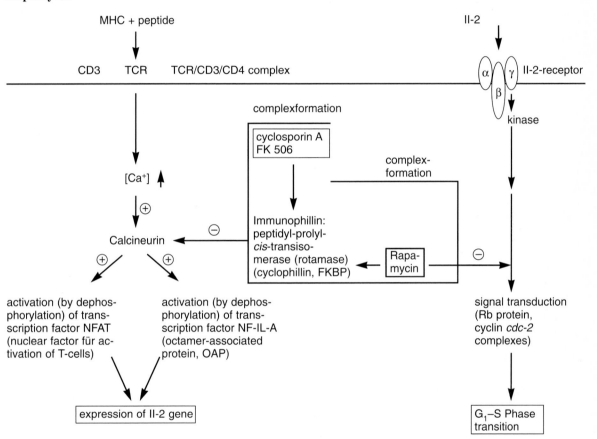

Wiederrecht et al. 1993, Clipstone et al. 1993, Flanagan et al. 1993, Albers et al. 1993.

Mycophenolic Acid

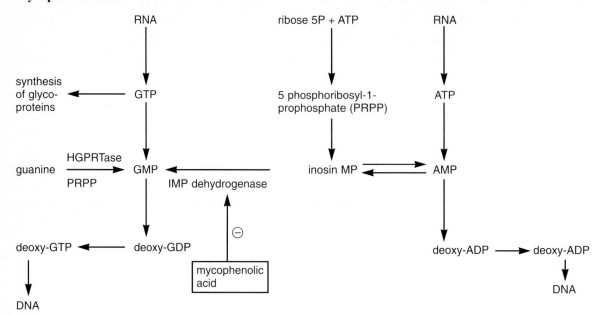

Allison et al. 1993, Natsumeda et al. 1993.

±15-Deoxyspergualin

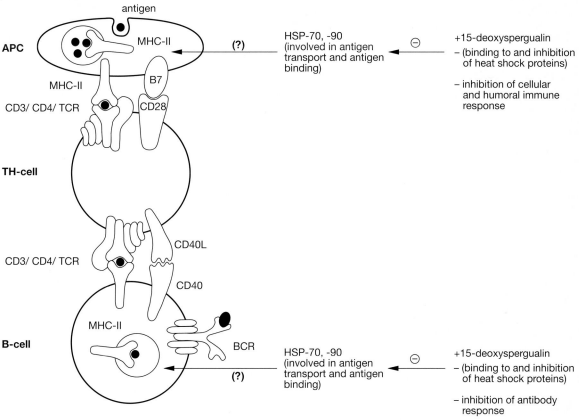

APC

antigen

MHC-II

MHC-II

CD3/ CD4/ TCR

B7

CD28

TH-cell

CD3/ CD4/ TCR

CD40L

CD40

B-cell

MHC-II

BCR

(?)

HSP-70, -90
(involved in antigen
transport and antigen
binding)

⊖

+15-deoxyspergualin
– (binding to and inhibition
of heat shock proteins)

– inhibition of cellular
and humoral immune
response

(?)

HSP-70, -90
(involved in antigen
transport and antigen
binding)

⊖

+15-deoxyspergualin
– (binding to and inhibition
of heat shock proteins)

– inhibition of antibody
response

Tepper et al. 1993, 1994; Nadler et al. 1993

cyclosporin A (CsA)

FK506

rapamycin

R₁=OH, R₂=OH Spergualin
R₁=H , R₂=OH Deoxyspergualin

Antibiotic and Xeno-biotic Immunosuppressive Compounds

Compound	Mode of action Biochemical	Cellular	References
6-Mercaptopurin (6-MP) (synthetic anti-metabolite)	– metabolization to 6-thio-inosinic acid (active drug) – decrease of purine sythesis by inhibition of Glutamine-5-phosphoribosyl pyrophos-phate aminotransferase	– inhibition of S phase of cell cycle	Chabner 1981
Azathioprine (AZA) (synthetic anti-metabolite)	– metabolization to 6-MP and to 6-thio-inosinic acid	– inhibition of S-phase of cell cycle	Chabner 1981
Corticosteroids (synthetic steroids, various derivatives)	– promotion of formation of lipocortin (inhibitor of phospholipase A_2) – reduced production of cytokines	– blockage of IL-1 secre-tion (macrophages) – reduction (number, func-tion) of T-cells, B-cell, macrophages	Snyder et al. 1982
Cyclosporin A (CyA) cyclic oligopeptide (MW 1203)	– inhibition of peptidylprolyl-isomerase (= rotamase = cyclo philin) and of transition of *cis-trans* rotamers of prolylamide linkages of peptides – cyclophilin-CyA complexes inhibit phosphatase activity of calcineurin, which activates transcription of IL-2 by dephos-phorylation of regulatory protein (NF-AT)	– inhibition of IL-2 secretion (T-cells) by blockage of TCR signal transduction (calcineurin) – inhibition of transition from G_0 to G_1	Britton et al. 1982 Borel et al. 1976 Hess et al. 1982 Schreiber 1991
FK506 (macrolide lactone)	– inhibition of cyclophilin (FK binding protein) – FK-cyclophilin complexes inhibit calcineurin	– inhibition of IL-2 secretion (T-cells) by blockage of TCR signal transduction (calcineurin) – inhibition of transition from G_0 to G_1 – inhibition of Fc ε receptor signaling on mast cells	Kino et al. 1987 Sigal et al. 1990 Liu et al. 1991 Liu et al. 1991 Alters et al. 1993

Compound	Mode of action Biochemical	Cellular	References
Rapamycin (macrolide lactone)	– inhibition of Cyclophilin – rapamycin-cyclophilin complexes inhibit calcineurin – inhibition of IL-2 induced expression of p34cdc2	– inhibition of IL-2 induced signal transduction – inhibition of transition from G_1 to S phase – inhibition of insulin receptor on hepatocyes	Vezina et al. 1975 Sigal et al. 1991 Dumont et al. 1990 Baumann et al.1992 Flanagan et al.1993 Albers et al. 1993
Mycophenolic acid (mofetil) (synthetic antimetabolite)	– inhibition of purine synthesis	– inhibition of S phase of cell cycle	Ohsugi et al. 1976 Allison et al. 1993
Brequinar sodium (Dup 785) (synthetic antimetabolite)	– inhibition of pyrimidine synthesis by blocking dihydro-oratate dehydrogenase	– inhibition of S phase of cell cycle	Murphy et al. 1991
Methotrexate (MTX) (synthetic antimetabolite)	– decrease of purine and thymidine synthesis by inhibition of Dihydrofolatereductase	– inhibition of S phase of cell cycle	Bertino et al. 1981
Cyclophosphamide- (synthetic alkylans)	– metabolization to the alkylating metabolite phosphorodiamide N mustard	– cell cycle independent inhibition of proliferation	Colvin et al. 1981
15-Deoxyspergualin (15-DOS) (spergualin derivative)	– binding to and inhibition of heat shock protein Hsp 70 (Hsp 70 involved in protein folding and processing) (Hypothesis)	– suppression of macrophage activity – inhibition of MHC-class II antigen expression – inhibition of effector phase of immune response – inhibition of B-cells	Umezawa et al.1981 Nadler et al. 1992 Dickneite et al. 1985, 1986, 1987 Morikawa et al.1992 Tepper et al. 1993
Discodermolide	– decrease of IL-2 receptor expression	– block at the G2-M interface	Longley et al. 1993

21.2.2 Monoclonal Antibodies

Mechanisms by which monoclonal antibodies can be immunosuppressive:
– Blocking the interaction between T-cells and other cells (T, B, APC, monocytes)
– Delivering signals to T-cells, which downregulate the normal T-cell function
– Activation induced death of T-cells (apoptosis).
– Direct inhibition of T-cells, followed by an inhibition of the corresponding ligand on the partner cell by anti-idiotype antibodies I, which is followed by amplification of the effect of the primary antibody by anti-idiotype antibody II.

Olive et al. 1993.

Major groups of cellular targets that can be used for immunomodulation by monoclonal antibodies (MAbs):
– The T-cell receptors (TCR) and/or its transduction system, the CD3 complex. Against the TCR, MAbs are available against either the constant region (common part of all receptors) or the variable region (esp. $V\beta$), allowing suppression of a specific (restricted) T-cell repertoire.

– The accessory molecules for interaction of the TCR:
  CD4 (ligand: MHC-class II)
  CD8 (ligand: MHC-class I)

– Other accessory adhesion molecules:
  CD2   (ligand: LFA3)
  LFA1 (ligand: ICAM-1)
  CD28 (ligand: B7-BBI)
  CD40 (ligand: CD40L)

– The major receptors for lymphokines:
  IL-2 receptor: p55 (α-chain)
              β75 (β-chain)
              β75 (γ-chain)
  IL-4 receptor
  IL-1 receptor

**Cellular Targets for
Immune Suppression
by Antibodies**

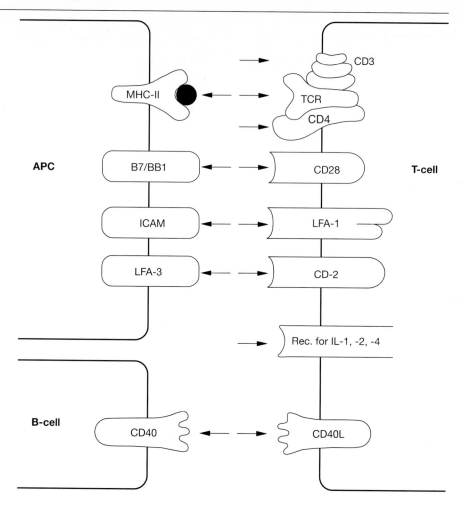

The most prominent immunosuppressive antibodies are specific for CD4.

The CD4 antigen is directly involved in the process of activation of T-cells through TCR recognizing antigenic peptide presented by MHC class II antigens (Biddison et al. 1982).

The CD4 antigen has functional abilities on the intracellular signal transduction following TCR/CD3 mediated T-cell activation (Schrezenmeier et al. 1988).

CD4 T-cells produce large amounts of proinflammatory cytokines, thereby prompting secondary cell types to become involved in the immune and inflammatory response (Ranges et al. 1988).

Monoclonal anti-CD4 antibodies have successfully been tested in:
- Allogeneic organ transplantation in primates (Jonker et al. 1987, Cosimi et al. 1990, Delmonico et al. 1992)
- Rheumatoid arthritis in man (Herzog et al. 1987, 1989; Reiter et al. 1991; Wendling et al. 1991; Van der Lubbe et al. 1991)
- Due to its way of action, human anti murine antibodies (HAMAs) in response of application of murine anti CD4 antibodies are low or absent (Olive et al. 1993).

22 Immune Reactions in Neoplasia

22.1 Overview

Basic assumptions for tumor immunotherapy:
– There exist qualitative or quantitative differences between tumor cells and (most) normal cells.

– The immune system is sufficiently equipped to identify these differences.

– The immune system can be stimulated or taught by antigen-specific or non-antigen-specific procedures to recognize these differences and to mediate tumor rejection.

Possible modes of tumor immunotherapy:
– Active, by stimulation or teaching the immune system
  * Antigen-specifically
    – At "early" stages by "tumor vaccines"
    – At "later" stages by stimulation/amplification of immune cells committed for tumor antigens
  * Non-antigen-specifically
    – By stimulation of cells responsible for the general defence system

– Passive, by substituting the immune system
  * Antigen-specifically
    – With antibodies specific for tumor antigens
    – With cells (autochthonous), sensitized in vitro for tumor antigens
  * Non-antigen-specifically
    – With interleukins and/or mediators which limit by their concentration the strength of the immune response

Possibilities of Tumor Immunotherapy

	Non antigen-specific	Antigen-specific	
	General defense system	Immune response specific for tumor antigens	
		Afferent pathway	Efferent pathway
	macrophages granulocyte natural killer cells	antigen presenting cells T-lymphocytes (T-help) B-lymphocytes	cytotoxic T-cells plasma cells/anti- bodies
Active therapy	immunostimulators (synthetic, bacterial) interleukins (IL-1, -2, -4, -6, G-CSF, GM-CSF, M-CSF)	tumor vaccines interleukins (IL-1, -2, -4, -6)	interleukins (IL-2, -4, -5, -6, -7, -8, -9, -10, -11, -12, -13)
	neutrophil activating peptides (NAP-1, -2, MGSA)	interleukin (IL-1, -2, TNF) secreting tumor cells (somatic gene therapy)	IFN γ
	TNF, IFNα, β, γ	tumor-specific monoclonal antibodies linked to in- terleukins (IL-1, -2, IFN)	IL-4 receptors
Passive therapy	(in vitro) lymphokine (IL-2), activated killer cells (LAK-cells)	interleukins (IL-1, -2, -3, -6)	(in vitro) propagated tumor infiltrating lymphocytes (TIL) monoclonal antibodies (naked or linked to effec- tor molecules such as – toxins – enzymes for pro- drug activation)

Antigens on Tumor Cells

Classification based on origin:
– Viral antigens
– Differentiation (oncofetal) antigens
– Oncogene products

Classification based on occurrence:
– Tumor-specific antigens (TSA), not on normal cells
  * Unique (patient, tumor)
  * Shared (patients, tumor types)
– Tumor-associated antigens (TAA), also on normal cells
  * Functional specific due to anatomical barriers
  * Tumor-selective due to big differences between tumor cells and normal cells

22.2 Details

22.2.1 Human Tumor Antigens Detected by Immune Responses

Tumor type	Antigen	Classifica-tion	Immune response	References
Melanoma	glycoprotein AU	unique	serum autoantibodies	Carey et al. 1976, 1979
Melanoma	glycoprotein FD (gp95, p97) (melanotransferrin)	unique	serum autoantibodies	Real et al. 1984, 1988 Furuhawa et al. 1989
Melanoma	glycoprotein gp75, localized in melanosomes	shared	serum autoantibodies	Mattes et al. 1983 Vijayasaradhi et al. 1990 Joughton et al. 1993
Melanoma	ganglioside AH (related to GD2)	shared	serum autoantibodies	Watanabe et al. 1982
Melanomas	gangliosides GM3, GM2 (OFA-I-1) GD3, GD2 (OFA-I-2) (O-acetyl-GD3) (O-acetyl-GD2) (GT3) Neu AC-GM3 Neu GC-GM3 Neu AC-GM3 Neu GC-GM3	shared	serum auto- and allogeneic antibodies human monoclonal antibodies	Schulz et al. 1984 Tai et al. 1983, 1984 Dippold et al. 1980 Lloyd 1990, 1993 Cahan et al. 1982 Yamaguchi et al. 1987, 1990 Furuhawa et al. 1989, 1988 Usuba et al. 1988 Pukel et al. 1982
Melanomas	oncofetal protein MAGE-1, -2, -3	shared	cytotoxic autologous T-cells	van der Bruggen et al. 1991
Neuro-blastoma	gangliosides GM3, GM2, GD2	shared	serum auto- and allogeneic antibodies	Schulz et al. 1984 Lloyd 1993
Astrocytomas (gliomas)	IV3 Neu AcLcOs14Cer	shared	serum auto- and allogeneic antibodies	Traylor et al. 1980 Wilstrand et al. 1993
Breast cancer ovarian cancer	20 aa repeat of the protein core of mucin	shared	cytotoxic autol. and allogeneic T-cells (TCR mediated, but no MHC restriction)	Barnd et al. 1989 Jerome et al. 1991

Tumor type	Antigen	Classification	Immune response	References
Ovarian cancer	Her2/neu peptides	shared	cytotoxic autologous T-cells	Ioannides et al. 1991
Breast cancer ovarian cancer	Neu Ac 2–6-(Neu AC 2-3) Galβ 1–3 Ga 1NAc carbohydrate chains in polymorphic epithelial mucin (PEh)	shared	serum auto- and allogeneic antibodies cytotoxic autologous T-cells	Zotter et al. 1988 Girling et al. 1989 Taylor-Papadimitriou et al. 1993 Jerome et al. 1991 Rughetti et al. 1993
Cervical cancer	E4, E6, E7 proteins of HPV-16 or HPV-18	shared, specific	serum autoantibodies	Gissmann et al. 1993
Lymphoma nasopharyngea carcinoma	EBNA LMP1, 2A, 2B	shared, specific	serum allogeneic antibodies	Thomas et al. 1990 Falk et al. 1990 Young et al. 1989
Lymphoma	EBV antigens (EBNA-4, -6)	shared, specific	cytotoxic autologous T-cells	Richinson et al. 1981 Misko et al. 1984 Gavioli et al. 1992
T-cell leukemia	HTLV-1	shared, specific	cytotoxic autologous T-cells	Mitsaya et al. 1983
Sarcoma	unknown	unique	cytotoxic autologous T-cells	Slovin et al. 1986
Colon cancer	Ras (p21) protein (mutated 12, 61)	shared	serum autologous antibodies	Cheever et al. 1993
Colon cancer	Ras (p21) protein (mutated 12, 61)	shared, specific	CD4+ T-cell response (autologous)	Gaudernack et al. 1993
Various carcinomas	T- and Tn-antigen	shared	serum autologous antibodies cytotoxic autologous T-cells	Springer et al. 1993

22.2.2 Viruses Associated with Cancer

Type of virus	Proven	Putative	Type of cancer	Protective vaccine Established	Research
Papova viridae (DNA)					
Simian virus (SV40)	monkey	man	carcinoma	+	
Papova virus (BK, JC)		man			
Polyoma virus	mouse				
Papilloma virus (skope)	rabbit other species		carcinoma		
Papilloma virus (HPV-16, -18, -31, -39, -45)		man	carcinoma		+
Herpes viridae (DNA)					
Marek disease virus	chicken		lymphoma	+	
Herpes simplex virus		man	carcinoma		+
Epstein Barr virus	man		lymphoma carcinoma		+
HEPA DNA virus (DNA)					
Woodchuck hepatitis virus	woodchuck				
Hepatitis B	man		carcinoma	+	
Retroviridae (RNA)					
Leukemia virus (MLV)	mouse		leukemia		
Leukemia virus (FLV)	cat		leukemia	+	
Leukemia virus (BLV)	cattle		leukemia		
Leukemia virus (HTLV-I, -II)	man		leukemia		+
Immunodeficiency virus					
Immunodeficiency simian (SIV)	monkey			+	
Immunodeficiency feline (FIV)	cat				+
Immunodeficiency human (HIV-1, -2)	man		sarcoma		+
Flaviridae					
Hepatitis C		man	carcinoma		+
Adenoviridae (DNA)					
Various types	mouse other species	man	carcinoma	+	

Hilleman 1993; Gissmann et al. 1993; Masucci et al. 1993.

22.2.3 Vaccines for Prophylaxis of Virus-Induced Tumors

Type of virus	Type of cancer	Species	Type of vaccine
			Established
Simian virus (SV40)	carcinoma	hamster	irradiated SV40 tumor cells viral T-antigen (recombinant)
Marek disease virus	lymphoma	chicken	Turkey herpes virus attenuated Marek disease virus
Feline leukemia virus	leukemia	cats	whole killed virus envelope gp70 glycoprotein
Simian immunodeficiency virus	leukemia sarcoma	monkey	whole killed virus
Hepatitis B virus	carcinoma	man	HBV surface antigen (isolated from carriers or by recombinant technology)
Adenovirus	carcinoma	man (animals)	whole killed virus
			Research
Epstein Barr virus	lymphoma, carcinoma	man	gp340 isolated from cell membranes of infected cells or by recombinant techniques gp340 in viral vector systems (vaccinia, adenovirus, varicella)
Hepatitis C	carcinoma	man	envelop proteins (recombinant technology)
Papilloma virus (HPV-16, -18, -31, -39, -45)	carcinoma	man (animals)	oncoproteins E6, -E7 + structural proteins L1, L2 (recombinant technology)

Hilleman 1993; Gissmann et al. 1993; Masucci et al. 1993.

Tumors Can Attract, Activate and Suppress Macrophages by Cytokines	Tumor-derived cytokine	Biological effect on macrophages	References
	Monocyte chemotactic protein 1 (MCP-1) (tumor-derived chemotactic factor, TDCF)	chemotaxis	Bottazi et al. 1983, 1992 Zachariae et al. 1990 Rollins et al. 1991
	Monocyte colony stimulating factor (M-CSF)	chemotaxis; downregulation of oxygen-radical formation; proliferation	Wang et al. 1988 Bottazi et al.
	Granulocye-macrophage colony stimulating factor (GM-CSF)	chemotaxis; proliferation; (adhesion to endothelial cells (increase of expression of adhesion molecules on EC) and diapedesis); inhibition of cytotoxicity	Fu et al. 1992 Sotomayor et al.
	Vascular permeability factor (VPF) (vascular endothelial growth factor)	chemotaxis (angiogenesis and diapedesis)	Dvorak et al. 1991
	Protein p15E	inhibition of chemotaxis	Wang et al. 1986

22.2.4 Tumors and Infiltrating Macrophages

Function of Tumor-Associated Macrophages (TAM)	Function	Biological effect on tumors	References
	Release of TNF, IL-1, IL-6	cytotoxic for tumor cells, regulation of growth	Mantovani et al. 1986 Fidler 1985
	Antibody-dependent cellular toxicity (ADCC)	cytotoxic for tumor cells, regulation of growth	Mantovani et al. 1986
	Release of PGE_2	local and systemic suppression of T-cell and NK-cell responses	Varesio et al. 1979

Function	Biological effect on tumors	References
Release of PDGF, EGF, and/or TGF-β	stimulation of tumor cell growth	Mantovani et al. 1986
Release of angiogenic factors (FGF, others)	stimulation of neovascularization at the tumor site	Polverini et al. 1984
Lysosomal enzymes (proteases, plasminogen activator, glycosidases, lipases)	destruction of thrombi, extracellular matrix, help for invasion	Mussoni et al. 1988
Generation of tissue factor	coagulation/fibrin deposition at the tumor site	Semeraro et al. 1990
Generation of oxygen radicals	cytotoxic for tumor cells	Mahoney et al. 1987
Expression of MHC-class II	antigen presentation to stimulate immune response	Peri et al. 1986

22.2.5 Tumors and Infiltrating Lymphocytes

Tumor-Infiltrating Lymphocytes (TIL)

Histological observations indicate that mononuclear cell infiltrations are directly related to improved prognosis (Underwood 1974, Joachim 1976, Svennevig et al. 1984, Watt et al. 1978, Lauder et al. 1972, Wolf et al. 1986).

Indications also exist that TIL are mediating nonspecific rather than tumor-specific interactions (Brocker et al. 1984).

Most tumor infiltrating mononuclear cells have a T-cell phenotype (Rowe et al. 1984; Whiteside et al. 1986, 1992).

TIL isolated from human solid tumors and cultured with IL-2 were heterogenous populations of mostly MHC-unrestricted effector cells (Whiteside et al. 1989, 1992).

In melanomas, however, TIL seem to be CTL (Itoh et al. 1986, Muul et al. 1987).

TIL, grown in IL-2 and reinjected seem to have a therapeutic effect superior to LAK-cells in murine tumor systems. Therapeutic results in patients are very modest and limited mostly to melanomas (Topalian et al. 1988, Rosenberg et al. 1989).

Clinical studies to treat tumor patients with tumor infiltrating lymphocytes (TIL)

– Most clinical studies have been done in melanoma.

– Melanoma seem to be sensitive for TIL. Response rate (CR, PR) varies considerably.

– Other solid tumors are less sensitive to TIL.

Tumor	No. of patients	Complete responses	Partial responses	References
Melanoma	6	0	1	Topalian et al. 1988
	20	1	10	Rosenberg et al. 1989
	13	0	3	Kradin et al. 1989
	5	1	1	Rosenberg et al. 1990
	20	1	4	Oldham et al. 1990
	55	2	22	Aebersold et al. 1991
Kidney	4	0	1	Topalian et al. 1988
	7	0	2	Rosenberg et al. 1989
Colon	1	0	0	Topalian et al. 1988
Lung	8	0	0	Kradin et al. 1989
Breast	1	0	1	Topalian et al. 1988

22.2.6 Tumor therapy with cytokines

Many clinical studies are in progress to evaluate the therapeutic effect on solid tumors of cytokines alone or in combination.

To date, $IFN\alpha$ and IL-2 were shown to be effective.

Combination of IL-2 with cytostatics or with $IFN\alpha$ improves significantly the therapeutic effect.

Tumors sensitive for treatment with IL-2 and/or $IFN\alpha$ seem to be:
- Renal cell carcinoma   IL-2, $IFN\alpha$
- Melanoma $IFN\alpha$, $IFN\alpha$ + IL-2, $IFN\alpha$ + cytostatics
- Kaposi sarcoma $IFN\alpha$
- Insulinoma $IFN\alpha$
- Gastrointestinal tumors   IL-2 + cytostatics
- Lung tumors (NSCLC)   IL-2 + cytostatics

Therapy with IL-2, IFNα

Tumor type	Cytokine	No. of patients	Response rate Mean (%)	Range (%)
Hairy cell leukemia	IFNα	293	72	62–89
CLL	IFNα	153	51	14–63
NHL	IFNα	40	50	44–54
Kaposi's sarcoma	IFNα	295	26	3–46
Renal cancer	IFNα	361	12	0–30
Renal cancer	IL-2	60	12	5–18
Renal cancer	IL-2 + LAK	86	33	16–50
	IL-2 + TIL	20	29	
Melanoma	IFNα	291	20	11–27
Melanoma	IL-2	18	0	0
	IL-2 + LAK	83	36	19–50
	IL-2 + TIL	33	39	23–55

Compilation of data by Taylor et al. 1992; Rosenberg et al. 1987, 1988; Dorr 1993; Lotze et al. 1991.

**Therapy with IL-2,
IFN-α, IFN-γ versus
IL-4, IL-6, TNF, IFN-β**

Cytokine	Tumor	Response rate (%)	Dose-limiting toxicities	References
IL-2	renal cell carcinoma (metastatic)	15–30	capillary leak syndrome	Lotze et al. 1991
IFNα	melanoma renal cell carcinoma Kaposi'ssarcoma insulinoma	16 14 45 83		Kirkwood et al. 1991 Stahl et al. 1992 Dewit et al. 1988 Erikson et al. 1987
IFNγ gamma	renal cell carcinoma	18		Renal Cancer Study Group 1987
IL-4	renal cell carcinoma, melanoma	0	capillary leak syndrome, gastric ulceration	Lotze et al. 1992
IL-6	various advanced stages	0 (?)	fever, chills, hepatotoxicity	Weber et al. 1993
TNF	various advanced stages	≈1	capillary leak syndrome, fever, chills, nausea	Spriggs et al. 1992
IFNβ	renal cell carcinoma	0		Rinehart et al. 1986

Therapy with IL-2, IFN-α in Combination With Other Drugs

Dose	Tumor	Other drug(s)	No. of patients Total	CR	All responses (%)	References
Interleukin-2						
700 U/m^2/12h	gastro-intestinal	mitomycin	33	0	30	Arinaga et al. 1992
18x10^6 U/m^2	melanoma	dacarbazine	18	2	22	Shiloni et al. 1989
4x10^6 U/m^2	melanoma	dacarbazine + cisplatin	13	1	38	Redman et al. 1991
6x10^5 U/kg/8h	melanoma	cisplatin	27	3	26	Demchach et al. 1991
12x10^6 U/m	lung (NSCLC) head+neck	cisplatin + 5-FU	18 11	0 2	39 55	Valone et al. 1991
(1–3)x10^6 U/m	various	doxorubicin	15	0	0	Bukowski et al. 1991
20x10^6 U	various	doxorubicin	16	0	31	Paciucci et al. 1991
700 U/m^2/12h	lung (NSCLC)	TNF (25–100 µg)	16	0	7	Yang et al. 1990
700 U/m^2/12h	various	TNF (120 µg)	31	0	6	Negrier et al. 1992
7.2x10^5 U/kg	various	IL-4 (20 µg/kg)	28	1	18	Lotze 1992
5x10^6 U/m	various	IFNβ (10x10^6 U/m^2)	32	0	3	Kriegel et al. 1988
5x10^6 U/m	various	IFNβ (2x10^6 U/m^2)	50	0	4	Paolozzi et al. 1989
5x10^6 U/m	various	IFNgamma (0.25 mg/m^2)	89	2	9	Margolin et al. 1992 Taylor et al. 1992 Viens et al. 1992
5x10^6 U/m^2, other doses	renal cell carcinoma	IFN-α (various doses)	342	17	23	Stahl et al. 1992

Dose	Tumor	Other drug(s)	No. of patients Total	CR	All responses (%)	References
IFNalpha						
5×10^6 U/m^2	various	IFNγ gamma	35	0	3	Creagan et al. 1988 Osanlo et al. 1989
5×10^6 U/m^2	melanoma	IL-2 (3×10^6 U/m^2) cisplatin, dacarbazine, vinblastine	30	6	57	Legha et al. 1992
6×10^6 U/m^2	melanoma	IL-2 (1.5×10^6 U/m^2) cisplatin, dacarbazine, darmustine, tamoxifene	74	11	55	Richards et al. 1992
9×10^6 U/m^2	melanoma	IL-2 (18×10^6 U/m^2) cisplatin	20	4	60	Khayat et al. 1992
3×10^6 U/m^2	melanoma	IL-2 (18×10^6 U/m^2) cisplatin, dacarbazine	12	3	83	Hamblin et al. 1991
Various doses	melanoma	dacarbazine	203	19	27	Garbe et al. 1992

Immunomodulation by Cytokines Expressed by a Vaccinia Vector In Vivo

Tumor therapy with cytokines may in future be improved by injection of cells transduced to express cytokines. The injection of vaccinia vectors expressing cytokines already has an immune modulating effect.

Cytokine expressed by vaccinia vector	Immunomodulation after injection of vaccinia vector	References
IL-1α	none	Ruby et al. 1991
IL-2	inhibition of vaccinia infection	Ramshaw et al. 1987
IL-5	enhancement of IgA response	Ruby et al. 1992
IL-6	enhancement of IgG1 response	Ruby et al. 1992
TNFα	inhibition of vaccinia infection	Sambhi et al. 1991
IFNα	inhibition of vaccinia infection	Kohonen Corish et al. 1990 Giavedoni et al. 1992

Tumor Cells Transduced to Express Cytokines Can Loose Tumorigenicity and Gain Immunogenicity

Cytokine expressed by vector	Transduced cell (vector)	Species treated	Route of application of transduced cells	Biological effect	References
IL-2	adenocarcinoma kidney carcinoma Mu-myeloma (X63) (RV-based vector) mouse fibrosarcoma (RV-based vector)	mouse	s.c.	immunogenicity + tumorigenicity –	Bash et al. 1993 Golumbek et al. 1991 Bubenik et al. 1991 Patel et al. 1992
IL-4	Mu-myeloma (X63) (RV-based vector) mouse fibrosarcoma (RV-based vector)	mouse	s.c. s.c.	immunogenicity Ø immunogenicity + tumorigenicity –	Bubenik et al. 1991 Tepper et al. 1989 Patel et al. 1992
G-CSF	Mu-adenocarcinoma (C-26)	mouse	s.c.	tumorigenicity – immunogenicity +	Colombo et al. 1991
IFN gamma	Mu-neuroblastoma (C1300) Mu-fibrosarcoma (CMS-5) Mu-adenocarcinoma (SP1)	mouse mouse mouse	s.c s.c. s.c.	tumorigenicity – immunogenicity + immunogenicity + immunogenicity +	Watanabe et al. 1989 Restifo et al. 1992 Gansbacher et al. 1990 Esumi et al. 1991
GM-CSF	adenocarcinoma	mouse	s.c.	immunogenicity +	Colombo et al. 1991
TNF alpha	Mu-sarcoma (MCA 205) Mu-plasmacytoma (J 558 L)	mouse	s.c. s.c.	immunogenicity + tumorigenicity – immunogenicity + tumorigenicity –	Asher et al. 1991 Blankenstein et al.1991

Therapy with Cells Transduced to Express Cytokines

Genes coding for	Cells transduced	Disease treated	Investigators (location)
TNF	TIL	melanoma	NIH (Rosenberg et al.)
TNF	tumor cells	solid tumors	NIH (Rosenberg et al.)
IL-2	TIL	solid tumors	NIH (Rosenberg et al.)
IL-2	neuroblastoma	brain tumors	Memphis (Brenner et al.)
IL-2	TIL	melanoma, kidney cancer	New York (Gilboa)
IL-4	TIL	solid tumors	Pittsburg (Lotze et al.)

22.2.7 Active Specific with "Tumor Vaccines"

Historical Approaches for Tumor Immuno-therapy in Man

Year	Kind of treatment	References
1902	autologous tumor cells	von Leiden et al.
1909	tumor cell homogenate	von Dungern
1911	extract from tumor tissue (autologous, allogenic)	Risley
1913	phenol treated tumor cells	Pinkuss
1922	tumor fragments (autologous)	Kellock et al.
1960	tumor homogenate, suspended in CFA	Finney et al.
1967	tumor cells covalently coated with rabbit IgG	Czajkowski et al.
1970	tumor extract, suspended in Bordetella pertussis vaccine or CFA	Hughes et al.
1971	tumor cells, irradiated	Currie et al.

Each trial stimulated numerous similar studies. No approach resulted in a significant, reproducable tumor therapeutic effect.

**Present Approaches
for Active Specific
Immunotherapy with
Tumor Vaccines**

Tumor	Kind of vaccine	Specific immune response		Efficacy	References
		Cellular	Humoral		

Autologous tumor cells

Tumor	Kind of vaccine	Cellular	Humoral	Efficacy	References
Melanoma (human)	dinitrophenyl conjugated to autologous irradiated tumor cells mixed with BCG + low dose cyclophosphamide	DTH CTL T-cell infil.	–	case reports: inflammation at the tumor site tumor regression in stage IV patients	Berd et al. 1993
Melanoma	autologous, irradiated tumor cells, treated in vitro with IFN gamma	DTH	–	case reports: local tumor regression	Wiseman et al. 1993
Colon carcinoma Duke C (human)	Newcastle disease virus infected autologous carcinoma cells irradiated	DTH	antibody	pilot study with matched control group: recurrence in 61% of patients, compared to 87% in control group	Schirrmacher et al. 1993 Liebrich et al. 1991
Colorectal carcinoma Duke C (human)	irradiated, autologous carcinoma cells mixed with BCG	DTH	–	prospective controlled study: no significant increase in survival	Hanna et al. 1993
Renal cancer	autologous, irradiated tumor cells + BCG	DTH	–	prospective controlled study: interim analysis: no significant increase in survival	Galligioni et al. 1993

Tumor	Kind of vaccine	Specific immune response		Efficacy	References
		Cellular	Humoral		

Allogeneic tumor cells: in mixture with immunostimulants

Tumor	Kind of vaccine	Cellular	Humoral	Efficacy	References
Melanoma (human)	three allogeneic irradiated melanoma cell lines (M10, M24, M101) expressing gangliosides (GM2, BD2, 0-acetyl GD3) glycoprotein (fetal Ag 69,5 kD, urine Ag 90 kD) and lipoprotein (M-TAA 180 kD) mixed with BCG + low dose cyclophosphamide	CTL DTH	IgG and IGM response and 0-ace tylated GD3	case reports, historical controls: increase in survival of stage IV patients ($<0,001$) median survival: control: 7,5 months treated: 23,1 months rate of 5 year survival: control: 6% treated: 26%	Ravindranath et al. 1989 Morton et al. 1993
Colon carcinoma (human)	Delta cell mixed with vibrio cholera neuraminidase (checker board vaccination)	DTH		prospective controlled study: increase in remission free survival	Rainer et al. 1981
				prospective controlled study: no therapeutic effect (62 patients)	Ulsperger et al. 1993

Allogeneic tumor cells: tumor cell lysates

Tumor	Kind of vaccine	Cellular	Humoral	Efficacy	References
Melanoma (human)	lysate after vaccinia virus infection of 4 melanoma cell lines (concentrated by ultracentrifugation)	DTH	antibodies	case reports: 50% response rate (48 patients stage I,II)	Wallack et al. 1986 Wallack et al. 1993
Melanoma (human)	lysate after vaccinia virus infection of melanoma cell line (supernatant after ultracentrifugation) + low dose cyclophosphamide	–	–	case reports: increase of survival (3x > historical controls)	Wallack et al. 1986 Hersey et al. 1993

Tumor	Kind of vaccine	Specific immune response		Efficacy	References
		Cellular	Humoral		
Melanoma (human)	homogenized (mechanically + freeze/thawing) allogeneic melanoma cell lines (M-1, M-2) mixed with Detox (monophosphoryl lipid A cell wall skeleton (*Mycobacterium phlei*) squalane oil and Tween 80)	CTL	anti-bodies	case reports: (historical and non-randomized control) 5% complete response 15% partial response (of 106 patients)	Mitchell et al. 1993

Allogeneic tumor cells: transfected cells

Tumor	Kind of vaccine	Cellular	Humoral	Efficacy	References
Cervical carcinoma (human)	transformed cells expressing HPV 16-E6 or E7 antigens	CTL (murine)	–	protection by transfer of specific CTL (murine)	Chen et al. 1991, 1992 Zhou et al. 1991 Meneguzzi et al. 1991
Breast carcinoma ovarian carcinoma (human)	B-cell lines (EBV), transfected with mucin (muc 1) expression vector and treated with phenyl-Ga1NAc to inhibit 0-linked glycosylation (truncated mucin expression)	CTL (in vitro)	–	–	Magarian-Blander et al. 1993
Breast carcinoma (murine)	mammary carcinoma cell line transfected with PEM expressing gene	–	–	protection against tumor challenge	Taylor-Papadimitriou et al. 1993
Melanoma (murine)	B7 transfected into tumor cells	–	–	tumorigenicity: reduced therapeutic effect: regression of established tumors	Townsend et al. 1993 Hellström et al. 1993 Razi-Wolf et al. 1992 Gimmi et al. 1991 Baskar et al. 1993 Ramarathinam et al. 1994
Sarcoma (murine)	syngeneic MHC-class II transfected into MHC-class II negative tumor cell	–	–	tumorigenicity: reduced	Ostrand-Rosenberg 1990

Tumor	Kind of vaccine	Specific immune response		Efficacy	References
		Cellular	Humoral		
Line 1 (murine)	highly tumorigenic Line 1 transfected to express IFNγ gamma and IL-2	CTL		tumorigenicity: reduced protection best with IFN gamma + IL-2 producing cell	McAdam et al. 1993
Plasmacytoma (murine)	plasmacytoma cell line transfected to produce IL-2, IL-4, IL-7, TNF or IFNγ gamma (murine system)	CD4+ T-cells (IL-7)	increase in CD4+ T-cells (IL-7)	protection by all cell lines, combinations of cell lines or single cell lines not superior to mixture of untransfected cell line + killed corynebacterium parvum	Hock et al. 1991, 1993
Melanoma (murine)	melanoma cell line (B16) transfected to produce IL-2, IL-4, IL-5, IL-6, GM-CSF, IFNγ gamma, IL-1RA, TNF, ICAM	–	–	tumorigenicity: only IL-2 transfected cells were completely rejected protection: only GM-CSF secreting cells were sufficiently effective	Dranoff et al. 1993
B-cell lymphoma (murine)	tumor cells transfected to produce IL-4 (murine)	–	–	reduced tumorigenicity	Tepper et al. 1989
Kidney carcinoma (murine)	tumor cells transfected to produce IL-2 (murine)	CTL	–	regression of established tumors	Golumbek et al. 1991
Neuroblastoma (murine)	tumor cells transfected to produce IFNγ gamma (murine)	CTL	–	reduced tumorigenicity	Watanabe et al. 1989
Sarcoma (murine)	tumor cells transfected to produce IFNγ gamma (murine)	CTL	–	–	Restifo et al. 1992
Adeno carcinoma (murine)	tumor cells transfected to produce GM-CSF	CTL	–	tumorigenicity: reduced	Colombo et al. 1991
Colon adeno carcinoma (murine)	tumor cells transfected with a vaccinia vector inserted with IL-2 gene (murine)	–	–	protection against tumor challenge	Bash 1993

Tumor	Kind of vaccine	Specific immune response		Efficacy	References
		Cellular	Humoral		
Lung carcinoma (murine)	tumor cells transfected to release IL-2, IL-6 or IFNγ gamma	CTL	–	tumorigenicity: reduced (no correlation with depletion of CD4+ T-cells) therapy: no effect with IL-2, IL-6, therapeutic effect with IFNγ gamma (no correlation with MHC-class I expression)	Porgador et al. 1993

Purified natural or synthesized tumor-associated antigens

Tumor	Kind of vaccine	Cellular	Humoral	Efficacy	References
Melanoma (human)	shed antigens from 4 melanoma cell lines (concentrated by ultracentrifugation)	CTL DTH	antibodies	case reports: increase of survival > 50% of historical controls	Bystryn 1993
Colon carcinoma (human)	TAA 32 kD of colon carcinoma cells	DTH		–	Hanna et al. 1993
Carcinoma (pancreas, colon, lung, others) (human)	synthetic peptide 5-16 of p21-Ras protein (position 12 = arginine)	CTL (murine)	–	–	Cheever et al. 1993 Jung et al. 1991
Breast carcinoma (human)	T/Tn antigen, isolated from 0 red blood cells absorbed to Ca3 (PO4) + 0,5 U typhoid vaccine	DTH	antibody	case reports: survival of 16 pat. (stage IV) > 5 years	Springer et al. 1993
Breast carcinoma (human)	synthetic sialyl-Tn-KLH (NANA α (2–6) GalNAc α-0-crotyl-KLH) mixed with monophosphoryl-lipid A and cell wall skeleton from *Mycobacterium phlei* (DeTox)	–	specific antibodies (IgM, IgG)	case reports: 17% partial response (12 pat.)	Longenecker et al. 1993 Fung et al. 1990

| Tumor | Kind of vaccine | Specific immune response | | Efficacy | References |
		Cellular	Humoral		
Melanoma (human)	GM1, GM2, GM3, GD2, GD3 adherent to salm. Minnesota	–	anti-bodies (IgM)	–	Livingston et al. 1989
Melanoma (human)	GM2 adherent to BCG + low dose of cyclophosphamide	–	anti-bodies (IgM)	–	Livingston 1993 Hamilton et al. 1993
Melanoma (human)	GM2 linked to KLH + adjuvant QS21	–	antibodies (IgM + IgG1)	–	Helling et al. 1993, 1994
Lung and colon carcinoma (human)	aa 109–145 of β-subunit of HCG, conjugated to diphtheria toxin, mixed with MDP + squalene/mannide monooleate	–	antibody (murine)	–	Triozzi et al. 1993
Melanoma (human)	GD3 incorporated into proteosomes, formed by outer membrane proteins from *Neisseria gonorrhoeae*	–	antibodies IgM + IgG1 (murine)	–	Livingston et al. 1993
Cervix carcinoma (human)	HPV-16 polio chimeric vaccine	in work	–	–	Gruber et al. 1993
Hepato carcinoma (human)	recombinant HCV S protein		–	–	Hilleman 1993
Breast carcinoma ovarian carcinoma pancreatic carcinoma (human)	24 aa peptide of epithelial mucin tandem repeat of polymorphic epithelial mucin 1 (PEM)	–	lymphocyte transformation (murine)	–	Taylor-Papadimitrou et al. 1993
Lymphoma nasopharyngeal carcinoma Hodgkin (human)	recombinant EBV gp	–	–	–	Hilleman 1993

Tumor	Kind of vaccine	Specific immune response		Efficacy	References
		Cellular	Humoral		
Cervical carcinoma (human)	immune stimulating complex (ISCOM), containing HPV 16-E6 or E7	–	–	–	McLean et al. 1993
Acute and chronic myelo- (human)	joining region of the *bcr-abl* chimeric fusion protein (210 kD)	CTL (murine)	–	–	Cheever et al. 1993 Chen et al. 1992, 1993

Vectors expressing tumor-associated antigens

Tumor	Kind of vaccine	Cellular	Humoral	Efficacy	References
Cervical carcinoma	vaccinia virus, expressing HPV 16-E6 or E7	–	–	–	Chen et al. 1992
Cervix carcinoma (human)	HPV-16 L1, L2, E2, E6, E7 genes inserted into listeria monocytogenes vector	–	–	–	Gruber et al. 1993
Cervix carcinoma (human)	HPV-16 L1 inserted into baculovirus vector	–	no specific antibodies	–	Gruber et al. 1993
AIDS	HIV-I *env* peptide in canary pox virus vector (Alvac)	CTL	–	–	Paoletti et al. 1993
Breast, lung colon (human)	p53 gene inserted into vaccinia virus vector	–	–	–	Ronen et al. 1992
Mammary carcinoma (murine)	MUC-1 gene coding for PEM inserted into vaccinia virus vector	–	–	protection against tumor challenge	Taylor-Papadimitriou et al. 1993
Melanoma (human)	p97 gene inserted into vaccinia virus vector	CTL (murine)	antibodies (murine)	protection against tumor challenge (mice) (monkeys)	Hu et al. 1988 Estin et al. 1988
Colon (human)	CEA gene inserted into vaccinia virus vector	CTL	antibodies (murine)	protection against tumor challenge (mice) immunogenicity (monkey)	Kaufman et al. 1991 Kantor et al. 1992, 1993

Tumor	Kind of vaccine	Immunogenicity		Efficacy in vivo	References
		In vitro	In vivo		
Breast (human)	epithelial tumor antigen (ETA) inserted into vaccinia virus vector	–	antibodies (rats)	protection against ETA positive *ras* transformed tumor cells (rats)	Harenveni et al. 1990
Breast (human)	human *HER2-neu* inserted into vaccinia virus vector	–	–	protection against human *HER2-neu* transfected tumor cells, but not against tumors expressing murine *HER2-neu*	Bernards et al. 1987

Antiidiotype antibodies mimicing tumor-associated antigens

Tumor	Kind of vaccine	Immunogenicity		Efficacy in vivo	References
		In vitro	In vivo		
Colon carcinoma (human)	antiidiotype MAb mimicing gp37 (Ab 1: 791 T/36) + Al(OH)3	lymphocyte proliferation		case reports: indication for increase in survival (6 of 12 patients)	Durrant et al. 1993
Colon carcinoma (human)	antiidiotype MAb mimicing CEA (Ab 1: T84.66)	–	antibody (rabbit)	–	Gaida et al. 1992
Colon carcinoma	MAB 17-1A	DTH	antiidiotype antibodies	case reports: 3 of 10 patients with complete responses	Fagerberg et al. 1993
Melanoma	antiidiotype antibodies mimicing GD2	cellular CTL	–	–	Morton et al. 1993
Melanoma	antiidiotype antibodies mimicing GM3	CTL	–	–	Morton et al. 1993
Melanoma	antiidiotype antibodies mimicing melanoma antigen 225.28	–	anti-antiidiotype antibodies	case reports: 1 complete response in 21 patients	Ferrone 1993
Hodgkin lymphoma	antiidiotype MAb mimicing CD30 antigen	–	antibodies	–	Renner et al. 1993
B-cell lymphoma	idiotype (BCR) GM-CSF fusion protein	–	antibodies	–	Tao et al. 1993

Tumor	Kind of vaccine	Immunogenicity In vitro	In vivo	Efficacy in vivo	References
T-cell lymphoma	antiidiotype antibodies (TCR)	DTH	antibody	case reports: complete responses in 2/4 patients	Chatterjee et al. 1993
B-cell lymphoma	antiidiotype antibodies (BCR) linked to key hole limpet hemocyanin in squalene and MDP	DTH	antibody	case reports: increase of time of remission free survival (8/8)	Hsu et al. 1993
B-cell lymphoma	vectors expressing idiotype (BCR)	–	–	–	Stevenson et al. 1994

New Adjuvant Formulations Used in Human Trials

Standard:
– Al(OH)$_3$ (= alhydrogel)

Under investigation*):
– Squalene in water dispersion stabilized with polysorbate 80 (Tween 80) and containing monophosphoryl lipid A.
– Liposomes containing dimyristoyl phosphatidylcholine, dimyristoyl phosphatidylglycerol, cholesterol, monophosphoryl lipid A. Liposomes are absorbed to Al(OH)$_3$.
– Squalene in water microfluidized emulsion stabilized with polysorbate 80 and sorbitan trioleate (MF59).
– MF59 also containing muramyltripeptide-phosphatidyl ethanolamine.
– Squalene in water microfluidized emulsion stabilized with polysorbate 80 and containing a nonionic block copolymer (L121) (SAF-M).
– SAF-M emulsion also containing threonyl muramyldipeptide.

*) Approved by the FDA-USA for clinical research of vaccines (HIV, others)

Alving et al. 1993.

22.2.8 Mechanisms by Which Tumor Cells Become "Immune Resistant"

Inhibition of the afferent pathway of immune response
- Release of tumor antigens; neutralisation of TCR (CD4+ T-cells) and BCR (review Sedlacek 1995)
- Increased expression of MHC-class II molecules (Eliott et al. 1989, Ruiz-Cabello et al. 1991, McDougall et al. 1994) no expression of B7 molecules (Hellström et al. 1993)
- Monostimulation of CD4+ T-cells, anergy and apoptosis of T-cells (Jenkins et al. 1991, Harding et al. 1992, Lenschow et al. 1993).
- Release of TGFβ, immunosuppression (Fargeas et al. 1992, Machold et al. 1993, Dupuy D'Angeac et al. 1991, Lord et al. 1993)
- Release of PGE2, stimulated by IL-1 and TNFα (Merluzzi et al. 1987), suppression of helper T-cells to secrete IL-2 and IFNgamma suppression of NK-cells (Uotila 1993)

Inhibition of the efferent pathway of immune response
- Change of epitope pattern of tumor-associated antigen (Ernst et al. 1986; Frankel et al. 1985; Knuth et al. 1989, 1991; Masucci et al. 1993)
- Release of tumor antigen, neutralisation of TCR (CD8+ T-cells) and antibodies
- Immune complex formation; suppression of B-cells by cross-linking BCR and Fc-receptors (Kalsi 1991)
- Downregulation or abnormal expression of MHC-class I molecules (Möller et al. 1987, 1991, 1992; Ottesen et al.1987; Tomita et al. 1990; Loncha et al. 1991; Cordon Cardo et al. 1991; Pantel et al. 1991; Hui et al. 1991; Wintzer et al. 1990)
- Downregulation of expression of ICAM-1 (Johnson et al. 1989, Gregory et al. 1988, Masucci et al. 1993, Murphy et al. 1993)
- Expression of inhibitors for complement factors and for membrane attack complex (MAC) formation (Parker 1992, Morgan et al. 1991, Porcel 1992, Agostin et al. 1992)
- Shedding, pinocytosis and degradation of MAC (Morgan et al. 1988, 1992)
- Release of proteases like Cathepsin B, D, L, collagenases I, II, IV, uPA, elastase (Burtin et al. 1984, Schmitt et al. 1992, Monsky et al. 1993, Schultz et al. 1994, Kao et al. 1986, Denhardt et al. 1987);
  Malignancy and metastatic potential closely correlates with the degree of enzyme release (Denhardt et al. 1987, Kane et al. 1989, Kwaan 1992); growth factors (IL-1, IL-6, TGFβ, TNFα) can stimulate tumor cells to an enhanced secretion of proteases (Brown et al. 1990, Collart et al. 1985, Monsky et al. 1993); tumor cells can express cytokines and growth factors (Krasagakis et al. 1993);
  Tumor cells express surface receptors for collagenases and uPA (Emonard et al. 1992, Moll et al. 1990, Zucker et al. 1990);
- Degradation of antibodies into Fab and Fc-fragments (Hamilton 1987, Shakib et al. 1980, Spiegelberg 1974); neutralisation of antigens and Fc-receptors (Sedlacek et al. 1979, 1987; Weissbarth et al. 1979; Debre et al. 1993).

Tumor cells can escape the control of the immune response by prostaglandin secretion:

— Tumor cells can form and release PGE2. Formation by tumor cells is stimulated by IL-1α, IL-1β, TNFα and histamine (Last-Barney et al. 1988, Merluzzi et al. 1987).
— PGE2 increases the level of cAMP (Goodwin et al. 1979), which leads to inhibition of:
  * Helper T-cells by:
    – inhibition of formation and expression of IL-2 and IL-2-rec. (Rappaport et al. 1982, Krause et al. 1991, Mary et al. 1987).
    – Decrease of formation of IFNgamma (Phipps et al. 1991)
  * Macrophages/monocytes by:
    – Inhibition of secretion of TNFα (Kunkel et al. 1988, Strieter et al. 1990)
  * NK-cells by:
    – Inhibition of binding to tumor cells (Goto et al. 1983, Ramstedt et al. 1985)
— PGE2 secretion by tumor cells is inhibited by inhibitors of cyclooxygenase indomethacin (Goodwin 1985).
— Inhibition of cyclooxygenase concomitantly leads to an enhanced production of leukotrienes. Leukotriene B_4 is chemotactic for leukocytes. Activated neutrophils can stimulate NK-cells (Samuelson 1983, Yang et al. 1984).
— In addition to PGE2, histamine may promote tumor growth.
  Histamine via binding to H_2 receptors (Dohlsten et al. 1987; Khan et al. 1985) can increase the level of cAMP, which leads to inhibition of:
  * Helper T-cells by inhibition of formation and expression of IL-2, IL-2-rec. and IFNgamma (Dohlsten et al. 1989; Khan et al. 1985)
  * Secretion of TNFα by macrophages/monocytes (Hotermans et al. 1991, Strieter et al. 1990)

Tumor Cells Can Suppress the Immune Response by Secretion of Prostaglandin E$_2$

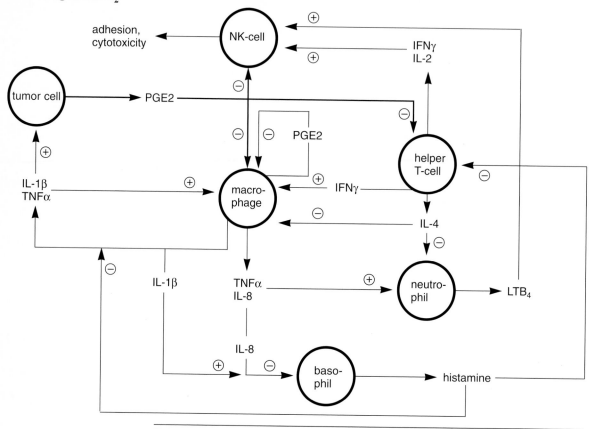

Uctila 1993, Falus et al. 1992, Ijzemans et al. 1989.

Role of MHC-class I on Tumor Cells and their Susceptibility to Cytotoxic Attack:

- CTL are specific for tumor-associated peptides presented by MHC-class I (murine P815).

  Lurguin et al. 1989

- MAb anti MHC-class I block CTL against.
  * All allogeneic human tumors
  * Only some autologous tumors

  Slovin et al. 1986
  Vanky et al. 1987

- IFN-α/γ induces MHC-class I in MHC-class I negative autologous tumor cells:
  * Increase CTL-mediated lysis
  * Can be blocked by MAb anti MHC-class I

  Vanky et al. 1989

– In melanoma CTL can lyze autologous tumors and   Darrow et al. 1989
  allogeneic tumors with shared MHC-class I. Lysis
  can be blocked by MAb anti MHC-class I.

– CTL, isolated from tumor infiltrating lymphocytes,   Itoh et al. 1988
  lyse autologous tumor cells.

– Lack of MHC-class I expression is correlated with low   Kärre et al. 1986
  or no CTL-mediated and high NK-mediated lysis;   Sturmhöfel et al. 1990
  IFN-treatment increases CTL and reduces NK cytolysis.

– Loss of MHC-class I expression is correlated with
  malignancy:
  * In B-cell lymphoma   Möller et al. 1987
  * In carcinomas   Ottesen et al. 1987
                                                          Tomita et al. 1990
                                                          Concha et al. 1991

– Loss of MHC-class I does not correlate with malignancy:
  * In carcinomas   Möller et al. 1991
                                                          Wintzer et al. 1990

Changes in Expression of MHC-I and MHC-II Antigens on Human Tumors (Primaries and Metastatic Nodules)	Expression level (% of positive tumors) of	
	MHC-I	MHC-II
Breast carcinoma	25–73	30
Ductal	47	27
Medullary	100	100
Lobular	22	33
Other	33	33
Metastatic nodules	5	
Benign lesions	100	100
Colorectal carcinoma	72–86	36–56
Mucinous	25	25
Nonmucinous	100	100
Adenoma	100	100
Metastatic nodules	50	
Gastric carcinoma	90	53
Endometrial carcinoma	50	25
Bronchial carcinoma	68	15
SCLC	0	0
NSCLC	72	?
Larynx carcinomas	80	12
Melanoma	72–90	25–56
B-cell lymphoma	56	?
Skin basaliomas	50	0
Neuroblastoma	20	10
Bladder carcinoma	67	
Metastatic nodules	0	
Renal carcinoma	100	
Metastatic nodules	40	
Corresponding normal tissues	≈100% (majority)	≈0% (exceptions: lymphoid tissues, areas of gastric and respiratory tract)

Eliott et al. 1989; Cordon-Cardo et al. 1991; Ruiz-Cabello et al. 1991; McDougall et al. 1990.

Mechanism of Abnormal Expression of MHC-Class I/β_2m	Downregulation	amplification of N-*myc* in neuroblastoma amplification of c-myc – in melanoma – in bronchial carcinoma	Versteeg et al. 1990 Versteeg et al. 1988 Marley et al. 1989
	Lack of β_2m expression	lack of β_2m translation after EBV-infection spontaneous loss of β_2m transcription – in colon carcinoma – in melanoma	Rosa et al. 1983 Momburg et al. 1989 D'Urso et al. 1991
	Defective assembly of MHC-class I and β_2m	lack of assembly in response to defect in supply of peptides into endoplasmic reticulum (ER) in B-cell leukaemia	DeMars et al. 1984
		deletions in transporter genes, responsible for transport of peptides from cytosol to ER	Deverson et al. 1990 Spies et al. 1990
		defect in assembly of MHC-class I and β_2m	Klar et al. 1989

22.2.9 Passive Therapy with Antibody Preparations

	Year	Reference	Preparation	Source	Specificity
Historical Approaches for Tumor Immuno-therapy in Man	1895	Hericourt and Richet	antisera	dogs, monkeys	immunized with espective tumor
	1901	Boeri	antisera	goat	immunized with respective tumor
	1958	Murray	IgG	horses	immunized with respective tumor
	1959	Buinauskas et al.	IgG	sheep	immunized with respective tumor
	1960	Sumner and Foraker	whole blood	man	patients with same type of tumor in regression
	1968	Laszlo et al.	sera	man	isoantibodies against lymphocytes (CLL)

	References	MAb	Disease	Response
Monoclonal Antibodies Specific for Leukemia-Associated Antigens Seem to Have a Therapeutic Effect	Miller et al. 1985, 1989	anti-idiotypic	B-cell lymphoma	1/13 CR
	Meeker et al. 1985			6/12 MR
	Garcia et al. 1985	anti-idiotypic	B-cell lymphoma	1/10 CR
				5/10 PR
	Rankin et al. 1985	anti-idiotypic	B-cell lymphoma	2/2 MR
	Hamblin et al. 1987	anti-idiotypic (chimeric)	follicular lymphoma	1/1 PR
	Bertram et al. 1986	T101	CTCL	1/8 CR
				1/8 PR
	Dillmann et al. 1986	T101	CTCL	4/10 MR
	Dillmann et al. 1986	T101	CLL	2/6 MR
	Miller et al. 1983	anti T-cell	CTCL	5/7 MR
	Ritz et al. 1981	anti CALLA	ALL	no response

CR, Complete response; PR, partial response (tumor reduction > 50%); MR, mixed response (tumor reduction < 50%), CTCL, chronic T-cell leukemia; CLL, chronic lymphatic leukemia; ALL, acute lymphatic leukemia; CALLA, common acute lymphatic leukemia antigen.

Most clinical studies with "naked" monoclonal antibodies specific for tumor-associated antigens do not seem to have a therapeutic effect on solid tumors.

Tumor	Summary of clinical data response rate (%)		
	Complete	Partial	Minimal
Colon carcinoma	0–10	0	0–20
Melanoma	0–10	0–20	0–20
Pancreatic carcinoma	0	0	0–8

Review Sedlacek et al. 1988, 1992.

Minimal residual diseases, however, might successfully be treated with monoclonal antibodies.

Colon carcinoma (Stage III) after surgery	n	Tumor-free after 5 years	Significance
Control group (untreated)	82	28	
Group treated with 900 mg MAb 17-1A	84	46	$(p = 0.002)$
Reduction in mortality rate		39%	

Schneider-Gädicke et al. 1993

The reduction in mortality rate in colon carcinoma induced by MAb (17-IA) is in the same range as the therapeutic effect of the combination of levamisole and 5-fluorouracil in stage III colon carcinoma (reduction in mortality rate compared to untreated control group 33%) (Riethmüller et al. 1993, Moertel et al. 1990).

22.2.10 Targeting Drugs with Monoclonal Antibodies to Malignant Cells

Historical Approaches for Tumor Immunotherapy in Man

Year	Author	
Proposals		
1900	Ehrlich	"magic bullet"
1948	Pressman and Keighley	antibodies as carriers for cytostatics and radionuclides
Experiments		
1951	Beierwaltes	131I-labeled antibodies for treatment of human melanoblastoma
1953	Pressman and Korngold	131I-labelled antibodies for detection of rat tumors
1958	Mathé et al.	aminopterin-conjugated antibodies for treatment of L1210 leukemia
1972	Ghose et al.	chlorambucil-conjugated antibodies for treatment of human melanoma

Stages of Action of an Immunotoxin

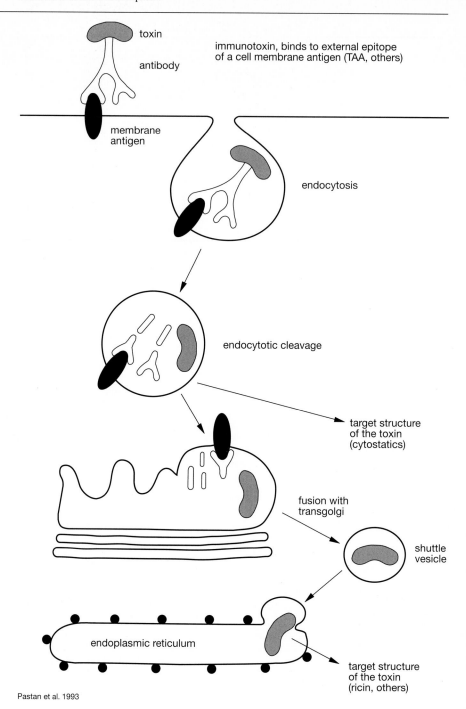

toxin

antibody

immunotoxin, binds to external epitope of a cell membrane antigen (TAA, others)

membrane antigen

endocytosis

endocytotic cleavage

target structure of the toxin (cytostatics)

fusion with transgolgi

shuttle vesicle

endoplasmic reticulum

target structure of the toxin (ricin, others)

Pastan et al. 1993

Clinical trials for systemic treatment of solid tumors with immunotoxins or immunoconjugates could not show any significant benefit for the patients but toxicities. The main reason for this failure is the low localisation rate of the antibody (in the average ≤0,01% of the given MAb/g tumor). Due to the low localisation rate the concentration of the immunotoxin or immunoconjugate at the tumor site is too low to eradicate the tumor. On the other hand, > 99% of the given immunotoxin localizes in normal tissues and causes toxicities. In consequence, there exists no therapeutic dose range (Sedlacek et al. 1992).

Tumor	Toxin-linked to Tu-MAb	CR	PR	MR	n	Dose-limiting toxicities	References
Melanoma	ricin A	0	0	0	22 46 6	hepatotoxicity edema weight gain	Spitler et al. 1987, 1988 Byers et al. 1989
Colon carcinoma	ricin A	0	0	0	17 7	hepatotoxicity edema neuropathy	Byers et al. 1989 Spitler et al. 1988
	ytrium 90	0	0	0	27	myelotoxicity	Haller et al. 1991
	neocarcino-statin	0	0	3	41	–	Takahashi et al. 1988
	vindesine	0	0	0	24	gastrointestinal toxicity	Rybak et al. 1991
	pseudomonas exotoxin	0	0	0	12	hepato toxicity	Rybak et al. 1991
Breast carcinoma	ricin A	0	0	0		hepatotoxicity edema, weight gain, neuropathy	Goud et al. 1989 Weiner et al. 1989
Various	mitomycin doxorubicin	0 0	0 0	0 0	43	thrombocytopenia anemia	Oldham et al. 1984 Oldham et al. 1984

CR, Complete response; PR, partial response; MR, minimal response; n, number of patients.

In contrast to solid tumors clinical studies in leukemias show that immunotoxins may have a therapeutic effect. Leukemic cells in blood and lymphoid organs can be reached by MAb and immunotoxins much better than cells within a solid tumor. This better accessibility of leukemic cells for MAbs and immunotoxins gives immunotoxins a chance to localize to leukemic cells to a degree sufficient to kill them. This therapeutic effect can be seen when the minimal toxic dose of the immunotoxin is applied.

Leukemia	Toxin-linked to Tu-MAb	CR	PR	MR	*n*	Dose-limiting toxicities	References
B-CLL	ricin A	0	0	0	5	–	Hertler et al. 1989
CLL	ricin A	0	0	0	4	–	Hertler et al. 1989
T-ALL	ricin A	0	0	1	6	–	Laurent et al. 1988
B-CLL B-ALL	ricin A	1	2	10	25	hepatotoxicity	Nadler et al. 1990
B-CLL B-ALL	ricin A	1	3	4	18	hepatotoxicity	Nadler et al. 1990
C-CLL	ricin A	2	4	10	36	hepatotoxicity thrombocytopenia edema	Blattler et al. 1991
B-Lymphoma	iodine-131	0	2	2	5	–	Goldenberg et al. 1991

CR, complete response; PR, partial response; MR, minimal response; *n*, number of patients.

22.2.11 Reasons for the Limited Success of Antibodies

Tumor cell
– Lack of tumor-specific antigen

– Low degree of expression of tumor antigens
  * Low amount per cell
  * Steric hindrance
  * Masking of antigens

– Qualitative and quantitative variation in the expression of antigens

– Release (shedding) of antigens and peripheral neutralization of antitumoral antibodies

– Release of proteases and degradation of antibodies

– Blockage of Fc-receptors of ADCC cells by shedded immune complexes or by Fc fragments arising through cleavage of antibodies by expressed proteases

– Inhibition of MAC formation by tumor cell associated inhibitors of complement; shedding and/or pinocytosis and degradation of MACs formed

Antibodies
– Insufficient specificity, affinity and quantity

– Insufficient potency to induce effector mechanisms for cytolysis (complement activation; ADCC)

Host
– Mechanical barrier limiting contact of tumor cells with antibodies

– Impaired convection and diffusion into tumor tissue due to high interstitial hydraulic and osmotic pressure inside the tumor

– Insufficient vascularization of or shunts and sinusoids in the tumor

– Absorption and enzymatic degradation of antibodies in lung, liver, spleen

– Qualitative or quantitative insufficiency of the complement system and/or ADCC cells

– Induction of immunosuppressive mechanisms by the antibodies

Sedlacek et al. 1988

Inhibition of antibody binding to the tumor cell and inhibition of complement dependent cytolysis by the tumor cell may be crucial factors why most antibodies are less effective in tumor therapy.

Modulation of antigens	decrease of the number or density of membrane antigens in response to antibody binding by internalization of the antigen-antibody complex	Gordon et al. 1981
Blockage of tumor antigens	cleavage of antibodies into (antigen binding) F(ab')2 and Fab fragments within the tumor tissue	Ran et al. 1970
Blockage of antibodies	shedding of tumor antigens by tumor cells	Nordquist et al. 1977 Steplewski et al. 1981
Blockage of ADCC	shedding of immune complexes and saturation of Fc-receptors	Baldwin et al. 1972
Blockage of complement mediated lysis by		
– Inhibition of C3/C5 convertase	decay accelerating factor (DAF) in the membrane of tumor cells	Cheung et al. 1988
– Proteolytic cleavage of C3b	protease p65 in the membrane of tumor cells	Ollert et al. 1990 Panneerselvam et al. 1986, 1987
	protease FI sensitized by plasma factor FH after its binding to surface bound C3b	Vogel 1991 Newman et al. 1985
	cofactor activity of CR1, CR2, and MCP	Vogel 1991 Dierich et al. 1988
– Restriction of the lytic complex C5b6789	restriction factor for cell lysis blocks homologous C8	Schönermark et al. 1986 Zalman et al. 1986
	CD59 and homologous proteins inhibit the lytic complex Holguin et al. 1989	Okada et al. 1988 Davies et al. 1989
– Removal of lytic complexes C5b6789	C5b6–9 complexes in the cell membrane are shed or internalized	Campbell et al. 1985 Carney et al. 1985

Function of
Complement Inhibitors

Target	Location Plasma	Membrane	Function
C1q, C1r, C1s	C1-INH		– inhibition of activation (C1q), dissociation of C1q from C1r2, C1s2, formation of complexes C1r C1s-CI-INH
	factor J		– inhibition of binding of C1q with C1rs C1s2
C4b2b (C3-convertase)	C4b-BP		– inhibition of C4b-C2 interaction, inactivation of C4b2b
	factor I		– enzymatic cleavage of C4b
		DAF	– accelerates inactivation of C4b2b
		CR1	– accelerates inactivation of C4b2b (cofactor for degradation of C4b), transport of IC by erythrocytes
		MCP	– cofactor for degradation of C4b
C3bBb (C3-convertase)	factor H		– accelerates inactivation of C3bBb
	factor I		– enzymatic cleavage of C3b
		CR1	– accelerates inactivation of C3bBb (cofactor for degradation of C3b, transport of IC by erythrocytes)
		DAF	– accelerates inactivation of C4b2b
		MCP	– cofactor for degradation of C3b
C3a, C4a, C5a	carboxy-peptidase N		– inactivation of anaphylatoxins by cleavage of arginin in the carboxy terminal position
C5b67	protein S		– inhibition of association of C5b67 with the cell membrane, binds the complex SC5b-9
	SP40/40		– inhibition of association of C5b67 with the cell membrane, formation of inactive SC5b6789 complexes
C8 (C5b678n9)		HRF	– binding to C8, inhibition of C8 to complex with C5b67 (acts on homologous MAC)
		MIP	– inhibition of polymerization of C9 (acts on homologous MAC)
		MIRL	– inhibition of polymerization of C9 (acts on homologous MAC)

Parker 1992; Morgan et al. 1992; Porcel 1992; Agostoni et al. 1992.

**Extremely Low
Localization Rate at the
Tumor Site of Tumor-
Specific Antibodies
after i.v. or Local
Injection**

Tumor	Localization rate (% injected dose/g tumor)	References
Intravenous injection of MAb		
Lymphoma (non-Hodgkin)	0.0002–0.009	Press et al. 1989
CLL	0.01	
Neuroblastoma	0.08	Miraldi et al. 1986
Colon	0.00004–0.01	Lohde et al. 1991
		Colcher et al. 1987
		Mach et al. 1980
		Farrands et al. 1982
		Beatty et al. 1986
		Armitage et al. 1985
		Sedlacek et al. 1988
Ovarian	0.006–0.009	Epenetos et al. 1986
		Powell et al. 1987
Melanoma	0.003–0.01	Larson et al. 1983
		Buraggi et al. 1985
Osteosarcoma	0.0003–0.0006	Greager et al. 1986
Adeno carcinoma	0.005–0.01	Haller et al. 1991
Breast (superficial metastases)	0.06–0.12	De Nardo et al. 1991
Intravesical injection of MAb		
Bladder carcinoma	0.0003–0.006	Bamias et al. 1991
Intraperitoneal injection of MAb		
Ovarian cancer	0.009–0.92	Lamki et al. 1991
		Hnatowich et al. 1988
		Haisma et al. 1987
		Ward et al. 1987
Peritoneal tumors	0.1–0.13	Malamitsi et al. 1988
Retro-peritoneal tumors	0.002	Malamitsi et al. 1988
Intrapleural injection of MAb		
Breast cancer (pleural tumor)	0.02	Malamitsi et al. 1988
Subcutaneous injection of MAb		
Melanoma	0.003–0.03 (i. lymph.)	Lotze et al. 1986
		Nelp et al. 1987

Compared to normal tissue the concentration of tumor-specific antibodies is increased at the tumor site by a factor of only 1.3–10.

Tumor type	Tumor/normal MAb tissue ratio (increase by a factor of)	References
Intravenous injection		
Colon carcinoma	1,1–10,1	Armstrong et al. 1985
Versus normal		Armitage et al. 1984
Colon mucosa	1.3–5	Mach et al. 1983, 1980
or serosa		
Local administration		
Intraperitoneal		
Ovarian carcinoma	3–25	Hnatowich et al. 1988
Versus normal serosa	1–10	Ward et al. 1987
Intravesical		
Bladder	8–19	Bamias et al. 1991
carcinoma versus		
normal bladder mucosa		

All trials to increase the localization rate of monoclonal antibodies at the tumor site by different measures were of minor success and insufficient.

Measure	Compound	Tumor	Species
Increase of blood flow	norepinephrine propanolol	solid tumors	man, mice
External beam irradiation	–	hepatoma	man, mice
Hyperthermia	–	melanoma	man
Local inflammation	IgG3 MAb specific for GD3 or GD2	melanoma neuroblastoma	man man
	TNFα, IL-1 or IL-2	thymoma	mice
	IL-2 conjugated to MAb specific for tumor necrotic antigen	solid tumors	rat
Increase of tumor antigen expression	IFNα	colon, breast melanoma, adenocarcinoma	man
	IFNβ	adenocarcinoma	man

Review: Sedlacek et al. 1988, 1992.

22.2.12 Pharmacokinetic Parameters for Antibodies

Pharmacokinetic Parameters that Influence the Localization Rate of Antibodies in Tumors

High interstitial hydraulic and osmotic pressure within the tumor impairs convection of monoclonal antibodies into the tumor tissue.

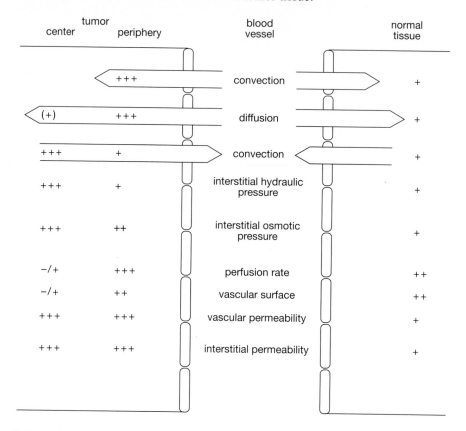

	tumor		blood vessel		normal tissue
	center	periphery			
convection		+++			+
diffusion	(+)	+++			+
convection	+++	+			+
interstitial hydraulic pressure	+++	+			+
interstitial osmotic pressure	+++	++			+
perfusion rate	−/+	+++			++
vascular surface	−/+	++			++
vascular permeability	+++	+++			+
interstitial permeability	+++	+++			+

Review: Sedlacek et al. 1992

Pharmacokinetic of Polyclonal Immunoglobulins in Man

Monoclonal antibodies are subject to the pharmacokinetic of immunoglobulins.

	IgG (IgG-1,-2,-4)	IgG3	IgM (19S)	IgM (7S)
Mean serum level	1,2 g/100 ml (IgG1 = 60–72%; IgG2 = 19–31%; IgGG4 = 7–4%)	5–8% of IgG	80–90 mg/100 ml	–
Total circulating pool	510 mg/kg	35 mg/kg		
Total body IgG pool	1.060 mg/kg	49 mg/kg		
Intravascular pool	48.2%	76%		
Catabolization rate/day	6.3%	10–18%	5%	
$t_{1/2\beta}$	21 days	7.5–9 days	2–9 days	5.6 days
Synthetic rate	32 mg/kg/day 2.2 g/person/day	4.7–7 mg/kg/day		
Protein exchange rate	26.7%/day	extremely low		
Plasma/interstitium	39%/day			

Review: Waldmann et al. 1969.

Comparison of Blood Half-Life Times of Antibodies in Tumor Patients After i.v. Injection

Compared to polyclonal human immunoglobulins, monoclonal antibodies have a significantly shortened half-life time in man, irrespective, whether they are of murine origin or humanized.

		$t_{1/2\beta}$
Polyclonal human	IgG (-1, -2, -4)	21 (18–25) days
	IgG3	7.5–9 days
	IgM (19S)	5 (2–9) days
	gM (5S)	5,6 days
	IgA	5–7 days
Monoclonal murine	Fab	18.7 h
	F(ab')2	19–27 h
	IgG1	18–60 h
	IgG2a	30–44 h
	IgG2b	22–62 h
Monoclonal chimeric (murine v, human c)	IgG1	24–185 h
	IgG4	42–250 h
	Fab	8 h
	F(ab')2	21 h
Monoclonal humanized dose/ (murine CDR, human v,c)	IgG1 24 h	5–20% of injected
		86 h

Review: Sedlacek et al. 1992.

Persistence of Monoclonal Antibodies (Specific for Tumor Antigens) in Blood, Normal Tissues and Tumorous tissues

Longer persistence of TuMAB in tumor tissues may give a chance for specific antibody mediated tumor therapy.

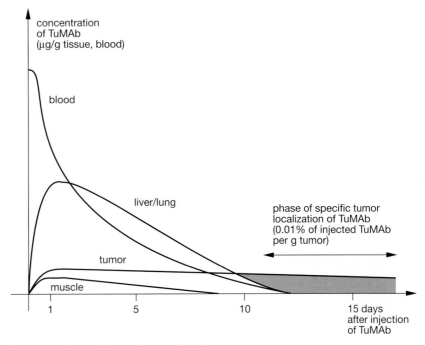

longer persistence in tumor tissue of TuMAb has been proven

– in nude mice, xenografted with human tumors

Colcher et al. 1983, 1984, 1987
Bosslet et al. 1990

– in tumor patients

Armtage et al. 1985
Begent et al. 1990, 1991

Strategy To Use the Longer Persistence of Tumor-Specific Antibodies at the Tumor Site for Specific Tumor Therapy

Biphasic treatment with TuMAB (phase I) and with nontoxic small MW ligand (phase II) which is toxified at the tumor site.

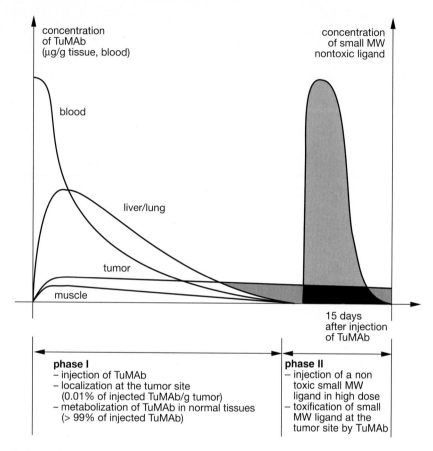

concentration of TuMAb (µg/g tissue, blood)

blood

liver/lung

tumor

muscle

concentration of small MW nontoxic ligand

15 days after injection of TuMAb

phase I
– injection of TuMAb
– localization at the tumor site
  (0.01% of injected TuMAb/g tumor)
– metabolization of TuMAb in normal tissues
  (> 99% of injected TuMAb)

phase II
– injection of a non toxic small MW ligand in high dose
– toxification of small MW ligand at the tumor site by TuMAb

Sedlacek et al. 1992

22.2.13 Antibody-Dependent Enzyme-Mediated Prodrug Therapy (ADEPT)

Synonym: immune-specific enzyme-mediated chemotherapy, ISEC

phase I

– tumor localization of antibody
  enzyme fusion protein (AEFP)
  (or conjugate)

AEFP =

– persistance of AEFP
  (or conjugate)
  at the tumor site after metabolization of AEFP in normal
  tissues

phase II

– injection of a nontoxic small
  MW prodrug in high dose =

– toxification of prodrug by
  enzymatic cleavage at the tumor
  site into toxic drug = ▲
  by AEFP bound to the
  tumor cell

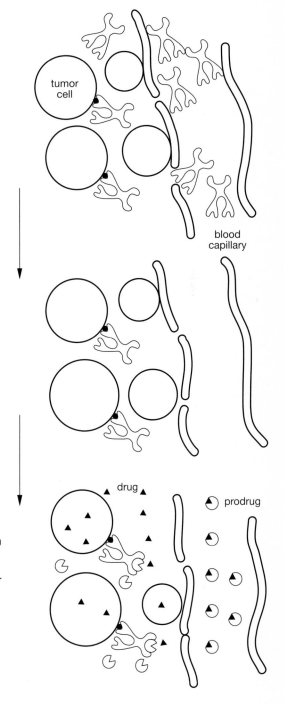

Parameters Critical for Effective ADEPT	Components	Parameters and goals
	Monoclonal antibodies	– specificity selective for the target cell – number of epitopes $>10^4$–10^5/cell – homologous distribution of epitopes through the target tissue (i.e. tumor) – high affinity ($>10^{10}$ l/mol) – no immunogenicity
	Enzyme	– not present or not active in normal blood or interstitium – high turnover rate under physiological conditions – no immunogenicity
	Monoclonal antibody enzyme fusion protein (or conjugate)	– molecular weight as low as possible – localization rate for target tissue at least equal to MAb – percolation and retention at the target tissue equal to or better than MAb – elimination from normal tissue enhanced – no immunogenicity
	Prodrug	– stable in vivo – slow penetration into cells (hydrophilic) – low molar toxicity – high distribution volume – long half-life time – specific cleavage into drug by enzyme fused (or conjugated) to monoclonal antibody
	Drug	– quick penetration into cells (lipophilic) – high molar toxicity – short half-life time – cytotoxicity not dependent on cell cycle phase

Sedlacek et al. 1992.

**Experimental ADEPT
Systems**

Antibody	Enzyme	Linkage	Prodrug/drug	Target	References
Rabbit IgG	glucose oxidase (*Aspergillus niger*)	chemical	L-peroxidase + KJ + glucose/toxic iodine + hydrogen peroxide	tumor cells	Philpott et al. 1973
Rabbit IgG	glucose oxidase (*Aspergillus niger*)	chemical	L-peroxidase + KJ + glucose/toxic iodine + hydrogen peroxide	bacteria	Knowles et al. 1973
Goat IgG	glucose oxidase (*Aspergillus niger*)	chemical	arsphenamine HCL + L-peroxidase + glucose/ toxic arsenical	tumor cells	Philpott et al. 1974
Rabbit IgG	alcohol dehydrogenase (horse liver)	chemical	allylalcohol/ acrolein	tumor cells	Philpott et al. 1979
Murine MAb	human urokinase	chemical	–	fibrin clots	Bode et al. 1985
Murine MAb	bacterial streptokinase/ human tPA urokinase	chemical or by rec. DNA	–	fibrin clots tumor cells	Haber et al. 1985
Murine MAb	carboxypeptidase G2 (bacterial)	chemical	*p*-*N*-bis 2-chlorethyl) aminobenzyol glutamic acid	tumor cells	Bagshawe et al. 1988
Murine MAb	cytosine deaminase (yeast)	chemical 5-FU	5-fluorocytosine/	tumor cells	Senter et al. 1989
Murine MAb	alkaline phosphatase	chemical	mitomycinphosphate etoposidphosphate	tumor cells	Senter et al. 1989
Murine MAb	glucose oxidase and lactoperoxidase	chemical	glucose + KJ/ toxic iodine and hydrogen peroxide	tumor cells	Stanislawski et al. 1989
Murine MAb	human urokinase	conjugation by rec. DNA	–	fibrin clots	Quertermous et al. 1990 Callewaert et al. 1990

Antibody	Enzyme	Linkage	Prodrug/drug	Target	References
Murine MAb	(bacterial) penicillin V-amidase	chemical	doxorubicin phenoxy-acetamine melphalan phenoxy-acetamide	tumor cells	Kerr et al. 1990
Human MAb	lysozyme	chemical	doxorubicin chitin taurine derivative/ doxorubicin	tumor cells	Bredehorst et al. 1990
Bispecific murine MAb	human alkaline phosphatase	antibody/ antigen binding	mitomycin phosphate/ mitomycin	tumor cells	Sahin et al. 1990
Murine MAb	β-lactamase (bacterial)	chemical	β-lactam derivative of cytostatics	tumor cells	Eaton et al. 1990
Murine MAb	β-lactamase aminopeptidase glycosidase	chemical	various cytostatic lactams	tumor cells	Chen et al. 1990
Humanized murine MAb (Fab fragment)	human β-glucuronidase	rec. DNA	doxorubicin glucuronide (F 826)	tumor cells	Bosslet et al. 1993 Jacquesy et al. 1992

Antitumoral Activity of Experimental ADEPT Systems

Prodrug	Enzyme conjugated to MAb	Drug	Tumor	Antigen specific anti tumor activity		
				In vitro activity	Tumor (human)	In vivo activity
p-N-bis (2-Chloroethyl)-amino benzoyl glutamic acid	carboxypeptidase G$_2$ *(Pseudomonas)*	chlor-ambucil derivative	n.t.	n.t.	chorion-carcinoma	complete regression
N-(p-Hydroxy-phenoxyacetamide) melphalan	penicillin V-amidase *(Fusarium oxysporum)*	melphalan	colon leukemia	–	n.t.	n.t.
N-(p-hydroxy-phenoxyacetamide) doxorubicin	penicillin V-amidase *(Fusarium oxysporum)*	ADM	colon leukemia	+	n.t.	n.t.
Etoposide phosphate	alkaline phosphatase (calf intestine)	etoposide	lung carcinoma colon carcinoma	+	colon carcinoma	complete regressions
Mitomycin phosphate	alkali phosphatase (calf intestine)	MMC	lung carcinoma	+	lung carcinoma	complete regressions
5-Fluorocytosine	cytosine deaminase *(Saccharomyces derevisiae)*	5-FU carcinoma	lung colon carcinoma	+	n.t.	n.t.
Doxorubicin glucuronide	human β-Glucuroni-dase	ADM	colon carcinoma	+	colon carcinoma	complete regressions

n.t. = not tested

Bagshawe et al. 1988, Kerr et al. 1990, Senter et al. 1990, Bosslet et al. 1994.

Arrangement of Complementarity Determining Regions in the Framework Regions of the Variable Chains of Antibodies

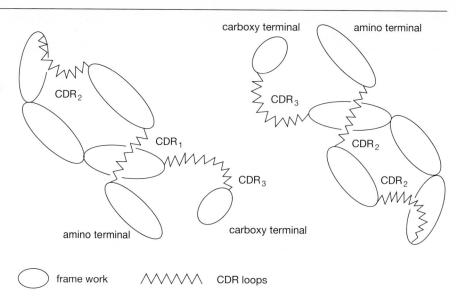

carboxy terminal   amino terminal

CDR$_2$

CDR$_3$

CDR$_1$

CDR$_2$

CDR$_3$

CDR$_2$

amino terminal   carboxy terminal

frame work   CDR loops

22.2.14 Antibody Engineering

**Possibilities to Engineer
Antibodies by DNA
Recombinant Techni-
ques**

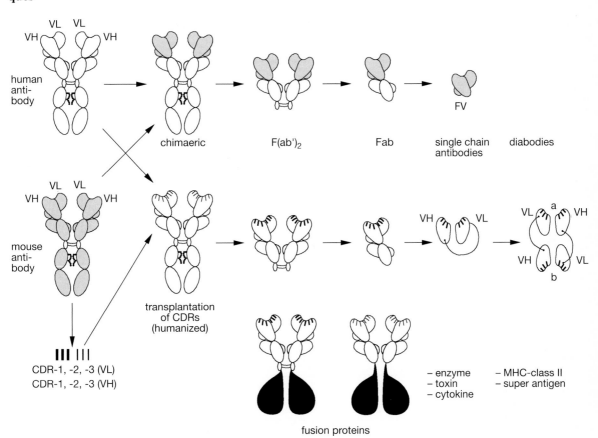

human anti-body

mouse anti-body

CDR-1, -2, -3 (VL)
CDR-1, -2, -3 (VH)

chimaeric

transplantation
of CDRs
(humanized)

F(ab')$_2$

Fab

single chain
antibodies

FV

diabodies

fusion proteins

– enzyme
– toxin
– cytokine

– MHC-class II
– super antigen

Bioengineered Antibodies Open New Perspectives for Tumor Immunotherapy

Antibody constructs		Improvement/goal	References
Chimeric antibodies	murine VL, VH-human CL, CH	– reduction of immunogenicity	Neuberger et al. 1984
	– CH of human IgG1	– increase of effector functions	Brüggemann et al. 1987
	– CH of human IgG4	– decrease of effector functions	van der Zee et al. 1986
Humanized antibodies	murine CDRs-human VL, VH (framework) human CH	– reduction of immunogenicity, construction of human like antibodies of specificities selected in murine systems	Riechmann et al. 1988
Fab F(ab')$_2$	VLCL-VHCH1; 2x(VLCL-VHCH1) – hinge region	– loss of Fc-mediated effector functions, short plasma half-life time, quick elimination	Skerra et al. 1988
FV	VL-VH	– reduction of nonspecific binding to non-target tissue; reduction of immunogenicity, reduced retention in the kidney (compared to Fab); may be very labile and (therefore) have reduced binding affinity	Huston et al. 1991 Riechmann et al. 1988
Single-chain antibodies (sFV)	VL linker VH	– stable FV by linker (14–28 aA in length) spanning the distance between C-terminus (V1) and N-terminus (V2) without perturbing normal domain structure and interdomain contacts	Huston et al. 1988, 1993
Immunotoxins	VL, VH linker *Pseudomonas* exotoxin	– fusion protein with unimpaired antibody binding affinity for targeting cytotoxicity	Chaudhary et al. 1989
Diabodies	VL(a) linker VH(b) VH(a) linker VL(b)	– stable FV by short linker; two heterodimers associate to a bispecific sFV	Holliger et al. 1993

Antibody constructs		Improvement/goal	References
Antibody enzyme protein	VL-CL, VH-CH1 hinge linker b-glucuronidase	– fusion protein wich unimpaired antibody binding affinity and enzyme activity for targeting enzyme activity to tumor cells for prodrug activation	Bosslet et al. 1992
Antibody cytokine protein	VH linker VL-IL-2	– fusion protein to target IL-2 to tumor cells	Savage et al. 1993
Antibody MHC-class I protein	VL-CL, VH-CH1 linker MHC class I	– fusion protein with unimpaired binding affinity for allogenisation by targeting foreign MHC-class I molecules to tumor cells to induce CTL response	Seemann et al. 1990
Antibody superantigen	VL-CL, VH-CH-1 staphylococcal entero-toxin A	– fusion protein with unimpaired antibody binding affinity to target super antigen to tumor cells to activate T-helper cells and to induce secretion of lymphotoxins	Kalland et al. 1993
Bispecific antibodies	VL(a)CL-VH(a)CH + VL(b)CL-VH(b)CH	– targeting of chelated Ytrium 90 or of cytotoxic T-cells to tumor cells – conjugation of toxins to antibodies by one specificity of the bispecific antibody	Bosslet et al. 1990 Fanger et al. 1992 Fanger et al. 1992

23 CNS and Immune Reactions

23.1 Overview

Interaction between the immune system and the CNS:

– Immune cells produce neuropeptides and neuronal hormones (CNS-mediators).

– Cells of the CNS produce immunomediators.

– Immune cells can be modulated by CNS mediators and hormones, the CNS by immune mediators.

– The consequence is a close communication between the immune system and the CNS.

– In consequence, the immune system can respond to cognitive stimuli (physical, emotional, chemical) and the CNS to noncognitive stimuli (infections, vaccination, tumor, others).

Interaction Between the Immune System and the CNS

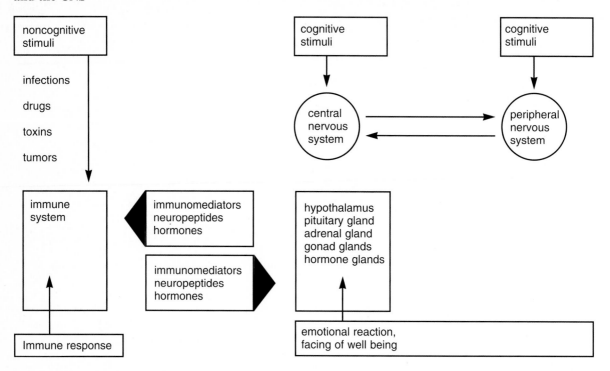

The Network of the CNS and the Immune

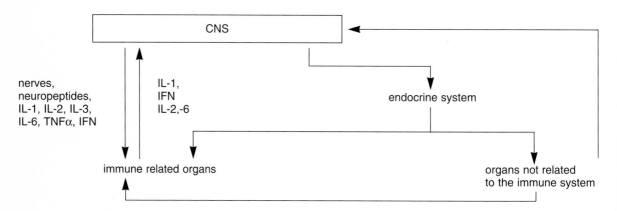

- Close association of nerves with lymphocytes and macrophages.
- Hormone receptors are on lymphocytes and macrophages.
- Neuropeptides are produced by immune cells in addition to CNS and influence both.
- Immune mediators influence the CNS, CNS expresses receptors for cytokines.
- Cytokines (IL-1,-2,-3,-6) are expressed by brain cells and hypothalamus, IL-1 is produced by pituitary gland.

Felten et al. 1988; Kasahara et al. 1993, Blalock 1994.

23.2 Details

23.2.1 Modulation of the Immune System by Neuropeptides

Neuropeptide	Pharmacology	Action on the immune system
Vasoactive intestinal polypeptide (VIP) (29 aa)	– vasodilatation – smooth muscle relaxation, inhibition of growth – increased salivary gland secretion	– potentiation of EGF induced growth of keratinocytes (other cells) – regulation of wound healing (Nilsson et al. 1985, Dalsgaard et al 1989)
Tachykinin substance P (11 aa)	– sensory neurotransmitter (relays pain signals) – vasodilatation – spasm of smooth muscle cells – hyperglycemia, inhibition of bile flow, enhanced salivation – enhanced natriuresis	– stimulation of T-cell proliferation – stimulation of proliferation of synovial cells, fibroblasts, keratinocytes, macrophages – stimulation of PGE2 release (Zachary et al. 1987, Payan et al. 1983, Lotz et al. 1987, Tanaka et al. 1988)
Endothelin (21 aa)	– vasoconstriction – increase in proliferation of vascular smooth muscle cells	– promotion of release of prostaglandins (Yoshizawa et al. 1990)
Bradykinin (9 aa)	– production of pain – smooth muscle contraction – vasodilatation – increase in vascular permeability	– stimulation of fibroblast proliferation – induction of PGE2 production (Owen et al. 1983)
β-Endorphin	– modulation of pain transmission	– stimulation of T-cell proliferation (Gillman et al. 1992)
α-Endorphin	– modulation of pain transmission	– suppression of B-cells (Blalock 1994)
ACTH (1-39)	– stimulation of adrenals (ACTH)	– suppression of B-cells (Blalock 1994)

Tachykinin Peptides in More Detail

Compounds	Structure	Receptor Type	Cell	Activity	References
Substance P	Arg-Pro-Lys-Pro-Glu-Glu-Phe-Phe-Gly-Leu-Met-NH$_2$	NK$_1$	dorsal horn spinal cord cells	transmitting pain from C fibers	Pernow 1953
			macrophages	release of IL-1, TNF	Lotz et al. 1988
			synovial cells collagenase proliferation	release of PGE2,	Lotz et al. 1987
			bronchial cells	mucus secretion	Rogers et al. 1989
			saliva glands	secretion	Snider et al. 1991
			T-cells	activation	Payan et al. 1983
			fibroblasts	proliferation	Nilsson et al. 1985
			keratinocytes	proliferation	Tanaka et al. 1988
			arterial smooth muscle cells	contraction	Nilsson et al. 1985
Neurokinin A	His-Lys-Thr.-Asp-Ser-Phe-Val-Gly-Leu-Met-NH$_2$	NK$_2$			Lowe 1992
Neurokinin B	Asp-Met-His-Asp-Phe-Val-Gly-Leu-Met-NH$_2$	NK$_3$			Lowe 1992

Neuroendocrine Hormones and Peptides Produced by Cells of the Immune System	Hormones and transmitters	Producing immune cells
	Releasing hormones	
	corticotropin releasing hormone (CRH)	thymocytes, splenic macrophages
	Luteinizing hormone releasing hormone (LHRH)	thymocytes
	Pituitary hormones	
	Adrenocorticotropic hormone (ACTH)	T-cells, B-cells, macrophages
	Thyroid-stimulating hormone (TSH)	T-cells
	Luteinizing hormone (LH)	lymphocytes (spleen)
	Follicle stimulating hormone (FSH)	lymphocytes (spleen)
	Growth hormone (GH)	T-cells, B-cells, macrophages
	Prolactin	T-cells
	Vasopressin	thymocytes
	Oxytocin	thymocytes
	Other neuropeptides	
	Vasoactive intestinal peptide (VIP)	mast cells, granulocytes
	Substance P (SP)	macrophages
	Atrial natriuretic factor (ANF)	macrophages
	β-endorphin	T-cells, B-cells, macrophages
	(Met) encephalins	T-cells
	Neuropeptide Y	megakaryocytes
	Other growth factors	
	Somatostatin	mast cells, granulocytes
	Parathyroid hormone related protein	T-cells
	Insulin-like growth factor (IGF-I)	T-cells, B-cells, macrophages

Blalock 1992, 1994; Smith et al. 1986, 1990; Lolait et al. 1984; Zurawaski et al. 1986, Webster et al. 1988.

23.2.2 IL-1 as a "Neuropeptide"

IL-1 is an important "neuropeptide" and the main cytokine, cross-linking the immune system, the CNS and endocrine organs.

Role of IL-1 in CNS:

- Produced by brain cells (neuronal cells, astrocytes) and pituitary cells (anterior lobe). IL-1β seems to be widespread in the brain whereas IL-1α appears to be confined to more discrete regions (anterior hypothalamus, hippocampus) (Koenig 1991, Busbrudge et al. 1991).
- Expression is increased by stress or after LPS injection (Rivest et al. 1993).
- Brain cells and pituitary cells express IL-1-receptors.

- Stimulates eicosanoid production in and proliferation of astrocytes (Hartung et al. 1989).
- Stimulates expression of nerve growth factor (NGF) by hippocampal neurons and glial cells (Friedman et al. 1990, Spranger et al. 1990).
- Stimulates CRH release by hypothalamic cells (paraventricular nucleus) (Rivier 1993).
- Stimulates ACTH and β-endorphin release in pituitary cells (Woloski et al. 1985, Bernton et al. 1987, Fagarasan et al. 1989, Fukuta et al. 1989).
- Stimulates vasopressin and oxytocin release in pituitary cells (Christensen et al. 1989, Naito et al. 1991, Hansen et al. 1992).
- Induces fever, stimulates thermogenesis (Dinarello 1988, Danscombe et al. 1989).
- Alterates slow wave sleep (Krüger et al. 1984).
- Reduces food intake (McCarthy et al. 1985).
- Induces analgesia (Nakamura et al. 1988).
- Stimulates the hypothalamic-pituitary-adrenocortical axis (Berkenbosch et al. 1987, Sapolsky et al. 1987).
- Inhibits the hypothalamic-pituitary-gonadal axis (Rivest et al. 1993, Rivier et al. 1989, Kalra et al. 1990).
- Inhibits LHRH and LH secretion in the hypothalamus or pituitary organ (Rivest et al. 1992, 1993).
- Inhibits steroidogenesis by Leydig's cells (Calkins et al. 1988, Fanser et al. 1989).
- Stimulates spermatogonial proliferation (Pollauen et al. 1989).
- Inhibits PGE2 release in the hypothalamus (Rivest et al. 1993).
- Elevates circulating level of insulin (Cornell et al. 1989).
- Inhibits release of thyroid hormone (Rettori et al. 1987).
- Inhibits gastric acid secretion (Saperas et al. 1990, Iehara et al. 1990).
- Induces acute phase glycoprotein synthesis (Blatteis et al. 1984).

23.2.3 Cytokines and Cytokine Receptors Expressed by Cells of the CNS and Endocrine Organs

Cells/tissues	Expression of		References
	Cytokine	Cytokine receptor	
Adrenal		IFNα-receptors	Blalock 1994
Testis (interstitial areas) Epididymis		IL-1-receptors	Tracey et al. 1988 Tahao et al. 1990 DeSouza 1993
Thyroid		IFNα-receptors	Blalock 1994
Hypothalamus (neuronal cells)	IL-1 (α, β) IL-2 IL-3 IL-6	IFNα-receptors IL-1-receptors (type I, type II) Breder et al. 1988 Koenig 1991 Busbridge et al. 1991	Menzies et al. 1992 Smith 1992 Spangelo et al. 1990
Pituitary cells (anterior lobe)	IL-1	IL-1-receptors (type I, type II) IL-6-receptors IL-2-receptors	Woloski et al. 1985 Paque et al. 1994 Parnet et al. 1993 Koenig et al. 1990 Marguette et al. 1990 Smith et al. 1989 Arzt et al. 1992 Tracey et al. 1988 DeSouza et al. 1989
Brain, neuronal cells (hippocampus		IL-1-receptors	Takao et al. 1990, 1992
Astrocytes	IL-1 (α, β) IL-3 IL-6 TNF IFN	IL-1-receptors	DeSouza et al. 1993 Fontana et al. 1982 Busbridge et al. 1991
Epithelial cells of choriod plexus		IL-1-receptors	Hartung et al. 1989

23.2.4 Communication of the CNS with the Immune System

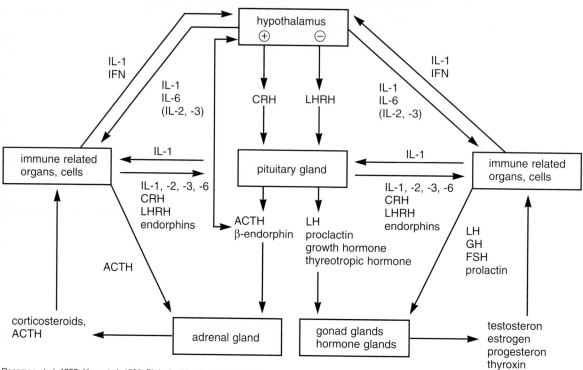

Roszman et al. 1992; Herz et al. 1980; Blalock 1994; Rivest et al. 1993.

23.2.5 Modulation of the Endocrine System by Immune Mediators

Target tissue	Stimulation By	Increase of	Inhibition By	Decrease of	References
Hypothalamus	IL-1β	CRH	thymosin β4	LHRH	Hall et al. 1992 Rivier 1993 Bateman et al. 1989
	(LPS)	IL-6	IL-1	LHRH PGE2	Spangelo et al. 1990 Kalra et al. 1990
Pituitary gland	IL-1β	IL-2 IL-6 prolactin GH (ACTH) β-endorphin vasopressin oxytocin	Thymosin β4 IL-1	LH prolactin GH LH FSH TSH	Nakatsuru et al. 1991 Hall et al. 1992 Marguette et al. 1990 Spangelo et al. 1991 Christensen et al. 1989 Naito et al. 1991 Rivest et al. 1993 Arzt et al. 1992 Karanth et al. 1991 Smith et al. 1989, 1992
	IL-2, -3, -6	ACTH			
Gonads	interferon	testosteron estrogen progesteron	IL-1β	testosteron estrogen progesteron	Hall et al. 1992 Calkins et al. 1988 Fauser et al. 1989
	IL-1β	LH-receptors			
Thyreoidea	interferon	thyroxine			Rettori et al. 1987 Hall et al. 1992
Adrenal gland	interferon	glucocortico-steroid			Blalock 1994
Pancreas	IL-1	insulin			Cornell et al. 1989

Interaction Between
the Immune System
and the Corticotrophic
Axis

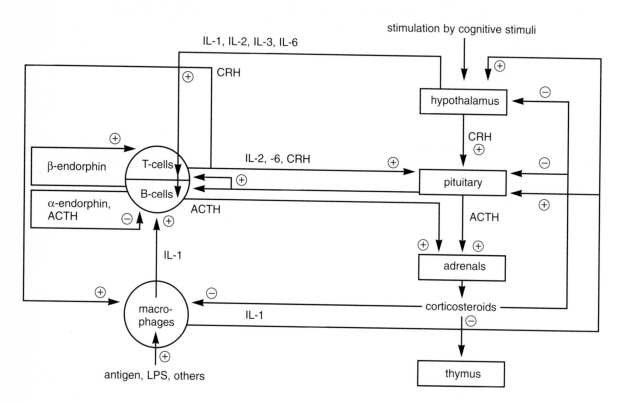

**Modulation of the
Corticotrophic Axis
by Immune "Related"
Means**

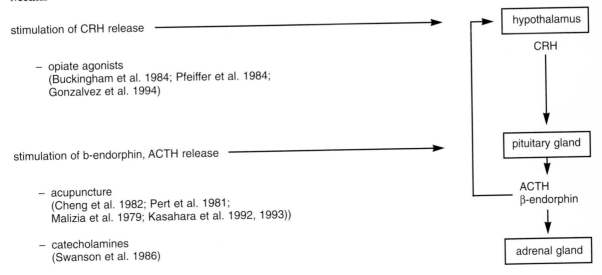

stimulation of CRH release

    – opiate agonists
      (Buckingham et al. 1984; Pfeiffer et al. 1984;
      Gonzalvez et al. 1994)

stimulation of b-endorphin, ACTH release

    – acupuncture
      (Cheng et al. 1982; Pert et al. 1981;
      Malizia et al. 1979; Kasahara et al. 1992, 1993))

    – catecholamines
      (Swanson et al. 1986)

hypothalamus
CRH
pituitary gland
ACTH
β-endorphin
adrenal gland

23.2.6 Hormonal Influence on Antibodies in Mucosal Tissues

Lacrimal gland/tears	Androgens	Increase of sIgA no effect on IgG	Sullivan et al. 1989
	insulin	support of androgens	
Uterus/vagina	estrogens/ progesterone	increase of sIGA	Wira et al. 1983, 1985
		increase of IgG	1980
Intestinum	secretin pancreozymin	increase of sIgA	Shah et al. 1983
		increase of IgG	
Peyer's patches	substance P somatostatin	increase of IgA	Stanisz et al. 1986
		no effect on IgG	
Mammary gland	estrogens progesterone	increase of sIgA	Weisz-Carrington et al. 1978
		increase of sIgA	

23.2.8 Immune Response and Epilepsy

Antigen-antibody immune complexes and autoimmune reactions may aggrevate brain damage and may cause epilepsy.

Immune reaction proposed in epilepsy

antibody ───▶◀───────────────────── infectious agent

− genetic predisposition
− IgA
− IgG$_2$

primary damage of the brain

− trauma
− tumor
− cerebrovascular disorders
− metabolic disorders
− anoxia

circulating Ag/Ab complexes

seizures

primary damage of blood brain barrier

secondary damage of blood brain barrier

exposure of CNS antigens

autoimmune reaction

genetic predisposition (HLA)

 possible targets for treatment with immunoglobulins:

− elimination of infectious agents
− elimination of Immune complexes
− suppression of autoimmune reaction

van Rijckevorsel-Harmant et al. 1988.

**Case Reports Indicate
to a Therapeutic Effect
of Polyclonal Immuno-
globulins in Epilepsy**

Type of epilepsy	Range of age	Dosage of immuno-globulin	Schedule of administration	No. of cases total/improved*	References
Infantile spasmus Lennox syndrome Myoclonic seizures Focal seizures	6 months 13 years	100 mg/kg	every 2 weeks for 12 weeks	18/9 (50%)	Arüzumi et al. 1983
Postencephalitis	1–6 years	100 mg/kg	every 2nd day 4 times	8/4 (50%)	Sandstedt et al. 1984
West syndrome Cryptogenic Symptomatic	6 months 12 years	100 mg/kg	every 2nd week 6–10 times	11/7 (64%)	Hibio et al. 1985
Postencephalitis West syndrome	1–12 years	400 mg/kg	every 2 weeks for 6 months	12/5 (42%)	Duse et al. 1986
Lennox syndrome Partial epilepsy	3–44 years	250 mg/kg	4 times during week 1 1 time at weeks 2 –3–6	20/8 (40%)	von Rijckevorsel et al. 1987, 1989
West syndrome Lennox syndrome Symptomatic epilepsy	1–12 years	400 mg/kg	daily during 5 days every 6 weeks for 6 months	23/5 (22%)	Echenne et al. 1991
Intractable seizures	20–48 years	1 g/kg	for 2 days daily	5/2 (40%	Schwartz et al. 1989
Malignant epilepsy	32–65 years	400 mg/kg	every 2 weeks for 6 months	18/13 (72%)	Sterio et al. 1990
Lennox syndrome	4–14 years	400 mg/kg	2 times weekly every 2 weeks for 6 months	10/2 (20%)	ILlum et al. 1990
West syndrome Lennox syndrome	6 months 10 years	400 mg/kg	daily for 5 days and then every 2 weeks for 3 months	15/13 (87%	van Engelen et al. 1992

* Improvement = reduction in number of seizures ≥50%.

24 Genetic Background of Apoptosis and Malignant Lymphocyte Growth

24.1 Apoptosis and Malignant Lymphocyte Growth

– The term apoptosis was proposed for a "mechanism of controlled cell deletion, which appears to play a complementary but opposite role to mitosis in the regulation of animal cell populations" (Kerr et al. 1972).

– Both apoptosis and cell proliferation are controlled by a network of genes. Result of this control is the balance between the rate of cell division and the rate of cell death.

– Uncontrolled growth observed in malignant tumors may be caused by cell populations increasing their rate of proliferation, decreasing their rate of cell death or both (Barr et al. 1994).

– Apoptosis plays a central role in the normal immune system. It occurs during lymphocyte and T-cell development as well as at later stages, after the interaction of lymphocytes with target antigens. Aberrant apoptosis induced by an imbalance in the activation of genes or by infectious organisms may be an essential cause either for malignant lymphocyte growth, for immune suppression or for autoimmune diseases.

– Uncontrolled apoptosis in population of nonproliferating, long-lived terminally differentiated cell types may be the pathophysiological pathway of many neurodegenerative and heart diseases.

**Apoptosis and Neo-
plasia Can Be Geneti-
cally Controlled by
Regulating Genes**

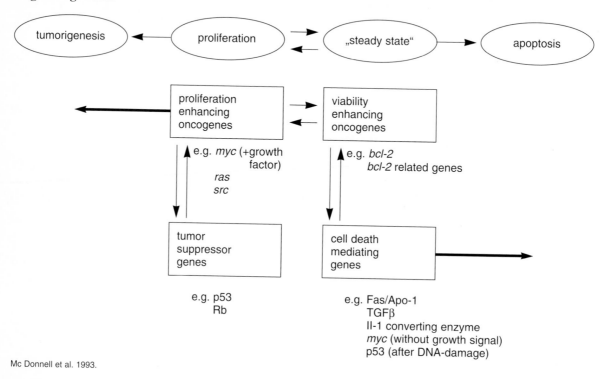

Mc Donnell et al. 1993.

Apoptosis of Cells

Definition: – apoptosis is the controlled "programmed" cell death

Morphology

Cellular:
– shrinkage of cells
– loose of contact with neighbouring cells and of specialized surface elements (i.e. microvilli, cell to cell junctions)
– surface convolution, formation of surface protuberances or "blebs"
– disaggregation of cell membrane bounded, condensed apoptotic bodies

Subcellular:
– dilatation of endoplasmatic reticulum
– crater-like cavities of ER, dilated cisternae fuse with the cell surface
– site to site aggregation of cytoskeletal filaments
– semicrystalline arrays of ribosomes

       – *mitochondria remain normal in structure for a very long*
       time (in contrast to cell necrosis)
       – condensation of nuclear chromatic into dense granular caps
       under the nuclear membrane, loss of nuclear pores in this
       region
       – dissociation of the nucleolus into osmiophilic particles

Tissue:
       – no inflammatory reaction
       – phagocytosis by macrophages or other adjacent viable cells
       – compacted organelles and condensed chromatin of the
       apoptotic cells are either visible or they are reduced to large
       nondescript lysosomal residual bodies within the phagocytic
       cells

Effector mechanism

Nuclear
change
       – activation of endogenous (Ca^{++} Mg^{++} dependent) nuclease
       – cleavage of chromatin between nucleosomes generating a
       series of fragments; this (nucleosomal site) fragments
       constitute the characteristic "ladder" on agarose gel electro-
       phoresis of the DNA of apoptotic cells

Plasmatic
change:
       – rise of free cytosolic Ca^{++} (McConkey et al. 1989)
       (blockage of Ca^{++} influx inhibit apoptosis)
       – new expression of a transglutaminase activity cross-linkage
       of cytoplasmic proteins by this enzyme
       – fluid leakage

Phagocytosis:
       – phagocytic cells recognize new molecular structures on the
       surface of the apoptotic cells
       – recognition can be blocked in vitro by *N*-acetylglucosamine
       (Duvall et al. 1985)
       – human macrophages phagocytose via their vitronectin
       receptor apoptotic human neutrophils (Savill et al. 1990),
       possibly via thrombospondin; phagocytosis via the vitro-
       nectin receptor does not induce release of cytokine, inflam-
       matory mediators or lysosomal enzymes (Wyllie 1992);
       this might explain the lack of inflammation associated with
       apoptosis.

Genetic
regulation:
       – c-*myc*, *bcl-2*, p53 and *ras* are involved in apoptosis
       – apoptosis is induced by
          * upregulation of c-*myc* and
             – withdrawal of growth factors
             – starvation (leukine deprivation or
             – S phase arrest (thymidine induced))
          * downregulation of *bcl-2*

	* modulation of *ras*
	* upregulation of p53
Pharma-cological induction:	– apoptosis is induced by
	* monostimulation of T-cells
	* monostimulation of B-cells
	* hormones (glucocorticoids, LH-RH, somatostatin, others
	* hormone deprivation (atrophia)
	* TNF
	* TGFβ
	* activation of Apo-1/Fas-receptor
	* cytostatics (Doxorubicin, Daunomycin)

Wyllie et al. 1980, 1992; Arends et al. 1991; Krammer et al. 1993; Reed 1994; Skladanowski et al. 1993; Debatin et al. 1990.

In a number of human diseases, dysregulation of apoptosis seems to be involved:

Cancer, lymphoma	– uncontrolled growth caused by cell populations:
	* increasing their rate of proliferation and/or
	* decreasing their rate of cell death
Immune system	– immune suppression, autoimmune or other hyper-reactive diseases, caused for example by:
	* induction of apoptosis of lymphocytes (i.e. apoptosis of CD4[+] T-cells by HIV infection)
	* induction of apoptosis of macrophages (i.e. *Shigella flexneri* infection)
	* increase of expression of Apo-1/Fas receptor on lymphocytes (i.e. HIV infection)
	* prevention of apoptosis by increased expression of soluble Apo-1/Fas receptors (i.e. systemic lupus erythematodes)
Neuro-degenerative diseases	– apoptotic death of neurons, observed in
	* Alzheimer disease (possibly induced by accumulation of β-amyloid)
	* multiple sclerosis, ataxia telangiectasia, stroke (mechanism unknown)
Heart disease	– apoptotic death of cardiomyocytes, observed in
	* doxorubicin induced cardiomyopathy
	* secondary necrosis following myocardial infarction
Accelerated aging	– possibly failure to maintain competence for adequate apoptosis

Barr et al. 1994.

Approaches to inhibit apoptosis:

- Costimulation
    * Costimulation of lymphocytes to prevent activation (TCR, BCR) induced death (i.e. B7/CD28 or CD40/CD40L)
    * Cross-linking of membrane receptors in mature cells

- Growth factors
    * TNF
    * Neurotrophin
    * Erythropoietin
    * Others

- Blockage of Apo-1/Fas-receptor cross-linking
    * Monovalent anti-Fas antibodies (Fab)
    * Soluble form of Apo-1/Fas receptor

- Upregulation of bcl-2

- Downregulation or mutation of p53

24.2 Mechanisms of Tumorigenesis

- Tumorigenesis is a multifactorial process.
- It requires the stepwise aquisition of multiple genetic lesions or alterations.
- Activation of oncogenes or inactivation of tumor suppressor genes represent such lesions.
- Tumors develop through several premalignant stages to full malignancy.
- To reach full malignancy, the synergistic effect of these genetic lesions and not their order is important, i.e. the products of activated oncogenes have to cooperate.
- Three or more pathways have to converge through the functional cooperation of several oncoproteins: stimulation of cell proliferation, inhibiton of apoptosis and independence of growth factors.
- Activation of oncogenes can occur via gene amplification, chromosomal translocations, insertion of viral transcriptional control elements near an oncogene, mutations and deletions, loss of a tumor suppressor gene, generation of fusion proteins after chromosomal translocation.

Hunter 1991.

Functions of the Main Cell-Derived Proto-oncogene Products

Class I: growth factors

sis	PDGF β-chain growth factor
int-2	FGF-related growth factor
hst (KS3)	FGF-related growth factor
FGF-5	FGF-related growth factor
int-1	growth factor?

Class 2: receptor and nonreceptor protein tyrosine kinases

src	membrane-associated nonreceptor protein tyrosine kinase
yes	membrane-associated nonreceptor protein tyrosine kinase
fgr	membrane-associated nonreceptor protein tyrosine kinase
lck	membrane-associated nonreceptor protein tyrosine kinase
fps/fes	nonreceptor protein tyrosine kinase
abl/bcr-abl	nonreceptor protein tyrosine kinase
ros	membrane-associated receptor-like protein tyrosine kinase
erbB	truncated EGF receptor protein tyrosine kinase
neu	receptor-like protein tyrosine kinase
fms	mutant CSF-1 receptor protein tyrosine kinase
met	soluble truncated receptor-like protein tyrosine kinase
trk	soluble truncated receptor-like protein tyrosine kinase
kit (W locus)	truncated stem cell receptor protein tyrosine kinase
ret	truncated receptor-like protein tyrosine kinase

Class 3: receptors lacking protein kinase activity

mas	angiotensin receptor

Class 4: membrane-associated G proteins

H-*ras*	membrane-associated GTP-binding/GTPase
K-*ras*	membrane-associated GTP-binding/GTPase
N-*ras*	membrane-associated GTP-binding/GTPase

class 5: cytoplasmic protein-serine kinases

raf/mil	cytoplasmic protein-serine kinase
pim-1	cytoplasmic protein-serine kinase
mos	cytoplasmic protein-serine kinase (cytostatic factor)
cot	cytoplasmic protein-serine kinase?

class 6: cytoplasmic regulators

crk	SH-2/3 protein that binds to (and regulates?) phosphotyrosine-containing proteins

Class 7: nuclear transcription factors

myc	sequence-specific DNA-binding protein
N-*myc*	sequence-specific DNA-binding protein
L-*myc*	sequence-specific DNA-binding protein
myb	sequence-specific DNA-binding protein
lyl-1	sequence-specific DNA-binding protein?

p53	mutant form may sequester wild-type p53 growth suppressor
fos	combines with c-*jun* product to form AP-1 transcription factor
jun	sequence-specific DNA-binding protein; part of AP-1
erbA	dominant negative mutant thyroxine (T$_3$) receptor
rel	dominant negative mutant NF-kB related protein
vav	GTP/GDP exchange factor for ras
ets	sequence-specific DNA-binding protein
ski	transcription factor?
evi-1	transcription factor?
gli-1	transcription factor?
maf	transcription factor?
pbx	chimeric E2A-homeobox transcription factor
Hox2.4	transcription factor?

Unclassified

dbl	cytoplasmic truncated cytoskeletal protein?
bcl-2	plasma membrane signal transducer?

Examples of Pairs of Cooperating Oncogenes in Experimental Hematopoietic Malignancies	**Tumor** · **Combination of activated oncogenes**

Tumor	Combination of activated oncogenes
Lymphoid progenitor pre-B- or B-lymphoma	*myc* / *bcl-2*
	myc / Ha-*ras*, N-*ras*
	myc / *raf*
	myc / *abl*
	myc / *pim-1*
	myc / *bcl-2*
Plasmacytoma	*myc* / v-*abl*

Adams and Cory 1991.

Immunophenotypic-Genomic Correlations in Malignant Lymphoid Diseases	Lymphoid tumors	Rearranged genes and/or combination of genes
	Acute lymphoblastic leukemia	
	Pre-B-cell	Prl, E2A
	B-cell (surface Ig$^+$)	Myc, Igh
		Igκ, Myc
		Myc, Igλ
		IL-3, Igh
	B-cell or B-myeloid	Abl, Bcr
	other	IFNα/β
	T-cell	Myc, Bcl-3
		Tal1/Ttg, Tcrδ
		Tcl2, Tcrδ
		Myc, Tcrα
		Igh, Tcrα
		Tcl1, Tcrα
		Tcl3, Tcrδ
		Tal1/Scl1, Tcrδ
		Tcrβ, Sup-T3
		Tcrβ, Tcl3
		Tcrγ
		Tcrβ, Lyl1
	Non-Hodgkin's lymphoma	
	B-cell	Myc, Igh
		Igκ, Myc
		Myc, Igl
		Igh, Bcl-2
		Bcl-1, Igh
	Chronic lymphocytic leukemia	
	B-cell	Bcl-1, Igh
		Igh, Bcl-3
		Igh
		Bcl-2, Igl
	T-cell	Myc, Tcrα
		Tcrα, Tcl1
	Multiple myeloma	
	B-cell	Bcl-1, Igh, Igh

Rowley 1991.

25 Somatic Gene Therapy

25.1 Overview

25.1.1 Opportunities and Risks

Somatic gene therapy involves treatment of somatic cells of a patient with recombinant nucleic acids to modulate expression of defined endogenous genes or to introduce and express certain exogenous genes. Treatment of somatic cells can be performed in vitro (with subsequent injection of such treated cells into the patient) or in vivo.

Mutations of autochthonous somatic cells by direct delivery, transfection or injection of:
– Expression constructs in:
   Viral vectors (adenovirus, adenovirus-associated viruses, retroviruses)
   Nonviral vectors (liposomes, bifunctional vectors)

– Blocking nucleic constructs in:
   Antisense mRNA   protected against de-
   Antisense DNA   gradation (nucleases)
   for triplex formation   by derivatisation
   Antisense mRNA with   (methylphosphate,
   nuclease activity   thiophosphate)
   (Ribozyme)

Targeting expression of genes for in vivo somatic gene therapy by
– Retroviral expression vectors with specificity for proliferating cells
– Tissue specific promotors
– Vectors or constructs with anti-sense or anti-gene information for cancer-specific mutations (oncogenes) or for viruses
– Vectors packaged into vehicles (virosomes, liposomes) carrying tissue-specific ligands for receptors exposed on target cell membrane.

Problems of somatic gene therapy:
– Safety and tolerability:
   Target cell specificity (random transfection rate)

Selectivity

Risk of recombination of viral vector with wild-type virus, resulting in replicative new virus (i.e. adenovirus based-vectors)

Tumorigenicity of transfected autochthonous cells

– Expression rate:

Low transfection rate due to low nuclear import rate

Low expression rate by insufficient promotor

Transcriptional extinction of transduced genes (i.e. by cytosine methylation)

Inconsistant expression

Uncontrolled modulation of expression rate

Uses of Somatic Gene Therapy

Disease	Conventional drug treatment	Gene therapy (aspired goal)
Monogenetic defects	continuous substitution of plasma proteins (expensive, risky) palliative, therapeutic effect limited	once or twice a year treatment
Autoimmune/ rheumatological/ allergical	palliative, therapeutic effect limited	new approaches to modulate the immune systems with its own mediators
Neurological	palliative with limited therapeutic effect or no effect	new approaches for causative treatment
Oncological	therapeutic effect limited/considerable toxicity	new approaches – for causative treatment – for more effective treatment
Infections	problem of drug resistance, considerable number of infections without possibility of vaccination	new approaches – for vaccination – to increase immune resistance
Cardiovascular	continuous application of antithrombotics	new approaches – for once or twice a year treatment – inhibition of intimal proliferation

25.1.2 Preconditions

– Life-threatening disease to be treated
– Gene cloned which is be inserted
– Precise targeting and regulation of new gene if required (technically not yet achieved)
– Suitable delivery systems for new gene available
– Resistance of inserted new gene to cellular switch off mechanisms
– Vector with potential suicide mechanism
– No significant safety problem and risk for the patient:
  * Pathogenicity of viral vector (recombination with wild virus)
  * Transfer of nonviral exogenous genetic material
  * Insertional mutagenesis and risk of cancer
  * Immune reaction to new epitopes on the expressed protein
  * Uncontrolled incorporation into cells (germ line, others)
  * No pathogenicity of viral vector (recombination with wild virus) for the staff
  * No pollution by infectious virus resulting from recombination of disabled vector with wild virus

Genetic Defects Being Potential Targets for Somatic Gene Therapy	Chromosome

1 Gaucher's disease, osteoporosis, hypertension, preeclampsia
2 Diabetes
3 Hemangioblastomas, pancreatic cancer, kidney cancer (VHL)
4 Huntington's disease
5 Renal cancer, colon cancer Polyposis (FAP)
6 Allergy (HLA); Ataxia
7 Cystic fibrosis
9 Malignant melanoma (pl6); Ataxia
10 Prostate cancer, obesity
11 Parkinson's disease, obesity, Wilm's kidney tumor (WT-1), sickle cell anemia, diabetes type I, allergy (Fc IgE-Rec. I)
12 Osteoporosis, diabetes, carcinomas (K-*ras*)
13 Retinoblastoma (RB I); Wilson's disease
14 Allergy (TCR-α); Alzheimer's disease (APP)
15 Baldness, Prader-Will neurological disease
16 Polycytic kidney disease
17 Carcinomas (p53), hypertension, neurofibromatosis (NF-1) STH deficiency, pressure palsy neuropathy, breast carcinomas (BRCA-1)
18 Amyloidosis, colon carcinomas (DCC)
19 Familial hypercholesterinaemia, myotonic dystrophia, Alzheimer's disease (ApoE) diabetes, pressure palsy, neuropathy
20 Polycystic kidney disease; familial Creutzfeld Jacob disease
21 Alzheimer's disease (APP), familial cerebral amyloid angiopathy
22 DiGeorge's syndrome; Neurofibromatosis (NF-2)
X Hemophilia, fragile X mental ratardation, muscular dystrophy (Duchenne)

FM9

Bertelsen et al. 1995.

25.1.3 Methods

– Gene addition therapy (new gene inserted, old gene present)
– Gene replacement or excision therapy (new gene inserted in place of old by homologous recombination)
– Transduction of autologous cells in vitro, injection of expressing cells
– Injection of new gene, transduction of cells in vivo
    * Systemic administration
    * Local administration (nasal, liver, spleen)

Gene Replacement or Excision Therapy (by Homologous Recombination)

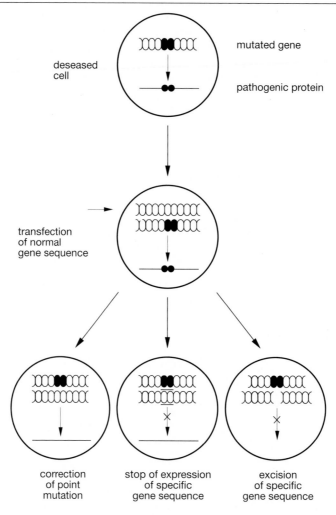

Huber 1994.

Gene Addition Therapy

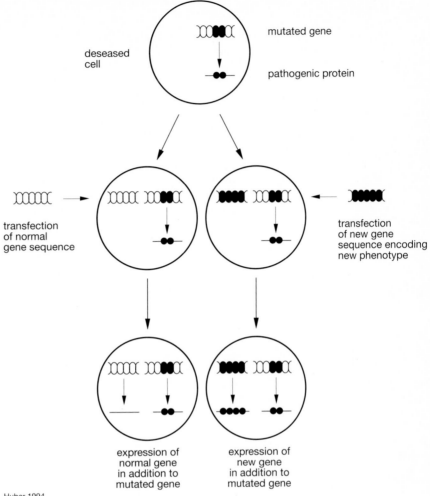

deseased cell

mutated gene

pathogenic protein

transfection of normal gene sequence

transfection of new gene sequence encoding new phenotype

expression of normal gene in addition to mutated gene

expression of new gene in addition to mutated gene

Huber 1994

Gene Transfer Technologies	Methods	Usefulness for gene therapy
	Chemical transfer	+ (in vitro)
	Electroporation	+ (in vitro)
	Microinjection into the nucleus	+ (in vitro)
	Scrape loading	+ (in vitro)
	Macroinjection into tissue	++ (in vivo, DNA-vaccines)
	Receptor-mediated delivery	++ (in vivo)
	Liposomal transfer	+++ (in vitro, in vivo)
	Viral transfer	
	– Retroviral vectors	++ (in vitro, in vivo)
	– Adenoviral vectors	++ (in vivo, lung tissue)
	– Adenoviral helped transfer of receptor mediated delivery	+++ (in vivo)

Somatic Gene Therapy

Retroviral vectors

Advantages	Disadvantages
– Well-known biology, small and simple genome	– Limited insert capacity for foreign DNA (6–8 kb)
– High transfection rate of replicating cells	– Infects only dividing cells
	– Often only transient expression
– Stable colinear integration into host genome	– Potentially mutagenic by random integration
	– May recombine with replication competent virus

Adenoviral vectors

Advantages	Disadvantages
– Well known biology	– No integration into host genome (only transient expression)
– High efficacy of in vivo infection of nonreplicating cells	– complicated vector design
	– limited insert capacity for foreign DNA (6–8 kb)
– Suitable for in vivo use (topical to the lung)	– Virus proteins may cause inflammatory reactions

Adenoassociated-virus vectors

Advantages	Disadvantages
– Small genome (5 kb)	– Biology not very well known
– Preferential integration into human chromosome 19	– Requires adeno virus as helper for replication
– Humans are natural hosts, nonpathogenic, nontoxic	– Limited insert capacity for foreign DNA ($\approx$ 4,5 kb)

Liposomes

Advantages	Disadvantages
– No infectious capability	– Low transduction efficiency
– Transfer of very large pieces of DNA (up to 150 kb)	– No specific targeting
– Low toxicity	– Only transient expression

Bifunctional (receptor-mediated) vectors

Advantages	Disadvantages
– No infectious capability	– Low transduction efficiency
– Transfer of very large pieces of DNA (up to 150 kb)	
– Low toxicity	– Only transient expression
– Targeting	

25.2 Details

25.2.1 Viral Transfer of Genes

Recombinant viral gene transfer vectors use the mechanisms, by which viruses transfer their genetic material to target cells.

Strategy for the design of such vectors is the incorporation of heterologous DNA sequences into the genome of the parent virus in such a way that the virion can deliver the incorporated heterologous nucleic acid sequences together with its endogenous nucleic acid sequences. This strategy imposes certain design limitations on the vector:

– The upper limit of foreign nucleic acid sequences which can be packaged in the virion capsid of recombinant retroviruses is on the order of 6–8 kb.

- In recombinant adenoviruses only 6-8 kb of heterologous DNA can practically be incorporated due to the problem that only a minority of viral genes can be deleted and/or provided in trans.
- The potential for interactions of viral and heterologous promotor elements may undermine the capacity to achieve specific regulation of the transferred gene.

Because the heterologous sequences are incorporated into a parent viral backbone, transfer of the heterologous DNA inevitably involves cotransfer of viral (retroviral or adenoviral) gene elements:

- For recombinant retroviruses the viral capacity to achieve host genome integration is retained with the recombinant vector. Moreover, viral promotor and enhancer elements are cotransferred as part of the vector design.
- Integration of the vector DNA occurs in a relatively random fashion and may cause safety problems:
  An insertion into an essential cellular gene would represent a potentially lethal event.
  An insertion of viral promotors in proximity to cellular oncogenes could activate these gene elements and lead to unregulated cellular proliferation.
  The integrated retroviral vector may recombine with wild type retrovirus coinfecting the modified cell and may result into replication competent recombinant virions. Such virions would have the potential to transfer the heterologous genes to sites where its expression could be deleterious.

Curiel 1994.

| **Retrovirus Mediated Transfer** | The unique replication cycle of retroviruses makes them useful as vectors for gene therapy. |

The unique replication cycle of retroviruses makes them useful as vectors for gene therapy.
- The parental virus attaches to a susceptible cell through a specific receptor and enters the cell.
- Within the cell the RNA genome of the retrovirus is copied to DNA by the virally encoded reverse transcriptase.
- The viral DNA is transported to the nucleus, where it is integrated into the host chromosome and is designated the provirus.
- The provirus is transcribed like endogenous DNA sequences and is stable in the chromosome during cell division.
- Unspliced and spliced transcripts are translated to produce the viral proteins.
- Some of the unspliced RNA is encapsidated into forming virions.
- Progeny virus is released from the cell by budding.

All retroviral genomes contain *cis*-acting sequences that direct the replication cycle:
- The long terminal repeats contain sequences involved in:
  Proviral transcription
  Reverse transcription
  Integration of the viral DNA into the host genome to form the provirus.
- Sequences between 5′LTR and *gag* direct the encapsidation of viral RNA into virion particles.

– *gag, pol* and *env* genes code for virion proteins and enzymes, including reverse transcriptase and integrase.

Retroviral vectors contain the *cis*-acting (LTR-associated) sequences of a retroviral vector; the *gag, pol* and *env* genes, however, are removed and replaced with
the coding sequences of a foreign gene.
– Such retroviral vectors are crippled and cannot replicate. For their multiplica-
tion they need replication proteins expressed from plasmids in helper or packaging cells.
– Helper plasmids are constructed to contain minimum sequence homology with
the retroviral vector in order to minimize the chance of recombination to form
a replication competent retrovirus. Such helper plasmids contain *gag-pol* and
env genes (together or separately), but the 5′LTR, the packaging and encapsidation signal are usually deleted and the 3′LTR is replaced with heterologous
promotors (i.e. SV 40 promotor).

Retroviral vectors are endowed with risks for safety due to
– A high level of genetic variability (around 5% of the proviruses resulting from
infection with vector RNA can be altered) mainly through
Errors during reverse transcriptions (deletions ± insertions, frameshifts, base
pair substitutions)
Copacking of vector RNA with cellular RNA, helper RNA or wild type retrovirus RNA, which gives a chance of genetic rearrangement by recombination
during reverse transcription. Potential products of recombination are a replication competent retrovirus, a novel viral vector that contains cellular sequences
or an altered vector
– Random integration of the vector provirus, which could
Inactivate a gene, essential for survival of the cell
Inactivate suppressor genes or activate expression of protooncogenes (since
transduced cells are diploid, inactivation of most suppressor genes would be
„silent“)

Boris-Lawrie et al. 1994.

Genomic Structure of a Retrovirus

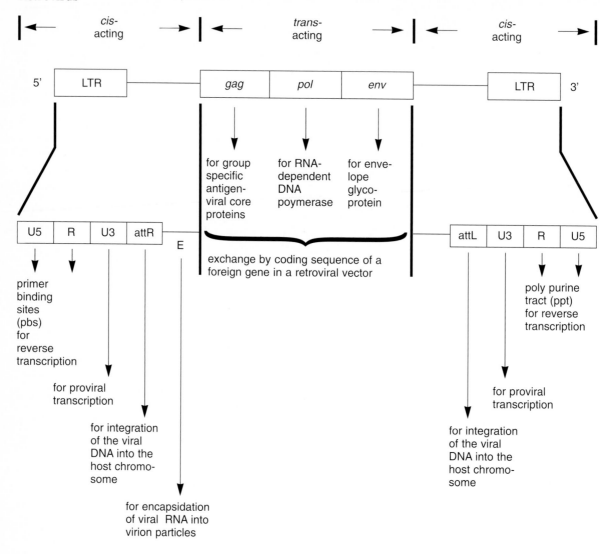

Boris-Lawrie et al. 1994.

Adenovirus Mediated Transfer

Adenovirus is a double stranded linear DNA virus with a naked protein capsid. There are 42 serotypes known to infect humans and to cause influenza-like illness, acute pharyngitis, conjunctivitis, pneumonia or gastrointestinal syndromes. Adenovirus serotype 5 is commonly used for the design of adenovirus vectors, which is as follows:
-   The E1a and E1b regions are deleted to prevent replication. They are substituted by the foreign gene.
-   The E3 region can be deleted to provide additional space for the insertion of exogenous DNA.
-   Up to 7,5 kb exogenous DNA can be inserted.

The (replication deficient) adenoviral vectors are propagated in a transformed human embryonic kidney cell line (293 cells) that expresses E1 proteins to allow the production of the replication deficient adenoviral vector in titers up to 10^{12} plaque forming units/ml.

Adenovirus enters cells by receptor-mediated endocytosis. Cell entry involves:
-   Initial binding to an uncharacterized cell surface receptor by the viral fiber protein. The internalization process involves the binding with the vitronectin receptor ($\alpha_2\beta_3$ integrin).
-   Internalization in clathrin coated pits and
-   Subsequently within cellular endosomes
-   Acidification of the endosome allows the virus to disrupt the cell vesicle (by means of capsid proteins in the peripontal region) and to achieve escape to the cell cytoplasm.
-   Ingress into the cytoplasm is followed by localization to the host nucleus and by translocation of the viral DNA.
-   Unlike retrovirus vectors, the genome of the adenovirus does not likely integrate into the host genome but instead functions episomally. This avoids potential problems inherent in random integration, but leads to transient gene expression.

Adenovirus can specifically facilitate entry of macromolecules (proteins, DNA) through its receptor mediated pathway. Cointernalization within the same endosome allows codelivery to the target cell cytosol through the ability of the adenovirus to disrupt cellular endosomes and to achieve nuclear localization.

Examples:
-   Adenovirus mixed to DNA complexed with bifunctional molecular conjugate enhance transduction rate by a factor of 1000 (Curiel 1991).
-   DNA complexed with bifunctional molecular conjugate and linked (via a monoclonal antibody) with their polylysin part to the hexon adenoviral capsid protein (into which a heterologous epitope was introduced by site directed mutagenesis) showed high efficiency gene transfer (Curiel 1994).
    This approach has significantly advantages:
    The size of the foreign DNA carried on the exterior of the virion is not limited
    DNA of any design can be incorporated into the complexes
    Since for the adenovirus the entry properties derive from capsid proteins, the integrity of viral genes is not essential.

Recombinant adenoviral virions, in which foreign DNA is integrated into the genome of the virion, take advantage of the adenovirus-specific receptor binding and vesicle escape mechanism. The disadvantages, however, are:
– The packaging constraints of the virus limit the size (6–8 kb) of the foreign DNA that can be transported.
– The specific regulation of the foreign DNA by heterologous promoter elements may be impaired by viral gene elements.
– Codelivery of viral gene elements to the host cell presents potential safety hazards.

Curiel 1994, Brody et al. 1994.

Genomic Structure of the Adenovirus (Type 5)

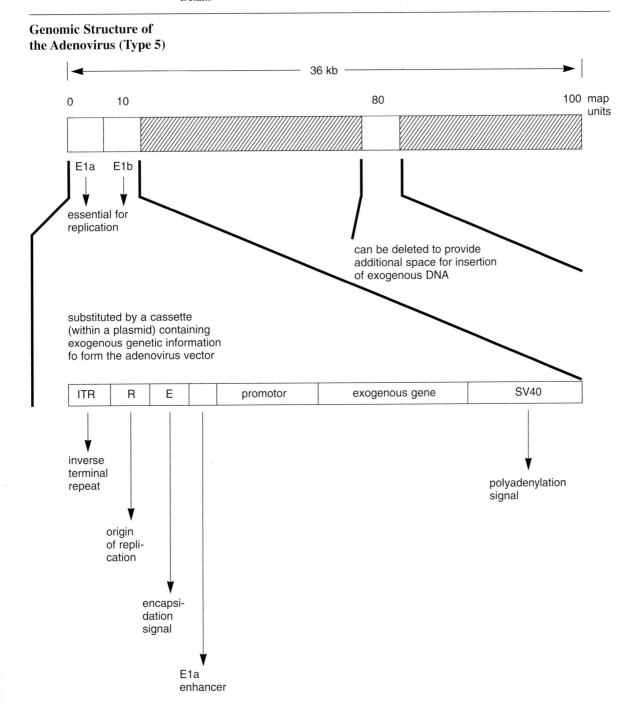

essential for replication

can be deleted to provide additional space for insertion of exogenous DNA

substituted by a cassette (within a plasmid) containing exogenous genetic information fo form the adenovirus vector

| ITR | R | E | | promotor | exogenous gene | SV40 |

inverse terminal repeat

origin of repli- cation

encapsi- dation signal

E1a enhancer

polyadenylation signal

Brody et al. 1994.

25.2.2 Liposomal Transfer of genes

Principle: – Cationic liposomes are complexed to negatively
             charged, naked DNA by simple mixing of both partners.
           – Resulting complex should have a net positive charge. Due to its
             positive charge the complex is easily bound to the negatively
             charged cell surface and taken up by the cells.

Advantage: – Simplicity (liposome preparation and use in transfection)
           – Ability to complex up to 100% of DNA (noncationic liposomes
             complex only small percentages)
           – Versatility in use with any type of naked DNA or RNA, with or
             without complexed proteins
           – No limitation of size of DNA (in contrast to viral vectors)
           – Ability to transfect many (although not all) different cell types
           – Superior transfection efficiency (in comparison to most nonviral
             methods of DNA delivery)
           – Safe for in vivo use, allowing repetitive use (no side effects, no
             immunogenicity)
           – Commercially available

Technique: – Lipofectin (prototype of most subsequent cationic liposome
             formulations) consists in equal amounts of:
             * synthetic cationic DOTMA
               (N-1-(2,3-dioleyloxy)propyl -N,N,N-trimethylammonium
               chloride
             * lipid dioleylphosphatidyl ethanolamine (DOPE)
             * mixture is sonicated, which produces small unilamellar
               vesicles with a size range of 50-200 nm in diameter
           – Mixing cationic liposomes with negatively charged DNA in
             aqueous solution produces a poorly characterized electrostatic-
             ally bound complex with a net positive charge at the optimal
             ratio of liposomes to DNA.
           – The positively charged complex bind efficiently to the negatively
             charged cell surface. Uptake of the complex follows, possibly
             through absorption-mediated endocytosis.
           – Complexes injected intravenously into mice localized mainly to
             the lung, heart and occasionally to the kidney. Tumor localiza-
             tion of DNA was detectable only with intratumoral injections.
             No toxicity could be found.

Farhood et al. 1994.

Liposomal Transfer of Genes

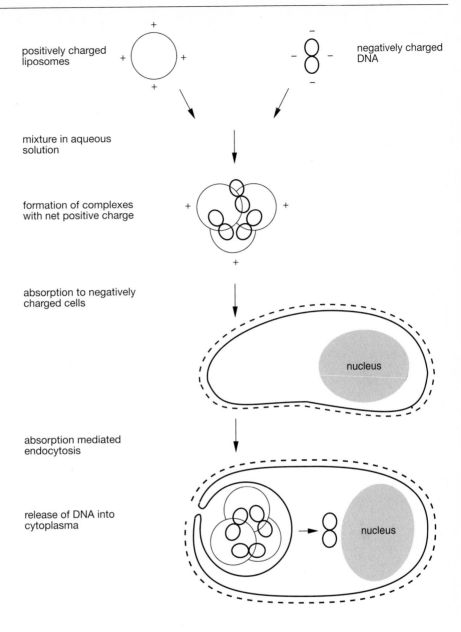

positively charged
liposomes

negatively charged
DNA

mixture in aqueous
solution

formation of complexes
with net positive charge

absorption to negatively
charged cells

nucleus

absorption mediated
endocytosis

release of DNA into
cytoplasma

nucleus

25.2.3 Receptor Mediated Transfer of Genes

Principle:
- A bifunctional molecular conjugate is used to bind DNA and to attach it to cell membrane receptors.
  * The DNA binding domain of the bifunctional molecule may be a cationic polylysine moiety.
  * The receptor binding domain of the bifunctional molecule may be a ligand for a receptor (i.e. transferrin).
- DNA in mixture with the bifunctional molecule form complexes. On the surface of such complexes the receptor binding domains of the bifunctional molecules are exposed.
- With their exposed receptor binding domains the complexes bind to the corresponding cell surface receptors and are internalized by the receptor mediated endocytosis pathway. Part of the internalized DNA escape from lysosomal degradation by penetration into the cytoplasm and achieve nuclear localization, where heterologous gene expression is effected.

Advantages:
- No safety problems associated with viral vectors and their potential to recombine with wild type viruses.
- High internalization (transfection) rate via receptor recirculation/metabolism.
- No vector associated toxicity due to membrane pertubation (DNA entry occurs via a physiologic internalization pathway).
- DNA can be delivered on a continuous or repetitive basis.
- Cell-specific delivery of nucleic acids via cell specific membrane receptors; examples (in vitro in vivo experiments):
  * Transferrin receptor of the liver (Zatloukal et al. 1992)
  * Asialoglycoprotein receptor of the liver (Wu et al. 1989)
  * IgA-receptors of lung epithelial cells (Ferkol et al. 1992)
  * Surfactant protein B-receptors in the lung (Baatz et al. 1992)

Disadvantages:
- Gene transfer from endosomes (receptor-mediated pathway) to nucleus often limited or absent due to:
  * lysosomal degradation of DNA bifunctional conjugate complexes.
  * no specific mechanism to escape the cell vesicle system.

Curiel 1994.

Receptor-Mediated
Transfer of Genes

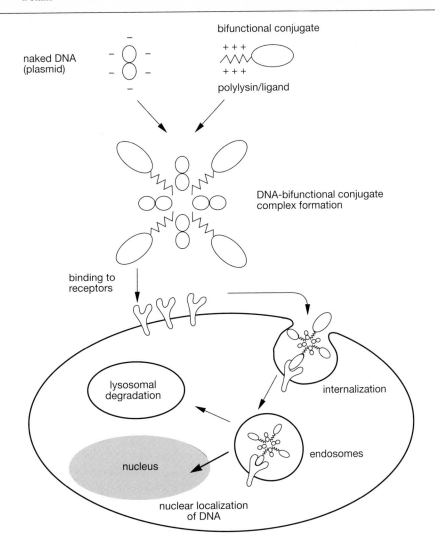

25.2.4 Experimental Therapeutic Approaches

Tumor Strategies
Diseases

Definition of pathogenic gene:
– A pathogenic gene producing an aberrant gene product which results in or contributes to neoplastic diseases has to be defined. Such pathogenic genes may
  arise by
    * Mutations (i.e. *ras* gene; codons 12, 13 or 61; p 53 gene, Rb gene)
    * Overexpression (i.e. *myc* gene)
    * Insertion (i.e. viral genes)

Gene replacement or excision therapy:
– Through homologous recombinant events

* The mutated sequence should be replaced with the normal sequence of the unmutated gene
* The expression of the pathogenic gene should be stopped by the in situ integration of stop codons or "nonsense" sequences into the internal domains of specific genes
* The integrated pathogenic genomic (viral) sequence could be excised.
– Homologous recombination has been demonstrated to take place in mammalian cells and used for generating "knock out" mice. However, since homologous recombination is a very rate event with the present technology, this approach is nearly impossible to apply for human somatic cell gene therapy at present.

Gene addition therapy:
– Through delivery of a complete copy of a normal gene to a particular target cell. The complete copy of a normal gene can
* Be randomly integrated into the genome of the target cell (no site specific integration)
* Remain extrachromosomal
– To replace important genetic information that has been "lost" through mutational events:
* Function of endogenous tumor suppressor genes in tumor cells can be regained
* Transduced normal cells seem to tolerate the expression of additional suppressor gene product, which seems to be the major advantage of gene addition therapy
* All tumor cells have to be transduced in vivo, expression of the administered tumor suppressor gene would have to be maintained for the natural life time of the cell (till to terminal differentiation state or apoptosis). The present gene transfer technology does not seem to fulfill these requirements.
– To create entirely new and unique phenotypes in the cancer cell:
* By genes that encode immune stimulatory proteins
* By genes that encode a toxin directly toxic to the tumor cells
* By genes that encode specific enzymes, which can produce toxic drugs at the tumor site when a nontoxic prodrug is administered
* Approaches which generate toxins or toxic drugs may have a "neighbouring cell effect" (cells neighbouring in the transduced tumor cell may be killed by the released toxin)
– Selective expression in the tumor cells of either suppressor genes or directly or indirectly acting toxin-producing genes can be achieved through the use of selective delivery systems
* use of retroviral vectors which transfect only dividing cells
* creation of chimeric genes where the expression of the administered gene is controlled by a tumor specific transcriptional regulatory sequence

Huber 1994.

Experimental approaches using in vitro transduced cells	– Transduction of tumor cells in vitro to produce cytokines (IL-1, IL-4, IL-6, IL-7, IL-12, IFNγ gamma, TNFα, G-CSF, GM-CSF): * Vaccination (experimental, clinical data) which such tumor cells does not seem to be more effective than conventional approaches (tumor cells in mixture with cytokines or *C. parvum,* BCG). – Transduction of tumor cells in vitro to express MHC-class II or B-7: * Vaccination (experimental data) induces a strong immune response. – Transduction of tumor infiltrating lymphocytes (TIL) to express cytokines (TNFα, IL-2) * TIL had problems to maintain expression of cytokines and to home to the tumor after systemic application. * Early enthusiastic clinical report of this approach could not be confirmed so far; clinical responses seem to be neither marked nor long lived. – Transduction of normal bone marrow cells to express high levels of the multidrug resistance (MDR) membrane protein: * in experimental studies reinjection of such bone marrow cells induced in tumor bearing mice resistance of the bone marrow against the toxicity of cancer chemotherapy.
In vivo experimental approaches for transduction	– Transduction of tumor cells in vivo: * To insert suppressor genes (wild type p 53; retinoblastoma gene (RB); adhesion molecules deleted in colorectal carcinoma (DCC), or * To block or replace oncogenes (c-*sis*, c-*erbB*, c-*ras*, c-*mos*, c-*myc*, others): * Tumor cells with defective suppressor genes can be repaired in vitro; repairment is associated with reduction of malignancy. – Oncogenes in tumor cells can be replaced in vitro (homologous recombination), such treated tumor cells have reduced malignancy – In vivo experiments suffer from insufficient targeting and insufficient transfection rate of the tumor cells – Transduction of tumor cells in vivo to express new enzyme for cleavage of prodrugs into cytostatic drugs: * Tumor selective expression is mediated by genes of promotors (transcriptional regulatory sequences) for a gene encoding a tumor associated antigen: carcinoembyronic antigen (CEA) colorectal cancer, part of other epithelial tumors

α-Fetoprotein (αFP)	hepatoma, germ cell tumors
neuron-specific enolase (NSE)	small cell lung cancer
prostate-specific antigen (PSA)	prostate cancer
thyroglobulin	thyroid follicular carcinoma
calcitonin	thyroid medullary carcinoma
tyrosinase	melanoma
polymorphic epithel-ial mucin (PEM)	breast cancer, pancreatic cancer
c-*erbB2*	breast cancer gastrointestinal cancer, pancreatic cancer
c-*erbB3*	breast cancer
c-*erbB4*	breat cancer gastrointestinal cancer
BCA-1	breast cancer

* Tumor selectivity of expression is increased by retroviral vectors, which transfect only deviding cells; ≈10–60% of tumor cells can be transfected in vivo (mice).

* Promotor genes are coupled to prodrug activating enzymes:

	cleavage of
cytosine deaminase	5-fluorocytosine to 5-fluorouracil
thymidine kinase	adenine arabinoside (ARA-A) to ARA-AMP
linamarase	amygdalin to cynamide

In vivo experiments (mice) show regression of human tumor xenografts. Transfected cells as well as neighbouring non-transfected cells are killed. About 2% of a solid tumor mass (xenografts) can be transduced in vivo.

Sikora 1994, Dalgleish 1994, Robbins et al. 1994, Huber et al. 1994, Gottesman et al. 1994, Howard et al. 1994, Hwu et al. 1994, Roemer et al. 1994.

Allergy and Asthma   Suitability   – Atopy and allergy affects 30% of Western populations
                             of clinical   – Is a complex genetic disease, which runs in families
                             indications   – No clear cut pattern of inheritance
                                            – Strong environmental component
                                            – Severe atopy is maternally inherited:
                                              * Linked to chromosome 11 (q 13)
                                              * Associated with chromosome 11 (q 13) is the gene for the β-chain of the Fc IgE RI receptor
                                              * Associated with severe allergy is the variant Leu 181/Leu 183 of the Fc IgE RI (present in 15% of asthmatics and in 4,5% of the general population)
                                            – Other genes which influence allergy:
                                              * HLA region on chromosome 6 (small effect)
                                              * TCR-α region on chromosome 14 (moderate effect)
                                            – It is questionable whether genes coding for interleukins (especially IL-4) on chromosome 5 are associated with allergies. Consequently, IL-4 seems to influence allergic reactions not in a specific, but in an unspecific way through its broad way of action.

                             Experimental   – Downregulation of the gene for the β-chain of Fc IgE RI
                             approaches   seems to be the only real approach so far:
                             for somatic   * Systemic injection of new gene and in vivo transduction of cells to reduce expression of Fc IgE RI has not been tested.
                             gene therapy   * In vitro transduction of cells to reduce expression of Fc IgE RI and injection of such transduced cells does not, however, seem to be a suitable approach.
                                            * In vitro transduction of cells to express proteins which block IL-4 (IL-4-receptors, IL-4 muteins) and injection of such transduced cells might be an approach indirectly to down modulate expression of Fc IgE RI expression.

Cookson 1992, 1993, 1994; Colleé et al. 1993; Moffatt et al. 1992; Sandford et al. 1993.

Immune Deficiencies   Suitability   – Severe combined immune deficiencies (SCID) of man
                             of clinical   comprise a syndrome that is characterized by absent cell
                             indications   mediated or humoral immunity and is usually fatal by 1–2 years of life.
                                            – SCID is caused by:
                                              * Defects in the gene for adenosine deaminase (ADA), an enzyme involved in purine metabolism ($\approx$ 25% of all SCID cases)
                                                – ADA-SCID is treated by allogeneic bone marrow transplantation (90% success rate using matched donors, 50–60% success rate using mismatched donors).

		– Injection of polyethylene glycol stabilized bovine ADA (PEG-ADA) leads to improvements in some patients (increase T-cell numbers, enhanced immune function).

       * Lack or deficiency of the γ-chain of the IL-2-receptor (in ≈ 30–35% of cases).

       * Defects in the gene for the NADPH-oxydase which impairs oxygen radical formation and results in defects of the extra- and intracellular killing mechanisms of phagocytic cells, leading to chronic granulomatous disease (CGD):

          – The recurrent and chronic bacterial and fungal infections in CGD can be treated with antibiotics (i.e. trimethoprim, sulfamethoxazole) and IFN gamma, but without significant change of the generally severely shortened life expectancy of affected individuals.

In vivo experimental approaches for transduction

– ADA-SCID is being treated in clinical experiments by autologous peripheral T-cells or bone marrow cells, transduced in vitro by retroviral vectors to express ADA:

    * Injection of transduced T-cells leads to a transient mitigation of the SCID symptoms; treatment has to be repeated at regular intervals.

    * Injection of transduced bone marrow cells may possibly be needed to be only performed once; treatment leads to mitigation of the SCID-symptoms.

– Cell lines derived from CGD-SCID patients were in vitro transduced by retroviral vectors to express NADPH; before starting clinical trials, technical problems have to be solved; these include:

    * Optimization of the expression of the transduced genes

    * Development of better gene delivery systems/ vectors

    * Introducing genes into pluripotent haemopoietic stem cells

Kinnon 1994.

Other Immune Diseases   **Suitability of clinical indications**

– Rheumatoid arthritis:

    * IL-1 may be involved in the initiation and/or progression

    * Autologous synovial cells, in vitro transduced by a retroviral vector to express IL-1-RA and reinjected into the rabbit knee joint became engrafted into the synovial lining

    * Such treatment inhibited arthritis, induced by the intraarticular injection of IL-1 into rabbits

Robbins et al. 1994.

Hemophilia	Suitability of clinical indications	– Tight regulation of the gene is not necessary. – Targeting to anatomical site is not required. – 10% of normal levels protects against minor bleedings. – The genes have been cloned. – Conventional treatment (substitution) very expensive.

Hemophilia A
- F VIII deficiency; recessive genetic disease, linked to chromosome X (tip of the long arm; close to genes for color vision, glucose 6 phosphate dehydrogenase, F IX).
- F VIII gene:
  * Spans about 190 000 base pairs.
  * Protein-coding regions are divided into 26 exons.
  * mRNA is about 9000 base pairs.
  * Specifies a protein of about 2351 aa.
  * Expressed mainly in liver cells.
  * Mutations are mostly caused by deletions.

Hemophilia B
- F IX deficiency; recessive genetic disease linked to chromosome X
- F IX gene:
  * Spans about 33 500 base pairs.
  * Protein coding regions are devided into 8 exons.
  * Specifies a protein of 461 aa.
  * Expressed mainly in liver cells.
  * Pre-F IX needs several modifications to be functionally active:
    - Certain glutamic acid residues have to be modified by the addition of an extra COOH group; this step requires the presence of vitamin K.
    - Aspartic acid residue at position 64 has to be hydroxylated in the β-position.
    - Two asparagine residues have to be glycosylated.
  * Functional defects mostly caused by point mutations.

Hemophilia C
- Factor XI deficiency
- Factor XI gene:
  * Spans about 23.000 base pairs,
  * Protein coding regions are devided into 15 exons,
  * Specifies a protein of 607 aa (monomer), each constitutes a single chain of a dimer with two identical subunits.
  * Functional defects could be referred to point mutations.

von Willebrand disease
- Deficiency in von Willebrand factor, encoded on chromosome 12
- von Willebrand factor gene:
  * Protein coding regions are devided into 52 exons.
  * specifies a protein (monomer) of 2050 aa.

* Monomers associate to the basic protomer with molecular weight of about 240 kDa.
* During biosynthesis in endothelial cells lining the blood vessels, the proteins are assembled first into dimers through carboxy-terminal disulfide interchange and then into multimers of higher order through N-terminal disulfide interchange in a step that depends on the presence of a very long propeptide.
* This long propeptide is excised from von Willebrand factor multimers during assembly and secreted separately; it consists of 763 aa and has no known function other than to promote multimer assembly; lack of long propeptide leads to unproper multimerization and poor function in platelet adhesion, although able to support factor VIII.

Experimental approaches using in vitro transduced cells	– F VIII gene: * Fibroblasts could be transduced by retroviral, adenoviral and nonviral (transferrin-transferrin receptor Transfection) vectors. After s.c. injection transduced fibroblasts expressed human F VIII for about 1 week only (reasons: transcriptional shut off, instability of mRNA). * Myoblasts could be transduced similarly as fibroblasts. After injection into liver or spleen (mouse system) expression lasted for several months. – F IX gene: * Fibroblasts and myoblasts could be transduced by retroviral, adenoviral and nonviral vectors. * After s.c. injection or injection into spleen or liver transduced cells expressed F IX for several months. * Experiments in man are ongoing.

Tuddenham 1991, 1994.

Neuromuscular Diseases	Suitability of clinical indications	– Some neuromuscular diseases have a genetic origin: * Spinal muscular atrophy * Leucodystrophics * Charcot-Marie tooth disease * Duchenne muscular dystrophy – Skeletal muscle fibres and nerve cells take up naked DNA (plasmid), retain them undegraded as episomal circular DNA (for months or even years) and express them throughout this time. – Integration of genes (i.e. introduced in a replication-defective retroviral vector) requires cell replication:

* Nerve cells are "end cells", i.e. their nuclei have left the mitotic cycle, entering G_0 and they do not devide after birth; thus, genetic modification of neurons can not include integration into the genome of the cell
* Multinucleated muscle fibres are also "end cells" in case of their damage, however, they can be repaired or replaced by the activation of myogenic satellite cells (myogenic stem cells), which lie between the muscle fibres and their surrounding basement membranes
* Myogenic satellite cells can proliferate and subsequently fuse with one another and with surviving portions of damaged muscle fibres, thereby restoring or replacing the syncytial structure; thus, myogenic satellite cells are able to integrate the new gene construct and to incorporate it into multinucleate muscle fibers.

Experimental approaches using in vitro transduced cells	– Duchenne muscular dystrophy is a lethal recessive monogenic disease of skeletal muscle: * Gene coding for dystrophin is mutated, function of mutated dystrophin is lost. * Myoblasts of the patients, transduced in vitro to express dystrophin and reinjected intramuscularly can mitigate the disease; clinical studies are running.

Dickson et al. 1993; Karpati et al. 1993; Partridge 1991, 1994.

Metabolic and Cardio-vascular Diseases	Suitability of clinical indications	– Gaucher's disease is caused by a genetic defect of the gene coding for glucocerebrosidase which hydrolyses glucosylceramide to glucose and ceramide. Deficiency leads to abnormal lysosomal storage of glucosylceramide primarily in macrophages. The disease is manifested by hepatosplenomegaly and painful bone lesions with or without neurological involvement. Conventional treatments include: * Enzyme replacement. Amount needed is very high and expensive. Dose reduction could be achieved by targeting the enzyme to macrophages (the oligosaccharide side chains were enzymatically cleaved by exoglycosidases to expose mannose residues for specific binding to mannose receptors). * Allogeneic bone marrow transplantation (limited availability, high risk procedure with considerable rate of mortality). – Familiar hypercholesterinaemia (FH) is caused by defects of the gene coding for the LDL-receptors of liver cells: * Heterozygotic gene defect (occurrence: 1/5000) leads to $\approx$50% acute myocard infarction beyond 50 years of age. * Homozygotic gene defect (occurrence: 1/1 million births) leads to $\approx$1000% acute myocard infarction at the age of 5–10 years.

* Conventional treatment is of minor success (removal of cholesterol by plasma exchange, liver transplantation).
– Thrombosis caused by increased fibrinogen or increased PAI-1 or decreased fibrinolysis (uPA, tPA, plasmin):
  * Conventional treatment by anticoagulants
– Reocclusions of arterial vessels by proliferating smooth muscle cells of the vessel wall:
  * No treatment available yet except angioplasty

Experimental approaches using in vitro transduced cells	– Homocygote FH has been treated in a clinical experiment by injection of autologous liver cells (≈15% of total liver tissue), transduced in vitro by a retroviral vector to express the LDL-receptor
	* Lipid-lowering effect was stable for >18 months (17% reduction of LDL-C, 30% improvement in LDL/HDL ratio).
	* Additional treatment with lovostatin (known to increase LDL receptor function) improved the therapeutic effect.
	* Side effects were not observed.
	* Improvement needed are:
	  – Improved expression of LDL-receptors.
	  – Safer (noninfectious) vectors.
	– Bone marrow cells from patients with Gaucher disease were transduced by an retroviral vector to express glucocerebrosidase (40-fold increase). Based on these results clinical studies are in preparation

In vivo experimental approaches for transduction	– Lowering of fibrinogen to reduce risk of thrombosis is going to be tried by antisense oligo DNA for the β-chain of fibrinogen (β-chain production is the rate limiting effect of synthesis of fibrinogen by liver cells): * Experiments are in a very early stage (promotor for the β-gene has been identified). – Reduction of PAI-1 may not be a suitable target to reduce risk of thrombosis: * PAI-1 transgenic mice developed venous thrombosis which resolved after a few weeks (possibly by feedback control of fibrinolysis). – Inhibition of local proliferation of smooth muscle cells of the vessel wall: * c-*myc* antisense oligo-DNA reduced c-*myc* expression and neointimal formation by 60–70% in rats (problem: suppression of reendothelialization) * gene transfer into cells of the vessel wall by local in vivo application (adeno virus vectors are prefered). Experimental studies are ongoing; whether this approach is superior to the local application of lipophilic cytostatics is questionable.

– Efficiency of transduction of endothelial cells is very low with retroviral or liposomal vectors. In contrast, adenoviral vectors transduce endothelial cells in vitro as well as in vivo very efficiently.

Humphries 1994, Robbins et al. 1994, Brody et al. 1994

Diseases of the Lung	Suitability of clinical indications	– Cystic fibrosis (CF) is an autosomal recessive monogenic disease of chromosome 7.

– Cystic fibrosis (CF) is an autosomal recessive monogenic disease of chromosome 7.
– Frequency:
  * Healthy gene carriers (heterozygotes): 1 in 22
  * Incidence of disease: 1 in 2000 (1 in 4 risk for children of couple of two healthy CF-carriers)
– Pathophysiology:
  * Genetic defect of the cystis fibrosis transmembrane regulator (CFTR); gene for CFTR resembles MDR-gene.
  * CFTR is an integral membrane protein with chloride transport function expressed in epithelial cells (1480 residue glycosylated molecule with 12 transmembrane and 3 intracytoplasmic domains).
  * CF patients have disturbed CFTR synthesis or processing resulting in impaired cellular chloride transport.
  * Dysfunction of epithelial function leads to
    – Pulmonal symptoms (coughing, mucous obstruction of airways, dyspnea, pneumonia)
    – Intestinal symptoms (voluminous fatty stools, subacute obstructions and abdominal pain)
    – General symptoms (enhanced appetite and underweight, male sterility, enhanced sweat chloride)
– No entirely satisfactory therapy available to date.
– CFTR gene has been cloned; molecular mechanism of disease has intensively been analysed in vitro and in vivo including transgenic CF mice.
– CFTR is effective at very low levels in normal lung cells; its overproduction is not toxic.
– Hereditary deficiency of α_1-antitrypsin reduces the inhibition of neutrophil elastase, accumulation of which damages the lung tissue and leads to pul monary emphysema
  * Continuous replacement of normal plasma derived α_1-antitrypsin is therapeutical effective.
  * Somatic gene therapy to introduce the normal α_1-antitrypsin cDNA into hepatocytes may be a long lasting therapeutic approach.

In vivo approaches for transduction	– Ion transport defect in CF cells can be corrected by transfection with and expression of wild type CFTR cDNA.
	– CFTR-gene has been incorporated into
	  * Adenovirus vector
	  * Liposomes
	– CFTR gene incorporated into vector or carrier has been given to patients (clinical experiments) by:
	  * Nasal administration: transient correction of chloride transport defect, no toxic effects (adenovirus vector, liposomes)
	  * Pulmonary administration: 1 case of severe transient inflammatory reaction (adenovirus vector)
	– The human α_1-antitrypsin gene incorporated into an adenoviral vector has been injected into the portal vein of adult rats; gene transfer and expression could be expressed in hepatocytes as well as by measurement of serum levels of human α_1-antitrypsin in rats.

Coutelle 1994, Brody et al. 1994.

22.2.5 Immunization with Polynucleotides

Vaccines Technical Approaches

The ability of polynucleotides to be introduced into cells in tissue culture by chemical means (i.e. with cationic lipids) and mechanically (by particle bombardment and electric shock) led to the developments of methods to deliver genetic material to somatic cells in vivo:
– Purified naked DNA without any vector system have been introduced:
  * Into skeletal muscle cells (Wolff et al. 1990).
  * Into cardiac muscle cells (Lin et al. 1990) by intramus cular injection.
  * Epidermal cells could be transfected by high velocity bom bardment with gold microparticles coated with DNA (Williams et al. 1991).
  * Bronchial epithelial cells by inhalation of an aerosol containing DNA complexed with cationic lipids (Stribling et al. 1992).
    Such transfected cells in vivo expressed the proteins encoded by the genetic material injected.
– The transfection rate could be enhanced when so-called facilitators (local anaesthetics) were injected at the same region and 24-h before injection of the polynucleotides (Wang et al. 1993).
– The expression rate could be enhanced when the DNA encoding the protein in question was driven by a strong viral promotor such as the RSV or CMV promotor (Wolff et al. 1990, Lin et al. 1990, Williams et al. 1991).
– Highest transfection and expression could be found after injection into muscle tissue, less expression in other tissues (Donnelly et al. 1994).
– Injected DNA constructs transfected individual muscle fibres (Wolff et al. 1990). Uptake of DNA by skeletal muscle cells seems to occur from T-tubules. Developing or regenerating muscle cells seem to take up DNA construct more efficiently than muscle fibres. The foreign DNA taken up by the muscle cells appears to remain episomal (Wolff et al. 1992, Wells et al. 1992, 1993).

Results
- Expression after i.m. injection of DNA constructs could be found in mice, rats, rabbits, dogs, cattle, chickens, fish and nonhuman primates (cynomolgus) (Donnelly et al. 1994).
- DNA sequences encoding for the following have been expressed in vivo; expression lasted for 4–20 months (Wolff et al. 1992):
    * Luciferase, chloramphenicol acetyl transferase, β-galacto sidase (Donnelly et al. 1994)
    * CD4 antigen (Wang et al. 1993)
    * Influenza A antigens (hemagglutinin, matrix protein, nucleoprotein) (Ulmer et al. 1993)
    * HIV antigens (gp120, gp160) (Wang et al. 1993)
    * Bovine herpes virus I antigen (g IV) (Cox et al. 1993)
    * Rabies virus antigen (surface glycoprotein; Donnelly et al. 1994)
    * IL-2, IL-4, TGF-β (Raz et al. 1993)
    * MHC-I antigens (Plautz et al.1993, Wahl et al.1992)
    * V genes of immunoglobulins (Hawkins et al. 1993)
    * Carcinoembryonic antigen (Conry et al. 1994)
- Expressed proteins induced a strong antibody response (predominantly of IgG type) and a strong cellular immune response (CD4+ and CD8+ T-cells) with CTL and ADCC.
- Cytokines (IL-2, IL-4, TGF-β) encoded by the DNA constructs and expressed by the myocytes modulated the immune response of the host (Raz et al. 1993).
- Intact, viable myoblasts or myocytes were required for induction of the immune response (Donnelly et al. 1994). Production of antigenic material by the transfected muscle cells seems to be sufficient to induce an immune response. Pretreatment of myoblasts with interferon gamma increased their expression of MHC-class I antigens and the immune response (Donnelly et al. 1994). The immune response seems to be both, MHC-class I and -class II restricted.
- There is lack of histological evidence of destruction of transduced muscle cells in injected tissues by the induced specific immune response (Wolff et al. 1990). It is assumed that the large size and the multinucleate structure of the myocytes make them resistant to lysis by cytotoxic (CTL, ADCC) cells (Donnelly et al. 1994).
- The immune response lasted for more than 6 months, CTL were found to persist for 1 year or more after immunization (Donnelly et al. 1994).
- The immune response was protective from a challenge with the specific virus (Donnelly et al. 1994).
- Tumor cells transfected to express the specific protein (CD4, HIV gp160, MHC-class I) demonstrated a reduced growth when they were transplanted into mice immunized with DNA constructs encoding for the corresponding protein (Wang et al. 1993, Plautz et al. 1993).

26 CD Terminology

CD Antigens

CD designation	Synonyms	Monoclonal antibodies	Molecular structure	Main cellular expression	Function(s)
CD1a	T6	VIT6, Leu6, NA1/34, T6	49 kDa; β_2 micro-globulin associated 1 IgSF domain	cortical thymocytes, dendritic cells (incl. Langerhans cells), B subsets	possible ligand for some T-cells (Antigenpresentation)
CD1b	–	WM-25, 4A76, NUT2	45 kDa; β_2 micro-globulin associated 1 IgSF domain	same as CD1a	same as CD1a
CD1c	–	L161, M241, 7C6, PHM3	43 kDa, β_2 micro-globulin associated 1 IgSF domain	same as CD1a	same as CD1a
CD2	T11, LFA-2, sheep red blood receptor	9.6, T11, 35.1	50 kDa, β_2 IgSF	T-cells, NK cells	adhesion molecule (binds LFA-3, CD58); T cell activation
CD3	T3, Leu-4	38,1; UCHT1, T3, Leu-4	composed of seven chains gp/p 26, 20, 16, 26, 20, 20 (γ, δ, ε, ζ, η) 1 IgSF each	T cells	signal transduction as a result of antigen recognition by T cells (T-cell receptor)
CD4	T4, Leu-3, L3T4 (mouse)	91.D6, T4, Leu-3	55 kDa, 4 IgSF domains	class II MHC-restricted T-cells; thymocytes	adhesion molecule (binds to class II MHC); signal transduction; HIV-receptor, on helper cells

CD designa-tion	Synonyms	Monoclonal antibodies	Molecular structure	Main cellular expression	Function(s)
CD5	T1, Lyt1, Leu-1	UCHT2, T101, HH9, AhG4, T1	67 kDa, 3 cysteine-rich extracellular domains	T cells, B cell subset	receptor for CD72, activation of TCR+ T-cells; (produce IL-10)
CD6	T12	T411, T12	100 kDa, 3 cysteine-rich extracellular domains	most T cells, some B cells	signal transduction
CD7	gp40	3A1, 4A, CL1.3, G3-7	40 kD, 1 IgbF domain + glycosylated hinge	T-cell precursors in fetal liver, thymus and bone marrow peripheral T-cells, stem cells	?
CD8 α-chain β-chain	T8, Leu-2, Lyt 2, T8/2	UCHT4, Leu2a, M236, UCHT4, T811, T8/2T8-5H7	composed of two 34 kDa chains; expressed as αα or α β dimer; 1 Ig domain per chain + glycosylated hinge	class I MHC-restricted thymocytes	adhesion (binds to class I) signal transduction on CTLs
CD9	–	CLB-thromb/8, PHN 200, FMC56	24 kDa	Pre-B and immature B cells, monocytes, platelets, eosinophils, activated T-cells	? role in platelet activation and aggregation
CD10	CALLA	J5, VILA1, BA-3	100 kDa, cysteine-rich extracellular domain	immature B+T and some mature B cells; lymphoid progenitors, granulocytes, cALL	structurally identical to neural endopeptidase (ence-phalinase); a Zn-metallopro-tease
CD11a	LFA-1 chain	2F12, CRIS-3, MHM24	180 kDa, associates with CD18 to form LFA-1 integrin (gp/180/95)	lymphocytes, granulocytes, monocytes, macrophages	adhesion (binds to ICAM-1)
CD11b	Mac-1, CR3, iC3b receptor chain	Mo1, 5A4.C5, LPM19C	180 kDa, associates with CD18 to form LFA-1 integrin (pg/155/95)	myeloid cells, NK-cells	adhesion; phagocytosis of iC3b-coated (opsonized) particles
CD11c	p150,95 CR4 α chain	B-Ly6, L29, BL-4H4	150 kDa, associates with CD18 to form gp150/95 integrin	myeloid cells, macrophages	adhesion; ? phagocytosis of iC3b-coated (opsonized) particles
CDw12	–	M67	? 90–120 kDa	monocytes, granulocytes, platelets	?

CD designation	Synonyms	Monoclonal antibodies	Molecular structure	Main cellular expression	Function(s)
CD13	–	My7, MCS-2, TÜK1, Mou28	150 kDa, type II glyco-protein	monocytes, granulocytes, fibroblasts, osteoclasts, renal cells, small intestine	aminopeptidase N; Zn-metalloprotease ? role in oxidative burst
CD14	Mo2	UCHM1, VIM13 MoP15, Mo2	55 kDa; GPI-linked	monocytes, B-cells, granulocyte subset	? role in oxidative burst; LPS receptor
CD15	Lewis X (Le^x)	My1, VIM-D5	branched pentasaccharide; two forms	granulocytes, monocytes	sialyted CD15 is ligand for CD62
CD16	Fc γ RIII	BW209/2, HUNK2, VEP13, Leu11c	50–65 kDa; GPI-linked and transmembrane, 2 IgSF domains	NK cells, granulocytes, macrophages	low-affinity Fc γ receptor: phagocytosis, ADCC, activation of NK cells
CDw17	LacCer	GO35, HuLym13	glycosphingolipide (lactosylceramide)	granulocytes, macrophages, platelets	exocytosis + packaging of granules
CD18	β-chain of LFA-1 family; inte-grin β$_2$ subunit	MHM23, M232, 11H6, CLB54	95 kDa, noncovalently linked to LFA-1 chains, CD11, CD11b or CD11c	leukocytes	see CD11a, CD11b, CD11c
CD19	B4	HD37, B4	95 kDa, 2 IgSF domains	B cells and B-precursors	? role in B cell proliferation
CD20	B1	IF5, B1	monomer forms 4 transmem-brane domains	all B cells	regulation of B-cell activation (Ca^{++} channel)
CD21	CR2, C3d receptor	B2, HB5	140 kDa, 15-16 extracel-lular CCP motive	mature B cells, FDC, epithelial cells, thymocytes	receptor for C3d and Epstein-Barr virus; ? role in B cell activation
CD22	BL-CAM	HD39, SHCL1, To15	135 kDa; homology to myelin-assoc. gp (MAG) β-form: 7 IgSF domains α-form: 5 IgSF domains	B cells	cell adhesion, CD45RO and CD 75 are ligands for CD22β
CD23	Fc ε RIIb blast-2	blast-2, MHM6	45–50 kDa, type II mem-brane protein, 1 lectin domain	activated B cells, macro-phages, eosinophils	low-affinity Fc ε receptor induced by IL-4

CD designation	Synonyms	Monoclonal antibodies	Molecular structure	Main cellular expression	Function(s)
CD24	–	VIBE3, BA-1	35–45 kDa, GPi linked sialoglycoprotein	B cells, granulocytes	role in the regulation of B-cell proliferation
CD25	TAC, P55, low-affinity IL-2 receptor (α-chain)	7G7/B6, 2A3, TAC	55 kDa, α-subunit, low affinity IL-2-rec., con- tains 2 CCP motives, asso- ciated with 75 kDa β-subunit	activated T and B cells, macrophages, monocytes	complexes with β-subunit to form high-affinity IL-2 re- cep- tor; T cell proliferation
CD26	–	134-2C2, TS145	120 kDa	activated T and B cells, macrophages epithelial cells, endothelial cells	serine peptidase (dipeptidyl- peptidase IV), function unknown
CD27	–	VIT14, S152, OKT18A, CLB-9FA	homodimer of 55 kDa chains; NGFR superfamily member, 2 cysteine-rich repeats in extracellular domain	most T cells; ? some plasma cells	? role in B cell growth
CD28	Tp44	9.3, KOLT2	S-S linked homodimer of 44 kDa chains, 2 IgSF domains	T cells (most CD4$^+$, some CD8$^+$ cells); plasma cells	T- and B-cell interaction T cell receptor for costimula- tor molecule(s), B7 is ligand
CD29	integrin β$_1$- subunit	K20, A-1A5	130 kDa; integrin β$_1$ chain; noncovalently associated with integrin α subunits 1–6 (= CD49 a–f); form the VLA	broad; platelets: GPIIa, T-cells	adhesion to extracellular matrix proteins, cell-cell adhesion (see CDw49)
CD30	Ki-1, Ber-H2 antigen	Ber-H2, HSR4, K-1	120 kDa, 5 cysteine-rich repeats; NGFR superfamily member	activated T and B cells, Reed-Sternberg cells in Hodgkin's disease	?
CD31	PECAM-1	SG134, TM3, HEC75, ES12F11	140 kDa, 5 IgSF domains	platelets; monocytes, granulo- cytes, B cells, endothelial cells	?; adhesion molecule
CDw32	Fc γ RIIA	CIKM5, 41H16, IV.3	40 kDa, 2 IgSF domains	macrophages, granulocytes, B cells, eosinophils, endothelial cells	Fc RII; Fc receptor for aggregated IgG; role in pha- gocytosis, ADCC
CD33	–	My9, H153, L4F3	67 kDa, 2 IgSF domains	monocytes, myeloid	?

CD designation	Synonyms	Monoclonal antibodies	Molecular structure	progenitor cells Main cellular expression	Function(s)
CD34	–	My10, Bl-3C5, ICH-3	105–120 kDa	precursors of hematopoietic cells; endothelial cells	?
CD35	CR1, C3b 4b receptor	T05, CB04, J3D3	polymorphic; four allotypes are 190 kDa; A allotype: 30 CCP motives	granulocytes, monocytes, erythrocytes, B-cells, T-cell subsets, FDC	binding and phagocytosis of C3b-coated particles and immune complexes
CD36	platelet gpIV OKM5 antigen	5F1, CIMeg1, ESIVC7	88 kDa	monocytes, platelets	receptor for plasmodium falciparum infection of erythrocytes
CD37	–	HD28, HH1, G28-1	TM4 superfamily member	B cells, some T cells	?
CD38	T10	HB7, T16	45 kDa, type II membrane glycoprotein	plasma cells, thymocytes, activated T cells, B-cells	?
CD39	–	AC2, G28-2	78 kDa	activated B cells, macrophages activated NK-cells, subsets of T-cells	?
CD40		G28-5	50 kDa, 4 cysteine-rich repeats, NGFR superfamily member	B cells, carcinomas	binds to CD40L, T-, B-cell interaction, role in B cell growth (costimulation), memory cell generation?
CD41	gpIIb of the gpIIbgpIIIa complex, IIb integrin	PBM6.4, CLB-thromb./7, PL273	integrin α-chain, expressed as a heterodimer with CD61	platelets, megakaryocytes	platelet aggregation and activation: receptor for fibrinogen, fibronectin (binds to R-G-D sequence)
CD42a	platelet gpIX	FMC25, BL-H6, GR-P	23 kDa, forms complex with gpIb (CD42b), LRG region	platelets, megakaryocytes	platelet adhesion, binding to von Willebrand factor
CD42b	platelet gpIbα	PHN89, AN51, GN287	dimer of 135 and 25 kDa chains, forms complex with gpIX (CD42a), LRG repeats	platelets, megakaryocytes	platelet adhesion, binding to von Willebrand factor receptor for Thrombin
CD42c	platelet gpIBβ		22 kDa	platelets	
CD 42d	GPV		85 kDA		

CD designation	Synonyms	Monoclonal antibodies	Molecular structure	Main cellular expression	Function(s)
CD43	Sialophorin, Leukosialin	OTH71C5, G19-1, MEM-59	95 kDa, highly sialylated	T cells, granulocytes, NK-cells, activated B-cells, platelets, plasma cells, stem cells	? role in T cell activation
CD44	Pgp-1, hermes antigen	GRHL-1, F10-44-2, 33-383, BRIC35	80–>100 kDa, highly glyco-sylated, numerous splice variants	T cell, granulocytes, brain B-cells, erythrocytes, mono-, cytes, epithelial cells, CNS, fibroblasts, smooth muscle cells, tumors	may function as homing receptor for matrix compo-nents (e.g. hyaluronate)
CD45	T200, leuko-cyte antigen (LCA), Ly, B220	T29/33, BMAC1, AB187	180–240 kDa, numerous splice variants	leukocytes, B220 in the B-cell specific isoform	role in signal transduction through T-cell receptor (tyrosine phosphatase)
CD45R	restricted forms of LCA (CD45)	G1-15, FB11-13, 73.5, PT17/26/16, UCHL1	CD45RO: 180 kD CD45RA: 220 kD CD45RB: 190, 205 and 220 kDa isoforms	CD45RO: memory T cells CD45RA: naive T cells CD45RB: B cells, subset of T cells	role in signal transduction (tyrosine phosphatase)
CD46	membrane cofactor protein (MCP)	HuLyM5, 122-2, J4B	56–66 kDa, 4 CCP motives	leukocytes, epithelial cells, fibroblasts, NK-cells, placenta, endothelial cells, platelets, spermatocytes	regulation of complement activation, CD46 binds to C3b or C4b
CD47	–	BRIC126, CIKM1, BRIC125	47–52 kDa, N-linked glycan	broad; Rh-associated; all hematopoietic cells	?
CD48	blast-1	WM68, LO-MN25, J4-57	41 kDa, 2 IgSF domains, GPi anchor	leukocytes, eosinophils, some epithelial cells	?
CDw49a	VLA α_1 chain		210 kDa, associates with β chain of VLA (CD29) to form VLA-1	T cells, monocytes, platelets	adhesion to collagen, laminin
CDw49b	VLA α_2 chain platelet gpIa	CLB-thromb./4, Gi14	170 kDa, associates with β chain of VLA (CD29) to form VLA-2	platelets, activted T cells, monocytes, some B cells	adhesion to extracellular matrix: receptor for collagen
CDw49c	VLA α_3 chain		dimer of 130 and 25 kDa, associates with β chain of VLA (CD29) to form VLA-3	T cells, some B cells, monocytes	adhesion to fibronectin, laminin

CD designation	Synonyms	Monoclonal antibodies	Molecular structure	Main cellular expression	Function(s)
CDw49d	VLA α_4 chain	B5G10, HP2/1, HP1/3	150 kDa, associates with β chain of VLA (CD29) to form VLA-4	T cells, monocytes, B cells, thymus	Peyer's patch homing receptor, binds to VCAM-1, adhesion to fibronectin
CDw49e	VLA α_5 chain		dimer of 135 and 25 kDa, associates with β chain of VLA (CD29) to form VLA-5	T cells, few B cells and monocytes	adhesion to fibronectin
CDw49f	VLA α_6 chain platelet GPIc	GoH3	150 kDa, associates with β chain of VLA (CD29) to form VLA-6	platelets, megakaryocytes, activated T cells	adhesion to extracellular matrix: receptor for laminin
CDw50	ICAM-3	101-1D2, 140-11	124 kDa, GPI-linked	leukocytes, monocytes, granulocytes	adhesion molecule
CD51	α chain of vitronectin receptor	13C2, 23C6, NKI-NKI-M9	140 kDa heterodimer, associates with β chain of vitronectin (CD61)	platelets, megarkaryocytes, monocytes	adhesion: receptor for vitronectin, fibrinogen, von Willebrand factor (binds R-G-D sequence)
CDw52	CAMPATH-1	097, YTH66.9, campath-1	21–28 kDa, short glycoprotein + GPi anchor	leukocytes	?
CD53	MRCOX-44	HI29, HI36, MEM-53, HD77	32–40 kDa, 4 TM domains TM 4 SF member	leukocyte, plasma cells, platelets, osteoclasts, osteoblasts	? transporter
CD54	ICAM-1	7F7, WEHI-CAMI	80–114 kDa, 5 IgSF domains	broad, many activated cells (cytokine-inducible)	adhesion: ligand for LFA-1 (CD11a/18) and Mac-1 (CD11b/CD18)
CD55	DAF (decay accelerating factor)	143-30, BRIC110, BRIC128, F2B7.2	70 kDa, GPI-linked, 4 CCP motives	broad	regulation of complement activation
CD56	Leu-19	NKH1, FP2-11.14, L185, Leu-19	135–220 kDa, 5 IgSF domains 2 fibronectin type III domain isoform of N-CAM	NK cells	homotypic adhesion, isoform of neural cell adhesion molecule

CD designation	Synonyms	Monoclonal antibodies	Molecular structure	Main cellular expression	Function(s)
CD57	HNK-1, Leu-7	L183, L187, Leu-7	110 kDa	NK cells, subset of T cells, B cells, brain	?
CD58	LFA-3	G-26, BRIC5, TS2/9	40–65 kDa, GPI-linked or TM domain, 2 IgSF domains	broad (leukocytes, epithelial cells)	adhesion: ligand for CD2
CD59	membrane inhibitor of reactive lysis	Y53.1, MEM43	18–20 kDa, GPI-linked 1 Ly-C sF domain	broad	regulation of complement (MAC) action
CDw60	–	M-T32, M-T21, M-T41	carbohydrate epitope (NeuAc-NeuAc-Gal)	subset of T cells, platelets; subset of monocytes	? co-stimulator
CD61	β chain of vitronectin receptor gpIIIa	Y2/51, CLB thromb/1, VIPL2, BL-E6	110 kDa, associates with α-chain of vitronectin receptor (CD51); associated with integrin β chain CD41	platelets, megakaryocytes, macrophages	adhesion: receptor for vitronectin, fibrinogen, von Willebrand factor platelet aggregation
CD62P	GMP-140 PADGEM	CLB-thromb/6; CLB-thromb/5; RUU-SP1,18,1	140 kDa, platelet granule protein that is translocated to cell surface upon activation, selectin family member	platelets, endothelial cells	neutrophil and monocyte adhesion to endothelium, platelets
CD62E	ELAM-1		115 kDa	endothelial cells	adhesion molecule to leukocytes
CD62L	LAM-1		75–80 kDa	leukocytes	adhesion molecule
CD63	–	RUU-SP2,28; CLB-gran12	53 kDa, present in platelet lysosomes, translocated to surface upon activation 4TM domains (TM4 family member)	activated platelets, monocytes, macrophages, granulocytes, T cells, B cells	neutrophil and monocyte adhesion to endothelium platelets
CD64	FcγRI	MAB32,2; Mab22	75 kDa, 3 IgSF domains	monocytes, macrophages	high-affinity Fc γ receptor: role in phagocytosis, ADCC, macrophage activation
CDw65	–	VIM2, HE10, CF4, VIM8	carbohydrate epitope (ceramide-dodecasaccharide 4c)	granulocytes, monocytes	? role in neutrophil activation

CD designation	Synonyms	Monoclonal antibodies	Molecular structure	Main cellular expression	Function(s)
CD66a	BGP-1	CLB gran 10, YTH 71.3	180–200 kDa phosphorylated glycoprotein, 4 IgSF domains	granulocytes, colonic epithelial cells	? homotypic adhesion
CD66b	CD67				
CD66c	NCA	various	90–85 kDA (reduced)	granulocytes	nonspecific cross-reacting antigen
CD66d	CGM1		30 kDa	granulocytes	?
CD66e	CEA	many	180–200 kDa (reduced)	granulocytes, colonic epithelial cells	carcinoembryonal antigen
CD67	CGM6 p100 (CD66b)	B13.9, G10F5, JML-H16	100 kDa, GPI-linked, 3 IgSF domains	granulocytes	?
CD68	macrosialin (mouse)	EBM11, Y2/131, Y-1/82A, Ki-M7, Ki-M6	110 kDa, (in cytoplasmic granules) cellular protein, weak surface expression, LGP family member	monocytes, macrophages	?
CD69	Leu-23	MLR3, L78, BL-Ac/p26, FN50	homodimer of 28–32 kDa chains, phosphorylated glycoprotein	activated B and T cells, macrophages, NK cells	?
CDw70	–	Ki-24, HNE51, HNC142	55, 75, 95, 100, 170 kDa (reduced)	activated T and B cells, Sternberg-Reed cells	?
CD71	T9, transferrin receptor	138-18.120-2A3, MEM-75, VIP-1, Nu-TfR2	95 kDa homodimer, type II membrane glycoprotein	activated T and B cells, macrophages, proliferating cells	receptor for transferrin; iron metabolism, cell growth
CD72	Lyb-2 (mouse)	S-HCL2, J3-109, BU-40, BU-41	heterodimer of 39 and 43 kDa chains, type II integral membrane protein	B cells	ligand for CD5
CD73		1E9.28.1, 7G2.2.11, AD2	69 kDa, GPI-linked	subsets of T and B cells endothelial and epithelial cells	ecto-5'-nucleotidase

CD designation	Synonyms	Monoclonal antibodies	Molecular structure	Main cellular expression	Function(s)
CD74	class II MHC-associated (γ chain)	LN2, BU-43, BU-45,	three protein species: 35, 41 and 33 kDa, type II integral membrane glyco-protein	B cells, monocytes, macro-phages, other MHC class II+ cells	associates with newly synthe-sized class II MHC mole-cules
CDw75	–	LN1, HH2, EBU-141	53 kDa and 87 kDa	mature B cells, weakly on sub-set of T-cells, epithelial cells	B-B-cell interaction
CD76	–	HD66, CRIS-4	(heterodimer of 67 and 85 kDa chains?)	mature B cells, subset of T cells epithelial cells	?
CD77	–	38.13, 424/4A11, 424/3D9	carbohydrate epitope (globotriasylceramide, Gb3)	germinal center B-cells, Burkitt lymphoma cells	lectin receptor
CDw78	Ba Leu-21	anti-Ba, Lo-pan Ba, 1588	?	B cells (macrophages)	?
CD 79a	Igα, mb-1		33, 40 kDa (reduced)	B-cells	part of B-cell receptor
CD79b	Igβ, B29		33, 40 kDa (reduced)	B-cells	part of B-cell receptor
CD 80	B7, BB1		60 kDa	B-cells, APC	costimulator for cooperation with helper T-cells
CD81	TAPA-1		22 kDa (serpentin-like protein)	B-cells	part of CR-2 complex
CD 82	R2, IA4, 4F9		50–53 kDa	B-cells	
CD 83	HB-15		43 kDa	B-cells	
CDw84	–		73 kDa	B-cells	
CD85	VMP-55, GH1/75		120, 83 kDa (reduced)	B-cells	
CD86	FUN-1, BU63		80 kDa	B-cells	
CD87	uPA-R		50–65 kDa (reduced)	myeloid cells, other cells, cancer cells	receptor for urokinase
CD88	C5a-R		42 kDa	granulocytes	receptor for C5a

CD designation	Synonyms	Monoclonal antibodies	Molecular structure	Main cellular expression	Function(s)
Cd89	Fcα-R		55–75 kDA (reduced)	granulocytes, lymphocytes	receptor for IgA
CDw90	Thy-1		25–35 kDa (reduced)	myeloid cells	
CD91	α2M-R		600 kDa	myeloid cells	receptor for α2m
CDw92			70 kDa	myeloid cells	
CDw93			120 kDa	myeloid cells	
CD94	KP43		43 kDa	NK-cells	
CD95	APO-1, FAS		42 kDa	lymphocytes, liver cells, other cells	receptor for induction of apoptosis
CD96	Tactile		160 kDa		
CD97			74, 80, 89 kDa (reduced)		
CD98	4F2, 2F3		80, 40 kDa (reduced)	T-cells	
CD99	E2, MIC2		32 kDa	T-cells	
CD100	BB18, A8		150 kDa	T-cells	
CDw101	BB27, Ba27		140 kDa	T-cells	
CD102	ICAM-2		60 kDa	various cells	adhesion molecule
CD103	HML-1		150, 25 kDa (reduced)	various cells	adhesion molecule
CD104	β_4 integrin cells		220 kDa		adhesion molecule
CD105	endoglin		95 kDa	endothelial cells	
CD106	VCAM-1, ICAM-110		100, 110 kDa (reduced)	endothelial cells	adhesion molecule
CD107a	LAMP-1		110 kDa	platelets	adhesion molecule
CD107b	LAMP-2		120 kDa	platelets	adhesion molecule
CDw108			80 kDa		adhesion molecule

CD designation	Synonyms	Monoclonal antibodies	Molecular structure	Main cellular expression	Function(s)
CDw109	8A3, 7D1		170, 150 kDa (redcued) 150 kDa	endothelial cells myeloid cells	receptor for M-CSF
CD115	CSF-R, M-CSF-R				
CDw116	GM-CSF-R, HGM-CSF-R		75–85 kDa (reduced)	myeloid cells	receptor for GM-CSF
CD117	SCFR, cKit		145 kDa	myeloid cells	receptor for SCF
CDw119	IFNγ-R		90 kDa	lymphocytes	receptor for IFN-γ
CD120a,b	TNF-R		55, 75 kDa	various cells	receptor for TNF
CDw121a b	IL-1-R type 1 type 2		80 kDa 68 kDa	monocytes; lymphocytes	receptors for IL-1
CD122	IL-2-Rβ		75 kDa	lymphocytes	receptor for IL-2
CDw124	IL-4-R		140 kDa	lymphocytes, granulocytes	receptor for IL-4
CD126	IL-6-R		80 kDa	lymphocytes	receptor for IL-6
CD127	IL-7-R		75 kDa	lymphocytes	receptor for IL-7
CD128	IL-8-R		58–67 kDa (reduced)	granulocytes	receptor for IL-8
CDw130	IL-6-R gp130 SIG		130 kDa	lymphocytes	receptor for IL-6

ADCC, antibody-dependent cell-mediated cytotoxicity; CCP, complement control protein; GP, glycoprotein; GMP, granule membrane protein; GPI, guanosine phosphatidylinositol; ICAM, intercellular adhesion molecule; IGSF, immunoglobulin superfamily; IL interleukin; Ig immunoglobulin; kDa, kilodalton; LFA, leukocyte function-associated antigen; LGP, lysosomal glycoproteins; LRG, Leu-rich motive; MAC, membrane attack complex; MHC, major histocompatibility complex; NGFR, nerve growth factor receptor; NK, natural killer; RGD, sequence Arg-Gly-Asp; TAC T, cell activation antigen; TM, transmembrane protein; VCAM, vascular cell adhesion molecule; VLA, very late antigen.

Compiled from Knapp et al. 1989; Abbas et al. 1991; Supplemented.

References

Aalberse R.C.; Dieges, P.H.; Knul-Bretlova, V.; Vooren, P.; Aalbers, M. and Van Leeuwen, J.: IgG4 as a blocking antibody. Clin. Rev. Allergy 1: 289–294, 1983.

Abbas, A.K.; Haber, S. and Rock, K.L.: Antigen presentation by hapten-specific B lymphocytes. II. Specificity and properties of antigen-presenting B lymphocytes and function of immunoglobulin receptors. J. Immunol. 135: 1661, 1985.

Abbas, A.K.; Lichtman, A.H. and Pober, J.S.: Cellular and molecular immunology., Wonsiewicz, M.J. (ed.), W.B. Saunders Company, USA, 1991.

Abraham, S.N. and Beachey E.H.: Host defenses against adhesion of bacterial to mucosal surfaces. In: Advances in Host Defense Mechanisms. Mucosal Immunology, eds. Gallin, J.I and Fauci A.S., Raven Press, New York, 4: 63–88, 1985.

Abrahams, S.; Philips, R.S. and Miner, R.A.: Inhibition of the immune response. Adv. Immunol. 8: 81, 1968.

Abramson, S.L. and Gallin, J.I.: IL-4 inhibits superoxide production by human mononuclear phagocytes. J. Immunol. 144: 625–631, 1990.

Accolla, R.S.; Auffray, C.; Singer, D.S. and Gaurdiola, J.: The molecular biology of MHC genes. Immunology Today 12: 97–99, 1991.

Acha-Orbea, H.; Mitchell, D.J.; Timmermann, L.; Wraith, D.C.; Tausch, G.S.; Waldor, M.K.; Zamvil, S.S.; McDevitt, H.O. and Steinman, L.: Limited heterogeneity of T cell receptors from lymphocytes mediating autoimmune encephalomyelitis allows specific immune intervention. Cell 54: 263–273, 1988.

Acsadi, G.; Dickson, G.; Love, D.R.; Jani, A.; Walsh, F.S.; Gurusinghe, A.; Wolff, J.A. and Davies, K.E.: Human dystrophin expression in mdx mice after intramuscular injection of DNA constructs. Nature 352: 815–818, 1991.

Acton, S.; Resnick, D.; Freeman, M.; Ekkel, Y.; Ashkenas, J. and Krieger, M.: The collagenous domains of macrophage scavenger and complement component C1q mediate their similar, but not identical binding specificities for polyanionic ligands. J. Biol. Chem. 268: 3530–3537, 1993.

Adler, S.; Baker, P.; Johnson, R.J.; Ochi, P.P. and Couser, W.G.: Complement membrane attack complex stimulates production of reactive oxygen metabolites by cultured rat mesangial cells. J. Clin. Invest. 77: 762–767, 1986.

Advenier, C.; Sarria, B.; Naline, E.; Puybasset, L. and Lagente, V.: Contractile activity of three endothelins (ET-1, ET-2 and ET-3) on the human isolated bronchus. Brit. J. Pharmacol. 100: 168–172, 1990.

Aebersold, P.; Hyatt, C.; Johnson, S.; Hines, K.; Korcak, L.; Sanders, M.; Lotze, M.; Topalian, S.; Yang, J. and Rosenberg, S.A.: Lysis of autologous melanoma cells by tumor-infiltrating lymphocytes: association with clinical response. J. Natl. Cancer Inst. 83: 932–937, 1991.

Aggarwal, A.; Kumar, S.; Jaffe, R.; Hone, A.; Gross, M. and Sadoff, J.: Oral salmonella: malaria circumsporozoite recombinants induce CDS + cytotoxic T cells. J. Exp. Med. 172: 1083–1090, 1990.

Agnello, V.: Lupus diseases associated with hereditary and acquired deficiencies of complement. Springer Semin Immunopathol. 9: 161–178, 1986.

Agosti, J.M.; Sprenger, J.K.; Lum, L.G.; Witherspoon, R.P.; Fisher, L.D.; Storb, R. and Henderson, W.R.jr.: Transfer of allergen-specific IgE-mediated hypersensitivity with allogeneic bone marrow transplantation. N. Engl. J. Med. 319: 1623–1628, 1988.

Agostoni, A.; Cicardi, M.; Gardinali, M. and Bergamaschini, L.: The complement System. Int. J. Immunopath. Pharmacol. 5: 123–130, 1992.

Aguet, M.; Dembic, Z. and Merlin, G.: Molecular cloning and expression of the human interferon-gamma receptor. Cell 55: 273, 1988.

Aharoni, R.; Teitelbaum, D.; Arnon, R. and Puri, J.: Immunomodulation of experimental allergic encephalitis by antibodies to the antigen-1ª complex. Nature 351: 147–150, 1991.

Ahearn, J.M. and Fearon, D.T.: Structure and function of the complement receptors, CR1 (CD35) and CR2 (CD21). Adv. Immunol. 46: 183–201, 1989.

Ahmadzaden, N.; Shingu, M.; Nobunaga, M. and Towara, T.: Relationship between leukotriene B4 and immunological parameters in rheumatoid synovial fluids. Inflammation 15: 497–503, 1991.

Ahmed, A.E.E.; Veitch, J. and Whaley, K.: Mechanism of action of an inhibitor of complement-mediated prevention of immune precipitation. Immunology 70: 139–144, 1990.

Akira, S.; Hirano, T.; Taga, T. and Kishimoto, T.: Biology of multifunctional cytokines: Il-6 and related molecules (Il-1 and TNF). FASEB J. 4: 2860–2867, 1990.

Alam, R.; Bodenburg, Y.; Forsythe, P.A.; Lett-Brown, M.A. and Grant, J.A.: Agonistic-antagonistic property of interleukin 8 on basophils: identification of Il-8 as a potent inhibitor of cytokine-induced histamine release. J. Allergy Clin. Immunol. 87: 241, 1991.

Alam, R.; Forsythe, P.A.; Stafford, S.; Lett-Brown, M.A. and Grant, J.A.: Macrophage inflammatory protein-1μ activates basophils and mast cells. J. Exp. Med. 176: 781, 1992.

Alam, R.; Lett-Brown, M.A.; Forsythe, P.A.; Anderson-Walters, D.J.; Kenamore, C.; Kormos, C. and Grant, J.A.: Monocyte chemotactic and activating factor is a potent histamine-releasing factor for basophils. J. Clin. Invest. 89: 723, 1992.

Albelda, S.M.: Biology of Disease. Role of integrins and other cell adhesion molecules in tumor progression and metastasis. Lab. Invest. 68: 4, 1993.

Albelda, S.M.: Biology of Disease. Role of integrins and other cell adhesion molecules in tumor progression and metastasis. Lab. Invest. 68: 4, 1993.

Albers, M.W.; Brown, E.J.; Tanaka, A.; Willimans, R.T.; Hall, F.L. and Schreiber, S.L.: An FKBP-Rapamycin-sensitive, cyclin-dependent kinase activity that correlates with the FKBP-Rapamycin-induced G1 arrest point in MG-63 cells. Immunosuppressive and Antiinflammatory Drugs, eds. Allison, A.C.; Lafferty, K.J. and Fliri, H., Annals of the New York Academy of Sciences 696: 54, 1993.

Alderuccio, F.; Toh, B.H.; Barnett, A.J. and Pedersen, J.S.: Identification and characterization of mitochondria autoantigens in progressive systemic sclerosis: identity with the 72,000 dalton autoantigen in primary biliary cirrhosis. J. Immun. 137: 1855–1859, 1986.

Alexander, H.R.; Doherty, G.M.; Buresh, C.M.; Venzon, D.J. and Norton, J.A.: A recombinant human receptor antagonist to interleukin-1 improves survival after lethal endotoxemia in mice. J. Exp. Med. 173: 1029–1032, 1991.

Alexander, H.R.; Sheppard, B.C.; Jensen, J.C.; Langstein, H.N.; Buresh, C.M.; Venzon, D.; Walker, E.C.; Fraker, D.L.; Stovroff, C. and Norton, J.A.: Treatment with recombinant human tumor necrosis factor-μ protects rats against the lethality, hypotension, and hypothermia of Gram-negative sepsis. J. Clin. Invest. 88: 34–39, 1991.

Allansmith, M.R. and Gillette, T.E.: Secretory component in human ocular tissues. Am. J. Ophthal. 89: 353–361, 1980.

Allison, A.C.; Kowalski, W.J.; Muller, C.D. and Eugui, E.M.: Mechanisms of action of mycophenolic acid. Immunosuppressive and Antiinflammatory Drugs, eds. Allison, A.C.; Lafferty, K.J. and Fliri, H., Annals of the New York Academy of Sciences 696: 63, 1993.

Allison, A.C. and Eugui, E.M.: The design and development of an immunosuppressive drug, mycophenolate mofetil. Springer Semin. Immunopathol. 14: 353–380, 1993.

Allison, R.C.; Hernandez, E.M.; Prasad, V.R.; Grisham, M.B. and Taylor, A.E.: Protective effects of O_2 radical scavengers and adenosine in PMA-induced lung injury. J. Appl. Physiol. 64: 2175–2182, 1988.

Alvin, C.R.; Detrick, B.; Richards, R.L.; Lewis, M.G.; Shafferman, A. and Eddy, G.A.: Novel adjuvant strategies for experimental malaria and AIDS vaccines. Specific Immunotherapy Of Cancer With Vaccines, eds. Bystryn, J.-C.; Ferrone, S. and Livingston P., The New York Academy of Sciences 690: 265, 1993.

Ameisen, J.C.; Capron, A.; Joseph, M.; Maclouf, J.; Vomg, H.; Pancrè, V.; Fournier, E.; Wallaert, B. and Tonnel, A.B.: Aspirin-sensitive asthma: abnormal platelet response to drugs inducing asthmatic attacks. Diagnostic and physiopathological implications. Int. Arch. Allergy Appl. Immunol. 78: 438–448, 1985.

Amin, A.R.; Coico, R.F.; Finkelman, F.; Siskind, G.W. and Thorbecke, G.J.: Release of IgD-binding factor by T cells under the influence of interleukin 2, interleukin 4, or cross-linked IgD. Proc. Natl. Acad. Sci. USA 85: 9179, 1988.

Anderson, C.L. and Looney R.J.: Human leukocyte IgG Fc receptors. Immunol. Today 7: 264–267, 1986.

Anderson, D.C.; Rothlein, R.; Marlin, S.D.; Krater, S.S. and Smith, C.W.: Impaired trans-endothelial migration by neonatal neutrophils: Abnormalities of Mac-1 (CD11b/CD18) -dependent adherence reactions. Blood 76: 2613–2621, 1990.

Anderson, D.C.; Butcher, E.C.; Gallatin, M.; Rosen, S.; Kishimoto, K.; Lasky, L.; Miyasaka, M.; Scollay, R.; Smith, C.W. and Haskard D.: Peripheral lymph node homing receptor (LECAM-1). Immunology Today 12: 216, 1991.

Andersson, M.; Paabo, S.; Nilsson, T. and Peterson, P.A.: Impaired intracellular transport of class I MHC antigens as a possible means for adenovirus to evade immune surveillance. Cell 43: 215, 1985.

Ando, B.; Wiedmer, T.; Hamilton, K.K. and Sims, P.J.: Complement proteins C5b-9 initiate secretion of platelet storage granules without increased binding of fibrinogen or von Willebrand factor to newly expressed cell surface GPIIb-IIIa. J. Biol. Chem. 263: 11907–11914, 1988.

Ando, B.; Wiedmer, T. and Sims, P.J.: The secretory release reaction initiated by complement proteins C5b-9 occurs without platelet aggregation through GPIIb-IIIa. Blood 73: 462–467, 1989.

Andrews, B.S.; Shadforth, M.; Cunningham, P. and Davis, J.S.: Demonstration of C1q receptor on the surface of human endothelial cells. J. Immunol. 127: 1075–1080, 1981.

Andrzejewski, C.; Rauch, J.; Lafer, E.; Stollar, B.D. and Schwartz, R.S.: Antigen-binding diversity and idiotypic crossreactions among hybridoma autoantibodies to DNA. J. Immun. 126: 226–231, 1981.

Andus, T.; Gross, V.; Cäsar, I.; Krumm, D.; Hosp, J.; David, M. and Schölmerich, J.: Activation of monocytes during inflammatory bowel disease. Pathobiology 59: 113, 1991.

Anhalt, G.J.; Labib, R.S.; Voorhees, J.J.; Beals, J.F. and Diaz, L.A.: Induction of pemphigus in neonatal mice by passive transfer of IgG from patients with the disease. New Engl. J. Med. 305: 1189–1196, 1982.

Aran, J.M.; Colomer, D.; Matutes, E.; Vives-Corrons, J.L. and Franco, R.J.: Presence of adenosine deaminase on the surface of mononuclear blood cells: immunochemical localization using light and electron microscopy. H. Histochem. Cytochem. 39: 1001–1008, 1991.

Arend, W.P.; Jolsin, F.G. and Massoni R.J.: Effects of immune complexes on production by human monocytes of Interleukin-1 or an Interleukin-1 inhibitor. J. Immunol. 134: 3868, 1985.

Arend, W.P.; Gordon, D.F.; Wood, W.M.; Janson, R.W.; Joslin, F.G. and Jameel, S.: Il-1β production in cultured human monocytes is regulated at multiple levels. J. Immunol. 143: 1881, 1989.

Arend, W.P.; Smith, F.F.; Janson, J.R.R. and Joslin, F.G.: IL-1 receptor antagonist and IL-1β production in human monocytes are regulated differently. J. Immunol. 147: 1530, 1991.

Arends, M.J. and Wyllie, A.H.: Apoptosis: mechanisms and roles in pathology. Int. Rev. Exp. Path. 32: 223–254, 1991.

Argilés, J.M.; López-Soriano, F.J.; Wiggins, D. and Williamson, D.H.: Comparative effects of tumour necrosis factor-alpha (cachectin), interleukin-1–beta, and tumour growth on amino acid metabolism in the rat in vivo. Absorption and tissue uptake of alpha-amino(1–14C)isobutyrate. Biochem. J. 261: 357–362, 1989.

Argilés, J.M.; Garcia-Martinez, C.; Llovera, M. and López-Soriano, F.J.: The role of cytokines in muscle wasting: Its relation with cancer cachexia. Med. Res. Rev. 12: 637–652, 1992.

Ariizumi, M.; Shiihara, H.; Hibio, S.; Ryo, S.; Baba, K.; Ogawa, K.; Suzuki, Y. and Momoki, T.: High dose gammaglobulin for intractable childhood epilepsy. Lancet II: 162–163, 1983.

Armitage, N.C.; Perkins, A.C.; Pimm, M.V.; Farrands, P.A.; Baldwin, R.W. and Hardcastle, J.C.: The localization of an antitumor monoclonal antibody (791T/36) in gastrointestinal tumors. Br. J. Surg. 71: 407, 1984.

Armitage, N.C.; Perkins, A.C.; Pimm, M.V.; Wastie, M.L.; Baldwin, R.W. and Hardcastle, J.D.: Imaging of primary and metastatic colorectal cancer using an 111In-labeled antitumor monoclonal antibody 791T.36. Nucl. Med. Commun. 6: 623, 1985.

Armitage, N.C.; Perkins, A.C.; Hardcastle, J.D.; Pimm, M.V.; Baldwin, R.W., in Baldwin, R.W., Byers, V.S. (eds.): Monoclonal antibody imaging in malignant and benign gastrointestinal diseases. Monoclonal Antibodies for Cancer Detection and Therapy. London, Academic, 129, 1985.

Armitage, R.J.; Fanslow, W.C.; Strockbine, L.; Sato, T.A.; Clifford, K.N.; Macduff, B.M.; Anderson, D.M.; Gimpel, S.D.; Davis-Smith, T.; Maliszewski, C.R.; Clark, E.A.; Smith, C.A.; Grabstein, K.H.; Cosman, D. and Spriggs, M.K.: Molecular and biological characterization of a murine ligand for CD40. Nature 357: 80, 1992.

Armitage, R.J.; Ziegler, S.F.; Friend, D.J.; Park, L.S. and Fanslow, W.C.: Identification of a novel low-affinity receptor for human interleukin-7. Blood 79: 1738–1745, 1992.

Armstrong, S.H.; Bronsky, D. and Hershman, J.: The persistence in the blood of the radioactive label of albumin, gamma globulins, and globulins of intermediate mobility. III. Comparison of die-away plots following oral and intravenous administration of the S35 label to the same subjects. J. lab. clin. Med. 46: 857–870, 1985.

Aronson, F.R.; Libby, P.; Brandon E.P.; Janicka, M.W. and Mier, J.W.: IL-2 rapidly induces natural killer cell adhesion to human endothelial cells: A potential mechanism for endothelial injury. J. Immunol. 141: 158–163, 1988.

Arsura, E.: Experience with intravenous immunoglobulin in myasthenia gravis. Clin. Immunol. Immunopathol. 53: 170, 1989.

Artandi, S.E.; Canifield, S.M.; Tao, M.-H.; Calame, K.L.; Morrison, S.L. and Bonagura, V.R.: Molecular analysis of IgM rheumatoid factor binding to chimeric IgG. J. Immunol. 146: 603, 1991.

Arya, S.K. and Gallo, R.C.: Transcriptional modulation of human T-cell growth factor gene by phorbol ester and interleukin I. Biochem 23: 6685–6690, 1984.

Arzt, E.; Stelzer, G.; Renner, U.; Lange, M.; Muller, O.A. and Stalla, B.K.: Interleukin-2 and interleukin-2–receptor expression in human corticotropic adenoma and murine pituitary cell cultures. J. Clin. Invest. 90: 1944–1951, 1992.

Asao, H.; Takeshita, T.; Nakamura, M.; Nagata, K. and Sugamuara K.: Interleukin 2 (IL-2)-induced tyrosine phosphorylation of IL-2 receptor p75. Exp. Med. 171: 637–644, 1990.

Asher, A.; Mule, J.; Kasid, A.; Restifo, N.; Salo, J.; Reichert, C.; Jaffe, G.; Fendly, B.; Kriegler, M. and Rosenberg, S.: Murine tumor cells transduced with the gene for tumor necrosis factor-alpha. Evidence for paracrine immune effects of tumor necrosis factor against tumors. J. Immunol. 146: 3227, 1991.

Assoian, R.K.; Komoriya, A.; Meyers, C.A.; Miller, D.M. and Sporn, M.B.: Transforming growth factor-ß in human platelets. Identification of a major storage site, purification, and characterization. J. Biol. Chem. 258: 7155–7160, 1983.

Assoian, R.K. and Sporn, M.B.: Type ß transforming growth factor in human platelets: release during platelet degranulation and action on vascular smooth muscle cells. J. Cell Biol. 102: 1217–1223, 1986.

Atalla, L.; Linker-Israeli, M.; Steinman, L. and Rao, N.A.: Inhibition of autoimmune uveitis by anti-CD4 antibody. Invest. Ophthalmol. Vis. Sci. 31: 1264–1270, 1990.

Atkinson, M.A.; Maclaren, N.K.; Scharp, D.; Lavy, P. and Riley, W.J.: 64.000 Mr autoantibodies as predictors of insulin-dependent diabetes. Lancet 335: 1357–1360, 1990.

Atkinson, M.A.; Kaufman, D.L.; Newman, D.; Tobin, A.J. and Maclaren, N.K.: Islet cell cytoplasmic autoantibody reactivity to glutamate decarboxylase in insulin-dependent diabetes. J. Clin. Invest. 91: 350–356, 1993.

Aubry, J.-P.; Pochon, S.; Graber, P.; Jansen, K.U. and Bonnefoy, J.-Y.: CD21 is a ligand for CD23 and regulates IgE production. Nature 358: 505, 1992.

Auerbach, R.; Kubai, L. and Sidky, Y.A.: Angiogenesis induction by tumors, embryonic tissues, and lymphocytes. Cancer Res. 36: 3435–3440, 1976.

Averill, F.J.; Hubbard, W.C.; Proud, D.; Gleich, G.J. and Liu, M.C.: Platelet activation in the lung after antigen challenge in a model of allergic asthma. Am. Rev. Respir. Dis. 145: 571–576, 1992.

Avraham, H.; Vannier, E.; Cowley, S.; Jiang, S.; Chi, S.; Dinarello, C.A.; Zsebo, K.M. and Groopman, J.E.: Effect of the stem cell factor, c-kit ligand on human megakaryocytic cells. Blood 79: 365, 1992.

Azuma, C.; Tanabe, T.; Konishi, M.; Kinashi, T.; Noma, T.; Matsuda, F.; Yaoita, Y.; Takatsu, K.; Hammarstroem, L.: Smith, C.I. et al.: Cloning of cDNA for human T-cell replacing factor (interleukin-5) and comparison with the murine homologue. Nuc. Acids Res. 14: 9149–9158, 1986.

Baatz, J.F.; Ciraolo, P.; Bruno, M.; Glasser, S.; Stripp, B. and Korfhagen, T.R.: Utilization of modified surfactant-associated protein B for delivery of DNA to airway cells in culture. Pediatr. Pulmonol. 8: 263, 1992.

Bacchetta, R.; Waal de, W.R.; Yssel, H.; Abrams, J.; Vries de, J.E.; Spits, H. and Roncarolo, M-G.: Host reactive CD4+ and CD8+ T cell clones isolated from a human chimera produce IL-5, IL-2, IFN-gamma and GM-CSF, but not IL-4. J. Immunol. 144: 902, 1990.

Bär, T. and Wolff, J.R.: The formation of a capillary basement membrane during internal vascularization of the rat's cerebral cortex. Z. Zellforsch mikrosk. Anat. 133–213, 1972.

Baeza, M.L.: Reddigari, S.R.; Kornfeld, D.; Ramani, N.; Smith, E.M.; Hossler, P.A.; Fischer, T.; Castor, C.W.; Gorevic, P.G. and Kaplan, A.P.: Relationship of one form of human histamine-releasing factor to connective tissue activating peptide-III. J. Clin. Invest. 85: 1516, 1990.

Bagby, G.J.; Plessala, K.J.; Wilson, L.A.; Thompson, J.J. and Nelson, S.: Divergent efficacy of antibody to tumor necrosis factor-μ in intravascular and peritonitis models of sepsis. J. Infect. Dis. 163: 83, 1991.

Bagshawe, K.D.; Jarman, M. and Springer, C.J.: Improvements relating to drug delivery systems. IPN: WO 88/07378, 1988.

Bagshawe, K.D.; Springer, C.J.; Searle, F.; Antoniw, P.; Sharma, S.K.; Melton, R.G. and Sherwood, R.F.: A cytotoxic agent can be generated selectively at cancer sites. Br. J. Cancer 58: 700–703, 1988.

Bahrami, S.; Redl, H.; Buurman, W.A. and Schlag, G.: Influence of the xanthine derivate HWA 138 on endotoxin-related coagulation disturbances: Effects in non-sensitized vs D-galactosamine sensitized rats. Thromb. Haemost. 68: 418–423, 1992.

Bahrami, S.; Redl, H.; Yu, Y.; Jiang, J.X.; Leichtfried, G. and Schlag, G.: Bactericidal/permeability-increasing protein (BPI) reduces lipopolysaccharid (LPS)-induced cytokine formation and mortality in rats. Circulatory Shock, Fourth Vienna Shock Forum in Association with the European Shock Society, May 9–13, Vienna, Austria (abstract), suppl. 1: 52–53, 1993.

Baird, A.; Mormede, P.; Ying, S.Y.; Wehrenberg, W.B.; Ueno, N.; Ling, N. and Guillemin, R.: A nonmitogenic pituitary function of fibroblast growth factor: regulation of thyrotropin and prolactin secretion. Proc. Natl. Acad. Sci. 82: 5545–5549, 1985.

Baird, A. and Ling, N.: Fibroblast growth factors are present in the extracellular matrix produced by endothelial cells in vitro: implications for a role of heparinase-like enzymes in the neovascular response. Biochem. Biophys. Res. Commun. 142: 428–435, 1987.

Baird, A.; Ueono, M.; Esch, F. and Ling, N.: Distribution of fibroblast growth factors (FGFs) in tissues and structure-function studies with synthetic fragments of basic FGF. J. Cell. Physiol. Suppl. 5: 101–106, 1987.

Baldwin, E.T.; Franklin, K.A.; Appella, E.; Yamada, M.; Matsushima, K.; Wlodawer, A. and Weber, I.T.: Crystallization of human interleukin-8. A protein chemotactic for neutrophils and T-lymphocytes. J. Biol. Chem. 265: 6851, 1990.

Baldwin, R.W.; Price, M.R. and Robbin, R.A.: Blocking of lymphocyte-mediated cytotoxicity for rat hepatoma cells by tumorspecific antigen-antibody complexes. Nature (New Biol.) 238: 185–187, 1972.

Balzereit, F.; Fathe-Moghadam, A.; Besinger, K.A. and Geursen, R.G.: Myasthenia gravis, humoral Diagnostik und Therapie einer Autoimmunerkrankung. Münchner Med. Wchschr. 39: 654–657, 1986.

Bamias, A.; Keane, P.; Krausz, T.; Williams, G. and Epenetos, A.A.: Intravesical administration of monoclonal antibodies in patients with superficial bladder carcinoma. 8th Int. Hammersmith Meeting, Greece, 1991.

Banchereau, J.; Defrance, T.; Galizzi, J.P.; Miossec, P. and Rousset F.: Human interleukin 4. Bull Cancer 78: 299–306, 1991.

Barbatis, C.; Woods, J.; Morton, J.A.; Fleming, K.A. and McGee, JO'D: Immunohistochemical analysis of HLA (A,B,C) antigens in liver disease using a monoclonal antibody. Gut 22: 985–991, 1981.

Barbin, G.; Manthorpe, M. and Varon, S.: Purification of the chick eye ciliary neuronotrophic factor. N. Neurochem. 43: 1468–1478, 1984.

Bard, J.B. and Ross, A.S.: LIF, the ES-cell inhibition factor, reversibly blocks nephrogenesis in cultured mouse kidney rudiments. Development 113: 193–198, 1991.

Barnathan, E.S.: Characterization and regulation of the Urokinase receptor of human endothelial cells. Fibrinolysis 6 (suppl. 1): 1–9, 1992.

Barnd, D.L.; Lan, M.S.; Metzgar, R.S. and Finn, O.J.: Specific, major histocompatibility complex-unrestricted recognition of tumor-associated mucins by human cytotoxic T cells. Proc. Natl. Acad. Sci. USA 86: 7159–7164, 1989.

Barr, P.J. and Tomei, L.D.: Apoptosis and its role in human disease. Bio/Technology 12: 487, 1994.

Barr, R.M.; Wong, E.; Mallet, A.I.; Olins, L.A. and Greaves, M.W.: The analysis of arachidonic acid metabolites in normal, uninvolved and lesional psoriatic skin. Prostaglandins 28: 57–65, 1984.

Barrett, P.A.; Butler, K.D.; Morley, J.; Page, C.P.; Paul, W. and White, A.M.: Inhibition by heparin of platelet accumulation in vivo. Thromb. Haemostas. 51: 366–370, 1984.

Barrett, P.A.; Butler, K.D.; Shand, R.A. and Wallis, R.B.: Intrathoracic platelet accumulation in the guinea-pig induced by intravenous administration of arachidonic acid – effect of cyclooxygenase and thromboxane synthetase inhibitors. Thromb. Haemostas. 56: 311–317, 1986.

Barton, B.E.; Jakaway, J.P.; Smith, S.R. and Siegel. M.I.: Cytokine inhibition by a novel steroid, mometasone furoate. Immunopharmacol. Immunotoxicol. 13: 251–261, 1991.

Bash, J.A.: Active specific immunotherapy of murine colon adenocarcinoma with recombinant vaccinia/Interleukin-2-infected tumor cell vaccines. Specific Immunotherapy Of Cancer With Vaccines, eds. Bystryn, J.-C.; Ferrone, S. and Livingston, P., The New York Academy of Sciences 690: 331, 1993.

Baskar, P.; Silberstein, D.S. and Pincus, S.H.: Inhibition of IgG-triggered human eosinophil function by IL-4. J. Immunol. 144: 2321–2326, 1990.

Baskar, S.; Nabavi, N.; Glimcher, L.H. and Ostrand-Rosenberg, S.: Tumor cells expressing major histocompatibility complex class II and B7 activation molecules stimulate potent tumor-specific immunity. Immunother. Emphasis Tumor Immunol. 14: 209–215, 1993.

Basset, P.; Bellocq, J.P.; Wolf, C.; Stoll, I.; Hutin, P.; Limacher, J.M.; Podhajcer, O.L.; Chenard, M.P.; Rio, M.C. and Chambon, P.: A novel metalloproteinase gene specifically expressed in stromal cells of breast carcinomas. Nature 348: 699–704, 1990.

Bataille, R.; Jourdan, M.; Zhang, YG. and Klein, B.: Serum levels of interleukin-6, a potent myeloma cell growth factor, as a reflection of disease severity in plasma cell dyscrasias. J. Clin. Invest. 84: 2008, 1989.

Bateman, A.; Singh, A.; Kral, T. and Solomin, S.: The immune-hypothalamic-pituitary-adrenal axis. Endocr. Rev. 10: 92–112, 1989.

Bauer, J. and Herrmann F.: Interleukin-6 in clinical medicine. Ann. Hematol. 62: 203, 1991.

Bauer, J.; Strauss, S.; Schreiter-Gasser, U.; Ganter U.; Schlegel, P.; Witt, I.; Yolk, B. and Berger, M.: Interleukin-6 and μ-2–macroglobulin indicate an acute-phase state in Alzheimer's disease cortices. FEBS Lett. 285: 111, 1991.

Baumann, G.: Molecular mechanism of immunosuppressive agents. Transplant. Proc. 24: 4–7, 1992.

Baumgartner, J.D.; Heumann, D.; Gerain, J.; Weinbreck, P.; Grau, G.E. and Glauser, M.P.: Association between protective efficacy of anti-lipopolysaccharide (LPS) antibodies and suppression of LPS-induced tumor necrosis factor alpha and interleukin 6: comparison of O side chain-specific antibodies with core LPS antibodies. J. Exp. Med. 171: 889–896, 1990.

Baxter, R.C.: The somatomedins: insulin-like growth factors. Adv. Clin. Chem. 25: 49–115, 1986.

Bayliss, M.: Mechanisms of cartilage damage, chondroprotection and biochemical monitoring. Rheumatoid Arthritis, Royal College of Physician, London, 17./18.6.1991.

Beall, C.J.; Mahajan, S. and Kolattukudy, P.E.: Conversion of monocyte chemoattractant protein-1 into a neutrophil attractant by substitution of two amino acids. J. Biol. Chem. 267: 3455–3459, 1992.

Beatty, J.D.; Duda, R.B.; Willis, L.E.; Sheibani, K.; Paxton, R.J. and Beatty, B.G.: Preoperative imaging of colorectal carcinoma with 111In-labeled anticarcinoembryonic antigen monoclonal antibody. Cancer Res. 46: 6494–6502, 1986.

Becherer, J.D. and Lambris, J.D.: Identification of the C3b receptor-binding domain in third component of complement. J. Biol. Chem. 263: 14586–14591, 1988.

Becherer, J.D.; Alsenz, J.; Servis, C.; Myones, B.L. and Lambris, J.D.: Cell surface proteins reacting with activated complement components. Complement Inflamm. 6: 142–165, 1989.

Becky Kelly, E.A.; Cruz, E.S.; Hauda, K.M. and Wassom, D.L.: IFN gamma and IL-5 producing cells compartmentalize to different lymphoid organs in Trichinella spiralis-infected mice. J. Immunol. 147: 306–314, 1991.

Begnet, R.H.J.; Ledermann, J.A.; Bagshawe, K.D.; Green, A.J.; Kelly, A.M.B.; Lane, D.; Secher, D.S.; Dewji, M.R. and Baker, T.S.: Phase I/II study of chimeric B72.3 antibody in radioimmunotherapy of colorectal carcinoma. Br. Ass. Canc. Res. Canc. Phax. 45: 487, 1990.

Begent, R.H.J.: Dosimetry in colorectal cancer. 6th Int. Conf. on Monoclonal Antibody Immunoconjugates for Cancer, San Diego, 1991.

Begent, R.H.J.; Ledermann, J.A.; Bagshawe, K.D.; Green, A.J.; Kelly, A.M.B.; Massoff, C.; Lane, D.; Baker, T.X.; Dewji, M.; Conlan, J. and Secher, D.S.: Dosimetry and immunogenicity of radioimmunotherapy with chimeric B72.3 antibody in colorectal cancer. 8th Int. Hammersmith Meeting, Greece, 1991.

Beierwaltes, W.H.: Effects of some 131I tagged antibodies in human melanoblastoma: Preliminary report. M. Mich. Med. Bull 20: 284, 1956.

Beijer, L.; Botting, J.; Crook, P.; Oyekan, A.O.; Page, C.P. and Rylander, R.: The involvement of platelet activating factor in endotoxin-induced pulmonary platelet recruitment in the guinea-pig. Br. J. Pharmacol. 92: 803–808, 1987.

Belizario, J.E. and Dinarello, C.A.: Interleukin 1, Interleukin 6, Tumor Necrosis Factor, and Transforming Growth Factor ß increase cell resistance to tumor necrosis factor cytotoxicity by growth arrest in the G1 phase of the cell cycle. Cancer Res. 51: 2379–2385, 1991.

Benacerraf, B.: Antigen processing and presentation. The biologic role of MHC molecules in determinant selection. J. Immunol., S17, suppl. 1988.

Ben-Chetrit, E.; Putterman, C. and Naprastek, Y.: Lupus refractory pleural effusion: transient response to intravenous immunoglobulins. J. Rheumatol. 18: 1635–1637, 1991.

Benjamin, D.; Knobloch, T.J. and Dayton, M.A.: Human B-cell interleukin-10: B-cell lines derived from patients with acquired immunodeficiency syndrome and Burkitt's lymphoma constitutively secrete large quantities of interleukin-10. Blood 80: 1289–1298, 1992.

Berd, D.; Maguire, H.C. jr. and Mastrangelo, M.J.: Treatment of human melanoma with a Hapten-modified autologous vaccine. Specific Immunotherapy Of Cancer With Vaccines, eds. Bystryn, J.-C.; Ferrone, S. and Livingston, P., The New York Academy of Sciences 690: 147, 1993.

Berger, M.; Wetzler, E.M. and Wallis, R.S.: Tumor necrosis factor is the major monocyte product that increases complement receptor expression on mature human neutrophils. Blood 71: 151–158, 1988.

Berk, B.C.; Alexander, R.W.; Brock, T.A.; Gimbrone, M.A. and Webb, R.C.: Vasoconstriction: a new activity for platelet-derived growth factor. Science 232: 87–90, 1986.

Berkenbosch, F.; Van Oers, J.; Del Rey, A.; Tilders, F. and Besedovsky, H.: Corticotropin-releasing factor-producing neurons in the rat activated by interleukin-1. Science 238: 524–526, 1987.

Bernard, G.R.; Lucht, W.D.; Niedermeyer, M.E.; Snapper, J.R.; Ogletree, M.L. and Brigham, K.L.: Effect of N-acetylcysteine on the pulmonary response to endotoxin in the awake sheep and upon in vitro granulocyte function. J. Clin. Invest. 73: 1722–1784, 1984.

Bernards, R.; Destree, A.; McKenzie, S.; Gordon, E.; Weinberg, R.A. and Panicali, D.: Effective tumor immunotherapy directed against an oncogene-encoded product using a vaccinia virus vector. Proc. Natl. Acad. Sci. USA 84: 6854–6858, 1987.

Bernton, E.W.; Beach, J.E.; Holaday, J.W.; Smallridge, R.C. and Fein, H.G.: Release of multiple hormones by a direct action of interleukin-1 on pituitary cells. Science 238: 519–521, 1987.

Berridge, M.J.; Heslop, J.P.; Irvine, R.F. and Brown, K.D.: Inositol trisphosphate formation and calcium mobilization in Swiss 3T3 cells in response to platelet-derived growth factor. Biochem. J. 222: 195–201, 1984.

Bertino, J.R.: Methotrexate: Molecular pharmacology. Cancer and Chemotherapy. III. Antineoplastic Agents, eds. Crooke, S.T. and Prestayko, A.W., Academic Press, New York, 311, 1981.

Bertram, J.H.; Gill, P.S.; Levine, A.M.; Boquiren, D.; Hoffmann, F.M.; Meyer, P. and Mitchell, M.S.: Monoclonal antibody T101 in T-cell malignancies: a clinical, pharmacokinetic and immunologic correlation. Blood 68: 752–761, 1986.

Berzofsky, J.A.: Epitope selection and design of synthetic vaccines. Molecular approaches to enhancing immunogenicity and cross-reactivity of engineered vaccines. Specific Immunotherapy Of Cancer With Vaccines, eds. Bystryn, J.-C.; Ferrone, S. and Livingston, P., The New York Academy of Sciences 690: 256, 1993.

Bessler, H.; Gilgal, R.; Djaldetti, M. and Zahavi, I.: Effect of pentoxifylline on the phagocytic activity, c-AMP levels and superanion production by monocytes and polymorphonuclear cells. J. Leukoc. Biol. 40: 747–754, 1986.

Beutler, B.; Milsark, I.W. and Cerami, A.C.: Passive immunization against cachectin/tumor necrosis factor protects mice from lethal effect of endotoxin. Science 229: 869, 1985.

Beutler, B. and Cerami, A.: Cachetin and tumor necrosis factor as two sides of the same biological coin. Nature 320: 584–588, 1986.

Beutler, B. and Cerami A.: The biology of cachectin/TNF – a primary mediator of the host response. Annu. Rev. Immunol. 7: 625–655, 1989.

Bevilacqua, G.; Sobel, M.E.; Liotta, L.A. and Steeg, P.S.: Association of low nm23 RNA levels in human primary infiltrating ductal breast carcinomas with lymph node involvement and other histopathological indicators of high metastatic potential. Cancer Res. 49: 5185–5190, 1989.

Bevilacqua, M.P.; Pober, J.S:; Wheeler, M.E.; Cotran, R.S. and Gimbrone, M.A.jr.: Interleukin I acts on cultured human vascular endothelial cells to increase the adhesion of polymorphonuclear leukocytes, monocytes and related leukocyte cell lines. J. Clin. Invest. 76: 2003–2011, 1985.

Bevilacqua, M.P.; Pober, J.S.; Mendrick, D.L.; Cotran, R.S. and Gimbrone, M.A. jr.: Identification of an iducible endothelial leukocyte adhesion molecule, ELAM-1. Proc. Natl. Acad. Sci. 84: 9238–9242, 1987.

Bevilacqua, M.P.; Stengelin, S.; Gimbroue, M.A. and Seed, B.: Endothelial leucocyte adhesion molecule 1: an inducible receptor for neutrophils and related to complement regulatory, proteins and lectins. Science 253: 1160–1165, 1989.

Beyers, A.D.; Spruyt, L.L. and Williams, A.F.: Molecular associations between the T-lymphocyte antigen receptor complex and the surface antigens CD2, CD4, or CD8 and CD5. Proc. Natl. Acad. Sci. USA 89: 2945–2949, 1992.

Bhardwaj, R.; Page, C.P.; May, G.R. and Moore, P.K.: Endothelium derived relaxing factor inhibits platelet aggregation in human whole blood and in the rat in vivo. Eur. J. Pharmacol. 157: 83–92, 1988.

Bhat, T.N.; Bentley, G.A.; Fischmann, T.O.; Boulot, G. and Poljak, R.J.: Small rearrangements in structures of Fv and Fab fragments of antibody D1.3 on antigen binding. Nature 347: 483–485, 1990.

Bhatt, H.; Brunet, L.J. and Stewart, C.L.: Uterine expression of leukemia inhibitory factor coincides with the onset of blastocyst implantation. Proc. Natl. Acad. Sci. 88: 11408–11412, 1991.

Bicknell, R. and Harris, A.L.: Novel growth regulatory factors and tumour angiogenesis. Eur. J. Cancer 27: 781–785, 1991.

Bicknell, R. and Harris, A.L.: Anticancer strategies involving the vasculature: vascular targeting and the inhibition of angiogenesis. Cancer Biol. 3: 399–407, 1992.

Biddison, W.E.; Rao, P.E.; Talle, M.A.; Goldstein, G. and Shaw, S.: Possible involvement of the OKT4 molecule in T-cell recognition of class II HLA antigens. J. Exp. Med. 156: 1065–1076, 1982.

Bieber, T.; Rieger, A.; Neuchrist, C.; Prinz, J.C.; Rieber, E.P.; Boltz-Nitulescu, G.; Scheiner, O.; Kraft, D.; Ring, J. and Stingl, G.: Induction of Fc R2/CD23 on human epidermal Langerhans cells by human recombinant interleukin 4 and gamma interferon. J. Exp. Med. 170: 309, 1989.

Bieber, T.; de la Salle, H.; Wollenberg, A.; Hakimi, J.; Chizzonite, R.; Ring, J.; Hanau, D. and de la Salle, C.: Human epidermal Langerhans cells express the high affinity receptor for Immunoglobulin E (Fc RI). J. Exp. Med. 175: 1285–1290, 1992.

Bierer, B.E.; Sleckman, B.P.; Ratnofsky, S.E. and Burakoff, S.J.: The biologic roles of CD2, CD4 and CD8 in T-cell activation. Annul. Rev. Immunol. 7: 579, 1989.

Biewenga, J.; Van Rees, E.P. and Sminia, T.: Short analytical review: Induction and regulation of IgA responses in the microenvironment of the gut. Clin. Immunol. Immunopath. 67: 1–7, 1993.

Bijsterbosch, M.K. and Klaus, G.G.B.: Cross-linking of surface immunoglobulin and Fc receptors and B lymphocytes inhibits stimulation of mositol phospholipid breakdown via the antigen receptors J. Exp. Med. 162: 1825–1836, 1985.

Billiau, A.: Interferon betasub 2 as a promotor of growth and differentiation of B cells. Immunology Today 8: 84–87, 1987.

Bischoff, S.C.; Brunner, T.; De Weck, A.L. and Dahinden, C.A.: Interleukin 5 modifies histamine release and leukotriene generation by human basophils in response to diverse agonists. J. Exp. Med. 172: 1577–1582, 1990.

Bjork, J.E.; Hedqiest, P. and Arfors, K.E.: Increase in vascular permeability induced by Leukotriene B4 and the role of polymorphonuclear leukocytes. Inflammation 6: 189–200, 1982.

Bjorkman, P.J.; Saper, M. Samraoui, B.; Bennett, W.; Strominger, J. and Wiley, D.: Structure of the human class I histocompatibility antigen HLA-A2. Nature 329: 506–512, 1987.

Bjorkman, P.J.; Saper, M.A.; Samraoui, B.; Bennet, W.S.; Strominger, J.L. and Wiley, D.C.: The foreign antigen binding site and T-cell recognition regions of class I histocompatibility antigens. Nature 329: 512–518, 1988.

Blaas, P.; Berger, B.; Weber, S.; Peter, H.H. and Hansch, G.M.: Paroxysmal nocturnal hemoglobinuria: enhanced stimulation of platelets by terminal complement components is related to the lack of C8bp in the membrane. J. Immunol. 140: 3045–3051, 1988.

Blackburn, W.D.jr.; Heck, L.W.; Loose, L.D.; Eskra, J.D. and Carty, T.J.: Inhibition of 5-lipoxygenase product formation and polymorphonuclear cell degranulation by tenidap sodium in patients with rheumatoid arthritis. Arthritis Rheum. 34: 204–210, 1991.

Blackmen, M.A.; Tigges, M.A.; Minie, M.E. and Koshland, M.E.: A model system for peptide hormone action in differentiation: Interleukin 2 induces a B lymphoma to transcribe the J chain gene. Cell 47: 609–617, 1986.

Blalock, J.E.: Production of peptide hormones and neurotransmitters by the immune system. Chem. Immunol. 52: 1–24, 1992.

Blalock, J.E.: The immune system. Our 6th sense. The Immunologist 2: 8, 1994.

Blanchette, V.; Kirby, M.A. and Turner, C.: Role if intravenous immunoglobulin G in autoimmune hematologic disorders. Sem. Hematol. 29/3: 72, 1992.

Blankenstein, T.; Qin, Z.; Uberla, K.; Muller, W.; Rosen, H.; Volk, H.-D. and Diamantstein, T.: Tumor suppression after tumor cell-targeted tumor necrosis factor alpha gene transfer. J. Exp. Med. 173: 1047–1052, 1991.

Blasi, F.: Surface receptors for urokinase plasminogen activator. Fibrinolysis 2: 73–84, 1988.

Blatteis, C.M.; Hunter, W.S.; Llonao, Q.J.; Ahokas, R.A. and Mashburn, T.A.: Activation of acute-phase responses by intrapreoptic injections of endogenous pyrogen in guinea pigs. Brain Res. Bull. 12: 689–696, 1984.

Blattler, W.A.: Blocked Ricin: A potent effector molecule for immunotoxin therapy. 6th Int. Conf. on Monoclonal Antibody Immunoconjugates, San Diego, 1991.

Blazquez, M.V.; Madueno, J.A.; Bonzalez, R.; Jurado, R.; Bachouchin, W.W.; Pena, J. and Munoz, E.: Selective decrease of CD26 expression in T cells from HIV infected individuals. J. Immunol. 149: 3073–3077, 1992.

Blottner, D.; Brueggemann, W. and Unsicker, K.: Ciliary neutotrophic factor supports target-deprived preganglionic sympathetic spinal cord neurons. Neurosci. Lett. 105: 316–320, 1989.

Bobak, D.A.; Gaither, T.G.; Frank, M.M. and Tenner, A.J.: Modulation of FcR function by complement subcomponent C1q enhances the phagocytosis of IgG-opsonized targets by human monocytes and culture-derived macrophages. J. Immunol. 138: 1150–1156, 1988.

Bockus, B.J. and Stiles, C.D.: Regulation of cytoskeletal architecture by platelet-derived growth factor, insulin and epidermal growth factor. Exp. Cell Res. 153: 186–197, 1984.

Bode, C.; Matsueda, G.R.; Hui, K.Y. and Haber, E.: Antibody-directed urokinase: a specific fibrinolytic agent. Science 229: 765, 1985.

Bodmer, W.F.; Browning, M.J.; Krausa, P.; Rowan, A.; Bicknell, D.C. and Bodmer, J.G.: Tumor escape from immune response by variation in HLA expression and other mechanisms. Specific Immunotherapy Of Cancer With Vaccines, eds. Bystryn, J.-C.; Ferrone, S. and Livingston, P., The New York Academy of Sciences 690: 42, 1993.

Boeri, D.G.: Europathologie: Recherches cliniques sur la respiration, sur le rire, sur le pleurer et sur le baillement des hémiplégiques. Gaz. heb. méd. Chir. 6: 73, 1901.

Bogdan, C.; Vodovotz, Y. and Nathan, C.: Macrophage deactivation by interleukin 10. J. Exp. Med. 174: 1549–1555, 1991.

Bogen, B.: Processing and presentation of immunoglobulin idiotypes to T cells. The Immunologist 1: 121, 1993.

Boguniewicz, M.; Jaffe, H.S.; Izu, A.; Sullivan, M.J.; York, D.; Geha, R.S. and Leung, D.Y.: Recombinant gamma interferon in treatment of patients with atopic dermatitis and elevated IgE levels. Am. J. Med. 88: 365–370, 1990.

Boitard, C.; Bendelac, A.; Richard, M.F.; Carnaud, C. and Bach, J.F.: Prevention of diabetes in nonobese diabetic mice by anti-I-A monoclonal antibodies: transfer of protection by splenic T cells. Proc Natl Acad Sci USA 85: 9719–9723, 1988.

Bomalaski, J.S.; Steiner, M.R.; Simon, P.L. and Clark, M.A.: Il-1 increases phospholipase A2 activity, expression of phospholipase A2–activating protein, and release of linoleic acid from the murine T helper cell line EL-4. J. Immunol. 148: 155, 1992.

Bone, R.C.: The pathogenesis of sepsis. Ann. Int. Med. 115: 457–469, 1991.

Bone, R.C.: Inhibitors of complement and neutrophils: a critical evaluation of their role in the treatment of sepsis. Intensive Care Medicine 20: 891, 1992.

Boni-Schnetzler, M. and Pilch, P.F.: Mechanism of epidermal growth factor receptor autophosphorylation and high-affinity binding. Proc. Natl. Acad. Sci. 84: 7832–7836, 1987.

Bonnefoy, J.Y.; Defrance T.; Peronne C.; Menetrier, C.; Pene J.; de Vries, J.E. and Bancherau J.: Human recombinant interleukin 4 induces normal B cells to produce soluble CD23/IgR binding factor analogous to that spontaneously released by lymphoblastoid B cell lines. Eur. J. Immunol. 18: 117, 1988.

Bonnefoy, J.-Y.; Shields, J. and Mermod, J.-J.: Inhibition of human interleukin 4–induced IgE synthesis by a subset of anti-CD23/Fc RII monoclonal antibodies. Eur. J. Immunol. 20: 139–144, 1990.

Bordin, S.; Kolb, W.P. and Page, R.C.: C1q receptors on cultured human gingival fibroblasts: analysis of binding properties. J. Immunol. 130: 1871–1875, 1983.

Bordin, S. and Page, R.C.: Role of platelet factors and serum complement in growth of fibroblasts with high-affinity C1q complement receptors. Journal of cellular and developmental Biology 24: 719–726, 1988.

Borel, J.F.: Comparative study of in vitro and in vivo drug effects on cell-mediated cytotoxicity. Immunology 31: 631–641, 1976.

Boris-Lawrie, K. and Temin, H.M.: The retroviral vector: replication cycle and safety considerations for retrovirus-mediated gene therapy. Annals of the New York Academy of Sciences 716: 59, 1994.

Borradori, L.; Gueissaz, F.; Frenk, E.; Rohner, R.; Scherz, R.; Lantin, J.P. and Spaeth, P.J.: Systemic lupus erythematosus associated with homozygous C2 deficiency. Apropos of a case report and literature review. Schweiz. Med. Wochenschr. 121: 418–423, 1991.

Borsos, T,; Chapuis, R.M. and Langone, J.J.: Distinction between fixation of C1 and the activation of complement by natural IgM anti-hapten antibody: effect of cell surface hapten density. Molec. Immun. 18: 863–868, 1981.

Bosslet, K. and Sedlacek, H.H.: Characterization of a colon carcinoma cell line for tumor immunotherapy. Cancer Detection and Prevention 12: 461–467, 1988.

Bosslet, K.; Hermentin, P.; Kuhlmann, L.; Steinstraesser, A.; Seemann, G. and Sedlacek, H.H.: Two-phase radioimmunotherapy using bispecific monoclonal antibodies (bs MAbs). Cancer Treatment Rev. 17: 355, 1990.

Bosslet, K.; Keweloh, H.C.; Hermentin, P.; Muhrer, K.H.; Sedlacek, H.H. and Schulz, G.: Percolation and binding of monoclonal antibody BW 494 to pancreatic carcinoma tissues during high dose immunotherapy and consequences for future therapy modalities. Br. J. Cancer 62: 37–39, 1990.

Bosslet, K.; Keweloh, H.C.; Hermentin, P.; Muhrer, K.H.; Sedlacek, H.H. and Schulz, G.: Percolation and binding of MAb BW 494 to pancreatic carcinoma tissues during high dose immunotherapy and consequences for future therapy modalities. Behring Inst. Mitt. 87: 68–75, 1990.

Bosslet, K.; Steinstraesser, A.; Hermentin, P.; Kuhlmann, L.; Bruynck, A.; Magerstaedt, M.; Seemann, G.; Schwarz, A. and Sedlacek, H.H.: Generation of bispecific monoclonal antibodies for two-phase radioimmunotherapy. Br. J. Cancer 63: 681, 1991.

Bosslet, K.; Czech, J.; Lorenz, P.; Sedlacek, H.H.; Schuermann, M. and Seemann, G.: Molecular and functional characterization of a fusion protein suited for tumor specific prodrug activation. Brit. J. Cancer 65: 234–238, 1992.

Bosslet, K.; Czech, J. and Hoffmann, D.: Tumor-selective prodrug activation by fusion protein-mediated catalysis. Cancer Res. 54: 2151–2159, 1994.

Bottazzi, B.; Polentarutti, N.; Acero, R.; Balsari, A.; Boraschi, D.; Ghezzi, P.; Salmona, M. and Mantovani, A.: Regulation of the macrophage content of neoplasms by chemoattractants. Science 220: 210–212, 1983.

Bottazzi, B.; Erba, E.; Nobili, N.; Fazioli, F.; Rambaldi, A. and Mantovani, A.: A paracrine circuit in the regulation of the proliferation of macrophages infiltrating murine sarcomas. J. Immunol. 144: 2409–2412, 1990.

Bottazzi, B.; Walter, S.; Govoni, D.; Colotta, F. and Mantovani, A.: Monocyte chemotactic cytokine gene transfer modulates macrophage infiltration, growth, and susceptibility to IL-2 therapy of a murine melanoma. J. Immunol. 148: 1280–12285, 1992.

Boucek, R.J. and Alvarez, T.R.: 5–Hydroxytryptamine: A cytospecific growth stimulator of cultured fibroblasts. Science 167: 898–899, 1970.

Bousso-Mittler, D.; Kloog, Y.; Wollbers, Z.; Bdolah, A.; Kochva, E. and Sokolovsky, M.: Functional endothelin/sarafotoxin recepotrs in the rat uterus. Biochem. Biophys. Res. Commun. 162: 952–957, 1989.

Boyd, F.T. and Massague, J.: Transforming growth factor-β inhibition of epithelial cell proliferation linked to the expression of a 53 kDa membrane receptr. J. Biol. Chem. 264: 2272–2278, 1989.

Boyer, V.; Desgranges, C.; Trabaud, M.A.; Fischer, E. and Kazatchkine, M.D.: Complement mediates human immunodeficiency virus type 1 infection of a human T cell line in a CD4- and antibody-independent fasion. J. Exp. Med. 173: 1151–1158, 1991.

Boyle, M.D.P.; Ohanian, S. and Borsos, T.: Lysis of tumor cells by antibody and complement VII. Complement-dependent 86Rb release – a non-lethal event. J. Immunol. 117: 1346–1350, 1976.

Boyle, M.D.P.; Ohanian, S. and Borsos, T.: Studies on the terminal stages of antibody-complement-mediated killing of a tumor cell. II. Inhibition of transformation of T* to dead cells by 3'5' cAMP. J. Immunol. 116: 1276–1279, 1976.

Brach, M.A.; Lowenberg, B.; Mantovani, L.; Schwulera, U.; Mertelsmann, R. and Herrmann, F.: Interleukin-6 (IL-6) is an intermediate in IL-1–induced proliferation of leukemic human magakaryoblasts. Blood 76: 10, 1990.

Brach, M.A. and Herrmann, F.: Interleukin 6: presence and future. Int. J. Clin. Lab. Res. 22: 143–151, 1992.

Brandley, B.K.; Swiedler, S.J. and Robbins, P.W.: Carbohydrate ligands of the LEC cell adhesion molecules. Cell 63: 861–863, 1990.

Brandt, J. Briddell, R.A. Srour, E.F.; Leemhuis, T.B. and Hoffman, R.: Role of c-kit ligand in the expansion of human hematopoietic progenitor cells. Blood 79: 634, 1992.

Brandtzaeg, P.: Mucosal and glandular distribution of immunoglobulin components: differential localization of free and bound SC in secretory epithelial cells. J. Immunol. 112: 1553–1559, 1974.

Brandtzaeg, P.: Transport model for secretory IgA and secretory IgM. Clin. Exp. Immunol. 44: 221–232, 1981.

Brandtzaeg, P.: Immunohistochemical characterization of intracellular J-chain and binding sites for secretory component (SC) in human immunoglobulin (Ig)-producing cells. Molec. Immun. 20: 941–966, 1983.

Bravo, R.: Synthesis of the nuclear protein cyclin (PCNA) and its relationship with DNA replication. Expl. Cell Res. 163: 287–293, 1986.

Bray, M.A.; Ford-Hutchinson, A.W. and Smith, M.J.H.: Leukotriene B4: An inflammatory mediator in vivo. Prostaglandins 22: 213–222, 1981.

Bray, M.A.: Prostaglandins and leukotrienes: fine tuning the immune response. ISI Atlas of Science, Pharmacology 101–106, 1987.

Bredehorst, R.; McCabe, R.; Pomato, N. and Vogel, C.W.: Site specific in vivo activation of therapeutic drugs. IPN: WO 90/07929, 1990.

Breder, C.D.; Dinarello, C.A. and Saper, C.B.: Interleukin-1 immunoreactive innervation of the human hypothalamus. Science 240: 321–324, 1988.

Breen, E.C.; Rezai, A.R.; Nakajima, K.; Beall, G.N.; Mitsuyasu, R.T.; Hirano, T.; Kishimoto, T. and Martinez-Maza, O.: Infection with HIV is associated with elevated IL-6 levels and production. J. Immunol. 144: 480, 1990.

Breitfeld, P.P.; Casanova, J.E.; McKinnon, W.C. and Mostov, K.E.: Deletions in the cytoplasmic domain of the polymeric immunoglobulin receptor differentially affect endocytotic rate and postendocytotic traffic. J. Biol. Chem. 265: 13750–13757, 1990.

Brennan, F.M.; Chantry, D.; Jackson, A.; Maini, R. and Feldmann, M.: Inhibitory effect of TNF alpha antibodies on synovial cell interleukin-1 production in rheumatoid arthritis. Lancet 2: 244–247, 1989.

Brenner, M.K.: Interleukin 2 and the treatment of leukemia and lymphoma. Leukemia and Lymphoma 5: 77–83, 1991.

Brenner, S.; Pepper, D.; Berns, M.W.; Tan, E. and Brinkley, B.R.: Kinetochore structure, duplication and distribution in mammalian cells: analysis by human autoantibodies from scleroderma patients. J. Cell Biol. 91: 95–102, 1981.

Briggs, D.C.; Donaldson, P.T.; Hayes, P.; Welsh, K.I.; Williams, R. and Neuberger, J.M.: A major histocompatibility complex class III allotype (C4B2) associated with primary biliary cirrhosis (PBC). Tissue Antigens 29: 141–145, 1987.

Brindley, L.L.; Sweet, J.M. and Goetzl, E.J.: Stimulation of histamine release from human basophils by human platelet factor 4. J. Clin. Invest. 72: 1218–1223, 1983.

Briscoe, D.M.; Schoen, F.J.; Rice, G.E.; Bevilacqua, M.P.; Ganz, P. and Pober, J.S.: Induced expression of endothelial-leukocyte adhesion molecules in human cardiac allografts. Transplantation 51: 537–539, 1991.

Brocke, S.; Brautbar, C.; Steinman, L.; Abramsky, O.; Rothbard, J.; Neumann, D.; Fuchs, S. and Mozes, E.: In vitro proliferative responses and antibody titres specific to human acetylcholine receptor synthetic peptides in patients with myasthenia gravis and relation to HLA class II genes. J Clin Invest 82: 1894–1900, 1988.

Brocker, E.B.; Kolde, G.; Steinhausen, D.; Peters, A. and Macher, E.: The pattern of the mononuclear infiltrate as a prognostic parameter in flat superficial spreading melanomas. J. Cancer Res. Clin. Oncol. 107: 48–52, 1984.

Brody, S.L. and Crystal, R.G.: Adenovirus-mediated in vivo gene transfer. Annals of the New York Academy of Sciences 716: 90, 1994.

Brown, E.J.: Complement receptors and phagocytosis. Curr. Opin. Immunol. 3: 76–82, 1991.

Brown, J.H.; Jardetzky, T.; Saper, M.A.; Samraoui, B.; Bjorkman, P.J. and Wiley, D.C.: A hypothetical model of the foreign antigen binding site of class II histocompatibility molecules. Nature 332: 845–850, 1988.

Brown, P.D.; Levy, A.T.; Margulies, I.M.; Liotta, L.A. and Stetler-Stevenson, W.G.: Independent expression and cellular processing of Mr 72,000 type IV collagenase and interstitial collagenase in human tumorigenic cell lines. Cancer Res. 50: 6184–6191, 1990.

Brown, T.J.; Rowe, J.M.; Liu, J.W. and Shoyab, M.: Regulation of Il-6 expression by oncostatin M. J. Immunol. 147: 2175–2180, 1991.

Browning, M.J. and Bodmer, W.F.: MHC antigens and cancer: implications for T-cell surveillance. Curr. Opin. Immunol. 4: 613–618, 1992.

Broxmeyer, H.E.; Williams, D.E.; Lu. L.; Cooper, S.; Anderson, S.L.; Beyer, G.S.; Hoffman, R. and Rubin Y.Y.: The suppressive influences of human tumor necrosis factor on bone marrow hematopoietic progenitor cells from normal donors and patients with leukemia: Synergism of tumour necrosis factor and interferon-gamma. J. Immunol. 136: 4487, 1986.

Broxmeyer, H.E.; Sherry, B.; Cooper, S.; Ruscetti, F.W.; Williams, D.E.; Arosio, P.; Kwon, B.S. and Cerami, A.: Macrophage inflammatory protein (MIP)-1 beta abrogates the capacity of MIP-1 alpha to suppress myeloid progenitor cell growth. J. Immunol. 147: 2586–2594, 1991.

Brueggeman, M.; Williams, G.T.; Binder, C.I.; Clark, M.R.; Walker, M.P.; Jeffrey, R.; Waldmann, H. and Neuberger, M.S.: Comparison of the effector functions of human immunoglobulin using a matched set of chimeric antibodies. J. Exp. Med. 166: 1351–1361, 1987.

Bubenik, J.; Lotzova, E.; Zeuthen, J.; Bubenikova, D.; Simova, J. and Indrova, M.: Gene therapy of cancer: use of interleukin-2 (IL-2) gene transfer in local immunotherapy. J. Exp. Clin. Cancer Rest. 10: 213, 1991.

Buckingham, J.C. and Cooper, T.A.: Differences in hypothalamo-pituitary-adrenocortical activity in the rat after acute and prolonged treatment with morphine. Neuroendocrinology 38: 411–417, 1984.

Budowle, B.; Reitnauer, P.J.; Barger, B.O.; Go, R.C.; Roseman, J.M. and Acton, R.T.: Properdin factor B in black type 1 (insulin-dependent) diabetic patients. Diabetologia 22: 483–485, 1982.

Bufler, P.; Stelter, F.; Krüger, C.; Schütt, C.; Riethmüller, G. and Engelmann, H.: Molecular mechanisms for the production of soluble CD14. Immunobiology 189: 38, 1993.

Buinauskas, P.; McCredie, J.A.; Brown, E.R. and Cole, W.H.: Experimental treatment of tumors with antibodies. Archs. Surg., Chicago 79: 432, 1959.

Bunting, S.; Simmons, P.M. and Moncada, S.: Inhibition of platelet activation by prostacyclin - possible consequences in coagulation and anticoagulation. Thromb. Res. 21: 89–102, 1981.

Buraggi, G.L.; Callegaro, L.; Mariani, G.; Turrin, A.; Cascinelli, C.: Attili, A.; Bombardieri, E.; Terno, G.; Plassio, G.; Dovis, M.; Mazzuca, N.; Natali, P.G.: Scassellati, G.A.; Rosa, U. and Ferrone, S.: Imaging with 131I-labeled monoclonal antibodies to a high-molecular-weight melanoma-associated antigen in patients with melanoma: efficacy of whole immunoglobulins and its F(ab')2 fragments. Cancer Res. 45: 3378, 1985.

Burdach, S.E.G.; Evers, K.G. and Geursen, R.G.: Treatment of acute idiopathic thrombocytopenic purpura of childhood with intravenous immunoglobulin G.: comperative efficacy of 7S and 5S preparations. J. Pediatr. 109: 770, 1986.

Burgess, W.H.; Mehlman, T.; Marshak, D.R.; Fraser, B.A. and Maciag, T.: Structural evidence that endothelial cell growth factor beta is the precursor of both endothelial cell growth factor alpha and acidic fibroblast growth factor. Proc. Natl. Acad. Sci. 83: 7216–7220, 1986.

Burgess, W.H. and Maciag, T.: The heparin-binding (fibroblast) growth factor family of proteins. Ann. Rev. Biochem. 58: 575–606, 1989.

Burrows, B.; Martinez, F.D.; Halonen, M.; Barbee, R.A. and Cline, M.G.: Association of asthma with serum IgE levels and skin-test reactivity to allergens. N. Engl. J. Med. 320: 271, 1989.

Burstein, S.A.; Mei, R. and Henthorn, J.: Recombinant human leukemia inhibitory factor (LIF) and interleukin-11 (IL-11) promote murine and human megakaryocytopoiesis in vitro. Blood 76: 450a, 1990 (abstr., suppl. 1).

Burtin, P.; Chavanel, G. and Fondaneche, M.C.: Proteases in human tumors. Bull Cancer 71: 474–480, 1984.

Burton, D.R.: Immunoglobulin G: Functional sites. Molec. Immunol. 22: 161–206, 1985.

Busbridge, N.J. and Grossman, A.B.: Stress and the single cytokine: Interleukin modulation of the pituitary-adrenal axis. Mol. Cell. Endocrinol. 82: C209–C214, 1991.

Bussel, J.B.; Kimberly, R.P.; Inman, R.D.; Schulman, I.; Cunningham-Rundles, C.; Cheung, N.; Smithwick, E.M.; O'Malley, J.; Barandun, S. and Hilgartner, M.W.: Intravenous gammaglobulin treatment of chronic idiopathic thrombocytopenic purpura. Blood 62: 480–486, 1983.

Bussolino, F.; Wang, J.M.; Defilippi, P.; Turrini, F.; Sanavio, F.; Edgell, G.J.; Aglietta, M.; Arese, P. and Mantovani, A.: Granulocyte- and granulocyte-macrophage-colony stimulating factors induce human endothelial cells to migrate and proliferate. Nature 337: 471–473, 1989.

Butler, K.D.; Pay, G.M.; Roberts, J.M. and White, A.M.: The effect of sulphinpyrazone and other drugs on the platelet response during the active arthus reaction in guinea pigs. Thromb. Res. 15: 319–340, 1979.

Butler, V.P. Jr. and Vaughan J.H.: Hemagglutination by rheumatoid factor of cells coated with animal gamma globulins. Proc. Soc. exp. biol. Med. 116: 585–593, 1964.

Buyon, J.P.; Shadick, N.; Berkman, R.; Hopkins, P.; Dalton, J.; Weissmann, G.; Winchester, R. and Abramson, S.B.: Surface expression of 165/95, the complement receptor CR3, as a marker of disease activity in systemic lupus erythematosus. Clin. Immunol. Immunopathol. 46: 141–149, 1988.

Byers, V.S.; Rodvien, R.; Grant, K.; Durrant, L.G.; Hudson, K.H.; Baldwin, R.W. and Scannon, P.J.: Phase I study of monoclonal antibody-Ricin A chain immunotoxin XomaZyme-791 in patients with metastatic colon cancer. Cancer Res. 49: 6153, 1989.

Bystryn, J.-C.: Immunogenicity and clinical activity of a polyvalent melanoma antigen vaccine prepared from shed antigens. Specific Immunotherapy Of Cancer With Vaccines, eds. Bystry, J.-C.; Ferrone, S. and Livingston, P., The New York Academy of Sciences 690: 190, 1993.

Cabrillat, H.; Galizzi, J.P.; Djossou, O.; Arai, N.; Yokota, T.; Arai, K. and Banchereau, J.: High affinity binding of human IL-4 to cell lines. Biochem. Biophys. Res. Commun. 149: 995–1001, 1987.

Cahan, L.D.; Irie, R.F.; Singh, R.; Cassidenti, A. and Paulsen, J.C.: Identification of a human neuroectodermal tumor antigen (OFA-I-2) as ganglioside GD2. Proc. Natl. Acad. Sci. USA 79: 7629–7633, 1982.

Cairns, J.; Flores-Romo, L.; Millsum, M.J.; Guy, G.R.; Gillis, S.; Ledbetter, J.A. and Gordon, J.: Soluble CD23 is related by B lymphocytes cycling in response to interleukin 4 and anti-Bp50 (CDw40). Eur. J. Immunol. 18: 349–353, 1988.

Calkins, J.H.; Sigel, M.M.; Nankin, H.R. and Lin, T.: Interleukin-1 inhibits Leydig cell steroidogenesis in primary culture. Endocrinology 123: 1605–1610, 1988.

Callewaert, D.M.: Suite selective plasminogen activator and method of making and using same. EPS: 0 146 050, 1990.

Cambier, J.C.; Justement, L.B.; Newell, K.; Chen, Z.Z.; Harris, L.K.; Sandoval, V.M.; Klemsz, M.J. and Ransom, J.T.: Transmembrane signals and intracellular "second messengers" in the regulation of quiescent B-lymphocyte activation. Immunol. Rev. 95: 37–57, 1987.

Camp, R.; Jones, R.R.; Brain, S.; Woolard, P. and Greaves, M.W.: Production of intraepidermal microabscesses by topical application of leukotriene B4. J. Invest. Dermatol. 84: 427–429, 1985.

Campbell, A.K. and Luzio, J.P.: Intracellular calcium as a pathogen in cell damage initiated by the immune system. Experientia 37: 110–112, 1981.

Campbell, A.K.; Daw, R.A.; Hallett, M.B. and Luzio, J.P.: Direct measurement of the increase in intracellular free Ca2+ concentration in response to the action of complement. Biochem. J. 194: 551–560, 1981.

Campbell, A.K.: Intracellular calcium: its universal role as regulator. Wiley, Chichester, 257, 304, 1982.

Campbell, A.K. and Morgan, B.P.: Monoclonal antibodies demonstrate protection of polymorphonuclear leukocytes against complement attack. Nature 317: 164–166, 1985.

Campbell, C.H. and Cunningham, D.D.: Binding sites for elastase on cultured human fibroblasts that do not mediate internalization. J. Cell Physiol. 130: 142–149, 1987.

Camussi, G.; Salvidio, G.; Biesecker, G.; Brentjens, J. and Andres G.: Heyman antibodies induce complement-dependent injury of rat glomerular visceral epithelial cells. J. Immunol. 139: 2906–2914, 1987.

Cannistra, S.A.; Vellenga, E.; Groshek, P.; Rambaldi, A. and Griffin, J.D.: Human granulocyte-monocyte colony-stimulating factor and interleukin 3 stimulate monocyte cytotoxicity through a tumor necrosis factor-dependent mechanism. Blood 71: 672–676, 1988.

Cannon, M.J.; Openshaw, P.J.M. and Askonas, B.A.: Cytotoxic cells clear virus but augment lung pathology in mice infected with respiratory syncytial virus. J. Exp. Med. 168: 1163–1168, 1988.

Caracciolo, D.; Valtieri, M.; Venturelli, D.; Peschle, C.; Gewirtz, A.M. and Calabretta, B.: Lineage-specific requirement of c-abl function in normal hematopoiesis. Science 245: 1107–1110, 1989.

Caracciolo, D.; Venturelli, D.; Valtieri, M.; Peschle, C.; Gewirtz, A.M. and Calabretta, B.: Stage-related proliferative activity determined c-myb functional requirements during normal human hematopoiesis. J. Clin. Invest. 85: 55–61, 1990.

Carbone, F.R. and Bevan, M.J.: Induction of ovalbumin-specific cytotoxic T cells by in vivo peptide immunization. J. Exp. Med. 169: 603–612, 1989.

Carey, T.E.; Takahashi, T.; Resnick, L.A.; Oettgen, H.F. and Old, L.J.: Cell surface antigens of human malignant melanoma. I. Mixed hemadsorption assays for humoral immunity to cultured autologous melanoma cells. Proc. Natl. Acad. Sci. USA 73: 3278–3282, 1976.

Carey, T.E.; Lloyd, K.O.; Takahashi, T.; Travassos, L.R. and Old, L.J.: AU cell-surface antigen of human malignant melanoma: Solubilization and partial characterization. Proc. Natl. Acad. Sci. USA 76: 2898–2902, 1979.

Carlos, T.M. and Harlan, J.M.: Membrane proteins involved in phagocyte anderence to endothelium. Immunological reviews 114: 5–29, 1990.

Carmassi, F.; Morale, M.; Puccetti, R.; Pistelli, F.; Palla, R.; Bevilacqua, G.; Viacava, P.; Antonelli, A. and Mariani, G.: Efficacy of intravenous immunoglobulin therapy in a case of autoimmune-mediated chronic active hepatitis. Clin. Exp. Rheumatol. 10: 13–17, 1992.

Carney, D.F.; Koski, C.L. and Shin, M.L.: Elimination of terminal complement intermediates from the plasma membrane of nucleated cells: the rate of disappearance differs for cells carrying C5b-7 or C5b-8 or a mixture of C5b-8 with a limited number of C5b-9. J. Immunol. 134: 1804–1809, 1985.

Carney, D.F.; Hammer, C.H. and Shin, M.L.: Elimination of terminal complement complexes in the plasma membrane of nucleated cells: influence of extracellular Ca2+. J. Immunol. 137: 263–270, 1986.

Carney, D.F.; Lang, T.I. and Shin, M.L.: Multiple signal messengers generated by terminal complement complexes and their role in terminal complex elimination. J. Immunol. 145: 623–629, 1990.

Carow, C.E.; Hangoc, G.; Cooper, S.H.; Williams, D.E. and Broxmeyer, H.E.: Mast cell growth factor (c-kit ligand) supports the growth of human multipotential progenitor cells with a high replating potential. Blood 78: 2216–2221, 1991.

Carpenter, G. and Cohen, S.: Epidermal growth factor. Ann. Rev. Biochem. 48: 192–216, 1979.

Carreer, F.M.J.: The C1 inhibitor deficiency. A review. Eur. J. Clin. Chem. Clin. Biochem. 30: 793–807, 1992.

Carreras, L.O.; Perez, G.N.; Vega, H.R. and Casavilla, F.: Lupus anticoagulant and recurrent fetal loss: successful treatment with gammaglobulin (letter). Lancet 2: 393–394, 1988.

Carroll, P.; Stafford, D.; Schwartz, R.S. and Stollar B.D.: Murine monoclonal anti-DNA auto-antibodies bind to endogenous bacteria. J. Immun. 135: 1086–1090, 1985.

Carter, R.H.; Spycher M.O.; Yin C.N.G.; Hoffman, R. and Fearon D.T.: Synergistic interaction between complement receptors type 2 and membrane IgM on B lymphocytes. J. Immunol. 141: 457, 1988.

Carter, R.H.; Spycher, M.O.; Ng, Y.C.; Hoffman, R. and Fearon, D.T.: Synergistic interaction between complement receptor type 2 and membrane IgM on B lymphocytes. J. Immunol. 141: 457–463, 1988.

Casanova, J.E.; Breitfeld, P.P.; Ross, S.A. and Mostov, K.E.: Phosphorylation of the polymeric immunoglobulin receptor required for its efficient transcytosis. Science 248: 742–745, 1990.

Catimel, B.; Leung, L.; El Ghissasi, H.; Mercier, N. and McGregor, J.L.: Human platelet glyco-protein IIIb bind to thrombospondin fragments bearing the carboxy, and/or the type I repeats (CSVTCG motif), but not to the amino-terminal heparin binding region. Biochem. J. 284: 231–236, 1992.

Caux, C.; Vanbervliet, B.; Dezutter-Dambuyant, C.; Massacrier, C.; Schmitt, D. and Banchereau, J.: In vitro generation of human dendritic cells. ENII Conf.: Integrated Function of Molecules of the Immune System. Les Embiez, France, 12th-16th, May 1993

Cavallo, T.; Sade, R.; Folkman, J. and Cotran, R.S.: Rapid induction of endothelial mitoses de-monstrated by autoradiography. J. Cell Biol. 54: 408, 1972.

Cawston, T.E.; Galloway, W.A.; Mercer, E.; Murphy, G. and Reynolds, J.J.: Purification of rab-bit bone inhibitor of collagenase. Biochem. J. 195: 159–165, 1981.

Cazenave, J.P.; Assimeh, S.N.; Painter, R.H.; Packham, M.A. and Mustard, J.F.: C1q inhibition of the interaction of collagen with human platelets. J. Immunol. 116: 162–163, 1976.

Celis, E.: T helper cells and autoantibodies in autoimmune disease. The Immunologist 1: 126, 1993.

Centrella, M.; McCarthy, T.L. and Canalis E.: Transforming growth factor ß is a bifunctional regulator of replication and collagen synthesis in osteoblast-enriched cell cultures from fetal rat bone. J. Biol. Chem. 262: 2869–2874, 1987.

Cerney, J.: Stimulation of bone marrow haemopoietic stem cells by a factor from activated T cells. Nature 249: 63–66, 1974.

Cerundolo, V.; Elliott, T.; Bastin, J.; Rammensee, H.-G. and Townsend, A.: The binding affinity and dissociation rates of peptides for class I major histocompatibility complex molecules. Eur. J. Immunol. 21: 2069–2076, 1991.

Ceuppens, J.L.; Bloemmen, F.J. and Van Wauwe, J.P.: T cell unresponsiveness to the mitogenic activity of OKT3 antibody results from a deficiency of monocyte Fc gamma receptors for mu-rine IgG2a and inability to cross-link the T3–Ti complex. J. Immunol. 135: 3882–3886, 1985.

Chabner, B.A.: Nucleoside Analogues. Cancer and Chemotherpy. III. Antineoplastic Agents, eds. Crooke, S.T. and Prestayko A.W., Academic Press, New York, 3, 1981.

Chabot, B.; Stephenson, D.A.; Chapman, V.M.; Besmer, P. and Bernstein, A.: The proto-onco-gene c-kit endocing a transmembrane tyrosine kinase receptor maps to the mouse W locus. Nature 35: 88–89, 1988.

Chan, C.C.; Nathaniel, D.J.; Yusco, P.Y.; Hall, R.A. and Ford-Hutchinson, A.W.: Inhibition of prostanoid-mediated platelet aggregation in vivo and in vitro by 3–hydroxymethyl-dibenzo(b,f)thiepin 5,5–dioxide (L-640,035). J. Pharmacol. Exp. Ther. 229: 276–282, 1984.

Chan, C.P.; Bowen-Pope, D.F.; Ross, R. and Krebs, E.G.: Regulation of glycogen synthase activity by growth factors. Relationship between synthase activation and receptor occupancy. J. Biol. Chem. 262: 276–281, 1987.

Chan, C.T.J.; Byfield, P.G.H.; Himsworth, R.L. and Shepherd P.: Human autoantibodies to thy-roglobulin are directed towards a restricted number of human specific epitopes. Clin. exp. Im-mun. 70: 516–523, 1987.

Chan, E.K.L. and Tan, E.M.: Human autoantibody-reactive epitopes of SS-B/La are highly con-served in comparison with epitopes recognized by murine monoclonal antibodies. J. exp. Med. 166: 1627–1640, 1987.

Chan, S.H.; Perussia, B.; Gupta, J.W.; Kobayashi, M.; Pospisil, M.; Young, H.A.; Wolf, S.F.; Young, D.; Clark, S.C. and Trinchieri, G.: Induction of Interferon-gamma production by natural killer cell stimulatory factor: characterization of the responder cells and synergy with other inducers. J. Exp. Med. 173: 869–879, 1991.

Chang, D.-M.; Baptiste, P. and Schur, P.H.: The effect of antirheumatic drugs on interleukin 1 (Il-1) activity and Il-1 and Il-1 inhibitor production by human monocytes. J. Rheumatol. 17: 1148–1157, 1990.

Chao, C.C.; Hu, S.; Close, K.; Choi, C.S.; Molitor, T.W.; Novick, W.J. and Peterson, P.K.: Cytokine release from microglia: differential inhibition by pentoxifylline and dexamethasone. J. Invest. Dis. 166: 847–853, 1992.

Chatterjee, M.; Mrozek, E.; Vaickus, L.; Oseroff, A.; Stoll, H.; Russell, D.; Kohler, H. and Foon, K.A.: Antiidiotype (Ab2) vaccine therapy for cutaneous T-cell lymphoma. Specific Immunotherapy Of Cancer With Vaccines, eds. Bystryn, J.-C.; Ferrone, S. and Livingston, P., The New York Academy of Sciences 690: p. 376, 1993.

Chaudhary, V.K.; Queen, C.; Junghans, R.F.; Waldmann, T.; Fitzgerald, D.J. and Pastan, I.: A recombinant immunotoxin consisting of two antibody variable domains fused to Pseudomonas exotoxin. Nature 339: 393–394, 1989.

Cheetham, J.J.; Chen, R.J.B. and Epand, R.M.: Interaction of calcium and cholesterol sulphate induces membrane destabilization and fusion: implications for the acrosome reaction. Biochim. Biophys. Acta 1024: 367–372, 1990.

Cheever, M.A.; Chen, W.; Disis, M.L.; Takahashi, M. and Peace, D.J.: T-cell immunity to oncogeneic proteins including mutated RAS and chimeric BCR-ABL. Specific Immunotherapy of Cancer with Vaccines, Bystryn, J.C.; Ferrone, S. and Livingston, P. (eds)., Annals of the New York Academy of Sciences 690: 1993.

Cheifetz, S.; Like, B. and Massague, J.: Cellular distribution of type I and type II receptors for transforming growth factor-ß. J. Biol. Chem. 261: 9972–9978, 1986.

Cheifetz, S.; Ling, N.; Guillemin, R. and Massague, J.: A surface component on GH3 pituitary cells that recognizes transforming growth factor-beta, activin, and inhibin. J. Biol. Chem. 263: 17225–17228, 1988.

Cheifetz, S.; Andres, J.L. and Massague, J.: The TGFß receptor type is a membrane proteoglycin. Domain structure of the receptor. J. Biol. Chem. 263: 16984–16991, 1988.

Chen, C.-J.; Banerjea, A.C.; Haglund, K.; Harmison, G.G. and Schubert, M.: Inhibition of HIV-1 replication by novel multitarget ribozymes. Antisense Strategies, eds. Baserga, R. and Denhardt, D.T., Annals of the New York Academy of Sciences 660: 271, 1992.

Chen, L.P.; Thomas, E.K.; Hu, S.L.; Hellstroem, I. and Hellstroem, K.E.: Human papillomavirus type 16 nucleoprotein is a tumor rejection antigen. Proc. Natl. Acad. Sci. USA 88: 110–114, 1991.

Chen, L.P.; Ashe, S.; Brady, W.A.; Hellstroem, I.; Hellstroem, K.E.; Ledbetter J.A.; McGowan, P. and Linsley P.S.: Costimulation of antitumor immunity by the B7 counterreceptor for the T lymphocyte molecules CD28 and CTLA-4. Cell 71: 1093–1102, 1992.

Chen, V.J.; Jungheim, L.N.; Meyer, D.L. and Shepherd, T.A.: Delivery of cytotoxic agents. Eur. Patent Appl. 0 382 411, 1990.

Chen, W.; Peace, D.J.; Rovira, D.K.; You, S.-G. and Cheever, M.A.: T cell immunity to the joining region of p210 bcr-abl protein. Proc. Natl. Acad. Sci. USA 89: 1468–1472, 1992.

Chen, W.; You, S.-G.; Disis, M.L. and Cheever, M.A.: Evaluation of the joining region segment of p210 bcr-abl chimeric protein as a potential leukemia-specific antigen to elicit class I MHC-restricted CTL responses. J. Cell Biochem. (abstr. suppl. 17D): 107 (abstr. NZ 203), 1993.

Cheng, C.M. and Hawiger, J.: Affinity isolation and characterization of immunoglobulin G Fc fragment-binding glycoprotein from human blood platelets. J. Biol. Chem. 254: 2165–2167, 1979.

Cheng, Q.; Zhou, D.; Wang, Y.; Tang, L. and Han, J.: Radioimmunoassay for ß-endorphin in the brain and pituitary as related to the effectiveness of acupuncture analgesia in the rat. Acupunct. Res. 7: 36–39, 1982.

Cher, D.J. and Mosmann, T.R.: Two types of murine helper T cell clones. II. Delayed type hypersensitivity is mediated by TH1 clones. J. Immunol. 138: 3688, 1987.

Chern, Y.; Spangler, R.; Choi, H.S. and Sytkowsi, A.J.: Erythropoietin activates the receptor in both Rauscher and Friend murine erythroleukemia cells. J. Biol. Chem. 266: 2009–2012, 1991.

Chesnut, R.W. and Grey, H.M.: Studies on the capacity of B cells to serve as antigen-presenting cells. J. Immunol. 126: 1075, 1981.

Cheung, N.K.; Walter, E.I.; Smith-Mensah, W.H.; Ratnoff, W.D.; Tykocinski, M.L. and Medof, M.E.: Decay-accelerating factor protects human tumor cells from complement-mediated cytotoxicity in vitro. J. Clin. Invest. 81: 1122–1128, 1988.

Chevalier, J. and Kazatchkine, M.D.: Distribution in clusters of complement receptor type one (CR1) on human erythrocytes. J. Immunol. 142: 2031–2036, 1989.

Chiang, T.M,; Gupta, R.C. and Kang, A.H.: Effect of the C1q on the soluble collagen-platelet interaction. Thrombosis Research 37: 605–612, 1985.

Chignard, M.; Lalau Keraly, C.; Nunez, D.; Coeffier, E. and Benveniste, J.: PAF-acether and platelets. In: MacIntyre, D.E. and Gordon, J.L. (eds.) Platelets in Biology and Pathology III, 289–315, Elsevier/North Holland Biomedical Press, Amsterdam, 1987.

Chihara, J.; Fukuda, K.; Yasuba, H.; Hishigami, N.; Sugihara, R.; Kubo, H. and Nakajima, S.; Platelet factor 4 enhances eosinophil IgG and IgE Fc receptor and has eosinophil chemotactic activity. Am. Rev. Respir. Dis. 137: 421, 1988.

Childs, C.B.; Proper, J.A.; Tucker, R.F. and Moses, H.L.: Serum contains a platelet-derived transforming growth factor. Proc. Natl. Acad. Sci. USA 79: 5312–5316, 1982.

Choi, H.S.; Wojchowski, D.M. and Sytkowski, A.J.: Erythropoietin rapidly alters phosphorylation of pp43, an erythroid membrane protein. J. Biol. Chem. 262: 2933–2936, 1991.

Choi, Y.; Herman, A.; DiGuisto, D.; Wade, T.; Marrack, P. and Kappler, J.: Residues of the variable region of the T-cell-receptor ß-chain that interact with S. aureus toxin superantigens. Nature 346: 471–473, 1990.

Chou, C.K.; Dull, T.J.; Russell, D.S.; Gherzi, R.; Lebwohl, D.; Ullrich, A. and Rosen, O.M.: Human insulin receptors mutated at the ATP-binding site lack protein tyrosine kinase activity and fail to mediate postreceptor effects of insulin. J. Biol. Chem. 262: 1842–1847, 1987.

Christadoss, P. and Dauphinee, M.J.: Immunotherapy for myasthenia gravis: a murine model. J. Immunol. 136: 2437–2440, 1986.

Christensen, J.D.; Hansen, E.W. and Fjalland, B.: Interleukin-1ß stimulates the release of vasopressin from rat neurohypophysis. Eur. J. Pharmacol. 171: 233–235, 1989.

Christinck, E.R.; Luscher, M.A.; Barber, B.H. and Williams, D.B.: Peptide binding to class I MHC on living cells and quantitation of complexes for CTL lysis. Nature 352: 67–70, 1991.

Chung, K.F. and Barnes, P.J.: PAF antagonists. Their potential therapeutic role in asthma. Drugs 35: 93–103, 1988.

Cikes, M.: Antigenic expression of an immune lymphoma during growth in vitro. Nature 225: 645–646, 1970.

Claesson, H.E.; Odlander, B. and Jakobsson, P-J.: Leukotriene B4 in the immune system. Int. J. Immunopharm. 14: 441–449, 1992.

Clark, R.A.: The human neutrophil respiratory burst oxidase. J. Infect. Dis. 161: 1140–1147, 1990.

Clark-Lewis, I. and Schrader, J.W.: Molecular structure and biological activities of P cell-stimulating factor interleukin-3. Lymphokines 15: 1–38, 1988.

Clipstone, N.A. and Crabtree, G.R.: Calcineurin is a key signaling enzyme in T lymphocyte activation and the target of immunosuppressive drugs Cyclosporin A and FK506. Immunosuppressive and Antiinflammatory Drugs, eds. Allison, A.C.; Lafferty, K.J. and Fliri, H., Annals of the New York Academy of Sciences 696: 20, 1993.

Clore, G.M.; Appella, E.; Yamada, M.; Matsushima, K. and Gronenborn, A.M.: Three-dimensional structure of interleukin 8 in solution. Biochemistry 29: 1689–1696, 1990.

Coffey, R.J.jr.; Kost, L.J.; Lyons, R.M.; Moses, H.L. and LaRusso, N.F.: Hepatic processing of transforming growth factor ß in the rat. Uptake, metabolism, and biliary excretion. J. Clin. Invest. 80: 750–757, 1987.

Coffman, R.L.; Ohara, J.; Bond, M.W.; Carty, J.; Zlotnick, A. and Paul, W.E.: B cell stimulatory factor-1 enhances the IgE response of lipopolysaccharide-activated B cells. J. Immunol. 136: 4538–4541, 1986.

Coffman, R.L. and Carty, J.: A T cell activity that enhances polyclonal IgE production and its inhibition by interferon-gamma. J. Immunol. 136: 949–954, 1986.

Coffman, R.L.; Lee, F.; Yokota, T.; Arai, K. and Mosmann T.R.: The effect of BSF 1 and IFN-gamma upon mouse immunoglobulin isotype expression. In UCLA Symposium: Immune Regulation by Characterized Polypeptides. G. Boldstein, J. Bach and H. Wigzell, eds. Alan Liss, New York, 523, 1987.

Coffman, R.L.; Seymour, B.W.; Lebman, D.A.; Hiraki, D.D.; Christiansen, J.A.; Shrader, B.; Cherwinski, H.M.; Savelkoul, H.F.; Finkelman, F.D.; Bond, M.W. and Mosman, T.R.: The role of helper T cell products in mouse B cell differentiation and isotpye regulation. Immunol. Rev. 102: 25–28, 1988.

Coffman, R.L.; Lebman, D.A. and Shrader, B.: Transforming growth factor ß specifically enhances IgA production by lipopolysaccharide-stimulated murine B lymphocytes. J. Exp. Med. 170: 1039–1044, 1989.

Cogan, D.G.: Vascularization of the cornea, its experimental induction by small lesions and a new theory of its pathogenesis. Archs. Ophthal. 41: 406, 1949.

Cohen et al. cited by Cohen, S., 1965.

Cohen, S.: The stimulation of epidermal proliferation by a specific protein (EGF). Dev. Biol. 12: 394–407, 1965.

Cohen, S.: Epidermal growth factor. In vitro Cell and Devel. Biol. 23: 239–246, 1987.

Colbran, R.J.; Schworer, C.M.; Hasimoto, Y.; Fong, Y-L.; Rich, D.P.; Smith, K.M. and Soderling, T.R.: Calcium/calmodulin dependent protein kinase II. Biochem. J. 258: 313–325, 1989.

Colcher, D.; Zalutsky, M.; Kaplan, W.; Kufe, D.; Austin, F. and Schlom, J.: Radiolocalization of human mammary tumors in athymic mice by a monoclonal antibody. Cancer Res. 43: 736, 1983.

Colcher, D.; Keenan, A.M.; Larson, S.M. and Schlom, J.: Prolonged binding of a radiolabeled monoclonal antibody (B72.3) used for the in situ radioimmunodetection of human colon carcinoma xenografts. Cancer Res. 44: 5744, 1984.

Colcher, D.; Carrasquillo, J.A.; Esteban, J.M.; Sugarbaker, P.; Reynolds, J.C.; Siler, K.; Bryant, G.; Larson, S.M. and Schlom, J.: Radiolabeled monoclonal antibody B72.3 localization in metastatic lesions of colorectal cancer patients. Nucl. med. Biol. 14: 251, 1987.

Colcher, D.; Esteban, J.M.; Carrasquillo, J.A.; Sugarbaker, P.; Reynolds, J.C.; Bryant, G.; Larson, S.M. and Schlom, J.: Quantitative analysis of selective radiolabeled monoclonal antibody localization in metastatic lesions of colorectal cancer patients. Cancer Res. 37: 1185, 1987.

Collart, M.A.; Belin, D.; Vassalli, J.D.; de Rosodo, S. and Vassalli, P.: Gamma interferon enhances macrophage transcription of the tumor necrosis factor/cachectin, interleukin-1 and urokinase genes which are controlled by short-lived repressors. J. Exp. Med. 164: 2113–2118, 1986.

Collée, J.M.; ten Kate, L.P.; de Vries, H.G.; Kliphuis, J.W.; Bouman, K.; Scheffer, H. and Gerritsen, J.: Allele sharing on chromosome 11q13 in sibs with asthma and atopy. Lancet 342: 936, 1993.

Coller, B.S.; Folts, J.D.; Smith, S.R.; Scudder, L.E. and Jordan, R.: Abolition of in vivo platelet thrombus formation in primates with monoclonal antibodies to the platelet GP11b/IIIa receptor. Correlation with bleeding time, platelet aggregation, and blockage of GPIIb/IIIa receptors. Circulation 80: 1766–1774, 1989.

Colombo, M.; Ferrari, G.; Stoppacciaro, A.; Parenza, M.; Rodolfo, M.; Mavilio, F. and Parmiani, G.: Granulocyte colony-stimulating factor gene transfer supresses tumorigenicity of a murine adeno carcinoma in vivo. J. Exp. Med. 173: 889–897, 1991.

Colombo, M.P. and Parmiani, G.: Tumor-cell-targeted cytokine gene therapy. Immunol. Today 12: 249–250, 1991.

Combe, N.; Cosso, B.; Clot, J.; Bonneau, M. and Sony, J.: Human placenta-cluted gammaglobulins in immunomodulating treatment of rheumatoid arthritis. Am. J. Med. 78: 920–928, 1985.

Concha, A.; Cabrera, T.; Ruiz-Cabello, F. and Garrido, F.: Can the HLA phenotype be used as a prognostic factor in breast carcinoma? Int. J. Cancer 6 (suppl.): 146–154, 1991.

Conley, M.E. and Delacroix, D.L.: Intravascular and mucosal immunoglobulin A: Two separate but related systems of immune defence? Ann. Intern. Med. 106: 892–899, 1987.

Conn, G.; Bayne, M.L.; Soderman, D.D.; Kwok, P.W.; Sullivan, K.A.; Palisi, T.M.; Hope, T.A. and Thomas, K.A.: Amino acid and cDNA sequences of a vascular endothelial cell mitogen that is homologous to platelet-derived growth factor. Proc. Natl. Acad. Sci. USA 87: 2628–2632, 1990.

Conn, G.; Sodermann, D.D.; Schaeffer, M.T.; Wile, M.; Hatcher, V.B. and Thomas, K.A.: Purification of a glycoprotein vascular endothelial cell mitogen from a rat glioma-derived cell line. Proc. Natl. Acad. Sci. USA 87: 1323–1327, 1990.

Connolly, D.T.; Heuvelman, D.M.; Nelson, R.; Olander, J.V.; Eppley, B.L.; Delfing, J.; Siegel, N.R.; Leimgruber, R. and Feder, J.: Tumor vascular permeability factor stimulates endothelial cell growth and angiogenesis. J. Clin. Invest. 84: 1478–1489, 1989.

Conrad, D.H.; Waldschmidt, T.J.; Lee, W.T.; Rao, M.; Keegan, A.D.; Noelle, R.J.; Lynch, R.G. and Kehry, M.R.: Effect of B cell stimulatory factor-1 (Interleukin-4) on Fc and Fcgamma receptor expression on murine B lymphocytes and B cell lines. J. Immun. 139: 2290–2296, 1987.

Conry, R.M.; LoBuglio, A.F.; Kantor, J.; Schlom, J.; Loechel, F.; Moore, S.E.; Sumerel, L.A.; Barlow, D.L.; Abrams, S. and Curiel, D.T.: Immune response to a carcinoembryonic antigen polynucleotide vaccine. Cancer Res. 54: 1164–1168, 1994.

Conti, P.; Barbacane R.C.; Panara, M.R.; Reale, M.; Placido, F.C.; Fridas, S.; Bongrazio, M. and Dempsey, R.A.: Human recombinant Interleukin-1 receptor antagonist (hrIL-1ra) enhances the stimulatory effect of Interleukin-2 on natural killer cell activity against Molt-4 target cells. Int. J. Immunopharmac. 14: 987–993, 1992.

Cookson, W.O.C.M.; Young, R.P.; Sandford, A.J.; Moffatt, M.F.; Shirakawa, T.; Sharp, P.A.; Faux, J.A.; Julier, C.; le Souef, P.N.; Nakamura, Y.; Lathrop, G.M. and Hopkin, J.M.: Maternal inheritance of atopic IgE responsiveness on chromosome 11q. Lancet 340: 381–384, 1992.

Cookson, W.O.C.M.: The genetics of asthma. In: Burr, M. The epidemiology of asthma. Monogr. Allergy. S. Karger and Co., Basel, 31: 171–189, 1993

Cookson, W.: Asthma - the impact of genetics. Gene Therapy - New Challenges for the Pharmaceutical Industry, London, September 15–16, 1994.

Cooper, J.A.; Bowen-Pope, D.F.; Raines, E.; Ross, R. and Hunter, T.: Similar effects of platelet-derived growth factor and epidermal growth factor on the phosphorylation of tyrosine in cellular proteins. Cell 31: 263, 1982.

Cooper, N.R.; Polley, M.J. and Oldstone, M.B.A.: Failure of terminal complement components to induce lysis of Moloney virus transformed lymphocytes. J. Immunol. 112: 866–868, 1974.

Cooper, N.R.; Bradt, B.N.; Rhim, J.S. and Menerow, G.R.: CR2 complement receptor. J. Invest. Dermatol. 94: 112–117, 1990.

Cordon-Cardo, C.; Fuks, Z.; Drobnjak, M.; Moreno, C.; Eisenbach, L. and Feldman, M.: Expression of HLA-A,B,C antigens on primary and metastatic tumor cell populations of human carcinomas. Cancer Res. 51: 6372–6380, 1991.

Corkill, M.M.; Kirkham, B.W., Haskard, D.O.; Barbatis, C.; Gibson, T. and Panayi, G.S.: Gold treatment of rheumatoid arthritis decreases synovial expression of the endothelial leukocyte adhesion receptor ELAM-1. J. Rheumatol. 1991, in press.

Corley, R.B.; Lund, F.E.; Randall, T.D.; King, L.B.; Doerre, S. and Woodland, D.L.: Mouse mammary tumor proviral gene expression in cells of the B lineage. Immunology 4: 287–296, 1992.

Cornacoff, J.B.; Hebert, L.A.; Smead, W.L.; VanAman, M.E.; Birmingham, D.J. and Waxman, F.J.: Primate erythrocyte-immune complex-clearing mechanism. J. Clin. Invest. 71: 236–247, 1983.

Cornell, R.P. and Schwartz, D.B.: Central administration of interleukin-1 elicits hyperinsulinemia in rats. Am. J. Physiol. 25: R772–R777, 1989.

Corvetta, A.; Della Bitta, R.; Gabrielli, A.; Spaeth, P.J. and Danieli, G.: Use of high-dose intravenous immunoglobulin in systemic lupus erythematosus: report of three cases. Clin. Exp. Rheumatol. 7: 295–299, 1989.

Cosimi, A.B.; Delmonico, F.L.; Kelly-Wright, J.; Wee, S.L.; Preffer, F.I.; Lolliffe, L.K. and Colvin, R.B.: Prolonged survival of nonhuman primate renal allograft recipients treated only with anti-CD4 monoclonal antibody. Surgery 180: 406, 1990.

Cotran, R.S.; Pober, J.S. Gibrone, M.A. jr.; Springer, T.A.; Wiebke, E.A.; Gaspari, A.A.; Rosenberg, S.A. and Lotze, M.T.: Endothelial activation during IL-2 immunotherapy: A possible mechanism for the vascular leak syndrome. J. Immunol. 140: 1883–1888, 1988.

Cotran, R.S. and Pober, J.S.: Endothelial activation: Its role in inflammatory and immune reactions, in Sinionescu, N.; Sinionescu, N. (eds): Endothelial cell Biology. New York, Plenum, 335–347, 1988.

Coulie, P. and Van Snick J.: Rheumatoid factors and secondary immune responses in the mouse. II. Incidence, kinetics and induction mechanisms. Euro. J. Immunol. 13: 895, 1983.

Coulie, P. and Van Snick, J.: Rheumatoid factor (RR) production during anamnestic immune response in the mouse. III. Activation of RF precursor cells is induced by their interaction with immune complexes and carrier-specific helper T cells. J. Exp. Med. 161: 88, 1985.

Coulie, P.; Weynants, P.; Muller, C.; Lehmann, F.; Herman, J.; Baurain, J.-F. and Boon, T.: Genes coding for antigens recognized on human tumors by autologous cytolytic T lymphocytes. Specific Immunotherapy Of Cancer With Vaccines, eds. Bystryn, J.-C.; Ferrone, S. and Livingston, P., The New York Academy of Sciences 690: 113, 1993.

Coutelier, J.-P.; Van der Logt, J.T.M.; Hessen, F.W.A.; Vink, A.; Warnier, G. and Van Snick J.: IgG2a restriction of murine antibodies elicited by viral infections. J. Exp. Med. 165: 64, 1987.

Coutelle, C.: Cystic fibrosis. Gene Therapy - New Challenges for the Pharmaceutical Industry, London, September 15–16, 1994.

Cox, G.J.M.; Zamb, T.J. and Babiuk, L.A.: Bovine herpes virus 1: immune responses in mice and cattle injected with plasmid DNA. J. Virol. 67: 5664–5667, 1993.

Cox, J.A.: Interactive properties of calmodulin. Biochem. J. 249: 612–629, 1988.

Crawford, R.M.; Finbloom, D.S.; O'Hara, J.; Paul, W.E. and Meltzer, M.S.: B cells stimulatory factor-1 (interleukin-4) activates macrophages for increased tumoricidal activity and expression of 1a antigens. J. Immunol. 139: 135–142, 1987.

Cross, M. and Dexter, T.M.: Growth factors in development, transformation, and tumorigenesis. Cell 64: 271–280, 1991.

Crum, R.; Szabo, S. and Folkman, J.: A new class of steroids inhibits angiogenesis in the presence of heparin or a heparin fragment. Science 230: 1375–1378, 1985.

Cunliffe, D.A. and Cox, K.O.: IgM-autoantibodies against autologous erythrocytes also react with isologous IgG (Fc). Nature 286: 720–722, 1980.

Curiel, D.T.; Agarwal, S.; Wagner, E. and Cotten, M.: Adenovirus enhancement of transferrin-polylysine-mediated gene delivery. Proc. Natl. Acad. Sci. USA 88: 8850–8854, 1991.

Curiel, D.T.: High-efficiency gene transfer mediated by adenovirus-polylysine-DNA complexes. Annals of the New York Academy of Sciences 716: 36, 1994.

Czech, M.P.: Signal transmission by the insulin-like growth factors. Cell 59: 235–238, 1989.

Czech, W.; Krutmann, J.; Budnik, A.; Kurrle, R.; Schöpf, E. and Kapp, A.: Expression of intercellular adhesion molecule 1 (ICAM-1) on normal human eosinophils - regulation by cytokines. Annual Meeting of the European Society for Dermatological Research, London (UK), April 4–7, 1992.

Daar, A.S.; Fuggle, S.V.; Fabre, J.W.; Ting, A. and Morris, P.J.: The detailed distribution of HLA-A,B,C antigens in normal human organs. Transplantation 38: 287–292, 1984.

Daddona, P.E.; Shewach, D.S.; Kelley, W.N.; Argos, P.; Markham, A.F. and Orkin, S.H.: Human adenosine deaminase: cDNA and complete primary amino acid sequence. J. Biol. Cehm. 259: 12101–12106, 1984.

Daeron, M.; Bonnerot, C.; Sandor, M.; Varin, N.; Hogarth, P.M.; Even, J. and Fridman, W.H.: Molecular mechanisms regulating the expression of murine T cell Fc gamma receptor II. Mol. Immunol. 25: 1143, 1988.

Daeron, M.; Bonnerot, C.; Latour S.; Benhamou, M. and Fridman W.H.: The murine αFc-gammaR gene product: identification, expression, and regulation. Mol. Immunol. 27: 1181, 1990.

Daha, M.R.; Miltenburg, A.M.M.; Hiemstra, P.S.; Klar-Mohamad, N.; Van Es, L.A. and Van Hisbergh, V.W.M.: The complement subcomponent C1q mediates binding of immune complexes and aggregates to endothelial cells in vitro. Eur. J. Immunol. 18: 783–787, 1988.

Daha, M.R.; Klar, N.; Hoekzema, R. and van Es, L.A.: Enhanced Ig production by human peripheral lymphocytes induced by aggregated C1q. J. Immunol. 144: 1227–1232, 1990.

Dalgleish, A.G.: Cancer Vaccines. Eur. J. Cancer 30A: 1029–1035, 1994.

Dalsgaard, C.-J.; Haultgardh-Nilsson, A.; Haegerstrand, A. and Nilsson, J.: Neuropeptides as growth factors. Possible roles in human diseases. Regul. Peptides 25: 1–9, 1989.

Damle, N.K.; Doyle, L.V.; Bender, J.R.; and Bradley, E.C.: Interleukin-2 activated human lymphocytes exhibit enhanced qadhesion to normal vascular endothelial cells and cause their lysis. J. Immunol. 138: 1779–1785, 1987.

Damle, N.K. and Doyle, L.V.: IL-2 activated human killer lymphocytes but not their secreted products mediate increase in albumin flux across cultured endothelial monolyers: Implications for vascular leak syndrome. J. Immunol. 142: 2660–2669, 1989.

Damle, N.K. and Doyle, L.V.: Distinct regulatory effects of IL-4 and TNFα during CD3–dependent and CD3–independent initiation of human T cell activation. Lymphokine Res. 8: 85–97, 1989.

Dang, N.H.; Torimoto, Y.; Deusch, K.; Schlossman, S.F. and Morimoto, C.: Comitogenic effect of solid-phase immobilized anti-1F7 on human CD4 T cell activation via CD3 and CD2 pathways. J. Immunol. 144: 4092–4100, 1990.

Dang, N.H.; Torimoto, Y.; Schlossman, S.F. and Moritomo, C.: Human CD4 helper T cell activation: Functional involvement of two distinct collagen receptors. 1F1 and VLA integrin family. J. Exp. Med. 172: 649–652, 1990.

D'Angeac, A.D.; Dornand, J.; Emonds-Alt, X.; Jullien, P.; Garcia-Sanz, J.E. and Erard, F.: Transforming growth factor type Beta 1 (TGF-ß1) down-regulates Interleukin-2 production and up-regulates Interleukin-2 receptor expression in a thymoma cell line. J. Cell. Physiol. 147: 460–469, 1991.

Dangl, J.L.; Wensel, T.G.; Morrison, S.L.; Stryer, L.; Herzenberg, L.A. and Oi, V.T.: Segmental flexibility and complement fixation of genetically engineered chimeric human rabbit and mouse antibodies. EMBO J. 7: 1989–1994, 1988.

Daniels, R.H.; Houston, W.A.; Petersen, M.M.; Williams, J.D.; Williams, B.D. and Morgan, B.P.: Stimulation of rheumatoid synovial cells by non-lethal complement membrane attack. Immunology 69: 237–242, 1990.

Daniels, R.H.; Williams, B.D. and Morgan, B.P.: Human rheumatoid synovial cell stimulation by the membrane attack complex and other pore-forming toxins in vitro; the role of calcium in cell activation. Immunology 71: 312–316, 1990.

Daniels, R.H.; Willimans, B.D. and Morgan, B.P.: Non-lethal complement membrane attack on cultured synovial cells induces G-protein and calcium-dependent PGE2 release and release of IL-6. Compl. Inflamm. 7: 137 (abstract), 1990.

Danscombe, M.J.; LeFeuvre, R.A.; Sagay, B.O.; Rothwell, N.J. and Stock, M.J.: Pyrogenic and thermogenic effects of interleukin-1 beta in the rat. Am J. Physiol. 256: E7–E11, 1989.

Da Prada, M.; Richards, J.G. and Kettler, R.: Amine storage organelles in platelets. In: Gordon, J.L. (ed.) Platelets in Biology and Pathology-2, Elsevier/North Holland Biomedical Press, Amsterdam, 107–145, 1981.

Darrow, T.L.; Slingluff, C.L. and Seigler, H.F.: The role of HLA class I antigens in recognition of melanoma cells by tumor-specific cytotoxic T lymphocyts: evidence for shared tumor antigens. J. Immunol. 142: 3329–3335, 1989.

Davidson, J. et al., 1991: cited by Tuffin, D.P., 1992.

Davies, A.G.; Simmons, D.L.; Hale, G.; Harrison, R.A.; Tighe, H. and Lachmann, P.J.: CD59, a Ly-9 like protein expressed in human lymphoid cells, regulates the action of the complement membrane attack complex on homologous cells. J. Exp. Med. 170: 637, 1989.

Davignon, D.; Martz, E.; Reynolds, T.; Kurzinger, K. and Springer T.A.: Lymphocyte function-associated antigen 1 (LFA-1): A surface antigen distinct from Lyt-2.3 that participates in T lymphocyte-mediated killing. Proc. Natl. Acad. Sci. USA 78: 4535–4539, 1981.

Davis, A.E. and Kenny, D.M.: Properdin factor D: effects on thrombin-induced platelet aggregation. J. Clin. Invest. 64: 721–728, 1979.

Davis, A.E. and Lachmann, P.J.: Bovine conglutinin is a collagen-like protein. Biochemistry 23: 2139–2144, 1984.

Davis, F.M.; Gossett, L.A.; Pinkston, K.L.; Liou, R.S.; Sun, L.K.; Kim, Y.W.; Chang, N.T.; Chang, T.W.; Wagner, K.; Bews, J.; Brinkmann, V.; Towbin, H.; Subramanian, N. and Heusser, C.: Can anti-IgE be used to treat allergy? Springer Semi Immunopathol. 15: 51–73, 1993.

Davis, J.M.; Meyer, J.D.; Barie, P.S.; Yurt, R.W.; Duhaney, R.; Dineen, P. and Shires, G.T.: Elevated production of neutrophil leukotriene B4 preceeds pulmonary failure in critically ill surgical patients. Surgery 170: 495–500, 1990.

Davis, S.; Aldrich, T.H.; Valenzuela, D.M.; Wong, V.V.; Furth, M.E.; Squinto, S.P. and Yancopoulos, G.D.: The receptor for ciliary neurotrophic factor. Science 253: 59–63, 1991.

Davitz, M.A.; Low, M.G. and Nussenzweig, V.: Release of decay-accelerating factor (DAF) from the cell membrane by phosphatidylinositol-specific phospholipase C (PIPLC): selective modification of a complement regulatory protein. J. Exp. Med. 163: 1150–1161, 1986.

Dean, J.H.; Cornacoff, J.B.; Barbolt, T.H.; Gossett, K.A. and LaBrie, T.: Pre-clinical toxicity of IL-4: A model for studying protein therapeutics. Int. J. Immunopharm. 14: 391–397, 1992.

Deb, S.; Jackson, C.T.; Subler, M.A. and Martin, D.W.: Modulation of cellular and viral promoters by mutant human p53 proteins found in cancer cells. J. Virol. 66: 6164–6170, 1992.

Debatin, K.M.; Goldmann, C.K.; Bamford, R.; Waldmann, T.A. and Krammer, P.H.: Monoclonal-antibody-mediated apoptosis in adult T-cell leukaemia. Lancet 335: 497–500, 1990.

Debré, M.; Bonnet, M.-C.; Fridman, W.-H.; Carosella, E.; Philippe, N.; Reinert, P.; Vilmer, E.; Kaplan, C.; Teillaud, J.-L. and Gruscelli, C.: Infusion of Fc gamma fragments for treatment of children with acute immune thrombocytopenic purpura. The Lancet 342: 945, 1993.

Dechanet, J.; Merville, P.; Miossec, P. and Banchereau, J.: Differentiation of human B lymphocytes into plasma cells. ENII Conf.: Integrated Function of Molecules of the Immune System. Les Embiez, France, 12th-16th May 1993.

Defize, L.H. and de Laat, S.W.: Structural and functional aspects of epidermal growth factor (EGF) and its receptor. Progress in Brain Research 69: 169–182, 1986.

DeForge, L.E.; Fantone, J.C.; Kenney, J.S. and Remick, D.G.: Oxygen radical scavengers selectively inhibit interleukin 8 in human whole blood. J. Clin. Invest. 90: 2123–2129, 1992.

Defrance, T.; Aubry, J.P.; Rousset, F.; Vanbervliet, B.; Bonnefoy, J.Y.; Arai, N.; Takebe, T.; Yokota, Y.; Lee, F.; Arai, K.; de Vries, J.E. and Banchereau, J.: Human recombinant Il-4 induces Fc receptors (CD23) on normal human B lymphocytes. J. Exp. Med. 165: 1459–1467, 1987.

Defrance, T.; Vanbervliet, B.; Aubry, J.P.; Takebe, Y,; Arai, N.; Miyajima, A.; Yokota, T.; Lee, T.; Arai, K.; de Vries, J.E. and Banchereau, J.: B cell growth promoting activity of recombinant human IL-4. J. Immunol. 139: 1135–1141, 1987.

Defrance, T.; Vanbervliet, B.; Aubry, J.P. and Banchereau, J.: Interleukin 4 inhibits the proliferation but not the differentiation of activated human B cells in response to IL-2. J. Exp. Med. 168: 1321–1337, 1988.

Defrance, T.; Vanbervliet, B.; Durand, I. and Banchereau, J.: Human IL-4 down-regulated the surface expression of CD5 on normal and leukemic B cells. Eur. J. Immunl. 19: 293–299, 1989.

Defreyn, G.; Deckmyn, H. and Vermylen, J.: A thromboxane synthetase inhibitor reorients endoperoxide metabolism in whole blood towards prostacyclin and prostaglandin E2. Thromb. Res. 26: 289–400, 1982.

DeKruyff, R.; Ju, S.; Laning, J.; Cantor, H. and Dorf, M.: Activation requirements of cloned inducer T cells. III. Need for two stimulator cells in the response of a cloned line to Mls determinants. J. Immunol. 137: 1109–1114, 1986.

DeKruyff, R.H.; Turner, T.; Abrams, J.S.; Palladino, M.A.jr. and Umetsu, D.T.: Induction of human IgE synthesis by CD4+ T cell clones. Requirement for interleukin 4 and low molecular weight B cell growth factor. J. Exp. Med. 170: 1477–1493, 1989.

Delacroix, D.L. and Vaerman, J.P.: Function of the human liver in IgA homeostasis in plasma. Ann. N.Y. Acad. Sci. 409: 383–401, 1983.

Delespesse, G.; Hofstetter, H. and Sarfati, M.: Low-affinity receptor for IgE (FcERIL.CD23) and its soluble fragments. Int. Arch. Allergy Appl. Immunol. 90: 41–44, 1989.

Delespesse, G.; Sarfati, M. and Peleman, R.: Influence of recombinant Il-4, IFN-alpha, and IFN-gamma on the production of human IgE-binding factor (soluble CD23). J. Immunol. 142: 134–138, 1989.

Delespesse, G.; Sarfati, M. and Hofstetter, H.: Human IgE-binding factors. Immunol. Today 10: 159, 1989.

Delli-Bovi, P.; Duratola, A.M.: Kern, F.G.; Greco, A.; Ittmann, M. and Basilico, C.: An oncogene isolated by transfection of Kaposi's sarcoma DNA encodes a growth factor that is a member of the FGF family. Cell 50: 729–737, 1987.

Delmonico, F.; Knowles, R.; Colvin, R.; Cavender, D.; Kawai, T.; Bedle, M.; Stroka, D.; Preffer, F.; Haug, C. and Cosimi, A.B.: Immunosuppression of cynomolgus renal allograft recipients with humanized IKT4A monoclonal antibodies (abstr.). Int. Congr. Transplantation, 1992.

Del Prete, G-F.; Tiri, A.; De Carli, M.; Mariotti, S.; Pinchera, A.; Chretien, I.; Romagnani, S. and Ricci, M.: High potential to tumor necrosis factor-μ (TNF-μ) production of thyroid-infiltrating T lymphocytes in Hashimoto's thyroiditis: a preculiar feature of destructive thyroid autoimmunity. Autoimmunity 4: 267, 1989.

Del Prete, G-F.; Tiri, A.; Maggi, E.; De Carli, M.; Macchia, D.; Parronchi, P.; Rossi, M.E.; Pietrogrande, M.C.; Ricci, M. and Romagnani, S.: Defective in vitro production of gamma-interferon and tumor necrosis factor-alpha by circulating T cells from patients with hyper-immunoglobulin E syndrome. J. Clin. Invest. 84: 1830–1835, 1989.

Del Prete, G.V.; Maggi, E.; Parronchi, P.; Chrétien, I.; Tiri, A.; Macchia, D.; Ricci, M.; Banchereau, J.; de Vries, J.E. and Romagnani, S.: IL-4 is an essential factor for the IgE synthesis induced in vitro by human T cell clones and their supernatants. J. Immunol. 140: 4193–4198, 1988.

DeMars, R.; Rudersdorf, R.; Chang, C.C.; Petersen, J.; Strandtmann, J.; Korn, N.; Sidwell, B. and Orr, H.T.: Mutations that impair a posttranscriptional step in expression of HLA-A and – B antigens. Proc. Natl. Acad. Sciences USA 82: 8183–8187, 1985.

DeNardo, S.J.; Warhoe, K.E.; O'Grady, L.F.; Gobuty, A.H.; Macey, D.J.; Hellstrom, I.; Hellstrom, K.E.; Kroger, L.E. and DeNardo, G.L.: Radioimmunotherapy in patients with metastatic breast cancer. 8th Int. Hammersmith Meeting, Greece, 1991.

Denhardt, D.T.; Greenberg, A.H.; Egan, S.E.; Hamilton, R.T.; Wright, R.T. and Wright, J.A.: Cysteine proteinase cathepsin L expression correlates closely with the metastatic potential of H-ras transformed murine fibroblasts. Oncogene 2: 55–59, 1987.

Denis, O.; Latinne, D.; Nisol, F. and Bazin, H.: Resting B cells can act as antigen presenting cells in vivo and induce antibody responses. Int. Immunol. 5: 71–78, 1993.

Denorory, M.C.; Yodoi, J. and Banchereau, J.: Interleukin 4 and interferons alpha and gamma regulate Fc epsilon R2 CD23 mRNA expression on normal human B cells. Mol. Immunol. 27: 129–134, 1990.

D'Ercole, A.J.; Stiles, A.D. and Underwood, L.E.: Tissue concentrations of somatomedin C: further evidence for multiple sites of synthesis and paracrine or autocrine mechanisms of action. Proc. Natl. Acad. Sci. 81: 935, 1984.

Derynck, R.; Goeddel, D.V.; Ullrich, A.; Gutterman, J.U.; Williams, R.D.; Bringman, T.S. and Berger, W.H.: Synthesis of messenger RNAs for transforming growth factors α and β and the epidermal growth factor receptor by human tumors. Cancer Res. 47: 707–712, 1987.

de Sauvage, F.J.; Hass, P.E.; Spencer, S.D.; Malloy, B.E.; Gurney, A.L.; Spencer, S.A.; Darbonne, W.C.; Henzel, W.J.; Wong, S.C.; Kunag, W-J.; Oles, K.J.; Hultgren, B.; Solberg, L.A.; Goeddel, D.V. and Eaton, D.L.: Stimulation of megakaryocytopoiesis and thrombopoiesis by the c-Mpl ligand. Nature 369: 533, 1994.

De Souza, E.B.; Webster, E.L.; Grigoriadis, D.E. and Tracey, D.E.: Corticotropin-releasing factor (CRF) and interleukin-1 (Il-1) receptors in the brain-pituitary-immune axis. Psychopharmacol. Bill. 25: 299–305, 1989.

De Souza, E.B.: Corticotropin-releasing factor and interleukin-1 receptors in the brain-endocrine-immune axis. Role in stress response and infection. Annals of the New York Academy of Sciences 697: 9, 1993.

Desreumaux, P.; Janin, A.; Colombel, J.F.; Prin, L.; Plumas, J.; Emilie, D.; Torpier, G.; Capron, A. and Capron, M.: Interleukin 5 messenger RNA expression by eosinophils in the intestinal mucosa of patients with coeliac disease. J. Exp. Med. 175: 293–296, 1992.

Deuel, T.F.; Senior, R.M.; Chang, D.; Griffin, G.L.; Heinrickson, R.L. and Kaiser, E.T.: Platelet factor 4 is chemotactic for neutrophils and monocytes. Proc. Natl. Acad. Sci. USA 78: 4584–4587, 1981.

Deuel, T.F.; Senior, R.M.; Huang, J.S. and Griffin, G.L.: Chemotaxis of monocytes and neutrophils to platelet-derived growth factor. J. Clin. Invest. 69: 1046–1049, 1982.

Deverson, E.V.; Gow, J.R.; Coadwell, W.J.; Monaco, J.J.; Butcher, G.W. and Howard, J.C.: MHC class II region encoding proteins related to the multidrug resistance family of transmembrane transporters. Nature 348: 738–741, 1990.

Devine, D.V.; Siegel, R.S. and Rosse, W.F.: Interactions of the platelets in paroxysmal nocturnal hemoglobinuria with complement. J. Clin. Invest. 79: 131–137, 1987.

Devine, D.V. and Rosse, W.F.: Regulation of the activity of platelet-bound C3 convertase of the alternative pathway of complement by platelet factor H. Proc. Natl. Acad. Scu. USA 84: 5873–5877, 1987.

Devine, D.V. and Kovacs, R.: Characterization of the C3dg receptor of human platelets. Compl. Inflamm. 6: 355, 1989.

Devine, D.V.: The effects of complement activation on platelets. Current Topics in Microbiology and Immunology 178, 1992.

Devos, R.; Plaetinck, G.; Van der Heyden, J.; Cornelis, S.; Vandekerckhove, J.; Fiers, W. and Tavernier, J.: Molecular basis of a high affinity murine interleukin-5 receptor. EMBO J. 10: 2133–2137, 1991.

de Vries, J.E.; Gauchat, J-F.; Aversa, G.G.; Punnonen, J.; Gascan, H. and Yssel, H.: Regulation of IgE synthesis by cyotkines. Curr. Op. Immunol. 3: 851–858, 1991.

de Waal, M.R.; Abrams, J.; Bennet, B.; Figdor, C. and de Vries, J.E.: Il-10 inhibits cytokine synthesis by human monocytes: an autoregulatory role of Il-10 produced by monocytes. J. Exp. Med. 174: 1209–1220, 1991.

de Waal, M.R.; Mihara, N.; Gauchat, J-F.; Johnson, K.; Kastelein, R. and de Vries, J.E.: IL-10 and viral IL-10 (v-IL-10) inhibit IL-4 induced IgE synthesis in the induction phase. Schweizerische Medizinische Wochenschrift 121 (suppl. 40/1) 60, 1991.

de Waal Melafyt, R.; Haanen, J.; Spits, H.; Roncarlo, M.G:; te Velde, A.; Figdor, C.; Johnson, K.; Kastelein, R.; Yssel, H. and de Vries, J.E.: Interleukin 10 (Il-10) and viral Il-10 strongly reduce antigen-specific human T cell proliferation by diminishing the antigen-presenting capacity of monocytes via downregulation of class II major histocompatibility complex expression. J. Exp. Med. 174: 915–924, 1991.

Dhar, R. and Ogra P.L.: Local immune responses. Br. Med. Bull. 41: 28–33, 1985.

Dickneite, G.; Walter, P.; Schorlemmer, H.U. and Sedlacek, H.H.: The immunosuppressive properties of 15–Deoxyspergualin and its effects on experimental skin and islet cell transplantation. In: Ishigami, J. (ed.): Recent advances in chemotherapy: Anticancer Section. University of Tokyo Press 949–950, 1986.

Dickneite, G.; Schorlemmer, H.U.; Walter, P. and Sedlacek, H.H.: Graft survival in experimental transplantation could be prolonged by the action of the antitumoral drug 15–Deoxyspergualin. Transplant. Proc. 18: 1295–1296, 1986.

Dickneite, G.; Schorlemmer, H.U.; Sedlacek, H.H.; Falk, W.; Ulrichs, K. and Müller-Ruchholtz, W.: Suppression of macrophage function and prolongation of graft survival by the new guanidinic-like structure, 15–Deoxyspergualin. Transplant. Proc. 19: 1301–1304, 1987.

Dickneite, G.; Schorlemmer, H.U. and Sedlacek, H.H.: Decrease of mononuclear phagocyte cell functions and prolongation of graft survival in experimental transplantation by (±)-15-Deoxyspergualin. Int. J. Immunopharmac. 9: 559–565, 1987.

Dickneite, G.; Schorlemmer, H.U.; Weinmann, E.; Bartlett, R.R. and Sedlacek, H.H.: Skin transplantation in rats and monkeys: evaluation of efficient treatment with 15-Deoxyspergualin. Transplant. Proc. 19: 4244–4247, 1987.

Dickneite, G.: Effects of combination of antithrombin III and HWA 138 in endotoxic shock (mouse). In: Hakim, J.; Mandell, G.L. and Novick, W.J. (ed.): Effects of Leukocyte Function; Karger, Basel, 1990.

Dickneite, G. and Pâques, E.P.: Reduction of mortality with antithrombin III in septicemic rats: A study of Klebsiella pneumoniae induced sepsis. Thromb. Haemost. 69: 98–102, 1993.

Dickson, C.; Smith, R.; Brookes, S. and Peters, G.: Proviral insertions within the int-2 can generate multiple anomalous transcripts but leave the protein-coding domain intact. J. Virol 64: 784–793, 1990.

Dickson, G. and Dunckley, M.: Human dystrophin gene transfer: genetic correction of dystrophin deficiency. In Partridge, T.A. (ed.), Molecular and Cell Biology of Muscular Dystrophy, London: Chapman and Hall, 283–302, 1993.

Dierich, M.P.; Schulz, T.F.; Eigentler, A.; Huemer, H. and Schwäble, W.: Structural and functional relationships among receptors and regulators of the complement system. Molec. Immunol. 25: 1043–1051, 1988.

Dierich, M.P.; Ebenbichler, C.F.; Marschang, P.; Füst, G.; Thielens, N.M. and Arlaud, G.J.: HIV and human complement: mechanisms of interaction and biological implication. Immunology Today 14: 435, 1993.

Dighiero, G.; Guilbert, B. and Avrameas, S.: Naturally occurring antibodies against nine common antigens in human sera. II. High incidence of monoclonal Ig exhibiting antibody activity against actin and tubulin and sharing antibody specificities with natural antibodies. J. Immun. 128: 2788–2797, 1982.

diGiovine, F. and Duff, G.W.: Interleukin 1: the first interleukin. Immunol. Today 11: 13, 1990.

Dillman, R.O.; Beauregard, J.; Ryan, K.P.; Hagan, P.L.; Clutter, M.; Amor, D.; Fricke, J.M.; Bartholomew, R.M.; Burnett, K.G.; Davis, G.S. et al.: Radioimmunodetection of cancer with the use of indium 111I-labeled monoclonal antibodies. NCI Monogr. 3: 33–36, 1987.

Dinarello, C.A. and Wolf, S.M.: Molecular basis of fever in humans. Am. J. Med. 72: 779–783, 1982.

Dinarello, C.A.: Biology of interleukin 1. FASEB J. 2: 108–115, 1988.

Dinerman, J.L. and Mehta, J.L.: Endothelial, platelet and leukocyte interactions in ischemic heart disease: insights into potential mechanisms and their clinical relevance. J. Am. Coll. Cardiol. 16: 207–222, 1990.

Dionne, C.A.; Crumley, G.; Bellot, F.; Kaplow, J.M.; Searfoss, G.; Ruta, M.; Burgess, W.H.; Jaye, M. and Schlessinger, J.: Cloning and expression of two distinct high-affinity receptors cross-reacting with acidic and basic fibroblast growth factors. EMBO J. 9: 2685–2692, 1990.

DiPersio, J.; Billing, P.; Kaufman, S.; Eghtesady, P.; Williams, R.E. and Gasson, J.C.: Characterization of the human granulocyte-macrophage colony-stimulating factor receptor J. Biol. Chem. 263: 1834, 1988.

Dippold, W.G.; Lloyd, K.O.; Li, L.T.C.; Ikeda, H.; Oettgen, H.F. and Old, L.J.: Cell surface antigens of human malignant melanoma: Definition of six antigenic systems with mouse monoclonal antibodies. Proc. Natl. Acad. Sci. USA 77: 6114–6118, 1980.

Djuric S.W.; Fretland D.J. and Penning T.D.: The leukotriene B4 receptor antagonists – A most discriminating class of antiinflammatory agent? Drugs of the Future 17: 819–830, 1992.

Dobson, D.E.; Kambe, A.; Block, E.; Dion, T.; Lu, H.; Castellot J.J.jr. and Speigelman, B.M.: 1–Butyryl-glycerol: A novel angiogenesis factor secreted by differentiating adipocytes. Cell 61: 223–230, 1961.

Docherty, A.J.P.; Lyons, A.; Smith, B.J.; Wright, E.M.; Stephens, P.E.; Harris, T.J.; Murphy, G. and Reynolds, J.J.: Sequence of human tissue inhibitor of metalloproteinases and its identity to erythroid-potentiating activity. Nature 318: 66–69, 1985.

Dohlsten, M.; Sjögren, H.O. and Carlsson, R.: Histamine acts directly on human T cells to inhibit interleukin-2 and interferon-gamma production. Cell Immunol. 109: 65, 1987.

Dohlsten, M.; Hedlung, G.; Fischer, H.; Sjögren, H.O. and Carlsson, R.: Proliferation of human CD4+45R+ and CD+45R- T helper cells is promoted by both Il-2 and Il-4 while interferon-gamma production is restricted to Il-2 activated CD4+45R- T cells. Immunol. Lett 20: 29, 1989.

Donehower, L.A.; Harvey, M.; Slagle, B.L.; McArthur, M.J.; Montgomery, C.A.; Beutel, J.S. and Bradley, A.: Mice deficient for p53 are developmentally normal but susceptible to spontaneous tumours. Nature 356: 215–221, 1992.

Donnelly, J.J.; Ulmer, J.B. and Liu, M.A.: Immunization with polynucleotides. The Immunologist 2: 20, 1994.

Donnelly, R.P.; Fenton, M.J.; Kaufmann, J.D. and Gerrard, T.L.: Il-1 expression in human monocytes is transcriptionally and posttranscriptionally regulated by Il-4. J. Immunol. 146: 3431, 1991.

Dorr, R.T.: Interferon-alpha in malignant and viral diseases. Drugs 45: 177–211, 1993.

Dow, C.A.; De-Aizpurua, H.J.; Pedersen, J.S.; Ungar, B. and Toh, B.H.: 65–70 kD protein identified by immunoblotting as the presumptive gastric microsomal autoantigen in pernicious anemia. Clin. exp. Immun. 62: 732–737, 1985.

Dower, S.K. and Urdal, D.L.: The interleukin-1 receptor. Immunology Today 8: 46–51, 1987.

Dower, S.K.; Wignall, J.M.; Schooley, K.; McMahan, C.J.; Jackson, J.L.; Prickett, K.S.; Lupton, S.; Cosman, D. and Sims, J.E.: Retention of ligand binding activity by the extracellular domain of the IL-1 receptor. J. Immun. 142: 4314–4320, 1989.

Downward, J.; Yarden, Y.; Mayes, E.; Scrace, G.; Totty, N.; Stockwell, P.; Ullrich, A.; Schlessinger, J. and Waterfield, M.D.: Close similarity of epidermal growth factor receptor and v-erb-B oncogene protein sequences. Nature 307: 521–527, 1984.

Doyle, C. and Strominger, J.L.: Interaction between CD4 and class II MHC molecules mediates cell adhesion. Nature 330: 256, 1987.

Drachman, D.B.; Adams, R.N.; Josifek, L.F. and Self, S.G.: Functional activities of autoantibodies to acetylcholine receptors and the clinical severity of myasthenia gravis. New. Engl. J. Med. 307: 769–775, 1982.

Dranoff, G.; Jaffee, E.; Lazenby, A.; Golumbek, P.; Levitsky, H.; Brose, K.; Jackson, V.; Hamada, H.; Pardoll, D. and Mulligan, R.C.: Vaccination with irradiated tumor cells engineered to secrete murine granulocyte-macrophage colony-stimulating factor stimulates potent, specific, and long-lasting anti-tumor immunity. Proc. Natl. Acad. Sci. USA 90: 3539–3543, 1993.

Drickamer, K.; Dordal, M.S. and Reynolds, L.: Mannose-binding proteins isolated from rat liver contain carbohydrate-recognition domains linked to collagenous tails. Complete primary structures and homology with pulmonary surfactant apoprotein. J. Biol. Chem. 261: 6878–6887, 1986.

Droller, M.; Lindgren, J.-A.; Claesson, H.-E. and Perlmann, P.: Production of prostaglandin E2 by bladder tumor cells in tissue culture and a possible mechanism of lymphocyte inhibition. Cell. Immun. 47: 261–273, 1979.

Dube, S.; Fisher, J.W. and Powell, J.S.: Glycosylation at specific sites of erythropoietin is essential for biosynthesis, secretion, and biological function. J. Biol. Chem. 263: 17516–17521, 1988.

Duff, G.: Cytokines as mediator of immunopathology. Rheumatoid Arthritis, Royal College of Physicians, London, 17./18.6.1991.

Dugas, B.; Renauld, J.C.; Pene, J.; Bonnefoy, J.Y.; Peti-Frere, C.; Braquet, P.; Bousquet, J.; Van Snick, J. and Mencia-Huerta, J.M.: Interleukin-9 potentiates the interleukin-4–induced immunoglobulin (IgG, IgM and IgE) production by normal human B lymphocytes. Eur. J. Immunol. 23: 1687–1692, 1993.

Dumont, F.J.; Staruch, M.J.; Koprak, S.L.; Melino, M.R. and Sigal, N.H.: Distinct mechanisms of suppression of murine T cell activation by the related macrolides FK-506 and rapamycin. J. Immunol. 144: 251–258, 1990.

Dunkley, M.L. and Husband, A.J.: The induction and migration of antigen-specific helper cells for IgA responses in the intestine. Immunol. 57: 379–385, 1983.

Dunlop, D.J. and Steward, W.P.: Recombinant human granulocyte macrophage colony-stimulating factor: current status of clinical trials and potential future applications. Anti-Cancer Drugs 2, 327–337, 1991.

Durrant, L.G.; Denton, G.W.L. and Robins, R.A.: Immunization with human monoclonal anti-idiotypic antibody in colorectal cancer. Specific Immunotherapy Of Cancer With Vaccines, eds. Bystryn, J.-C.; Ferrone, S. and Livingston, P., The New York Academy of Science 690: 334, 1993.

D'Urso, C.M.; Wang, Z.; Cao, Y.; Takate, R.; Zeff, R.A. and Ferrone, S.: Lack of HLA class I antigen expression by cultured melanoma cells FO-1 due to a defect in ß2m gene expression. J. Clin. Invest. 87: 284–292, 1991.

Duse, M.; Tiberti, S.; Plebani, A.; Avanzini, M.A.; Gardenghi, M.; Menegati, E.; Monafo, V. and Ugazio, A.G.: IgG2 deficiency and intractable epilepsy of childhood. Monogr. Allergy 20: 128–134, 1986.

Duvall, E.; Wyllie, A.H. and Morris, R.G.: Macrophage recognition of cells undergoing programmed cell death. Immunology 56: 351–358, 1985.

Dvorak, H.F.; Nagy, J.A. and Dvorak, A.M.: Structure of solid tumors and their vasculature: implications for therapy with monoclonal antibodies. Cancer Cells 3: 77–85, 1991.

Dyke, R.J.; McBride, H.; George, A.J.T.; Hamblin, T.J. and Stevenson, F.K.: Idiotypic vaccination against B-cell lymphoma leads to dormant tumor. Cell Immunol. 132: 70–83, 1991.

Dykman, T.R.; Cole, J.L.; Iida, K. and Atkinson, J.P.: Polymorphism of human erythrocyte C3b/C4b receptor. Proc. Natl. Acad. Sci. USA 80: 1698–1702, 1983.

Dykman, T.R.; Hatch, J.A. and Atkinson, J.P.: Polymorphism of the human C3b/C4b receptor. Identification of a third allele and analysis of receptor phenotypes in families and patients with systemic lupus erythematosus. J. Exp. Med. 159: 691–703, 1984.

Dykman, T.R.; Hatch, J.A.; Aqua, M.S. and Atkinson, J.P.: Polymorphism of the C3b/C4b receptor (CR1): characterization of a fourth allele. J. Immunol. 134: 1787–1789, 1985.

Eaton, D.L. and Baker J.B.: Phorbol esters and mitogens stimulate human fibroblast secretions of plasmin-activatable plasminogen activator and protease nexin, an antiactivator/antiplasmin. J. Cell Biol. 97: 323–328, 1983.

Eaton, M.A.W.; Alexander, R.P. and Pratt, A.J.: Immunoconjugates and prodrugs and their use in association for drug delivery. IPN WO 90/11782, 1990.

Echenne, B.; Dulac, O.; Parayre-Chanaz, M.J.; Chiron, C.; Taillebois, L.; Cognot, C.; Andary, M.; Clot, J. and Baldy-Moulinier, M.: Treatment of infantile spasms with intravenous gamma-globulins. Brain and Development 13: 5, 1991.

Echtenacher, B.; Falk, W.; Mannel, D.N. and Krammer, P.H.: Requirement of endogenous tumor necrosis factor/cachectin for recovery from experimental peritonitis. J. Immunol. 145: 3762, 1990.

Ehlers, S. and Smith, K.A.: Differentiation of T cell lymphokine gene expression. The in vitro acquisition on T cell memory. J. Exp. Med. 173: 25–36, 1991.

Ehrlich, P.: A general review of the recent work in immunity; in Collected papers of Paul Ehrlich, vol. 2: Immunology and cancer research, 442, Pergamon Press, London, 1956.

Eilat, D.; Steinberg, A.D. and Schechter, A.N.: The reaction of SLE antibodies with native, single-stranded RNA: radioassay and binding specificities. J. Immun. 120: 550–557, 1978.

Elliott, B.E.; Carlow, D.A.; Rodrick, A-M. and Wade, A.: Perspectives on the role of MHC antigens in normal and malignant cell development. Advances in Cancer Res. 53: 181, 1989.

Emilie, D.; Touitou, R.; Raphael, M.; Peuchmaur, M.; Devergnee, O.; Rea, D.; Coumbraras, J.; Crevon, M.-C.; Edelman, L.; Joab, I. and Galanaud, P.: In vivo production of interleukin-10 by malignant cells in AIDS lymphomas. Eur. J. Immunol. 22: 2937–2942, 1992.

Emonard, H.P.; Remacle, A.G.; Noel, A.C.; Grimaud, J.A.; Stetler-Stevenson, W.G. and Foidart, J.M.: Tumor cell surface-associated receptor for the Mr 72,000 type IV collagenase. Cancer Res. 52: 5845–5848, 1992.

Emslie-Smith, A.M.; Arahata, K. and Engel, A.G.: Major histocompatibility complex class I antigen expression, immunolocalization of interferon subtypes, and T cell-mediated cytotoxicity in myopathies. Human Immunol. 20: 224–231, 1989.

Endo, T. and Kobata, A.: Structure and function of the carbohydrate chains of immunoglobulin G. Mod. Media 32: 432–433, 1989.

Endo, T.; Kochibe, N. and Kobata, A.: Structural study of the carbohydrate moieties of two human immunoglobulin subclasses (IgG2 and IgG4). Glycoconjugate J. 6: 57–67, 1989.

Endres, S.; Fuller, H.J.; Sinha, B.; Stoll, D.; Dinarello, C.A.; Gerzer, R. and Weber, P.C.: Cyclic nucleotides differentially regulate the synthesis of tumor necrosis factor α and interleukin-1β by human mononuclear cells. Immunology 172: 56–60, 1991.

Engerman, R.L.; Pfaffenbach, D. and David, M.D.: Cell turnover of capillaries. Lab. Invest. 17: 738, 1967.

Engler, R.: Consequences of activation and adenosine-mediated inhibtion of granulocytes during myocardial ischemia. Fed. Proc. 46: 2407–2412, 1987.

Epenetos, A.A.; Carr, D.; Johnson, P.M.; Bodmer, W.F. and Lavender, J.P.: Antibody-guided radiolocalisation of tumor in patients with testicular or ovarian cancer using two radioiodinated monoclonal antibodies to placental alkaline phosphatase. Br. J. Radiol. 59: 117, 1986.

Erdei, A. and Reid, K.B.M.: The C1q receptor. Mol. Immunol. 25: 1067–1073, 1988.

Ermak, T.H.; Steger, H.J. and Pappo, J.: Phenotypically distinct subpopulations of T cells in domes and M-cell pockets of rabbit gut-associated lymphoid tissues. Immunol. 71: 530–537, 1990.

Ernsberger, U.; Sendtner, M. and Rohrer, H.: Proliferation and differentiation of embryonic chick sympathetic neurons: effects of ciliary neurotrophic factor. Neuron 2: 1275–1284, 1989.

Esch, F.; Baird, A.; Ling, N.; Ueno, N.; Hill, F.; Denoroy, L.; Klepper, R.; Gospodarowicz, D.; Boehlen, P. and Guillemin, R.: Primary structure of bovine pituitary basic fibroblast growth factor (FGF) and comparison with the amino-terminal sequence of bovine brain acidic FGF. Proc. Natl. Acad. Sci USA 82: 6507–6511, 1985.

Esch, F.; Ueno, N.; Baird, A.; Hill, F.; Denoroy, I.; Ling, N.; Gospodarowicz, R. and Guillemin, R.: Primary structure of bovine brain acidic fibroblast growth factor (FGF). Biochem. Biophys. Res. Commun. 133: 554–562, 1985.

Eskandari, M.K.; Bolgos, G.; Miller, C.; Nguyen, D.T.; DeForge, L.E. and Remick, D.G.: Antitumor necrosis factor antibody therapy fails to prevent lethality after cecal ligation and puncture or endotoxemia. J. Immunol. 148: 2724–2730, 1992.

Espada, J.: Langton, A.A. and Dorado, M.: Human erythropoietin: studies on purity and partial characterization. Biochim. Biophys. Acta. 285: 427–435, 1972.

Essner, R.; Rhoades, K.; McBride W.H.; Morton, D.L. and Economou, J.S.: IL-4 down-regulates IL-1 and TNF gene expression in human monocytes. J. Immunol. 142: 3857–3861, 1989.

Estin, C.D.; Stevenson, U.S.; Plowman, G.D.; Hu, S.L.; Sridhar, P.; Hellström, I.; Brown, J.P. and Hellström, K.E.: Recombinant vaccinia virus vaccine against the human melanoma antigen p97 for use in immunotherapy. Proc. Natl. Acad. Sci. USA 85: 1052–1056, 1988.

Esumi, N.; Hunt, B.; Itaya, T. and Frost, P.: Reduced tumorigenicity of murine tumor cells secreting gamma-interferon is due to nonspecific host responses and is unrelated to class I major histocompatibility complex expression. Cancer Res. 51: 1185–1189, 1991.

Ettinghausen, S.E.; Puri, R.K. and Rosenberg, S.A.: Increased vascular permeability in organs mediated by the systemic administration of lymphokine-activated killer cells and recombinant interleukin-2 in mice. J. Natl. Cancer Inst. 80: 177–188, 1988.

Eugui, E.M.; Delustro, B.; Rouhafza, S.; Wilhelm, R. and Allison, A.C.: Coordinate inhibition by some antioxidants of TNFα, Il-1β and Il-6 production by human peripheral blood mononuclear cells. Immunosuppressive and Antiinflammatory Drugs, eds. Allison, A.C.; Lafferty, K.J. and Fliri, H., Annals of the New York Academy of Sciences 696: 171, 1993.

Evans, G.F.; Snyder, Y.M.; Butler, L.D. and Zuckerman, S.H.: Differential expression of interleukin-1 and tumor necrosis factor in murine septic shock models. Circ. Shock. 29: 279, 1989.

Everson, M.P.; Brown, C.B. and Lilly, M.B.: Interleukin-6 and granulocyte macrophage colony-stimulating factor are candidate growth factors for chronic myelomonocytic leukemia cells. Blood 74: 1472, 1989.

Fagarasan, M.O.; Eskay, R. and Axelrod, J.: Interleukin-1 potentiates the secretion of β-endorphin induced by secretagogues in a mouse pituitary cell line (ArT-20)- Proc. Natl. Acad. Sci. USA 86: 2070–2073, 1989.

Fagerberg, J.; Frödin, J.-E.; Ragnhammar, P.; Steinitz, M.; Wigzell, H. and Mellstedt, H.: Immunization effect of monoclonal antibodies against tumor-associated antigens during cancer treatment. Specific Immunotherapy Of Cancer With Vaccines, eds. Bystryn, J.-C.; Soldano, F. and Livingston, P., The New York Academy of Sciences 690: 337, 1993.

Fairman, R.P.; Glauser, F.L.; Merchant, R.E.; Bechard, D. and Fowler, A.A.: Increase of rat pulmonary microvascular permeability to albumin by recombinant interleukin-2. Cancer Res. 47: 3528–3532, 1987.

Faist, E.; Markewitz, A.; Fuchs, D.; Lang, S.; Zarius, S.; Schildberg, F.W.; Wachter, H. and Reichart, B.: Immunomodulatory therapy with thymopentin and indomethacin: Successful restoration of Interleukin-2 synthesis in patients undergoing major surgery. Annals of Surgery 214: 264–273, 1991.

Falk, K.; Erbnerg, I.; Sakthivel, R.; Davis, J.; Christensson, B.; Luka, J.; Okano, M.; Grierson, H.L.; Klein, G. and Purtilo, D.T.: Expression of Epstein-Barr virus-encoded proteins and B-cell markers in fatal infectious mononucleosis. Int. J. Cancer 46: 976–984, 1990.

Falo, L.D.; Benacerraf, B. and Rock, K.: Phospholipase treatment of accessory cells that have been exposed to antigen selectively inhibits antigen-specific Ia-restricted, but not allospecific, stimulation of T lymphocytes. Proc. Natl. Acad. Sci. USA 83: 6994–6997, 1986.

Falo, L.D.; Haber, S.I,; Hermann, S.; Benacerraf, B. and Rock, K.L.: Characterization of antigen association with accessory cells: specific removal of processed antigens from the cell surface by phospholipases. Proc. Natl. Acad. Sci. USA 84: 522–526, 1987.

Falus, A. and Meretey, K.: Histamine: an early messenger in inflammatory and immune reactions. Immunol. Today 13: 154, 1992.

Fanger, M.W.; Shen, L.; Graziano, R.F. and Guyre, P.M.: Cytotoxicity mediated by human Fc receptors for IgG. Immunol. Today 10: 92, 1989.

Fanger, M.W.: Bispecific Antibodies. Critical Rev. Immunol. 12: 101–124, 1992.

Fanslow, W.C.; Sims, J.E.; Sassenfeld, H.; Morrissey, P.J.; Gillis, S.; Dower, S.K. and Widmer, M.B.: Regulation of alloreactivity, in vivo by a soluble form of the interleukin-1 receptor. Science 248: 739–742, 1990.

Fargeas, C.; W, C.Y.; Nakajiama, T.; Cos, D.; Nutman, T. and Delespesse, G.: Differential effect of transforming growth factor β on the synthesis of Th1- and Th2-like lymphokines by human T lymphocytes. Eur. J. Immunol. 22: 2173–2176, 1992.

Farhood, H.; Gao, X.; Son, K.; Yang, Y.Y.; Lazo, J.S.; Huang, L.; Barsoum, J.; Bottega, R. and Epand, R.M.: Cationic liposomes for direct gene transfer in therapy of cancer and other diseases. Annals of the New York Academy of Sciences 716: 23, 1994.

Farina, P.R.; Deleon, R.; Graham, A.; Grob, P.; David, E.; Barton, R.; Ksiazek, J.; Rothlein, R.; Mainolfi, E. and Matsushima, K.: Monocyte-derived neutrophil chemotactic factor MDNCF a stimulator of neutrophil function. FASEB J. 3: A1333, 1989.

Farrands, P.A.; Perkins, A.C.; Pimm, M.V.; Hardy, J.D.; Embleton, M.J.; Baldwin, R.W. and Hardcastle, J.D.: Radioimmunodetection of human colorectal cancers by an antitumor monoclonal antibody. Lancet 2: 397, 1982.

Farrar, W.L.; Thomas, T.P. and Anderson, W.B.: Altered cytosol/membrane enzyme redistribution on interleukin-3 activation of protein kinase C. Nature 315: 235–237, 1985.

Faull, R.J. and Russ, G.R.: Tubular expression of intercellular adhesion molecule-1 during renal allograft rejection. Transplantation 48: 226–230, 1989.

Fauser, B.C.J.M.; Galway, A.B. and Hsueh, A.J.: Inhibitory actions of interleukin-1β on steroidogenesis in primary cultures of neonatal rat testicular cells. Acta Endocrinol. (Copenh.) 120: 401–408, 1989.

Favre, C.; Saeland, S.; Caux, C.; Duvert, V. and de Vries, J.E.: IL-4 has basophilic and eosinophilic cell growth-promoting activity on cord blood cells. Blood 75: 67–73, 1990.

Fearon, D.T.: Regulation of the amplification C3 convertase of human complement by an inhibitory protein isolated from human erythrocyte membrane. Proc. Natl. Acad. Sci. USA 76: 5867–5871, 1979.

Feeley, T.W.; Minty, B.D.; Scudder, C.M.; Jones, J.G.; Royston, D. and Teng, N.N.H.: The effect of human antiendotoxin monoclonal antibodies on endotoxin-induced lung injury in the rat. Am. Rev. Respir. Dis. 135: 665–670, 1987.

Fehr, J.; Hofmann, V. and Kappeler, U.: Transient reversal of thrombocytopenia in idiopathic thrombocytopenic purpura by high-dose intravenous gammaglobulin. N. Engl. J. Med. 306: 1244, 1982.

Feigen, L.G. et al., 1991: cited by Tuffin , D.P. et al. 1992.

Feletou, M. and Vanhoutte, P.M.: Endothelium-dependent hyperpolarization of canine coronary smooth muscle. Brit. J. Pharmacol. 93: 515–524, 1988.

Felten, S.Y.; Felten, D.L.; Bellinger, D.L. and Olschowka, J.A.: Noradrenergic and peptidergic innervation of lymphoid organs. In Neuroimmunoendocrinology, 2nd rev. edn (ed. Blalock, J.E.) 25–41, 1988. Chemical immunology, Vol. 52, Karger, Basel.

Feng, Y.J.; Shalts, E.; Xia, L.; Rivier, J.; Rivier, C.; Vale, W. and Ferin, M.: An inhibitory effect of interleukin-1α on basal gonadotropin release in the ovariectomized rhesus monkey: Reversal by a CRH antagonist. Endocrinology 128: 2077–2082, 1991.

Fenton, M.J.: Review; Transcriptional and post-transcriptional regulation of Interleukin 1 gene expression. Int. J. Immunopharmac. 14: 401–411, 1992.

Ferkol, T.; Davis, P.; Kaetzel, C. and Hanson, R.: Targeted gene delivery to respiratory epthelial cells. Pediatr. Pulmonol. (abstr.), 1992.

Ferrante, A.; Seow, W.K.; Rowan-Kelly, B. and Thong, Y.H.: Tetrandrine, a plant alkaloid, inhibits the production of tumor necrosis factor α (cachectin) by human monocytes. Clin. Exp. Immunol. 80: 232–235, 1990.

Ferrara, N. and Henzel, W.J.: Pituitary follicular cells secrete a novel heparin-binding growth factor specific for vascular enothelial cells. Biochem. Biophys. Res. Commun. 161: 851–855, 1989.

Ferrara, N.; Winer, J. and Henzel, W.J.: Pituitary follicular cells secrete an inhibitor of aortic endothelial cell growth: identification as leukemia inhibitory factor. Proc. Natl. Acad. Sci. 89: 698–702, 1992.

Ferrone, S.; Cooper, N.R.; Pellegrino, M.A. and Reisfeld, R.A.: Interaction of histocompatibility (HLA) antibodies and complement with synchronized human lymphoid cells in continuous culture. J. Exp. Med. 137: 55–68, 1973.

Ferrone, S.: Human tumor-associated antigen mimicry by anti-idiotypic antibodies, immunogenicity and clinical trials in patients with solid tumors. Specific Immunotherapy Of Cancer With Vaccines, eds. Bystryn, J.-C.; Ferrone, S. and Livingston, P., The New York Academy of Sciences 690: 214, 1993.

Festenstein, H.: Immunogenetic and biological aspects of in vitro lymphocyte allotransformation (MLR) in the mouse. Transplant. Rev. 15: 62–88, 1973.

Fett, J.W.; Strydom, D.J.; Lobb, R.R.; Alderman, E.M.; Bethune, J.L.; Riordan, J.F. and Vallee, B.L.: Isolation and characterization of angiogenin, an angiogenic protein from human carcinoma cells. Biochem. 24: 5480–5486, 1985.

Fibbe, W.E.; Schaafsma, M.R.; Falkenburg, J.H.F. and Willemze, R.: The biological activities of Interleukin-1. Blut 59: 147–156, 1989.

Fidler, I.J.: Macrophages and metastasis - a biological approach to cancer therapy. Cancer Res. 45: 4714–4726, 1985.

Finbloom, D.S.; Hoover, D.L. and Wahl, L.M.: The characteristics of binding of human recombinant interferon-gamma to its receptor on human monocytes and human monocyte-like cell lines. J. Immunol. 135: 300–305, 1985.

Finch, P.W.; Rubin, J.S.; Miki, T.; Ron, D. and Aaronson, S.A.: Human KGF is FGF-related with properties of a paracrine effector of epithelial cell growth. Science 245: 752–755, 1989.

Fink, M.P.; Rothschild, H.R.; Deniz, Y.F. and Cohn, S.M.: Complement depletion with Naje haje cobra venom factor limits prostaglandin release and improves visceral perfusion in porcine endotoxic shock. J. Trauma 29: 1076–1084, 1989.

Finkelman, F.D.; Katona, I.M.; Urban, J.F.; Snapper, C.M.; Ohara, J. and Paul, W.E.: Suppression of in vivo polyclonal IgE response by monoclonal antibody to the lymphocyte B cell stimulatory factor-1. Proc. Natl. Acad. Sci. USA 83: 9675, 1986.

Finkelman, F.D.; Katona, I.M.; Mosmann, T.R. and Coffman, R.L.: IFN-gamma regulates the isotypes of Ig secreted during in vivo humoral immune responses. J. Immunol. 140: 1022–1027, 1988.

Finkelman, F.D.; Holmes, J.; Katona, I.M.; Urban, jr., J.F.; Beckmann, J.P.; Park, L.S.; Schooley, K.A.; Coffman, R.L.; Mosmann, T.R. and Paul, W.E.: Lymphokine control of in vivo immunogloublin isotype selection. Annu. Rev. Immunol. 8: 303–333, 1990.

Fiorentino, D.F.; Bond, M.W. and Mosmann, T.R.: Two types of mouse T helper cell. IV. Th2 clones secrete a factor that inhibits cytokine production by Th1 clones. J. Exp. Med. 170: 2081–2095, 1989.

Fisch, P.; Malkovski, M.; Kovats, S.; Sturm, E.; Braakamn, E.; Klein, S.B.; Voss, S.D.; Morrisey, L.W.; DeMars, R.; Welch, W.J.; Bolhuis, R.L.H. and Sondel P.M.: Recognition by human V9/V2T cells of a GroEL homolog on Daidi Burkitt's lymphoma cells. Science 250: 1269–1272, 1990.

Fischer, E.; Delibrias, C. and Kazatchkine, M.D.: Expression of CR2 (the C3dg/EBV receptor, CD21) on normal human peripheral blood T lymphocytes. J. Immunol. 146: 865–869, 1991.

Flanagan, M. and Crabtree, G.R.: Rapamycin inhibits p34cdc2 expression and arrests T lymphocyte proliferation at the G1/S transition. Immunosuppressive and Antiinflammatory Drugs, eds. Allison, A.C.; Lafferty, K.J. and Fliri, H., Annals of the New York Academy of Sciences 696: 31, 1993.

Fleischer, B. and Schrezenmeier, H.: T cell stimulation by staphylococcal entertoxins. Clonally variable response and requirement for major histocompatibility complex class II molecules on accessory or target cells. J. Exp. Med. 167: 1697, 1988.

Fleischer, B.; Schrezenmeier, H. and Conradt, P.: T lymphocyte activation by staphylococcal enterotoxins: role of class II molecules and T cell surface structures. Cell Immunol. 120: 92–101, 1989.

Fleischer, B.: Superantigene: Schock und Immunsuppression als Folge der T-Zell-Stimulation. Gelbe Hefte 4: 141, 1991.

Fleury, S.; Lamarre, D.; Meloche, S.; Ryu, S.E.; Cantin, C.; Hendrickson, W.A. and Sekaly, R.P.: Mutational analysis of the interaction between CD4 and class II MHC: class II antigens contact CD4 on a surface opposite the gp120–binding site. Cell 66: 1037, 1991.

Flexner, C.; Hugin A. and Moss, B.: Prevention of vaccinia virus infection in immunodeficient mice by vector-directed Il-2 expression. Nature 330: 259–262, 1987.

Florini, J.R.; Robert, A.B.; Ewton D.Z.; Falen, S.L.; Flanders, K.C. and Sporn, M.B.: Transforming growth factor-ß: a very potent inhibitor of myoblast differentiation, identical to the differentiation inhibitor secreted by Buffalo rat liver cells. J. Biol. Chem. 261: 16509–16513, 1986.

Florkiewicz, R.A. and Sommer, A.: Human basic fibroblast growth factor gene encodes four polypeptides: three initiate translation from non-AUG codons. Proc. Natl. Acad. Sci. USA 86: 3978–3981, 1989.

Floros, J.; Steinbrink, R.; Jacobs, K.; Phelps, D.; Kriz, R.; Recny, M.; Sultzman, L.; Jones, S.; Taeusch, H.W.; Frank, H.A. and Fritsch, E.F.: Isolation and characterization of cDNA clones for the 35–kDa pulmonary surfactant-associated protein. J. Biol. Chem. 261: 9029–9033, 1986.

Folkman, J.; Merler, E.; Abernathy, C. and Williams, G.: Isolation of a tumor factor responsible for angiogenesis. J. Exp. Med. 113: 275, 1971.

Folkman, J.: Tumor angiogenesis. Adv. Cancer Res. 19: 331, 1974.

Folkman, J.; Langer, R.; Linhardt, R.H.; Haudenschild, C. and Taylor, S.: Angiogenesis inhibition and tumor regression caused by heparin or a heparin fragment in the presence of cortisone. Science 221: 719–725, 1983.

Folkman, J.: How is blood vessel growth regulated in normal and neoplastic tissue? Cancer Res. 46: 467–473, 1986.

Folkman, J. and Klagsbrun, M.: Angiogenic factors. Science 239: 442, 1987.

Fontana, A.; Kristense, F.; Dubs, R.; Gemsa, D. and Weber, E.: Production of prostaglandins E and an interleukin-1 like factor by cultured astrocytes and C glioma cells. J. Immunol. 129: 2413–2419, 1982.

Forbes, C.; Pensky, J. and Ratnoff, O.: Inhibition of activated Hageman factor and activated plasma thromboplastin antecedent by purified serum C1 inactivator. J. Lab. Clin. Med. 76: 809–815, 1970.

Forth, W.; Henschler, D. and Rummel, W.: Allgemine und spezielle Pharmakologie und Toxikologie. Bibliographisches Institut-Wissenschaftsverlag, Mannheim 1980.

Fox, D.A.; Hussey, R.E.; Fitzgerald, K.A.; Acuto, O.; Poole, C.; Palley, L.; Daley, F.J.; Schlossman, S.F. and Reinherz E.L.: Ta1, a novel 105KD human T cell activation antigen defined by a monoclonal antibody. J. Immunol. 133: 1250–1256, 1984.

Fox, E.A. and Riordan, J.F.: The molecular biology of angiogenin. In: Chien S (ed): Molecular biology of the cardiovascular system. Amsterdam, Elsevier, 285: 139–154, 1990.

Fox, J.E.B. and Boyles, J.K.: The membrane skeleton - a distinct structure that regulates the function of cells. Bioessays, 8: 14–18, 1988.

Frackelton, A.R. jr.; Tremble, P.M. and Williams, L.T.: Evidence for the platelet-derived growth factor-stimulated tyrosine phosphorylation of the platelet-derived growth factor receptor in vivo. Immunopurification using a monoclonal antibody to phosphotyrosine. J. Biol. Chem. 259: 7909, 1984.

Francoeur, A.M.; Peebles, C.L.; Heckman, K.J.; Lee, J.C. and Tan, E.M.: Identification of ribosomal protein autoantigens. J. Immun. 135: 2378–2384, 1985.

Francoeur, A.M.; Peebles, C.L.; Gompper, P.T. and Tan, E.M.: Identification of Ki (Ku,p70/p80) autoantigens and analysis of anti-Ki autoantibody reactivity. J. Immun. 136: 1648–1653, 1986.

Frank, M.M.: Complement in the pathophysiology of human disease. N. Engl. J. Med. 316: 1525–1530, 1987.

Frank, M.M. and Fries, L.F.: The role of complement in inflammation and phagocytosis. Immunol. Today 12: 322–326, 1991.

Frankel, A.E.; Ring, D.B.; Tringale, F. and Hsieh-Ma, S.T.: Tissue distribution of breast cancer-associated antigens defined by monoclonal antibodies. J. Biol. Resp. Modif. 4: 273, 1985.

Franks, A.K.; Kujawa, K.I.; and Yaffe, L.J.: Experimental elimination of tumor necrosis factor in low-dose endotoxin models has variable effects on survival. Infect. Immun. 59: 2609, 1991.

Fraser, J.D.; Straus, D. and Weiss, A.: Signal transduction events leading to T-cell lymphokine gene expression. Immunol. Today 14: 357, 1993.

Frater-Schröder, M.; Risau, W.; Hallmann, R.; Gautsch, P. and Böhlen, P.: Tumor necrosis factor type μ, a potent inhibitor of endothelial cell growth in vitro, is angiogenic in vivo. Proc. Natl. Acad. Sci. 84: 5277–5281, 1987.

Frazer, I.H.; Mackay, I.R.; Jordan, T.W.; Whittingham, S. and Marzuki, S.: Reactivity of anti-mitochondrial autoantibodies in primary biliary cirrhosis: definition of two novel mitochondrial autoantigens. J. Immun. 135: 1739–1745, 1985.

Freeman, G.J.; Freedman, A.S.; Segil, J.M.; Lee, G.; Whitman, J.F. and Nadler, L.M.: B7, a new member of the Ig superfamily with unique expression on activated and neoplastic B cells. J. Immunol. 143: 2714–2722, 1989.

Freeman, G.J.; Gray, G.S.; Gimmi, C.C.; Lombard, D.B.; Zhou, L-J.; White, M.; Fingeroth, J.C.; Gribben, J.G. and Nadler, L.M.: Structure, expression, and T-cell costimulatory activity of the murine homologue of the human B lymphocyte activation antigen B7. J. Exp. Med. 174: 625–631, 1991.

Frei, K.; Malipiero, U.V.; Leist, T.P.; Zinkernagel, R.M.; Schwab, M.E. and Fontana, A.: On the cellular source and function of interleukin 6 produced in the central nervous system in viral diseases. Eur. J. Immunol. 19: 689–694, 1989.

French, M.: Serum IgG subclasses in normal adults. Monogr. Allergy 19: 100–107, 1986.

Frendl, G.: Interleukin 3: from colony-stimulating factor to pluripotent immunoregulatory cytokine. Int. J. Immunopharmac. 14: 421–430, 1992.

Freudenberg, M.A.; Keppler, D and Galanos, C.: Requirement for lipopolysaccharide-responsive macrophages in galactosamine-induced sensitization to endotoxin. Infect. Immun. 51: 891, 1986.

Fridman, W.H. and Golstein, P.: Immunoglobulin-binding factor present on and produced by thymus-processed lymphocytes (T cells). Cell. Immunol. 11: 424, 1974.

Fridman, W.H.; Gresser, I.; Bandu, M.T.; Aguet, M. and Neauport-Sautes, C.: Interferon enhances the expression of Fc receptors. J. Immun. 124: 2436–2441, 1980.

Friedman, W.J.; Larkfors, L.; Ayer-LeLievre, C.; Ebendal, T.; Olson, L. and Persson, H.: Regulation of ß-nerve growth factor expression by inflammatory mediators in hippocampal cultures. J. Neurosci. Res. 27: 374–388, 1990.

Fries, L.F.; Gordon, D.M.; Richards, R.L.; Egan, J.E.; Hollingdale, M.R.; Gross, M.; Silverman, C. and Alving, C.R.: Liposomal malaria vaccine in humans: A safe and potent adjuvant strategy. Proc. Natl. Acad. Sci. USA 89: 358, 1992.

Friesel, R.; Komoriay, A. and Maciag, T.: Inhibition of endothelial cell proliferation by gamma-interferon. J. Cell Biol. 104: 689–696, 1987.

Froesch, E.R.; Schmidt, C.; Schwander, J. and Zapf, J.: Actions of insulin-like growth factors. Ann. Rev. Physiol. 47: 443–467, 1985.

Fu, X.Y.; Cai, J.P.; Chin, H.Y.; Watson, G.A. and Lopez, D.M.: Regulation of leukocyte binding to endothelial tissues by tumor-derived GM-CSF. Int. J. Cancer 50: 585–588, 1992.

Fujisaku, A.; Harley, J.B.; Frank, M.B.; Gruner, B.A.; Frazier, B. and Holers, V.M.: Genomic organization and polymorphisms of the human C3d/Epstein-Barr virus. J. Biol. Chem. 264: 2118–2125, 1989.

Fukata, J.; Usui, T.; Naito, Y.; Nakai, Y. and Imura, H.: Effects of recombinant human interleukin-1μ, -1ß, 2 and 6 on ACTH synthesis and release in the mouse pituitary tumour cell line AtT-20. J. Endocrinol. 122: 33–39, 1989.

Fung, P.Y.S.; Madey, M.; Koganty, R.R. and Longenecker, B.M.: Active specific immunotherapy of a murine mammary adenocarcinoma using a synthetic tumor-associated glycoconjugate. Cancer Res. 50: 4308–4314, 1990.

Furchgott, R.F. and Zawadzki, J.V.: The obligatory role of endothelial cells in the relaxation of arterial smooth muscle by acetylcholine. Nature 8london) 288: 373–376, 1980.

Furchgott, R.F.; Khan, M.T. and Jothianandan, D.: Comparison of endothelium dependent relaxation and nitric oxide induced relaxation in rabbit aorta. Fed. Proc. 46: 385 (abstract), 1987.

Furchgott, R.F. and Vanhoutte, P.M.: Endothelium-derived relaxing and contracting factors. FASEB J. 3: 2007, 1989.

Furukawa, K.; Yamaguchi, H.; Oettgen, H.F.; Old, L.J. and Lloyd, K.O.: Analysis of the expression of N-glycolylneuraminic acid-containing gangliosides in cells and tissues using two human monoclonal antibodiess. J. Biol. Chem. 263: 18507–18512, 1988.

Furukawa, K.; Yamaguchi, H.; Oettgen, H.F.; Old, L.J. and Lloyd, O.O.: Two human monoclonal antibodies reacting with the major gangliosides of human melanomas and comparison with corresponding mouse monoclonal antibodies. Cancer Res. 49: 191–196, 1989.

Furukawa, K.S.; Furukawa, K.; Real, F.X.; Old. L.J. and Lloyd, K.O.: A unique antigenic epitope of human melanoma is carried on the common melanoma glycoprotein gp95/p97. J. Exp. Med. 169: 585–590, 1989.

Furukawa, K. and Kobata, A.: IgG galactosylation - its biological significance and pathology. Molecular Immunology 28: 1333–1340, 1991.

Furusho, K.; Kamiye, T.; Nakano, H.; Kiyosawa, N.; Shinomiya, K.; Hayashidera, T.; Tamura, T.; Hirose, O.; Manabe, Y.; Yokoyama, T. et al.: High-dose intravenous gammaglobulin for Kawasaki disease. Lancet 2: 1055–1058, 1984.

Furutani, Y.; Nomura, H.; Notake, M.; Oyamada, Y.; Fukui, T.; Yamada, M.; Larsen, C.G.; Oppenheim, J.J. and Matsushima, K.: Cloning and sequencing of the cDNA for human monocyte chemotactic and activating factor (MCAF). Biochem. Biophys. Res. Commun. 159: 249–255, 1989.

Fuse, A.; Kakuda, H.; Shima, Y.; Damme, J.v.; Billiqu, A. and Sato, T.: Interleukin 6, a possible autocrine growth and differentiation factor for the human megakaryocytic cell line, CMK. Br. J. Haematol. 77: 32, 1991.

Fussey, S.P.M.; Ali, S.T.; Guest, J.R.; James, O.F.W.; Bassendine, M.F. and Yeaman, S.J.: Reactivity of primary biliary cirrhosis sera with Escherichia coli dihydrolipoamide acetyltransferase (E2p): characterization of the main immunogenic region. Prod. natn. Acad. Sci. USA 87: 3987–3991, 1990.

Gaida, F.J.; Fenger, U.; Wagener, C. and Neumaier, M.: A monoclonal anti-idiotypic antibody bearing the image of an epitope specific to the human carcinoembryonic antigen. Int. J. Cancer 51: 459–465, 1992.

Gajewski, T.F. and Fitch, F.W.: Anti-proliferative effect of IFN-gamma in immune regulation. I. IFN-gamma inhibits the proliferation of Th2 but not Th1 murine HTL clones. J. Immunol. 140: 4245, 1988.

Gajewski, T.F.; Pinnas, M.; Wong, T. and Fitch, F.W.: Murine TH1 and TH2 clones proliferate optimally in response to distinct antigen-presenting cell populations. J. Immunol. 146: 1750, 1991.

Galandrini, R.; Albi, N.; Tripodi, G.; Zarcone, D.; Terenzi, A.; Moretta, A.; Grossi, C.E. and Velardi, A.: Antibodies to CD44 trigger effector functions of human T cell clones. J. Immunol. 150: 4225–4235, 1993.

Galizzi, J-P.; Gabrillat, H.; Rousset, F.; Menetrier, C.; De Vries, J.E. and Banchereau, J.: IFN-gamma and prostaglandin E2 inhibit Il-4–induced expression of Fc epsilon R2/CD23 on B lymphocytes through different mechanisms without altering binding of Il-4 to its receptor. J. Immunol. 141: 1982–1988, 1988.

Galizzi, J-P.; Castle, B.; Djossou, O.; Harada, N.; Cabrillat, H.; Ait Yahia, S.; Barrett, R.; Howard, M. and Banchereau, J.: Purification of a 130–kDa T cell glycoprotein that binds human IL-4 with high affinity. J. Biol. Chem. 265: 439–444, 1990.

Galligioni, E.; Francini, M.; Quaia, M.; Carbone, A.; Spada, A.; Sacco, C.; Favaro, D.; Santarosa, M.; Carmignani, G.; DiDonna, D.; Mazza, G.; Viggiano, S.; Fiaccevento, G.; Dal Bo, V. and Talamini, R.: Randomized study of adjuvant immunotherapy with autologous tumor cells and BCG in renal cancer. Specific Immunotherapy of Cancer with Vaccines, Bystryn, J.C.; Ferrone, S. and Livingston, P. (eds.), Annals of the New York Academy of Sciences 690: 1993.

Gallin, J.I.: Degranulating stimuli decrease the negative surface charge and increase the adhesiveness of human neutrophils. J. Clin. Invest. 65: 298–306, 1980.

Galloway, A.: Matrix metalloproteinases as mediators of tissue degradation. Rheumatoid Arthritis, Royal College of Physicians, London, 17./18.6.1991.

Galron, R.; Kloog, Y.; Bdolah, A. and Sokolovsky, M.: Functional endothelin/sarafotoxin receptors in rat heart myocytes: Structure-activity relationships and receptor subtypes. Biochem. Biophys. Res. Commun. 163: 936–943, 1989.

Gamett, D.C.; Tracy, S.E. and Robinson, H.L.: Differences in sequences encoding the carboxyl-terminal domain of the epidermal growth factor receptor correlate with differences in the disease potential of viral erbB genes. Proc. Natl. Acad. Sci. 83: 6053–6057, 1986.

Gansbacher, B.; Bannerji, R.; Daniels, B.; Zier, K.; Cronin, K. and Gilboa, E.: Retroviral vector-mediated gamma-interferon gene transfer into tumor cells generates potent and long lasting antitumor immunity. Cancer Res. 50: 7820–7825, 1990.

Ganser, A.; Lindenmann, A.; Seipelt, G.; Ottmann, O.G.; Herrmann, F.; Eder, M.; Frisch, H.; Schulz, G.; Mertelsmann, R. and Hoelzer, D.: Effects of recombinant human interleukin-3 in patients with normal hematopoiesis and in patients with bone marrow failure. Blood 76: 666, 1990.

Ganser, A.; Lindemann, A.; Seipelt, G.; Ottmann, O.G.; Herrmann, F.; Eder, M.; Frisch, J.; Schulz, G.; Mertelsmann, R. and Hoelzer, D.: Clinical effects of recombinant interleukin-3. Am. J. Clin. Oncol. 14: 51–63, 1991.

Garcia, D.L.; Anderson, S.; Rennke, H.G. and Brenner, B.M.: Anemia lessens and its prevention with recombinant human erythropoietin worsens glomerular injury and hypertension in rats with reduced renal mass. Proc. Natl. Acad. Sci. 85: 6142–6146, 1988.

Garcia-Penarrubia, P.; Bankhurst, A.D. and Koster, F.T.: Prostaglandins from human T suppressor/cytotoxic cells modulate natural killer antibacterial activity. J. Exp. Med. 170: 601, 1989.

Garrett, T.P.J.; Saper, M.A.; Bjorkman, P.J.; Strominger, J.L. and Wiley, D.C.: Specificity pockets for the side chains of peptide antigens in HLA-Aw68. Nature 342: 692–696, 1989.

Gascan, H.; Anegon, I.; Praloran, V.; Naulet, J.; Godard, A.; Soulillou, J.P. and Jacques, Y.: Constitutive production of human interleukin for DA cells/leukemia inhibitory factor by human tumor cell lines derived from various tissues. J. Immunol. 144: 2592–2598, 1990.

Gascan, H.; Gauchat, J.-F.; Roncarolo, M.G.; Yssel, H.; Spits, H. and de Vries, J.E.: Human B cell clones can be induced to proliferate and to switch to IgE and IgG4 synthesis by IL-4 and a signal provided by activated CD4+ T cell clones. J. Exp. Med. 173: 747–750, 1991.

Gascan, H.; Gauchat, J.-F.; Aversa, G.; van Vlasselaer, P. and de Vries, J.E.: Anti-CD40 monoclonal antibodies or CD4+ T cell clones and IL-4 induce IgG4 and IgE switching in purified human B cells via different signalling pathways. J. Immunol. 147: 8–13, 1991.

Gasson, J.C.; Weisbart, R.H.; Kaufman, S.E.; Clark, S.C.; Hewick, R.M.; Wong, G.G. and Golde, D.W.: Purified human granulocyte-macrophage colony-stimulating factor: Direct action on neutrophils. Science 226: 1339, 1984.

Gasson, J.C.; Kaufman, S.E.; Weisbart, R.H.; Tomonaga, M. and Golde, D.W.: High-affinity binding of granulocyte-macrophage colony-stimulating factor to normal and leukemic human myeloid cells. Proc. Natl. Acad. Sci. USA 83: 669, 1986.

Gasson, J.C.: Molecular physiology of granulocyte-macrophage colony-stimulating factor. Blood 77: 1131–1145, 1991.

Gately, M.K.; Desai, B.B.; Wolitzky, A.G.; Quinn, P.M.; Dwyer, C.M.; Podlaski, F.J.; Familletti, P.C.; Sinigalia, F.; Chizzonite, R.; Gubler, U. and Stern, A.S.: Regulation of human lymphocyte proliferation by a heterodimeric cytokine, Il-12 (cytotoxic lymphocyte maturation factor). J. Immunol. 147: 874–882, 1991.

Gatenby, P.A.; Barbosa, J.E. and Lachmann, P.J.: Differences between C4A and C4B in the handling of immune complexes: The enhancement of CR1 binding is more important than the inhibition of immunoprecipitation. Clin. Exp. Immunol. 79: 158–163, 1990.

Gauchat, J-F.; Aversa, G.; Gascan, H. and de Vries, J.E.: Modulation of Il-4 induced germline RNA synthesis in human B cells by tumor necrosis factor-μ, anti-CD40 monoclonal antibodies or transforming growth factor-ß correlates with levels of IgE production. Int. Immunol. 4: 397–406, 1992.

Gauchat, J.-F.; Aubry, J.-P.; Mazzei, G.; Life, P.; Jomotte, T.; Elson, G. and Bonnefoy, J.-Y.: Human CD40–ligand: molecular cloning, cellular distribution and regulation of expression by factors controlling IgE production. FEBS 315: 259–266, 1993.

Gaudernack, G.; Gedde-Dahl, T.; Fossum, B.; Olsen, B.H.; Eriksen, J.A. and Thorsby, E.: Oncogene derived peptides. A new class of tumor rejection antigens. J. Cell Biochem. Suppl. 17D: 109 (abstr. NZ 208), 1993.

Gauldie, J.; Richards, C.; Harnish, D.; Lansdorp, P. and Baumann, H.: Interferon beta 2/B-cell stimulatory factor type 2 shares identity with monocyte-derived hepatocyte-stimulating factor and regulates the major acute phase protein response in liver cells. Proc. Natl. Acad. Sci. 84: 7251–7255, 1987.

Gaulton, G.N. and Eardley, D.D.: Interleukin 2–dependent phosphorylation of interleukin 2 receptors and other T cell membrane proteins. J. Immuno. 136: 2470–2477, 1986.

Gavioli, R.; De Campos-Lima, P.-O.; Kurilla, M.G.; Kieff, E.; Klein, G. and Masucci, M.G.: Recognition of the EBV encoded nuclear antigens EBNA-4 and EBNA-6 by HLA A11 restricted cytotoxic T-lymphocytes. Implications for the down-regulation of HLA A11 in Burkitt's lymphoma. Proc. Natl. Acad. Sci. USA 89: 5862–5866, 1992.

Gearing, D.P.0 and Bruce, A.G.: Oncostatin M binds the high-affinity leukemia inhibitory factor receptor. New Biol. 4: 61–65, 1992.

Gelehrter, T.D. and Sznycer-Laszuk, R.: Thrombin induction of plasminogen activator-inhibitor in cultured endothelial cells. J. Clin. Invest. 77: 165–169, 1986.

Geppert, T.D.; Davis, L.S.; Gur, H.; Wacholtz, M.C. and Lipsky, P.E.: Accessory cell signals involved in T cell activation. Immunol. Rev. 117: 5–66, 1990.

Gergely, J.; Sarmay, G. and Rajnavölgyi, E.: Regulation of antibody production mediated by Fc gamma receptors, IgG binding factors, and IgG Fc-binding autoantibodies. Crit. Rev. Biochem. Molec. Biol. 27: 191–225, 1992.

Germain, R.N.; Bakke, O.; Bonney, E.; Catellino, F.; Layet, C.; Rinker, A.G.; Sadegh-Nasseri, S. and Romagnoli, P.: The regulation of MHC class II intracellular folding and transport by invariant chain and peptide controls the class II presentation pathway. Towards Selective Immunotheray of Autoimmune Diseases, Opening Symposium, Milan, Italy, September 9–11, 1993.

Gerrard, T.L.; Dyer, D.R.; Zoon, K.C.; zur Nedden, D. and Siegel, J.P.: Modulation of class I and class II histocompatibility antigens on human T cell lines by IFN-gamma. J. Immunol. 140: 3450–3455, 1988.

Gersten, D.M.; Bijwaard, K.E.; Law, L.W. and Hearing, V.J.: Homology of the B50 murine melanoma antigen to the Ro/SS-A antigen of human systemic lupus erythematosus and to calcium-binding proteins. Biochim. Biophys. Acta 1096: 20–25, 1991.

Ghebrehiwet, B.; Habicht, G.S. and Beck, G.: Interaction of C1q with its receptor on cultured cell lines induces an anti-proliferative response. Clin. Immunol. Immunopathol. 54: 148–160, 1990.

Ghebrehiwet, B. and Peerschke, E.I.B.: The C1q-R participates in immunoregulation and signal transduction. Behring Inst. Mitt. 93: 236–240, 1993.

Ghose, T.; Norvell, S.T.; Guclu, A.; Cameron, D.; Bodurtha, D. and MacDonald, A.S.: Immuno-chemotherapy of cancer with chlorambucil-carrying antibody. Br. Med. J. 3: 495, 1972.

Giacomini, P.; Tecce, R.; Gambari, R.; Sacchi, A.; Fisher, P.B. and Natali, P.G.: Recombinant human IFN-gamma, but not IFN-alpha or IFN-beta, enhances MHC-and non-MHC-encoded glycoproteins by a protein synthesis-dependent mechanism. J. Immunol. 140: 3037, 1988.

Giavedoni, L.D.; Jones, L.; Gardner, M.B.; Gibson, H.L.; Ng, C.T.L.; Barr, P.J. and Yilma, T.: Vaccinia virus recombinants expressing chimeric proteins of human immunodeficiency virus and gamma interferon are attenuated for nude mice. Proc. Natl. Acad. Sci. USA 89: 3409–3413, 1992.

Gigli, I.; Mason, J.W.; Coman, R.W. and Austen, K.F.: Interaction of plasma kallikrein with the C1 inhibitor. J. Immunol. 104: 574–581, 1970.

Gilman, S.C.; Schwartz, J.M.; Milner, R.J.; Bloom, F.E. and Feldman, J.D.: ß-Endorphin enhances lymphocyte proliferative responses. Proc. Natl. Acad. Sci USA 79: 4226, 1982.

Gimenez-Gallego, G.; Rodkey, J.; Bennet, C.; Rios-Candelore, M.; DiSalov, J. and Thomas, K.: Brain-derived acidic fibroblast growth factor: complete amino acid sequence and homologies. Science 230: 1385–1388, 1985.

Gimmi, C.D.; Freeman, G.J.; Gribben, J.G.; Sugita, K.; Freedman, A.S.; Morimoto, C. and Nadler, L.M.: B-cell surface antigen B7 provides a costimulatory signal that induces T-cells to proliferate and secrete interleukin 2. Proc. Natl. Acad. Sci. USA 88: 6575–6579, 1991.

Ginsberg, M.H.; Loftus, J.; Ryckwaert, J.J.; Pierschbacher, M.D.; Pytela, R.; Ruoslahti, E. and Plow, E.F.: Immunochemical and amino-terminal sequences comparison of two cytoadhesins indicate they contain similar or identical beta subunits and distinct alpha subunits. J. Biol. Cehm. 262: 5437–5440, 1987.

Girasole, G.; Jilka, R.L.; Passeri, G.; Boswell, S.; Boder, G. and Williams, D.C.: 17 beta-estradiol inhibits interleukin-6 production by bone marrow-derived stromal cells and osteoblasts in vitro: a potential mechanism for the antiosteoporotic effect of estrogens. J. Clin. Invest. 89: 883–891, 1992.

Girling, A.; Bartkova, J.; Burchell, J.; Gendler, S.; Gillett, C. and Taylor-Papadimitriou, J.: A core protein epitope of the polymorphic epithelial mucin detected by the monoclonal antibody SM-3 is selectively exposed in a range of primary carcinomas. Int. J. Cancer 43: 1072–1076, 1989.

Giroir, B.P.: Mediators of septic shock: New approaches for interrupting the endogenous inflammatory cascade. Crit. Care Med. 21: 780–789, 1993.

Gissmann, L.; Jochmus, I.; Nindl, I. and Müller, M.: Immune-response to genital papillomavirus infections in women - prospects for the development of a vaccine against cervical cancer. Specific Immunotherapy Of Cancer With Vaccines, eds. Bystryn, J.-C.; Ferrone, S. and Livingston, P., The New York Academy of Sciences 690: 80–85, 1993.

Glass, J.; Lavidor, L.M. and Robinson, S.H.: Use of cell separation and short-term culture techniques to study erythroid cell development. Blood 46: 705–711, 1975.

Glenn, K.; Bowen-Pope, D.F. and Ross, R.: Platelet-derived growth factor. III. Identification of a platelet-derived growth factor receptor by affinity labeling. J. Biol. Chem. 257: 5172–5176, 1982.

Glynne, R.; Powis, S.H.; Beck, S.; Kelly, A.; Kerr, L.-A. and Trowsdale, J.A.: Proteosome-related gene between the two ABC transporter loci in the class II region of the human MHC. Nature 353: 357–360, 1991.

Go, N.F.; Castle, B.E.; Barrett, R.; Kastelein, R.; Dang, W.; Mosmann, T.R.; Moore, K.W. and Howard, M.: Interleukin 10, a novel B cell stimulatory factor: unresponsiveness of X chromosome-linked immunodeficiency B cells. J. Exp. Med. 172: 1625–1631, 1990.

Godard, A.; Heymann, D.; Raher, S.; Anegon, I.; Peyrat, M.A.; Le Mauff, B.; Mouray, E.; Gregoire, M.; Virdee, K.; Soulillou, J.P. et al.: High and low affinity receptors for human interleukin for DA cells/leukemia inhibitory factor on human cells. J. Biol. Chem. 267: 3214–3222, 1992.

Goetzl, E.J. and Pickett, W.C.: The human PMN leucocyte chemotactic activity of complex hydroxy-eicosatetraenoic acids (Hetes). J. Immunol. 125: 1789–1791, 1980.

Gogusev, J.; Teutsch, B.; Morin, M.T.; Mongiat, F.; Haguenau, F.; Suskind, G. and Rabotti, G.F.: Inhibition of HLA class I antigen and mRNA expression induced by Rous sarcoma virus in transformed human fibroblasts. Proc. Natl. Acad. Sciences USA 85: 203–207, 1988.

Goldberg, B. and Green, H.: The cytotoxic action of immune gamma globulin and complement on Krebs ascites tumor cells. I. Ultrastructural studies. J. Exp. Med. 109: 505–510, 1959.

Goldberg, D.; Morel, P.; Chatenoud, L.; Boitard, C.; Menkes, C.J.; Bertoye, P-H.; Revillard, J.-P. and Bach, J-F.: Immunological effects of high dose administration of anti-CD4 antibody in rheumatoid arthritis patients. J. Autoimmun. 4: 617–630, 1991.

Goldberg, G.I.; Wilhelm, S.M.; Kronberger, A.; Bauer, E.A.; Grant, G.A. and Eisen, A.Z.: Human fibroblast collagenase. Complete primary structure and homology to an oncogene transformation-induced rat protein. J. Biol. Chem. 261: 6600–6605, 1986.

Goldenberg, D.M.: Targeting, dosimetry, and radioimmunotherapy of B-cell lymphomas with 131I-labeled LL2 (EPB-2) monoclonal antibody. 6th Int. Conf. on Monoclonal Antibody Immunoconjugates, San Diego, 1991.

Goldman, M.; Druet, P. and Gleichmann, E.: TH2 cells in systemic autoimmunity: insights from allogeneic diseases and chemically-induced autoimmunity. Immunol. Today 12: 223, 1991.

Goldstein, I.M.; Brai, M.; Osler, A.G. and Weissmann, G.: Lysosomal enzyme release from human leukocytes: Mediation by the alternate pathway of complement activation. J. Immunol. 111: 33, 1973.

Goldstein, R.; Arnett, F.C.; McLean, R.H.; Bias, W.B. and Duvic, M.: Molecular heterogeneity of complement component C1–null and 21–hydroxylase genes in systemic lupus erythematosus. Arthritis Rheum. 31: 736–744, 1988.

Goldwasser, E.: Erythropoietin and the differentiation of red blood cells. Fed. Proc. 34: 2285–2292, 1975.

Golumber, P.; Lazenby, A.; Levitsky, H.; Jaffee, E.; Karasuyama, H.; Baker, M. and Pardoll, D.: Treatment of established renal cancer by tumor cells engineered to secrete Interleukin-4. Science 254: 713–716, 1991.

Gomez-Sanchez, C.E.; Cozza, E.N.; Foecking, M.F.; Chiou, S. and Ferris, M.W.: Endothelin receptor subtypes and stimulation of aldosterone secretion. Hypertension 15: 744–747, 1990.

Gonzalez, M.E.; Thurmond-Anderle, G.M.E.; Kalmaz, G.D.; Bessman, D.J.; Lisse, J.R. and Daniels, C.: Intravenous immunoglobulin therapy in a patient with systemic lupus erythematosus. Clin. Immunol. Immunopathol. 53: S181–S182, 1989.

Gonzalvez, M.L.; Milanes, M.V. and Vargas, M.L.: Effects of acute and chronic administration of - and -opioid agonists on the hypothalamic-pituitary-adrenocortical (HPA) axis in the rat. Eur. J. Pharmac. 200: 155–158, 1991.

Good, D.J.; Polverini, P.J.; Rastinejad, F.; Le Beau, M.M.; Lemons, R.S.; Frazier, W. and Bouck, N.P.: A tumor suppressor-dependent inhibitor of angiogenesis is immunologically and functionally indistinguishable from a fragment of thrombospondin. Proc. Natl. Acad. Sci. USA 87: 6624–6628, 1990.

Goodnow, C.C.; Crosbie, J.; Adelstein, S.; Lavoie, T.B.; Smith-Gill, S.J.; Brink R.A.; Pritchard-Briscoe, H.; Witherspoon, J.S.; Loblay, R.H.; Raphael, K.; Trent, R.J. and Basten, A.: Altered immunoglobulin expression and functional silencing of self-reactive B lymphocytes in transgenic mice. Nature 334: 676, 1988.

Goodwin, J.S.; Kaszubowski, P.A. and Williams, R.C.: Cyclic adenosine monophosphate response to prostaglandin E2 in subpopulations of human lymphocytes. J. Exp. Med. 150: 1260, 1979.

Goodwin, J.S.: Immunologic effects of nonsteroidal anti-inflammatory drugs. Med. Clin. North Am. 69: 793, 1985.

Goodwin, R.G.; Lupton, S.; Schmierer, A.; Hjerrild, K.J.; Jerzy, R.; Clevenger, W.; Gillis, S.; Cosman, D. and Namen, A.E: Human interleukin 7: molecular cloning and growth factor activity on human and murine B-lineage cells. Proc. Natl. Acad. Sci. 86: 302–306, 1989.

Goodwin, R.G.; Friend, D.; Ziegler, S.F.; Jerzy, R.; Falk, B.A.; Gimpel, S.; Cosman, D.; Dower, S.K.; March, C.J.; Namen, A.E. et al.: Cloning of the human and murine interleukin-7 receptors: demonstration of a soluble form and homology to a new receptor superfamily. Cell 60: 941–951, 1990.

Goodwin, R.G.; Anderson, D.; Jerzy, R.; Davis, T.; Brannan, C.I.; Copeland, N.G.; Jenkins, N.A. and Smith, C.A.: Molecular cloning and expression of the type 1 and type 2 murine receptors for tumor necrosis factor. Molec and Cell Biol. 11: 3020–3026, 1991.

Gordon, D.; Bray, M.A. and Morley, J.: Control of lymphokine secretion by prostaglandins. Nature 262: 401–402, 1976.

Gordon, J. and Stevenson, G.T.: Antigenic modulation of lymphocytic surface immunoglobulin yielding resistance to complement-mediated lysis. Immunol. 42: 13, 1981.

Gordon, J.; Robinson, D.F. and Stevenson, G.T.: Antigenic modulation of lymphocytic surface immunoglobulin yielding resistance to complement-mediated lysis. Immunol. 42: 7, 1981.

Gordon, J.; Millsum, M.J.; Guy, G.R. and Ledbetter, J.A.: Resting B lymphocytes can be triggered directly through the CDw40 (Bp50) antigen. J. Immunol. 140: 1425–1430, 1988.

Gordon, J.; Flores-Romo, L.; Cairns, J.A.; Millsum, M.J.; Lane, P.J.; Johnson, G.D. and MacLennan, I.C.M.: CD23: a multi-functional receptor/lymphokine? Immunol. Today 10: 153, 1989.

Gospodarowicz, D.; Neufeld, G. and Schweigerer, L.: Fibroblast growth factor. Mol. Cell. Endocrin. 46: 187–204, 1986

Gospodarowicz, D.; Neufeld, G. and Schweigerer, L.: Molecular and biological characterization of fibroblast growth factor, an angiogenic factor which also control the proliferation and differentiation of mesoderm and neuroectoderm derived cells. Cell Differ. 19: 1–17, 1986.

Gospodarowicz, D.; Ferrara, N.; Schweigerer, L. and Neufeld, G.: Structural characterization and biological functions of fibroblast growth factor. Endocr. Rev. 8: 95–114, 1987.

Gosselin, E.J.; Tony, H.P. and Parker, C.C.: Characterization of antigen processing and presentation by resting B lymphocytes. J. Immunol. 140, 1408, 1988.

Goto, T.; Herberman, R.B.; Maluish, A. and Strong, D.M.: Cyclic AMP as a mediator of prostaglandin E-induced suppression of human natural killer cell activity. J. Immunol. 130: 1350, 1983.

Gottesman, M.; Germann, U.A.; Aksentijevich, I.; Sugimoto, Y.; Cardarelli, C.O. and Pastan, I.: Gene transfer of drug resistance genes: implications for cancer therapy. Annals of the New York Academy of Sciences 716, 126, 1994.

Gottlieb, D.J.; Brenner, M.K.; Heslop, H.E.; Bello-Fernandez, C.; Galazka, A. and Prentice, H.G.: Effects of recombinant interleukin 2 administration on cytotoxic function following high dose chemoradiotheray for haematologic malignancy. Blood 74: 2337, 1989.

Gould, B.J.; Borowitz, M.J.; Groves, E.S.; Carter, P.W.; Anthony, D.; Weiner, L.M. and Frankel, A.E.: Phase I study of an anti-breast cancer immunotoxin by continuous infusion: report of a targeted toxic effect not predicted by animal studies. J. Natl. Cancer Inst. 81: 775, 1989.

Gould, R.J.; Polokoff, M.A.; Friedman, P.A.; Huang, T.F.; Holt, J.C.; Cook, J.J. and Niewiaroski, S.: Disintegrins: a family of integrin inhibitory proteins from viper venoms. Proc. Soc. Exp. Biol. Med. 195: 168–171, 1990.

Gould, R.J.; Hartman, G.D.; Chang, C.T.C.; Egbertson, M.S.; Halczenko, W.; Laswell, W.L.; Lynch, R.J.; Manno, P.D.; Smith, R.L. et al.: Selective non-peptide antagonists of platelet alpha-IIB-beta-3. J. Cell Biochem., suppl., 16F: 174, 1992.

Grabstein, K.H.; Namen, A.E.; Shanebeck, K.; Voice, R.F.; Reed, S.G. and Widmer, M.B.: Regulation of T cell proliferation by Il-7. J. Immunol. 144: 3015–3020, 1990.

Graham, G.J.; Wright, E.G.; Hewick, R.; Wolpe, S.D.; Wilkie, N.M. and Donaldson, D.; Lorimore, S. and Pragnell, I.B: Identification and characterization of an inhibitor of haemopoietic stem cell proliferation. Nature 344: 442–444, 1990.

Grand, R.J.A.; Rowe, M.; Byrd, P.J. and Gallimore, P.H.: The level of expression of class-I MHC antigens in adenovirus-transformed human cell lines. Int. J. Cancer 40: 213–219, 1987.

Granowitz, E.V.; Clark, B.D.; Vannier, E.; Callahan, M.V. and Dinarello, C.A.: Effect of interleukin-1 (Il-1) blockade on cytokine synthesis: I. Il-1 receptor antagonist inhibits Il-1-induced cytokine synthesis and blocks the binding of Il-1 to its type II receptor on human monocytes. Blood 79: 2356–2363, 1992.

Grau, G.E.; Fajardo, L.F.; Piguet, P.F.; Allet, B.; Lambert, P.H. and Vassalli, P.: Tumor necrosis factor (cachectin) as an essential mediator in murine cerebral malaria. Science 237: 1210–1212, 1987.

Gravallese, E.M.; Darling, J.M.; Ladd, A.L. and Glimcher, L.H.: Localisation of collagenase and stromelysin mRNA production in rheumatoid synovium. J. of Cell Biochem. suppl. 15E, 181, 1991.

Gray, D.; Kosco, M. and Stockinger, B.: Novel pathways of antigen presentation for the maintenance of memory. Int. Immunol. 3: 141, 1991.

Gray, D. and Matzinger, P.: T cell memory is short lived in the absence of antigen. J. Exp. Med. 174: 969, 1991.

Gray, D. and Skarvall, H.: B-cell memory is short-lived in the absence of antigen. Nature 336: 70, 1988.

Gray, D.; Jainandunsing, S.; Kallberg, E. and Leanderson T.: Affinity maturation of immune responses: molecules and microenvironments. ENII Conf.: Integrated Function of Molecules of the Immune System. Les Embiez, France, 12th-16th May 1993.

Gray, P.W.; Aggarwal, B.b.; Benten, C.V.; Bringman, T.S.; Henzel, W.J.; Jarrett, J.A.; Leung, D.W.; Moffat, B.; Ng, P.; Svedersky, L.P. et al.: Cloning and expression of cDNA for human lymphotoxin, a lymphokine with tumor necrosis activity. Nature 312: 721–724, 1984.

Gray, P.W.; Leong, S.; Fennie, E.H.; Farrar, M.A.; Pingel, J.T.; Fernandez-Luna, J. and Schreiber, R.D.: Cloning and expression of the cDNA for the murine interferon gamma receptor. Proc. Natl. Acad. Sci. 86: 8497–8501, 1989.

Greager, J.A.; Brown, J.M.; Pavel, D.G.; Garcia, J.L.; Blend, M. and Das Gupta, T.K.: Localization of human sarcoma with radiolabeled monoclonal antibody. Cancer Immunol. Immunother. 23: 148, 1986.

Green, D. and Kwaan, H.C.: An acquired factor VIII inhibitor responsive to high-dose gamma-globulin. Thromb. Haemost. 58: 1005–1007, 1987.

Green, H. and Goldberg, B.: The action of antibody and complement on mammalian cells. Ann. NY Acad. Sci. 87: 352–361, 1960.

Greenman, R.L.; Schein, R.M.H.; Martin, M.A.; Wenzel, R.P.; Mac Intyre, N.R.; Emmanuel, G.; Chmel, H.; Kohler, R.B.; McCarthy, M.; Plouffe, J. et al.: A controlled clinical trial of E5 murine monoclonal IgM antibody to endotoxin in the treatment of gram-negative sepsis. JAMA 266: 1097–1102, 1991.

Gregory, C.C.; Murray, R.J.; Edwards, C.F. and Rickinson, A.B.: Downregulation of cell adhesion molecules LFA-3 and ICAM-1 in Epstein-Barr virus-positive Burkitt's lymphoma underlies tumor cell escape from virus-specific T cell surveillance. J. Exp. Med. 167: 1811–1824, 1988.

Gregory, H.: Isolation and structure of urogastrone and its relationship to epidermal growth factor. Nature 257: 325–327, 1975.

Gregory, H.; Young, J.; Schroeder, J.M.; Mrowietz, U. and Christophers, E.: Structure determination of a human lymphocyte derived neutrophil activating peptide (LYNAP). Biochem. Biophys. Res. Commun. 151: 883–890, 1988.

Greig, R.G.: CSAIDs: Cytokine suppressive antiinflammatory drugs. An emerging concept. Rheumatoid Arthritis, Conference Documentation, London (UK), June 17–18, 1991.

Gresele, P.; Deckmyn, H.; Nenci, G.G. and Vermylen, J.: Thromboxane synthase inhibitors, thromboxane receptor antagonists and dual blockers in thrombotic disorders. Trends in Pharmacol. Sciences 12: 158–163, 1991.

Gresele, P.: The platelet in asthma. Int conf. on: The platelet in health & disease. Royal College of Physicians, London, 132, 1992.

Griffiths, G.M.; Berek, C.; Kaartinen, M. and Milstein, C.: Somatic mutation and maturation of the immune response to 2–phenyloxazolone. Nature 321: 271, 1984.

Grob, P.M.; David, E.; Warren, T.C.; DeLeon, R.P.; Farina, P.R. and Homon, C.A.: Characterization of a receptor for human monocyte-derived neutrophil chemotactic factor/interleukin-8. J. Biol. Chem. 265: 8311–8316, 1990.

Groothoff, J.W. and VanLeeuwen, E.F.: High-dose intravenous gammaglobulin in chronic systemic juvenil arthritis. Brit. Med. J. 296: 1362, 1988.

Grossman, N. and Leive, L.: Complement activation via the alternative pathway by purified Salmonella lipopolysaccharide is affected by its structure but not its O-antigen length. J. Immunol. 132: 376–385, 1984.

Grossmann, R.M.; Krueger, J.; Yourish, D.; Granell-Piperno, A.; Murphy, D.P.; May, L.T.; Kupper, T.S.; Sehgal, P.B. and Gottlieb, A.B.: Interleukin-6 is expressed at high levels in psoriatic skin and stimulates proliferation of cultured human keratinocytes. Proc. Natl. Acad. Sci. USA 85: 6367, 1989.

Grotendorst, G.R.; Seppa, H.E.J.; Kleinman, H.K. and Martin, G.R.: Attachment of smooth muscle cells to collagen and their migration toward platelet-derived growth factor. Proc. Natl. Acad. Sci. USA 78: 3669–3672, 1981.

Grotendrost, G.R.; Chang, T.; Seppae, H.E.; Kleinman, H.K. and Martin, G.R.: Platelet-derived growth factor is a chemoattractant for vascular smooth muscle cells. J. Cell Physiol. 113: 261–266, 1982.

Grove, R.I.; Mazzucco, C.E.; Radka, S.F.; Shoyab, M. and Kiener, P.A.: Oncostatin M up-regulates low density lipoprotein receptors in HepG2 cells by a novel mechanism. J. Biol. Chem. 266: 18194–18199, 1991.

Gruber, J. and Cole, J.S.: Vaccines for human cancers of viral etiology. Specific Immunotherapy Of Cancer With Vaccines, eds. Bystryn, J.-C.; Ferrone, S. and Livingston, P., The New York Academy of Sciences 690: 311, 1993.

Gubler, U.; Chua, A.O.; Schoenhout, D.S.; Dwyer, C.M.; McComas, W.; Motyka, R.; Nabavi, N.; Wolitzky, A.G.; Quinn, P.M.; Familletti, P.C. and Gately, M.K.: Coexpression of two distinct genes is required to generate secreted bioactive cytotoxic lymphocyte maturation factor. Proc. Natl. Acad. Sci. USA 88: 4143–4147, 1991.

Guerrero, R.; Velasco, F.; Rodriguez, M.; Lopez, A.; Rojas, R.; Alvarez, M.A.; Villalba, R.; Rubio, V.; Torres, A. and del Castillo, D.: Endotoxin-induced pulmonary dysfunction is prevented by C1–esterase inhibitor. J. Clin. Invest. 91: 2754–2760, 1993.

Guilbert, B.; Dighiero, G. and Avrameas S.: Naturally occurring antibodies against nine common antigens in human sera. I. Detection, isolation and characterization. J. Immun. 128: 2779–2787, 1982.

Guilly, M.N.; Danon, F.; Brouet, J.C.; Bornens, M. and Courvalin J.C.: Autoantibodies to nuclear lamin B in a patient with thrombopenia. Eur. J. cell Biol. 43: 266–272, 1987.

Gyongyossy-Issa, M.I.C. and Devine, D.V.: Human platelet responses to ADP agonist are decreased by homolgous C3a. Compl. Inflamm. 6: 340, 1989.

Haak-Frendscho, M.; Arai, N.; Arai, K.; Baeza, M.L.; Finn, A. and Kaplan, A.P.: Human recombinant granulocyte-macrophage colony-stimulating factor and interleukin 3 cause basophil histamine release. J. Clin. Invest. 82: 17–20, 1988.

Haba, S. and Nisonoff, A.: Inhibition of IgE synthesis by anti-IgE: Role in long-term inhibition of IgE synthesis by neonatally administered soluble IgE. Proc. Natl. Acad. Sci. USA 87: 3363–3367, 1990.

Habenicht, A.J.; Dresel, H.A.; Goerig, M.; Weber, J.A.; Stoehr, M.; Glomset, J.A.; Ross, R. and Schettler, G.: Low density lipoprotein receptor-dependent prostaglandin synthesis in Swiss 3T3 cells stimulated by platelet-derived growth factor. Proc. Natl. Acad. Sci. 83: 1344–1348, 1986.

Haber, E. and Matsueda, G.R.: Method and use for site-specific activation of substances. EPA o 187 658, 1986.

Habicht, G.S.; Beck, G. and Ghebrehiwet, B.: C1q inhibits the expression of B lymphoblastoid cell line Interleukin 1 (Il-1). J. Immunol. 138: 2593–2597, 1987.

Habicht, G.S.; Beck, G. and Ghebrehiwet, B.: Characterization of C1q-induced inhibitors of interleukin. Complement 4: 163, 1987.

Hack, C.E.; Nuijens, J.H.; Felt-Bersma, R.J.F.; Schreuder, W.O.; Eerenberg-Belmer, A.J.M.; Paardekooper, J.; Bronsveld, W. and Thijs, L.G.: Elevated plasma levels of the anaphylatoxins C3a and C4a are associated with a fatal outcome in sepsis. Am. J. Med. 86: 20–26, 1989.

Hack, C.E.; Voerman, H.J.; Eisele, B.; Keinecke, H.-O.; Nuijens, H.J.; Eerenberg, A.J.M.; Ogilvie, A.; Strack van Schijndel, R.J.M.; Delvos, U. and Thijs, L.G.: C1–esterase inhibitor substitution in sepsis. Lancet 339: 378, 1992.

Häyry, P.: Chronic allograft arteriosclerosis: an update. Int. Confcerence on New Trends in Clinical and Experimental Immunosuppression. Geneva, Switzerland, February 10–13, 1994.

Hagan, P.; Poole, S. and Bristow, A.F.: Immunosuppressive activity of corticotrophin-releasing factor. Imhibition of interleukin-1 and interleukin-6 production by human mononuclear cells. Biochem J. 281: 251–254, 1992.

Haisma, H.J.; Moseley, K.R.; Battaile, A.; Zurawski, V.R. and Knapp, R.C.: Biodistribution, pharmacokinetics and imaging of I-131–labeled OC125 in patients with ovarian carcinoma. Br. J. Cancer 56: 519, 1987.

Hajjar, K.A. and Hamel, N.M.: Identification and characterization of human endothelial cell membrane binding sites for tissue plasminogen activator and urokinase. J. Biol. Chem. 265: 2908–2916, 1990.

Hakem, R.; le Bouteiller, P.; Barad, M.; Trujillo, M.; Mercier, P.; Wietzerbin, J. and Lemonnier, F.A.: IFN-mediated differential regulation of the expression of HLA-B7 and HLA-A3 class I genes. J. Immunol. 142: 297–305, 1989.

Hall, N.R.S.; O'Grady, M.P. and Menzies, R.A.: Thymic regulation of the hypothalamic-pituitary-gonadal axis. Int. J. Immunopharm. 14: 353–359, 1992.

Hall-Angerás, M.; Angerás, U.; Zamir, O.; Hasselgren, P.O. and Fischer, J.E.: Interaction between corticosterone and tumor necrosis factor stimulated protein breakdown in rat skeletal muscle, similar to sepsis. Surgery 180: 460–466, 1990.

Hallberg, T.; Dohlstein, M. and Baldetorp, B.: Demonstration of histamine receptors on human platelets by flow cytometry. Scand. J. Haematol. 32: 113–118, 1984.

Haller, D.G.: A phase I trial of 90Y labeled monoclonal antibody (MoAb) B72.3 (CYT-103–90Y) in refractory adenocarcinomas. 6th Int. Conf. on Monoclonal Antibody Immunoconjugates for Cancer, San Diego, 1991.

Hallett, M.B.; Luzio, P.J. and Campbell, A.K.: Stimulation of Ca2+ dependent chemiluminescence in rat polymorphonuclear leucocytes by polystyrene beads, and the non-lytic action of complement. Immunology 44: 569–577, 1981.

Hallmann, R.; Jutila, M.A.; Smith, C.W.; Anderson, D.C.; Kishimoto, T.K. and Butcher, E.C.: The peripheral lymph node homing receptor, LECAM-1 is involved in CD18–independent adhesion of human neutrophils to endothelium. Biochem. Biophys. Res. Comm. 174: 236–243, 1991.

Halpern, M. and Schwartz, S.: Regulation of the low affinity IgE Fc receptor (CD23) in atopic dermatitis. Int. Arch. Allergy Immunol. 100: 197–200, 1993.

Hamada, A. and Greene, B.M.: C1q enhancement of IgG-dependent eosinophil-mediated killing of Schistosomula in vitro. J. Immunol. 138: 1240–1245, 1987.

Hamada, F.; Aoki, M.; Akiyama, T. and Toyoshima, K.: Association of immunoglobulin G Fc receptor II with Src-like protein-tyrosine kinase Fgr in neutrophils. Proc. Natl. Acad. Sci. USA 90: 6305–6309, 1993.

Hamann, A.; Jablonski, D.; Duijvestijn, A.; Butcher, E.C.; Baisch, H.; Harder, R. and Thiele, H.G.: Evidence for an accessory role of LFA-1 in lymphocyte-high endothelium interaction during homing. J. Immunol. 140: 693–699, 1988.

Hamblin, T.J.; Catton, A.R.; Glennie, M.J.; MacKenzie, M.R.; Stevenson, F.K.; Watts, H.F. and Stevenson, G.T.: Initial experience in treating human lymphoma with a chimeric univalent derivative of monoclonal anti-idiotype antibody. Blood 69: 790, 1986.

Hamid, Q.; Azzawi, M.; Ying, S.; Moqbel, R.; Wardlaw, A.J.; Corrigan, C.J.; Bradley, B.; Durham, S.R.; Collins, J.V.; Jeffery, P.K.; Quint, D.J. and Kay, A.B.: Expression of mRNA for interleukin-5 in mucosal bronchial biopsies from asthma. J. Clin. Invest. 87: 1541, 1991.

Hamilton, B.W.; Helling, F.; Lloyd, K.O. and Livingston, P.O.: Ganglioside expression on human malignant melanoma assessed by quantitative immune thin layer chromatography. Int. J. Cancer 53: 566–573, 1993.

Hamilton, J.A.; Leizer, T.; Piccoli, D.S.; Royston, K.M.; Butler, D.M. and Croatto, M.: Oncostatin M stimulates urokinase-type plasminogen activator activity in human synovial fibroblasts. Biochem. Biophys. Res. Commun. 180: 652–659, 1991.

Hamilton, R.G.: Human IgG subclass measurements in the clinical laboratory. Clin. Chem. 33: 1707–1725, 1987.

Hammer, J.; Valsasnini, P. and Sinigaglia, F.: Promiscuous and allele-specific anchors in HLA-DR binding peptides. ENII Conf.: Integrated Function of Molecules of the Immune System. Les Embiez, France, 12th-16th May 1993.

Hancock, W.W.; Pleau, M.E. and Kobzik, L.: Recombinant granulocyte-macrophage colony-stimulating factor down-regulates expression of IL-2 receptor on human mononuclear phagocytes by induction of prostaglandine. J. Immun. 140: 3021–3025, 1988.

Hann, L.E.; Allansmith, M.R. and Sullivan, D.A.: Impact of aging and gender on the Ig-containing cell profile of the lacrimal gland. Acta Ophthal. 66: 87–92, 1988.

Hann, L.E.; Tatro, J. and Sullivan, D.A.: Morphology and function of lacrimal gland acinar cells in primary culture: Invest. Ophthal. Vis. Sci. 30: 145–158, 1989.

Hanna, M.G.; Ransom, J.H.; Pomato, N.; Peters, L.; Bloemena, E.; Vermorken, J.B. and Hoover, H.C.: Active specific immunotherapy of human colorectal carcinoma with an autologous tumor cell/bacillus Calmette-Guérin vaccine. Specific Immunotherapy Of Cancer With Vaccines, eds. Bystryn, J.-C.; Ferrone, S. and Livingston, P., The New York Academy of Sciences 690: 135, 1993.

Hannestad, K.: IgM rheumatoid factors reacting with nitrophenyl groups and denatured deoxyribonucleic acid. Ann. N.Y. Acad. Sci. 168: 63–75, 1969.

Hannestad, K. and Stollar, B.D.: Certain rheumatoid factors react with nucleosomes. Nature 275: 671, 1979.

Hannum, C.H.; Wilcox, C.J.; Arend, W.P.; Renneke, G.J.; Dripps, D.J.; Heimdal, P.L.; Armes, L.G.; Sommer, A.; Eisenberg, S.P. and Thompson, R.C.: Interleukin-1 receptor antagonist activity of a human interleukin-1 inhibitor. Nature 343: 336–340, 1990.

Hansch, G.M.; Seitz, M.; Marinotti, G.; Betz, M.: Hauterberg, E.W. and Shin, M.L.: Macrophages release arachidonic acid, prostaglandin E2, and thromboxane in response to late complement components. J. Immunol. 133: 2145–2150, 1984.

Hansch, G.M.; Seitz, M. and Betz, M.: Effect of the late complement components C5b-9 on human monocytes: release of prostanoids, oxygen radicals and of a factor inducing cell proliferation. Int. Arch. Allergy Appl. Immunol. 82: 317–320, 1987.

Hansch, G.M.: The homologous species restriction of complement attack: structure and function of the C8–binding protein. In: Podack, E.R. (ed.) Cytotoxic effector mechanisms. Springer Berlin, 109–118 (Current topics in microbiology and immunology, vol. 140), 1988.

Hansch, G.M.; Betz, M.; Gunther, J.; Rother, K.O. and Sterzel, B.: The complement membrane attack complex stimulates the prostanoid production of cultured glomerular mesangial cells. Int. Arch. Allergy Appl. Immunol. 85: 87–93, 1988.

Hansch, G.M.; Torbohm, I. and Rother, K.: Chronic glomerulonephritis: inflammatory mediators stimulate the collagen synthesis in glomerular epithelial cells. Int. Arch. Allergy Appl. Immunol. 88: 139–143, 1989.

Hansen, E.W. and Christensen, J.D.: Endotoxin and interleukin-1ß induces fever and increased plasma oxytocin in rabbits. Pharmacol. & Toxicol. 70: 389–391, 1992.

Hardin, J.A. and Thomas, J.O.: Antibodies to histones in systemic lupus erythematosus: localization of prominent autoantigens on histones H1 and H2b. Proc. natn. Acad. Sci. USA 80: 7410–7414, 1983.

Harding, F.A.; McArthur, J.G.; Gross, J.A.; Raulet, D.H. and Allison, J.P.: CD28–mediated signalling co-stimulates murine T-cells and prevents induction of anergy in T-cell clones. Nature 356: 607–609, 1992.

Hareuveni, M.; Gautier, C.; Kieny, M.P.; Wreschner, D.; Chambon, P. and Lathe, R.: Vaccination against tumor cells expressing breast cancer epithelial tumor antigen. Proc. Natl. Acad. Sci. USA 87: 9498–9502, 1990.

Harnett, M. and Rigley, K.: The role of G-proteins versus protein tyrosine kinases in the regulation of lymphocyte activation. Immunol. Today 13: 482, 1992.

Harper; J.W.; Strydom, D.J. and Lobb, R.R.: Human class 1 heparin-binding growth factor: structure and homology to bovine acidic brain fibroblast growth factor. Biochemistry 25: 4097–4103, 1986.

Harper, K.; Balzano, C.; Rouvier, E.; Mattei, M.-G.; Luciani, M.-F. and Golstein, P.: CTLA-4 and CD28 activated lymphocyte molecules are closely related in both mouse and human as to sequence, message expression, gene structure, and chromosomal location. J. Immunol. 147: 1037–1044, 1991.

Harriman, G.R.; Kunimoto, D.Y.; Elliott, J.F.; Paetkau, V. and Strober, W.: The role of Il-5 in IgA B cell differentiation. J. Immunol. 140: 3033–3039, 1988.

Harriman, G.R.; Lycke, N.Y.; Elwood, L.J. and Strober, W.: T lymphocytes that express CD4 and the µß-T cell receptor but lack Thy-1: Preferential localization in Peyer's patches. J. Immunol. 145: 2406–2414, 1990.

Hart, C.E.; Forstrom, J.W.; Kelly, J.D.; Seifert, R.A.; Smith, R.A.; ross, R.; Murray, M.J. and Bowen-Pope, D.F.: Two classes of PDGF receptor recognize different isoforms of PDGF. Science 240: 1529–1531, 1988.

Hart, P.H.; Vitti, G.V.; Burgess, D.R.; Whitiy, G.A.; Piccoli, D.S. and Hamilton, J.A.: Potential anti-inflammatory effects of IL-4: suppression of human monocyte tumor necrosis factor, IL-1 and prostaglandin E2. Proc. Natl. Acad. Sci. USA 86: 3803–3807, 1989.

Hart, P.H.; Whitty, G.A.; Piccoli, D.S. and Hamilton, J.A.: Control by IFN-gamma and PGE2 of TNFµ and Il-1 production by human monocytes. Immunology 66: 376, 1989.

Hartman, A.B.; Mallett, C.P.: Srinivasappa, J.; Prabhakar, B.S.; Notkins, A.L. and Smith-Gill, S.J.: Organ reactive autoantibodies from non-immunized adult Balb/c mice are polyreactive and express non-biased VH gene usage. Mol. Immunol. 26: 359, 1989.

Hartung, H.-P.; Schafer, B.; Heeininger, K. and Toyka, K.Y.: Recombinant interleukin-1β stimulates eicosanoid production in rat primary culture astrocytes. Brain Res. 489: 113–119, 1989.

Haskard, D.O.: Integrins and other intercellular adhesion molecules. Rheumatoid Arthritis, Conference Documentation, London (UK), June 17–18, 1991.

Haskard, D.: Overview of adhesion molecules in disease (abstract). Cell Adhesion Molecules in Cancer and Inflammation, London, IBC, 1991.

Haslam, R.J.: Signal transduction in platelets; implications for drug development. Int. Conf. on: The platelet in health & disease. Royal College of Physicians, London, 1, 1992.

Hasty, K.A.; Pourmotabbed, T.F.; Goldberg, G.I.; Thompson, J.P.; Spinella, D.G.; Stevens, R.M. and Mainardi, C.L.: Human neutrophil collagenase. A distinct gene product with homology to other matrix metalloproteinases. J. Biol. Chem. 265: 11421–11424, 1990.

Hatekeyama, M.; Tsudo, M.; Minamoto, S.; Kono, T.; Doi, T.; Miyata, T.; Miyasaka, M. and Taniguchi T.: Interleukin-2 receptor ß chain gene: generation of three receptor forms by cloned human μ and ß chain cDNAs. Science 252: 1523–1528, 1989.

Hatekeyama, M.; Knon, T.; Kobayashi, N.; Kawahara, A.; Levin, S.D.; Perlmutter, R.M. and Taniguchi, T.: Interaction of the IL-2 receptor with the src-family kinase p56lck: Identification of novel intermolecular association. Science 252: 1523–1528, 1991.

Hauptmann, G.: Frequency of complement deficiencies in man, disease associated and chromosome assignment of complement genes and linkage groups. Complement 6: 74–80, 1989.

Havell, E.A.: Production of tumor necrosis factor during murine listeriosis. J. Immunol. 139: 4225, 1987.

Hawgood, S.; Benson, B.J.; Schilling, J.; Damm, D.; Clements, J.A. and White, R.T.: Nucleotide and amino acid sequences of pulmonary surfactant protein SP 18 and evidence for cooperation between SP 18 and SP 28–36 in surfactant lipid adsorption. Proc. Natl. Acad. Sci. USA 84: 66–70, 1987.

Hawkins, R.E.; Winter, G.; Hamblin, T.J.; Stevenson, F.K. and Russell, S.J.: A genetic approach to idiotypic vaccination. J. Immunother. 14: 273–278, 1994.

Haynes, J.; Seibert, A.; Bass, J.B. and Taylor, A.E.: U74500A inhibition of oxidant-mediated lung injury. Am. J. Physiol. 259: 144, 1990.

Hebell, T.; Ahearn, J.M. and Fearon, D.T.: Suppression of the immune response by a soluble complement receptor of B lymphocytes. Science 254: 102–105, 1991.

Hebert, L.A.; Cosio, F.G.; Birmingham, D.J. and Mahan, J.D.: Biologic significance of the erythrocyte complement receptor: a primate perquisite. J. Lab. Clin. Med. 118: 301–308, 1991.

Hebert, L.A.; Cosio, F.G. and Birmingham, D.J.: The role of complement system in renal injury. Seminars in Nephrology 12: 408–427, 1992.

Hedlund, G.; Dohlsten, M.; Lando, P.A. and Kalland, T.: Staphylococcal enterotoxins direct and trigger CTL killing of autologous HLA-DR+ mononuclear leukocytes and freshly prepared leukemia cells. Cell. Immunol. 129: 426–434, 1990.

Hedlund, G.; Dohlsten, M.; Petersson, C. and Kalland, T.: Superantigen-based tumor therapy: in vivo activation of cytotoxic T cells. Cancer Immunol. Immunother. 36: 89–93, 1993.

Heeg, K.; Miethke, T.; Bader, P.; Bendigs, S.; Wahl, C. and Wagner, H.: CD4/CD8 coreceptor-independent costimulator dependent triggering of SEB-reactive murine T cells. Cur. Top. Microbiol. Immunol. 174: 93, 1991.

Heldin, C.H.; Wasteson, A. and Westermark, B.: Interaction of platelet-derived growth factor with its fibroblast receptor. J. Biol. Chem. 257: 4216–4221, 1982.

Heldin, C.H. and Roennstrand, L.: Characterization of the receptor for platelet-derived growth factor on human fibroblasts. Demonstration of an intimate relationship with a 185,000–Dalton substrate for the platelet-derived growth factor-stimulated kinase. J. Biol. Chem. 258: 10054–10061, 1983.

Helene, C.; Thuong, N.T. and Harel-Bellan, A.: Control of gene expression by triple helix-forming oligonucleotides. Antisense Strategies, eds. Baserga, R. and Denhardt, D.T., Annals of the New York Academy of Sciences 660: 27, 1992.

Helfgott, D.C.; Tatter, S.B.; Santhanam, E.; Clarick, R.H.; Bhardwaj, N.; May, L.T. and Sehgal, P.B.: Multiple forms of IFN-ß2/IL-6 in serum and body fluids during the acute bacterial infection. J. Immunol. 142: 948, 1989.

Heller, R.A.; Song, K.; Onasch, M.A.; Fischer, W.H.; Chang, D. and Ringold, G.M.: Complementary DNA cloning of a receptor for tumor necrosis factor and demonstration of a shed form of the receptor. Proc. Natl. Acad. Sci. 87: 6151–6155, 1990.

Helling, F.; Adluri, S.; Calves, M.; Koganty, R.R.; Oettgen, H.F. and Livingston, P.O.: Increased immunogenicity of GM2 conjugates with KLH and used with adjuvants in patients with melanoma. Proc. Am. Assoc. Cancer Res. 34: 491, 1993.

Helling, F.; Calves, M.; Shang, Y.; Oettgen, H.F. and Livingston, P.O.: Construction of immunogenic GD3–conjugate vaccines. Specific Immunotherapy of Cancer with Vaccines, Bystryn, J.C.; Ferrone, S. and Livingston, P. (eds)., Annals of the New York Academy of Sciences 690: 396–397, 1993.

Helling, F.; Shang, A.; Calves, M.; Zhang, S.; Ren, S.; Yu, R.K.; Oettgen, H.F. and Livingston, P.O.: GD3 vaccines for melanoma: superior immunogenicity of keyhole limpet hemocyanin conjugate vaccines. Cancer Res. 54: 197–203, 1994.

Hellström, K.E.; Hellström, I.; Linsley, P. and Chen, L.: On the role of costimulation in tumor immunity. Specific Immunotherapy Of Cancer With Vaccines, eds. Bystryn, J.-C.; Ferrone, S. and Livingston, P., The New York Academy of Sciences 690: 225, 1993.

Hemler, M.E.; Huang, C.; Takada; Schwarz, L.; Strominger, J.L. and Clabby, M.L.: Characterization of the cell surface heterodimer VLA-4 and related peptides. J. Biol. Chem. 262: 11478–11485, 1989.

Henson, P.M. and Pinckard, R.N.: Basophil-derived platelet-activating factor (PAF) as an in vivo mediator of acute allergic reactions: demonstration of specific desensitization of platelets to PAF during IgE-induced anaphylaxis in the rabbit. J. Immunol. 119: 2179–2184, 1977.

Henson, P.M. and Ginsberg, M.H.: Immunological reactions of platelets. In: Gordon, J.L. (ed.) Platelets in Biology and Pathology-2, Elsevier/North Holland Biomedical Press, Oxford, 265–308, 1981

Herbelin, A.; Machavoine, F.; Schneider, E.; Papiernik, M. and Dy, M.: Il-7 is requisite for Il-1–induced thymocyte proliferation. Involvement of Il-7 in the synergistic effects of granulocyte-macrophage colony-stimulating factor or tumor necrosis factor with Il-1. J. Immunol. 148: 99–105, 1992.

Herd, C.M.: Pharmacological modulation of PAF-induced platelet accumulation in the pulmonary circulation of the rabbit. Br. J. Pharmacol. 102: 175P, 1991.

Herd, C.M. and Page, C.P.: Methods for assessing anti-platelet drugs. Int. Conf. on: The platelet in health & disease. Royal College of Physicians, London, 1992.

Hericourt, J. and Richet, C.: Physiologie Pathologique - de la serotherapie dans le traitement du cancer. C. r. hebd. Seanc. Acad. Sci. Paris 121: 567, 1885.

Herlyn, M. and Malkowicz S.B.: Biology of disease. Regulatory pathways in tumor growth and invasion. Laboratory Investigations 65: 292, 1991.

Herman, A.; Kappler, J.W.; Marrack, P. and Pullen, A.M.: Superantigens: Mechanism of T-cell stimulation and role in immune responses. Annu. Rev. Immunol. 9: 745–772, 1991.

Herold, M. and Mur, E.: sICAM-1 levels in patients with rheumatoid arthritis. WMW 4: 1992.

Heron, I.; Hokland, M. and Berg, K.: Enhanced expression of ß2–microglobulin and HLA antigens on human lymphoid cells by interferon. Proc. Natl. Acad. Sciences USA 75: 6215–6219, 1978.

Herrmann, F.; Oster, W.; Meuer, S.C.; Lindemann, A. and Mertelsmann, R.H.: Interleukin 1 stimulates T lymphocytes to produce granulocyte-monocyte colony-stimulating factor. J. Clin. Invest. 81: 1415–1418, 1988.

Herrmann, T.; Maryanski, J.L.; Romero, P.; Fleischer, B. and Mac Donald, H.R.: Activation of MHC class I-restricted CD8+ CTL by microbial T cell mitogens. Dependence upon MHC class II expression of the target cells and Vß usage of the responder T cells. J. Immunol. 144: 1181–1186, 1990.

Hersey, P.: Evaluation of vaccinia viral lysates as therapeutic vaccines in the treatment of melanoma. Specific Immunotherapy Of Cancer With Vaccines, eds. Bystryn, J.-C.; Ferrone, S. and Livingston, P., The New York Academy of Sciences 690: 167, 1993.

Hershey, G.K.; McCourt, D.W. and Schreiber, R.D.: Ligand-induced phosphorylation of the human interferon-gamma receptor. Dependence on the presence of a functionally active receptor. J. biol. Chem. 265: 17868–17875, 1990.

Hertler, A.A.; Schlossman, D.M.; Borowicz, M.J.; Blythman, H.E.; Casellas, P. and Frankel, A.E.: An anti-CD5 immunotoxin for chronic lymphocytic leukemia: Enhancement of cytotoxicity with human serum albumin-monensin. Int. J. Cancer 43: 215, 1989.

Herz, A.; Höllt, V.; Przewtocki, R.; Osborne, H.; Gramsch, C. and Duka, T.: Functional aspects of endorphins. In: Progress in Biochemical Pharmacology (eds. Levy, A.; Heldman, E.; Vogel, Z. and Gutman, Y.), 16: 11–21, 1980. Karger, Basel.

Herzog, C.; Walker, C.; Pichler, W.; Aeschlimann, A.; Wassmer, P.; Stockinger, H.; Knapp, W.; Rieber, P. and Müller, W.: Monoclonal anti-CD4 in arthritis. Lancet II: 1461–1462, 1987.

Herzog, C.; Walker, C.; Müller, W.; Rieber, P.; Reiter, C.; Riethmüller, G.; Wassmer, P.; Stockinger, H.; Madic, O. and Pichler, W.J.K.: Anti-CD4 treatment of patients with rheumatoid arthritis. I. Effect on clinical course and circulating T-cells. J. Autoimmun. 2: 627–642, 1989.

Hess, A.D.; Tutschka, P.J. and Santos, G.W.: CsA inhibits the production of T lymphocyte growth factors in secondary mixed lymphocyte responses but does not inhibit the responses of primed lymphocytes to TCGF. J. Immunol. 128: 355–359, 1982.

Heyman, B.; Nose, M. and Weigle, W.O.: Carbohydrate chains on IgG2b: a requirement for efficient feedback immunosuppression. J. Immunol. 134: 4018, 1985.

Hibi, M.; Murakami, M.; Saito, M.; Hirano, T.; Taga, T. and Kishimoto, T.: Molecular cloning and expression of an IL-6 signal transducer, gp130. Cell 1149, 1990.

Hibio, S.; Michihiro, N.; Ogawa, K.; Goto, K.; Suzuki, H.; Shihara, H.; Ariizumi, M. and Baba, K.: Clinical effects and serum globulin changes following non-treated immunoglobulin administration in West syndrome. Brain Dev. 7: 183, 1985.

Hickey, K.A.; Rubanyi, G.; Paul, R.J. and Highsmith, R.F.: Characterization of coronary vasoconstrictor produced by cultured endothelial cells. Amer. J. Physiol. 248: 550–556, 1985.

Hickman, C.J.; Crim, J.A.; Mostowski, H.S. and Siegel, J.P.: Regulation of human cytotoxic T lymphocyte development by Il-7 J. Immunol. 145: 2415–2420, 1990.

Hidou, M. and Vivant, O.J.F.: Intérêt des immunoglobulines par voie veineuse. Un cas de syndrome de Guillain-Barré. Rev. Neurol. (Paris) 148: 706–708, 1992.

Hilgartner, M.W. and Bussel, J.: Use of intravenous gammaglobulin for the treatment of autoimmune neutropenia of childhood and autoimmune hemolytic anemia. Am. J. Med. 83: 25, 1987.

Hill, A.D.K.; Redmond, H.P.; Croke, D.T.; Grace, P.A. and Bouchier-Hayes, D.: Cytokines in tumour therapy. Br. J. Surg. 79: 990–997, 1992.

Hill, J.; Lindsay, T.F.; Ortiz, F.; Yeh, C.G.; Hechtman, H.B. and Moore, F.D.: Soluble complement receptor type 1 ameliorates the local and remote organ injury after intestinal ischemia-reperfusion in the rat. J. Immunol. 149: 1723–1728, 1992.

Hillarby, M.C.; Clarkson, R.; Grennan, D.M.; Bate, A.S.; Ollier, W.; Sanders, P.A.; Chattophadhyay, C.; Davis, M.; O'Sullivan, M.M. and Williams, B.: Immunogenetic heterogeneity in rheumatoid disease as illustrated by different MHC associations (DG, Dw and C4) in articular and extra-articular subsets. Br. J. Rheumatol. 30: 5–9, 1991.

Hilleman, M.R.: The promise and the reality of viral vaccines against cancer. Specific Immunotherapy Of Cancer With Vaccines, eds. Bystryn, J.-C.; Ferrone, S. and Livingston, P., The New York Academy of Science 690: 6, 1993.

Hilton, D.J.; Nicola, N.A. and Metcalf, D.: Specific binding of murine leukemia inhibitory factor to normal and leukemic monocytic cells. Proc. Natl. Acad. Sci. 85: 5971–5975, 1988.

Hinshaw, L.B.; Tekamp-Olson, P.; Chang, A.C.; Lee, P.A.; Taylor, F.B.jr.; Murrray, C.K.; Peer, G.T.; Emerson, T.E.jr.; Passey, R.B. and Kuo, G.C.: Survival of primates in LD100 septic shock following therapy with antibody to tumor necrosis factor (TNF-µ). Circ. Shock. 30: 279, 1990.

Hirano, T.; Matsuda, T.; Turner, M.; Miyasaka, N.; Buchan, G.; Tang, B.; Sato, K.; Shimizu, M.; Maini, R.; Feldman, M. and Kishimoto, T.: Excessive production of interleukin6/B-cells stimulatory factor-2 in rheumatoid arthritis. Eur. J. Immunol. 18: 1797, 1988.

Hirano, T.: Interleukin 6 (IL-6) and its receptor: their role in plasma cell neoplasia. Int. J. Cell. Cloning 9: 166, 1991.

Hirano, T.: Interleukin-6 and its relation to inflammation and disease. Clin. Immunol. Immunopath. 62: 60, 1992.

Hirschhorn, R.: Adenosine deaminase deficiency. In Rosen FS, Seligmann M (eds.). Immunodeficiency reviews, vol. 2, London: Howard, 175–198, 1990.

Hiti-Harper, J.; Wohl, H. and Harper, E.: Platelet factor 4: an inhibitor of collagenase. Science 199: 991–992, 1978.

Hivroz, C.; Le Deist, F.; Partisetti, M.; Buc, H.A.; Rieux-Laucat, F.; Chocquet, D. and Fischer, A.: Abnormal signal transduction in primary T-cell immunodeficiencies. ENII Conf.: Integrated Function of Molecules of the Immune System. Les Embiez, France, 12th-16th May 1993.

Hivroz, E.; Valle, A.; Brouet, J.C.; Banchereau, J. and Grillot-Courvalin, C.: Regulation by interleukin 2 of CD23 expression of leukemic and normal B cells: Comparison with interleukin 4. Eur. J. Immunol. 19: 1025–1030, 1989.

Hnatowich, D.J.; Chinol, M.; Siebecker, D.A.; Gionet, M.; Griffin, T.; Doherty, P.W.; Hunter, R.E. and Kase, K.R.: Patient biodistribution of intraperitoneally administered Yttrium-90-labeled antibody. J. Nucl. Med. 29: 1428–1434, 1988.

Hobson, B. and Denekamp, J.: Endothelial proliferation in tumors and normal tissues: Continuous labeling studies. Br. J. Cancer 49: 405–413, 1984.

Hock, H.; Dorsch, M.; Diamantstein, T. and Blankenstein, T.: Interleukin 7 induces CD4+ T cell-dependent tumor rejection. J. Exp. Med. 174: 1291–1298, 1991.

Hock, H.; Dorsch, M.; Kunzendorf, U.; Überla, K.; Qin, Z.; Diamantstein, T. and Blankenstein, T.: Vaccinations with tumor cells genetically engineered to produce different cytokines: effectivity not superior to a classical adjuvant. Cancer Res. 53: 714–716, 1993.

Hockel, M.; Jung, W.; Vaupel, P.; Rabes, H.; Khaledpour, C. and Wissler, J.H.: Purified monocyte-derived angiogenic substance (angiotropin) induces controlled angiogenesis associated with regulated tissue proliferation in rabbit skin. J. Clin. Invest. 82: 1075–1090, 1988.

Hoffman, M.K. and Kappler, J.W.: Two distinct mechanisms of immune suppression by antibody. Nature 272: 64–65, 1978.

Hoffman, T.; Lee, Y.L.; Lizzio, E.F.; Tripathi, A.K.; Jessop, J.J.; Taplits, M.; Abrahamsen, T.G.; Carter, C.S. and Puri, J.: Absence of modulation of monokine production via endogenous cyclooxygenase or 5-lipoxygenase metabolites: MK-886 (3-(-1-(4-chlorobenzyl)-3–t-butyl-thio-5-isopropylindol-2yl)-2,2-dimethylpropanoic acid), indomethacin, or arachidonate fail to alter immunoreactive interleukin-1ß, or TNF-µ production by human monocytes in vitro. Clin. Immun. Immunother. 58: 399–408, 1991.

Hoffmann, A.; Heck, M.M.S.; Bordwell, B.J.; Rothfield, N.F. and Earnshaw, W.C.: Human autoantibody to topoisomerase II. Expl. Cell Res. 180: 409–418, 1989.

Hofman, F.M.; Brock, M.; Taylor, C.R. and Lyons, B.: IL-4 regulates differentiation and proliferation of human precursor B cells. J. Immunol. 141: 1185–1190, 1988.

Hogg, N.: Leukocyte integrin activation. Proc. Cell adhesion molecules in cancer and inflammation (abstract). London Roy Coll obstet Gynec. 5, 1991.

Hokland, M.; Larson, D.; Heron, I. and Plessner, T.: Corticosteroids decrease the expression of ß2–microglobulin and histocompatibility antigens on human peripheral blood lymphocyts in vitro. Clin. Exp. Immunol. 44: 239–246, 1981.

Holguin, M.H.; Wilcox, L.A.; Bernshaw, N.J.; Rosse, W.F. and Parker, C.J.: Relationship between the membrane inhibitor of reactive lysis (MIRL) and the erythrocyte (E) phenotypes of paroxysmal nocturnal hemoglobinuria (PNA). Compl. Inflamm. 6: 346, 1989.

Holliger, P.; Prospero, T. and Winter, G.: "Diabodies": small bivalent and bispecific antibody fragments. Proc. Natl. Acad. Sci. USA 90: 6444–6448, 1993.

Hollstein, M.; Sidransky, D.; Vogelstein, B. and Harris, C.C.: p53 mutations in human cancers. Science 253: 49–53, 1991.

Holman, H.R.; Deicher, H.R.G. and Kunkel, H.G.: The LE cell and the LE serum factors. Bull. N.Y. Acad. Med. 35: 409–418, 1959.

Holmes, W.E.; Lee, J.; Kuang, W.J.; Rice, G.C. and Wood, W.I.: Structure and functional expression of a human interleukin-8 receptor. Science 253: 1278–1280, 1991.

Holmsen, H. and Weiss, H.J.: Secretable storage pools in platelets. Annu. Rev. Med. 30: 119–134, 1979.

Honda, M.; Yamamoto, S.; Cheng, M.; Yasukawa, K.; Suzuki, H.; Saito, T.; Osugi, Y.; Tokunaga, T. and Kishimoto, T.: Human soluble Il-6 receptor: its detection and enhanced release by HIV infection. J. Immunol. 148: 2175–2180, 1992.

Hoon, D.S.B.; Morisaki, T.; Uchiyama, A.; Hayashi, Y.; Foshag, L.J.; Nizze, A.J. and Morton, D.L.: Augmentation of T-cell response with a melanoma cell vaccine expressing specific HLA-A antigens. Specific Immunotherapy Of Cancer With Vaccines, eds. Bystryn, J.-C.; Ferrone, S. and Livingston, P., The New York Academy of Sciences 690: 343, 1993.

Hopkins, S.J.; Humphreys, M.; Kinnaird, A.; Jones, D.A. and Kimber, I.: Production of interleukin-1 by draining lymph node cells during the induction phase of contact sensitization in mice. Immunology 71: 493–496, 1990.

Horneff, G.; Burmester, G.R.; Emmrich, F. and Kalden, J.R.: Treatment of rheumatoid arthritis with an anti-CD4 monoclonal antibody. Arthritis Rheum. 34: 129–140, 1991.

Horneff, G.; Winkler, T.; Kalden, J.R.; Emmrich, F. and Burmester, G.R.: Human anti-mouse antibody response induced by anti-CD4 monoclonal antibody therapy in patients with rheumatoid arthritis. Clin. Immunol. Immunopathol. 59: 89–103, 1991.

Horneff, G.; Emmrich, F. and Burmester, G.R.: Advances in immunotherapy of rheumatoid arthritis: clinical and immunological findings following treatment with anti-CD4 antibodies. Br. J. Rheumat. 32 (suppl. 4): 39–47, 1993.

Horohov, D.W.; Crim, J.A.; Smith, P.L. and Siegel, J.P.: IL-4 (B cell-stimulatory factor 1) regulates multiple aspects of influenza virus-specific cell-mediated immunity. J. Immunol. 141: 4217–4223, 1988.

Horwitz, A.H.; Chang, C.P.; Better, M.; Hellström, K.E. and Robbinson, R.R.: Secretion of functional antibody and Fab fragment from yeast cells. Proc. Natl. Acad. Sci. USA 85: 8678–8682, 1988.

Hosoda, K.; Nakao, K.; Hiroshi-Arai; Suga, S.; Ogawa, Y.; Mukoyama, M.; Shirakami, G.; Saito, Y.; Nakanishi, S. and Imura, H.: Cloning and expression of human endothelin-1 receptor cDNA. FEBS Lett. 287: 23–26, 1991.

Hotermans, G.; Bury, T. and Radermecker, M.F.: Effect of histamine on tumor necrosis factor production by human monocytes. Int. J. Allergy Appl. Immunol. 95: 278, 1991.

Houghton, A.N.; Vijayasaradhi, S.; Bouchard, B.; Naftzger, C.; Hara, I. and Chapman P.B.: Recognition of autoantigens by patients with melanoma. Specific Immunotherapy Of Cancer With Vaccines, eds. Bystryn, J.-C.; Ferrone, S. and Livingston, P., The New York Academy of Sciences 690: 59, 1993.

Houle, J.J.; Leddy, J.P. and Rosenfield, S.I.: Secretion of the terminal complement proteins, C5–C9, by human platelets. Clin. Immunol. Immunopathol. 50: 385–393, 1989.

Hourcade, D. and Atkinson, J.P.: The regulators of complement activation (RCA) gene cluster. Prog. Immunol. VII: 171–177, 1989.

Hovanessian, A.G.; Krust, B.; Jacotot, E. and Callebaut, C.: Entry of HIV into CD4+ cells requires the T cell activation antigen CD26. Abstract, 8th Cent. Gardes Meeting, Paris, October 25–27, 1993.

Hovi, T.; Saksela, O. and Vaheri A.: Increased secretion of plasminogen activator by human macrophages after exposure to leucocyte interferon. FEBS Lett. 129: 233–236, 1981.

Howard, B.; Burrascano, M.; McCallister, T.; Chong, K.; Gangavalli, R.; Severinsson, L.; Jolly, D.J.; Darrow, T.; Vervaert, C.; Arbdel-Wahab, Z.; Siegler, H.F. and Barber, J.R.: Retrovirus-mediated gene transfer of the human gamma-IFN gene: a therapy for cancer. New York Academy of Sciences 716, 167, 1994.

Howard, M. Farrar, J.; Hilfiker, M.; Johnson, B.; Takatsu, K.; Hamaoka, T. and Paul, W.E.: Identification of a T cell-derived B cell growth factor distinct from interleukin 2. J. Exp. Med. 155: 914–923, 1982.

Howard, M.; Farrar, J.; Hilfiker, M.; Johnson, B.; Takatsu, K.; Hamaoka, T. and Paul, W.E.: Identification of a T-cell derived B cell growth factor distinct from IL-2. J. Exp. Med. 155: 914–921, 1982.

Howard, M. and Paul, W.E.: Regulation of B cell growth and differentiation by soluble factors. Ann. Rev. Immunol. 1: 307, 1983.

Howell, M.D.; Winters, S.T.; Olee, T.; Powell, H.C.: Carlo, D.J. and Brostoff, S.W.: Vaccination against experimental allergic encephalomyelitis with T cell receptor peptides. Science 246: 668–670, 1989.

Hsieh, C.S.; Macatonia, S.; Tripp, C.; Wolf, S.; O'Garra, A. and Murphy, K.: Development of Th1 CD4+ T cells through Il-12 produced by Listeria-induced macrophages. Science 260: 547–549, 1993.

Hsu, F.J.; Kwak, L.; Campbell, M.; Liles, T.; Czerwinski, D.; Hart, S.; Syrengelas, A.; Miller, R. and Levy, R.: Clinical trials of idiotype-specific vaccine in B-cell lymphomas. Specific Immunotherapy of Cancer with Vaccines, Bystryn, J.C.; Ferrone, S. and Livingston, P. (eds)., Annals of the New York Academy of Sciences 690: 1993.

Hu, S.L.; Plowman, G.D.; Sridhar, P.; Stevenson, U.S.; Brown, J.P. and Estein, C.D.: Characterization of a recombinant vaccinia virus expressing human melanoma-associated antigen p97. J. Virol. 62: 176–180, 1988.

Huber, B.E.: Gene therapy strategies for treating neoplastic disease. Annals of the New York Academy of Sciences 716: 6, 1994.

Huber, B.E.; Richards, C.A. and Austin, E.A.: Virus-directed enzyme/ prodrug therapy (VDEPT): selectively engineering drug sensitivity into tumors. New York Academy of Sciences 716, 104, 1994.

Huber, M.; Beutler, B. and Keppler, D.: Tumor necrosis factor μ stimulates leukotriene production in vivo. Eur. J. Immunol. 18: 2085–2088, 1988.

Huck, S.; Fort, P.; Crawford, S.M.; Tao, M.-H.; Calame, K.L.; Morrison, S.L. and Bonagura, V.A.: Molecular analysis of IgM rheumatoid factor binding to chimeric IgG. J. Immunol. 146: 603, 1991.

Hui, K.; Grosveld, F. and Festenstein, H.: Rejection of transplantable AKR leukaemic cells following MHC DNA-mediated cell transformation. Nature 311: 750–752, 1984.

Hui, K.M.; Sim, B.C.; Foo, T.T. and Oei, A.A.: Promotion of tumor growth by transfecting antisense DNA to suppress endogenous Il-2Kk MHC gene expression in AKR mouse thymoma. Cell Immunol. 136: 80–94, 1991.

Humm, J.L.: Dosimetric aspects of radiolabeled antibodies for tumor therapy. J. nucl. Med. 27: 1490, 1986.

Humphrey, J.H. and Jaques, R.: The release of histamine and 5–hydroxy-tryptamine (serotonin) from platelets by antigen-antibody reactions (in vitro). J. Physiol. 128: 9–27, 1955.

Humphries, R.G.; O'Connor, S.G. and Tomlinson, W.: Different inhibition of collagen and ADP-induced platelet aggregation by prostacyclin in vivo. Br. J. Pharmacol. 96: 167, 1989.

Humphries, R.G.: Tomlinson, W.; O'Connor, S.E. and Leff, P.: Inhibition of collagen- and ADP-induced platelet aggregation by substance P in vivo: involvement of endothelium-derived relaxing factor. J. Cardiovasc. Pharmacol. 16: 292–297, 1990.

Humphries, S.: Molecular therapeutics in the prevention and treatment of cardiovascular disease. Gene Therapy - New Challenges for the Pharmaceutical Industry, London, September 15–16, 1994.

Huston, J.S.; Levinson, D.; Mudgett-Hunter, M.; Tai, M.-S.; Novotny, J.; Margolies, M.N.; Ridge, R.J.; Bruccoleri, R.; Haber, E.; Crea, R. and Oppermann, H.: Protein engineering of antibody binding sites: Recovery of specific activity in an anti-digoxin single-chain Fv analogue produced in Escherichia coli. Proc. Nat. Acad. Sci. USA 85: 5879–5883, 1988.

Huston, J.S.; Tai, M.-S.; Mudgett-Hunter, M.; McCartney, J.; Warren, F.; Haber, E. and Oppermann, H.: Protein engineering of single-chain Fv analogues and fusion proteins. In: Molecular Design and Modeling: Concepts and Applications, part B, edited by J.J. Langone, Methods in Enzymology 203: 46–88, 1991.

Huston, J.S.; McCartney, J.; Tai, M.-S.; Mottola-Hartshorn, C.; Jin, D.; Warren, F.; Keck, P. and Oppermann, H.: Medical application of single-chain antibodies. Intern. Rev. Immunol. 10: 195–217, 1993.

Hwu, P. and Rosenberg, S.A.: The use of gene-modified tumor-infiltrating lymphocytes for cancer therapy. New York Academy of Sciences 716: 188, 1994.

Hynes, R.O.: Integrins, a family of cell surface receptors. Cell 48: 549–555, 1987.

Ichijo, H.; Rönnstrand, L.; Miyagawa, K.; Ohashi, H.; Heldin, C-H. and Miyazono, K.: Purification of transforming growth factor-beta 1 binding proteins from porcine uterus membranes. J. Biol. Chem. 266: 22459–22464, 1991.

Ichijo, H.; Hellman, U.; Wernstedt, C.; Gonez, L.J.; Claesson-Welsh, L.; Heldin. C-H. and Miyazono, K.: Molecular cloning and characterization of Ficolin, a multimeric protein with fibrinogen- and collagen-like domains. J. Biol. Chem. 268: 14505–14513, 1993.

Idzerda, R.L.; March, C.J.; Mosley, B.; Lyman, S.D.; Vanden Bos, T.; Gimpel, S.D.; Din, W.S.; Grabstein, K.H.; Widmer, M.B.; Park, L.S.; Cosman, D. and Beckmann, P.M.: Human IL-4 receptor confers biological responsiveness and defines a novel receptor superfamily. J. Exp. Med. 171: 861–873, 1990.

Ignarro, L.J.; Byrns, R.E. and Wood, K.S.: Biochemical and pharmacological properties of endothelium-derived relaxing factor and its similarity to nitric oxide radical. Vasodilation: Vascular Smooth Muscle, Peptides, Autonomic Nerves and Endothelium. P.M. Vandhoutte (Ed.) Raven Press: New York, 427–436, 1988.

Ignotz, R.A. and Massague, J.: Type ß transforming growth factor controls the adipogenic differentiation of 3T3 fibroblasts. Proc. Natl. Acad. Sci. USA 82: 8530–8534, 1985.

Ihle, J.N.; Keller, J.; Oroszlan, S.; Henderson, L.E.; Copeland, T.D. and Fitch, F.: Biological properties of homogenous interleukin 3. J. Immunol. 131: 282–287, 1983.

Ijzermans, J.N.M. and Marquet, R.L.: Interferon-gamma: a review. Immunobiology 179: 456, 1989.

Ikeda, K.; Sannoh, T.; Kawasaki, N.; Kawasaki, T. and Yamishina, I.: Serum lectin with known structure activates complement through the classical pathway. J. Biol. Chem. 262: 7451–7454, 1987.

Ikeda, Y.; Handa, M.; Kawano, K.; Kamata, T.; Murata, M.; Araki, Y.; Anbo, H.; Kawai, Y.; Watanabe, K.; Itagaki, I. et al.: The role of von Willebrand factor and fibrinogen in platelet aggregation under varying shear stress. J. Clin. Invest. 87: 1234–1240, 1991.

Illum, N.; Taudorf, K.; Heilmann, C.; Smith, T.; Wulff, K.; Mansa, B. and Platz, P.: Intravenous immunoglobulin: a single-blind trial in children with Lennox-Gastaut syndrome. Neuropediatrics 21: 87–90, 1990.

Imai, Y.; Singer, M.S.; Fennie, C.; Lasky, L.A. and Rosen, S.D.: Identification of a carbohydrate-based endothelial ligand for a lymphocyte homing receptor. J. Cell Biol. 113: 1213–1221, 1991.

Imamuara, N. and Kuramoto, A.: Natural killer cell activity is not dependent on the CD3Ti T cell receptor antigen complex. Blood 72: 1837, 1988.

Imamura, T.; Tokita, Y. and Mitsui, Y.: Identification of a heparin-binding growth factor-1 nuclear translocation sequence by deletion mutation analysis. J. Biol. Chem. 267: 5676–5679, 1992.

Imbach, P.; Barandun, S.; d'Apuzzo, V. et al.: High-dose intravenous immunoglobulin for idiopathic thrombocytopenic purpura in childhood. Lancet 1: 1228–1231, 1981.

Inaba, K.; Bhardwaj, N.; Cameron, P.; O'Doherty, U. and Steinman, R.: The handling of antigens and infectious agents by the dendritic cell system. ENII Conf.: Integrated Function of Molecules of the Immune System. Les Embiez, France, 12th-16th May 1993.

Inoue, A.; Yanagisawa, M.; Kimura, S.; Kasuya, Y.; Miyauchi, T.; Goto, K. and Masaki, T.: The human endothelin family: Three structurally and pharmacologically distinct isopeptides predicted by three separate genes. Proc. Natl. Acad. Sci. USA 86: 2863–2867, 1989.

Ioachim, H.L.: The stroma reaction of tumors: An expression of immune surveillance. J. Natl. Cancer Inst. 57: 465–475, 1976.

Ioannides, C.G.; Freedman, R.S.; Platsoucas, C.D.; Rashed, S. and Kim, Y.P.: Cytotoxic T cell clones isolated from ovarian tumor-infiltrating lymphocytes recognize multiple antigenic epitopes on autologous tumor cells. J. Immunol. 146: 1700–1707, 1991.

Ip, N.Y.; Li, Y.P.; van de Stadt, I.; Panayotatos, N.; Alderson, R.F. and Lindsay, R.M.: Ciliary neurotrophic factor enhances neuronal survival in embryonic rat hippocampal cultures. J. Neurosci. 11: 3124–3134, 1991.

Ip, N.Y.; Nye, S.H.; Boulton, T.G.; Davis, S.; Tag, T.; Li, Y.; Birren, S.J.; Yasukawa, K.; Kishimoto, T.; Anderson, D.J. et al.: CNTF and LIF act on neuronal cells via shared signaling pathways that involve the Il-6 signal transducing receptor component gp130. Cell 69: 1121–1132, 1992.

Isakson, P.C.; Pure, E.; Vitetta, S. and Krammer, P.H.: T cell-derived B cell differentiation factor(s). Effect on the isotype switch of murine B cells. J. Exp. Med. 155: 734–748, 1982.

Isenman, D.E. and Young, R.J.: The molecular basis of the difference in immune hemolytic activity of the Chido and Rodgers isotype of human complement component C4. J. Immunol. 132: 3018–3027, 1984.

Ishibashi, T.; Kimura, H.; Shikama, Y.; Uchida, T.; Kariyone, S.; Hirano, T.; Hishimoto, T.; Takatsuki, F. and Akiyama, Y.: Interleukin 6 is a potent thrombopoietic factor in vivo in mice. Blood 74: 1241, 1989.

Ishibashi, T.; Kimura, H.; Uchida, T.; Kariyone, S.; Freise, P. and Burstein, S.A.: Human interleukin 6 is a direct promoter of maturation of megarkaryocytes in vitro. Proc. Natl. Acad. Sci. USA 86: 5953, 1989.

Ishizaka, A.; Wu, Z.; Stephens, K.E.; Harada, H.; Hogue, R.S.; O'Hanley, P.T. and Raffin, T.A.: Attenuation of acute lung injury in septic guinea pigs by pentoxifylline. Am. Rev. Respir. Dis. 138: 376–382, 1988.

Ishizaka, K.: IgE-binding factors and regulation of the IgE antibody response. Annu. Rev. Immunol. 6: 513, 1988.

Ishizaka, K. and Ishizaka, T.: Allergy. In: Paul, W.E. (ed.) Fundamental Immunology, 2nd. edn. Raven Press, New York, 867–888, 1989.

Itoh, K.; Tilden, A.B. and Balch, C.M.: Interleukin 2 activation of cytotoxic T lymphocytes infiltrating into human metastatic melanomas. Cancer Res. 46: 3011–3017, 1986.

Itoh, K.; Platsucas, C.D. and Balch, C.M.: Autologous tumor-specific cytotoxic T lymphocytes in the infiltrate of human metastatic melanomas: activation by interleukin-2 and autologous tumor cells and involvement of the T cell receptor. J. Exp. Med. 168: 1419–1441, 1988.

Iwasaki, T.; Uehara, Y.; Graves, L.; Rachie, N. and Bomsztyk, K.: Herbimycin A blocks Il-1-induced NF-kappa B DNA-binding activity in lymphoid cell lines. FEBS Let. 298: 240–244, 1992.

Jabara, H.H.; Fu, S.M.; Geha, R.S. and Vercelli, D.: CD40 and IgE: synergism between anti-CD40 monoclonal antibody and Interleukin 4 in the induction of IgE synthesis by highly purified human B cells. J. Exp. Med. 172: 1861–1864, 1990.

Jackson, C.G.; Ochs, H.D. and Wedgwood, R.J.: Immune response of a patient with deficiency of the fourth component of complement and systemic lupus erythematosus. New Engl. J. Med. 300: 1124–1129, 1979.

Jacobs, C.A.; Baker, P.E.; Roux, E.R.; Picha, K.S.; Toivola, B.; Waugh, S. and Kennedy, M.K.: Experimental autoimmune encephalomyelitis is exacerbated by Il-1µ and suppressed by soluble Il-1 receptor. J. Immunol. 146: 2983–2989, 1991.

Jacobs, R.F. and Tabor, D.R.: Immune cellular interactions during sepsis and septic injury. Crit. Care Clinics 5: 9–25, 1989.

Jacobsen, E.B.; Caporale, L.H. and Thorbecke, G.J.: Effect of thymus cell injections on germinal centre formation in lymphoid tissues of nude (thymusless) mice. Cell Immunol. 12: 416, 1974.

Jacquesy, J.C.; Gesson, J.P.; Monneret, C.; Mondon, M.; Renoux, J.B.; Florent, J.C.; Koch, M.; Tillequin, F.; Sedlacek, H.H.; Gerken, M. and Kolar, C.: EP 511917, WO 92 19639.

Jahn, B.; von Kempis, J. and Hansch, G.M.: Induction of prostaglandin E2 (PGE2) and collagenase synthesis in human synovial fibroblast-like cells (SFC) by terminal complement components C5b-9. Compl. Inflamm. 7: 138 (abstract), 1990.

Janeway, C.; Lerner, E.; Jason, J. and Jones, B.: T lymphocytes responding to mls-locus antigens are lyt-1+2– and I-A restricted. Immunogenetics 10: 481–497, 1980.

Janeway, C.A.: Selective elements for the Vß region of the T cell receptor: Mls and the bacterial toxic mitogens. Adv. Immunol. 50: 1–53, 1991.

Jasin, H.E.; Lightfoot, E.; Kavanaugh, A.; Rothlein, R.; Faanes, R.B. and Lipsky, P.E.: Successful treatment of chronic antigen-induced arthritis in rabbits with monoclonal antibodies to leukocyte adhesion molecules. Arthritis Theum. 33 (suppl.), S34 (abstr.), 1990.

Jaye, M.; Howk, R.; Burgess, W.; Ricca, G.A.; Chiu, I.M.; Ravera, M.W.; O'Brient, S.J.; Modi, W.S.; Maciag, T. and Drohan, W.N.: Human endothelial cell growth factor: cloning, nucleotide sequences, and chromosome localization. Science 233: 541–545, 1986.

Jenkins, M.K.; Pardoll, D.M.; Mizuguchi, J.; Chused, T.M. and Schwartz, R.H.: Molecular events in the induction of a nonresponsive state in interleukin 2–producing helper T-lymphocyte clones. Proc. Natl. Acad. Sci. USA 84: 5409, 1987.

Jenkins, M.K.; Pardoll, D.M.; Mizuguchi, J.; Quill, H. and Schwartz, R.H.: T-cell unresponsiveness in vivo and in vitro: Fine specificity of induction and molecular characterization of the unresponsive state. Immunol. Rev. 95: 113, 1987.

Jenkins, M.K.; Taylor, P.S.; Norton, S.D. and Urdahl, K.B.: CD28 delivers a costimulatory signal involved in antigen-specific Il-2 production by human T-cells. J. Immunol. 147: 2461–2466, 1991.

Jennings, J.C.; Mohan, S.; Linkhart, T.A.; Widstrom, R. and Baylink, D.J.: Comparison of the biological actions of TGF beta-1 and TGF beta-2: differential activity in endothelial cells. J. Cell Physiol. 137: 167–172, 1988.

Jerome, K.R.; Barnd, D.L.; Bendt, L.M.; Boyer, C.M.; Taylor-Papadimitriou, J.; McKenzie, I.F.C.; Bast, R.C. and Finn, O.J.: Cytotoxic T-lymphocytes derived from patients with breast adenocarcinoma recognise an epitope present on the protein core of a mucin molecule preferentially expressed by malignant cells. Cancer Res. 51: 2908–2916, 1991.

Jetten, A.M. and Goldfarb, R.H.: Action of epidermal growth factor and retinoids on anchorage-dependent and -independent growth of non-transformed rat kidney cells. Cancer Res. 43: 2094–2099, 1983.

Jiao, S.S.; Williams, P.; Berg, R.K.; Hodgeman, B.A.; Liu, L.J.; Repetto, G. and Wolff, J.A.: Direct gene transfer into nonhuman primate myofibers in vivo. Human Gene Ther. 3: 21–33, 1992.

Jilg, W.; Voltz, R.; Markert-Hahn, C.; Mairhofer, H.; Münz, I. and Wolf, H.: Expression of class I major histocompatibility complex antigens in Epstein-Barr virus-carrying lymphoblastoid cell lines and Burkitt lymphoma cells. Cancer Res. 51: 27–32, 1991.

Jochum, M.; Lander, S.; Heimburger, N. and Fritz, H.: Effect of human granulocytic elastase on isolated human antithrombin III. Hoppe-Seyler's Z Physiol. Chem. 362: 103–112, 1981.

Jochum, M.; Inthorn, D.; Machleidt, W.; Waydhas, C. and Fritz, H.: Influence of proteinase inhibitor therapy on the release of cellular proteinases, cytokines and soluble adhesion molecules in acute inflammation. Circ. Shock, suppl. 1: 41, 1993.

Johannsen, R.; Sedlacek, H.H. and Seiler, F.R.: Adjuvant effect of vibrio cholerae neuraminidase on the in vitro and in vivo immune response. Proceedings: Vienna, Nov. 9–12, 1977. Immunotherapy of Malignant Diseases, pp. 244–259, Ed. Rainer, H.; Schattauer Verlag, Stuttgart 1978.

Johnson, E.; Irons, J.; Patterson, R. and Roberts, M.: Serum IgE concentration in atopic dermatitis. J. Allergy Clin. Immunol. 54: 94, 1974.

Johnson, J.P.; Stade, B.G.; Holzmann, B.; Schwable, W. and Riethmüller, G.: De novo expression of intercellular adhesion molecule I in melanoma correlates with increased risk of metastasis. Proc. Natl. Acad. Sci. USA 86: 641–644, 1989.

Johnson, K.J. and Ward, P.A.: Acute immunologic pulmonary alveolitis. J. Clin. Invest. 54: 349–356, 1974.

Johnson, K.J.; Fantone, J.C.; Kaplan, J. and Ward, P.A.: In vivo damage of rat lungs by oxygen metabolites. J. Clin. Invest. 67: 983–991, 1981.

Johnston, G.I.; Cook, R.G. and McEver, R.P.: Cloning of GMP-140 a granule membrane protein of platelets and endothelium sequence similarities to proteins involved in cell adhesion and inflammation. Cell 56: 1033–1044, 1989.

Johnston, R.B.: Monocytes and macrophages. N. Engl. J. Med. 318: 747–752, 1988.

Jonker, M.; Nooij, F.J.M. and Steinhof, G.: Effects of CD4 and CD8 specific monoclonal antibodies "in vivo" on T cells and their relation to the allograft response in rhesus monkeys. Transplant. Proc. 19: 4308, 1987.

Jordan, S.C.: Intravenous gammaglobulin therapy in systemic lupus erythematosus and immune complex disease. Clin. Immunol. Immunpathol. 53: 164, 1989.

Joseph, M.: Platelets as inflammatory cells. Int. Conf. on: The platelet in health & disease. Royal College of Physicians, London, 1992.

Jung, S. and Schluesner, H.J.: Human T lymphocytes recognize a peptide of single point-mutated, oncogenic Ras proteins. J. Exp. med. 173: 273–276, 1991.

Kärre, K.; Ljunggren, H.G.; Piontek, G. and Kiessling, R.: Selective rejection of H-2–deficient lymphoma variants suggests alternative immune defence strategy. Nature 319. 675–678, 1986.

Kahan, A.; Charriaut-Marlangue, C.; Kahan, A.; Barel, M.; Menkes, C.J.; Amor, B. and Frade, R.: Increased expression of Epstein-Barr virus receptor on lymphoblastoid cell lines from subsets of patients with rheumatoid arthritis. J. Rheumatol. 13: 1024–1027, 1986.

Kakiuchi, T.; Chesnut, R.W. and Grey, H.M.: B cells as antigen-presenting cells: the requirement for B cell activation. J. Immunol. 131: 109, 1983.

Kaliner, M. and Austen, K.F.: Adenosine 3'5'-monophosphate: inhibition of complement mediated cell lysis. Science 183: 659–661, 1974.

Kalland, T.; Dohlstein, M.; Lind, P.; Sundstedt, A.; Abrahmsen, L.; Hedlund, G.; Björk, P.; Lando, P.A. and Björklund, M.: Monoclonal antibodies and superantigens: a novel therapeutic approach. Med. Oncol. & Tumor Pharmacother. 10: 37–47, 1993.

Kalli, K.R.; Hsu, P.; Bartow, T.J.; Ahearn, J.M.; Matsumoto, A.K.; Klickstein, L.B. and Fearon, D.T.: Mapping of the C3b-binding site of CR1 and construction of a (CR1)2–F(ab')2 chimeric complement inhibitor. J. Exp. Med. 174: 1451–1460, 1991.

Kalra, P.S.; Sahu, A. and Kalra, S.P.: Interleukin-1 inhibits the ovarian steroid-induced luteinizing hormone surge and release of hypothalamic luteinizing hormone-releasing hormone in rats. Endocrinology 126: 2145–2152, 1990.

Kalsi, J.K. and Hall, N.D.: Feedback regulation of antibody production: a role in rheumatoid arthritis? Annals of the Rheumatic Diseases 50: 833–835, 1991.

Kane, S.E. and Gottesman, M.M.: The role of cathepsin L in malignant transformation. Semin Cancer Biol. 1: 127–136, 1990.

Kang, S.-M.; Beverly, B.; Tran, A.-C.; Brorson, K.; Schwartz, R.H. and Lenardo, M.J.: Transactivation by AP-1 is a molecular target of T cell clonal anergy. Science 257: 1134–1138, 1992.

Kantor, J.; Irvine, K.; Abrams, S.; Kaufman, H.; DiPietro, J. and Schlom, J.; Antitumor activity and immune responses induced by a recombinant carcinoembryonic antigen-vaccinia virus vaccine. J. Natl. Cancer Inst. 84: 1084–1091, 1992.

Kantor, J.; Irvine, K.; Abrams, S.; Snoy, P.; Olsen, R.; Greiner, J.; Kaufman, H.; Eggensperger, D. and Schlom, J.: Immunogenicity and safety of a recombinant vaccinia virus vaccine expressing the carcinoembryonic antigen gene in a nonhuman primate. Cancer Res. 52: 6917–6925, 1992.

Kantor, J.; Abrams, S.; Irvine, K.; Snoy, P.; Kaufman, H. and Schlom, J.: Specific immunotherapy using a recombinant vaccinia virus expressing human carcinoembryonic antigen. Specific Immunotherapy Of Cancer With Vaccines, eds. Bystryn, J.-C.; Ferrone, S. and Livingston, P., The New York Academy of Sciences 690: 370, 1993.

Kao, R.T. and Stern, R.: Elastases in human breast carcinoma cell lines. Cancer Res. 46: 1355–1358, 1986.

Kaplan, A.P.; Haak-Frendscho, M.; Fauci, A.; Dinarello, C. and Halbert, E.: A histamine-releasing factor from activated human mononuclear cells. J. Immunol. 135: 2027, 1985.

Kaplan, A.P. and Silverberg, M.: The coagulation-kinin pathway of human plasma. Blood 70: 1–15, 1987.

Kaplan, B.S.; Uni, S.; Aikawa, M. and Mahoud, A.A.F.: Effector mechanism of host resistance in murine Giardiasis: specific IgG and IgA cell-mediated toxicity. J. Immun. 134: 1975–1981, 1985.

Kaplan, G.; Cohn, Z.A. and Smith K.A.: Rational immunotherapy with Interleukin 2. Bio/Technology 10: 157, 1992.

Kapp, A.; Czech, W.; Kurrle, R.; Borckhaus, M.; Krutmann, J. and Zeck-Kapp, G.: Normal human eosinophils are activated by tumor necrosis factors (TNFα and β) and express the 55 kD and 75 kD TNF-receptor. Annual Meeting of the European Society for Dermatological Research, London (UK), April 4–7, 1992.

Kappler, J.W.; Staerz, U.; White, J. and Marrack, P.C.: Self-tolerance eliminates T cell specific for Mls-modified products of the major histocompatibility complex. Nature 332: 35–40, 1988.

Kapsenberg, M.L.; Wierenga, E.A.; Bos, J.D. and Jansen, H.M.: Functional subsets of allergen-reactive human CD4+ T lymphocytes. Immunol. Today 12: 392–395, 1991.

Karanth, S. and McCann, S.M.: Anterior pituitary hormone control by interleukin-2. Proc. Natl. Acad. Sci USA 88: 2961–2965, 1991.

Karjalainen, J.; Martin, J.M.; Knip, M.; Ilonen, J.; Robinson, B.; Savilahti, E.; Akerblom, H.K. and Dosch, H.-M.: A bovine albumin peptide as a possible trigger of insulin-dependent diabetes mellitus. N. Engl. J. Med. 327: 302–327, 1992

Karpati, G. and Acsadi, G.: The potential for gene therapy in Duchesse muscular dystrophy and other genetic muscle diseases. Muscle & Nerve 16: 1141–1153, 1993.

Kasahara, T.; Wu, Y.; Sakurai, Y. and Oguchi, K.: Suppressive effect of acupuncture on delayed type hypersensitivity to trinitrochlorobenzene and involvement of opiate receptors. Int. J. Immunopharmac. 14: 661–665, 1992.

Kasahara, T.; Amemiya, M.; Wu, Y. and Oguchi, K.: Involvement of central opioidergic and nonopioidergic neuroendocrine systems in the suppressive effect of acupuncture on delayed type hypersensitivity in mice. Int. J. Immunopharmac. 15: 501–508, 1993.

Kasiewski, C.J. et al., 1991: cited by Tuffin, D.P., 1992.

Kast, W.M.; Offringa, R.; Peters, P.J.; Voordouw, A.C.; Meloen, R.H.; Van der Eb, A.J. and Meljef, C.J.M.: Eradication of adenovirus E1–induced tumors by E1A-specific cytotoxic T lymphocytes. Cell 59: 603–614, 1989.

Kato, Y. and Gospodarowicz, D.: Sulfated proteoglycin synthesis by confluent cultures of rabbit costal chondrocytes grown in the presence of fibroblast growth factor. J. Cell Biol. 100: 477–485, 1985.

Katz, D.H.; Hamaoka, T.; Dorf, M.E. and Benacerraf, B.: Cell interactions between histoincompatible T and B lymphocytes. The H-2 gene complex determines successful physiologic lymphocytes interactions. Proc. Natl. Acad. Sci. USA 70: 2624–2628, 1973.

Katz, S.A.; Vencatachalam, M.; Crouch, R.K.; Heffner, J.E.; Halushka, P.V.; Wise, W.C. and Cook, J.A.: Catalase pretreatment attenuates oleic acid-induced edema in isolated rabbit lung. J. Appl. Physiol. 65: 1301–1306, 1988.

Kaufman, D.; Erlander, M.; Clare-Salzler, M.; Atkinson, M.; Maclaren, N. and Tobin, A.: Autoimmunity to two forms of glutamate decarboxylase in insulin-dependent mellitus. J. Clin. Invest. 89: 283–292, 1992.

Kaufman, H.; Schlom, J. and Kantor, J.: A recombinant vaccinia virus expressing human carcinoembryonic antigen (CEA). Int. J. Cancer 48: 900–907, 1991.

Kauser, K.; Stekiel, W.J.; Rubanyi, G.M. and Harder, D.R.: Mechanism of action of EDRF on pressurized arteries: Effect on K+ conductance. Circ. Res. 65: 199–204, 1989.

Kaushansky, K.; Lin, N. and Adamson, J.W.: Interleukin 1 stimulates fibroblasts to synthesize granulocyte-macrophage and granulocyte colony-stimulating factors. Mechanism for the hematopoietic response to inflammation. J. Clin. Invest. 81: 92–97, 1988.

Kaveri, S.V.; Dietrich, G.; Hurez, V. and Kazatchkine, M.D.: Intravenous immunoglobulins (IVIg) in the treatment of autoimmune diseases. Clin. Exp. Immunol. 86: 192, 1991.

Kawabe, T.; Maeda, Y.; Takami, M. and Yodoi, J.: Human Fc epsilon RII and IgE-binding factor: Triangular network with Il-2 and Il-4. Res. Immunol. 141: 82–85, 1990.

Kawai, K.; Takano, K.; Hizuka, N. and Shizume, K.: Properties and concentration of somatomedin A in various rat tissues. Endocrinol. Jpn. 26: 559–565, 1979.

Kawakami, M.; Pekala, P.H.; Lane, M.D. and Cermai, A.: Lipoprotein lipase suppression in 3T3–L1 cells by an endotoxin-induced mediator from exudate cells. Proc. Natl. Acad. Sci. 79: 912–916, 1982.

Kawakami, Y.; Rosenberg, S.A. and Lotze, M.T.: IL-4 promotes the growth of tumor-infiltrating lymphocytes cytotoxic for human autologous melanoma. J. Exp. Med. 168: 2183–2191, 1988.

Kawakami, Y.; Custer, M.C.; Rosenberg, S.A. and Lotze, M.T.: Il-4 regulates IL-2 induction lymphokine-activated killer activity from human lymphocytes. J. Immunol. 142: 3452–3459, 1989.

Kawamoto, T.; Sato, J.D.; Le, A.; Polikoff, J.; Sato, G.H. and Mendlsohn, J.: Growth stimulation of A431 cells by epidermal growth factor: identification of high-affinity receptors for epidermal growth factor by an anti-receptor monoclonal antibody. Proc. Natl. Acad. Sci. 80: 1337–1341, 1983.

Kawanishi, H.; Saltzmann, L.E. and Strober, W.: Mechanisms regulating IgA class-specific immunoglobulin production in murine gut-associated lymphoid tissues. I. T cells derived from Peyer's patches that switch sIgM B cells to sIgA B cells in vitro. J. Exp. Med. 157: 433–450, 1983.

Kawasaki, E.S.; Ladner, M.B.; Wang, A.M.; Van Arsdell, J.; Warren, M.K.; Coyne, M.Y.; Schwickart, D.L.; Lee, M.; Wilson, K.J.; Boosman, A.; Stanley, E.R.; Ralph, P. and Mark, D.F.: Molecular cloning of a complementary DNA encoding human macrophage-specific colony-stimulating factor (CSF-1). Science 230: 291, 1985.

Kay, A.B.; Ying, S.; Varney, V.; Gaga, M.; Durham, S.R.; Moqbel, R.; Wardlaw, A.J. and Hamid, Q.: Messenger RNA expression of the cytokine gene cluster, interleukin 3 (IL-3, IL-4, IL-5, and granulocyte/ macrophage colony-stimulating factor, in allergen-induced late-phase cutaneous reactions in atopic subjects. J. Exp. Med. 173: 775, 1991.

Keck, P.J.; Hauser, S.D.; Krivi, G.; Sanzo, K.; Warren, T.; Feder, J. and Connolly, D.T.: Vascular permeability factor, an endothelial cell mitogen related to PDGF. Science 246: 1308–1312, 1989.

Kehrl, J.H.; Wakefield, L.M.; Roberts, A.B.; Jakowiew, S.; Alvarez-Mon, M., Derynck, R.; Sporn, M.B. and Fauci, A.S.: Production of transforming growth factor ß by human T lymphocytes and its potential role in the regulation of T cell growth. J. Exp. Med. 163: 1037, 1987.

Kehrl, J.H.; Taylor, A.S.; Delsing, G.A.; Roberts, A.B.; Sporn, M.B. and Fauci, A.S.: Further studies of the role of transforming growth factor ß in human B cell function. J. Immunol. 143: 1868, 1989.

Keller, T.; McGrath, K.; Newland, A.; Gatenby, P.; Cobcroft, R. and Gibson, J.: Indications for use of intravenous immunoglobulin. Recommendations of the Australasian Society of Blood Transfusion consensus symposium. Med. J. Australia 159: 204, 1993.

Kenny, D.M. and Davis, A.E.: Association of alternative complement pathway components with human blood platelets: secretion and localization of factor D and beta-1H globulin. Clin. Immunol. Immunopathol. 21: 351–363, 1981.

Kerjaschki, K.; Schulze, M.; Binder, S.; Kain, R.; Ojha, P.P.; Susani, M.; Horvat, R.; Baker, P.J. and Couser, W.G.: Transcellular transport and membrane insertion of the C5b-9 membrane attack complex of complement by glomerular epithelial cells in experimental membranous nephropathy. J. Immunol. 143: 546–552, 1989.

Kern, S.E.; Pietenpol, J.A.; Thiagalingam, S.; Seymour, A.; Kinzler, K.W. and Vogelstein, B.: Oncogenic forms of p53 inhibit p53–regulated gene expression. Science 256: 827–830, 1992

Kerr, D.E.; Senter, P.D.; Burnett, W.V.; Hirschberg, D.L.; Hellström, I. and Hellström, K.E.: Antibody-penicillin-V-amidase conjugates kill antigen-positive tumor cells when combined with Doxorubicin phenoxyacetamide. Cancer Immunol. Immunother. 31: 202, 1990.

Kerr, J.F.R.; Wyllie, A.H. and Currie, A.R.: Apoptosis: a basic biological phenomenon with wide-ranging implications in tissue kinetics. Br. J. Cancer 26: 239–257, 1972.

Keski-Oja, J.; Blasi, F.; Leof, E.B. and Moses, H.L.: Regulation of the synthesis and activity of urokinase plasminogen activator in A549 human lung carcinoma cells by transforming growth factor-ß. J. Cell Biol. 106: 451–459, 1988.

Khan, M.M.; Sansoni, P.; Engleman, E.G. and Melmon, K.L.: Pharmacologic effects of autacoids on subsets of T-cells. J. Clin. Invest. 75: 1578, 1985.

Khayat, D.; Geffrier, C.; Yoon, S.; Scigliano, E.; Soubran, C.; Weil, M. and Unkeless, J.C.: Soluble circulating Fc-gamma receptor in human serum, a new ELISA assay for specific and quantitative detection. J. Immunol. 100: 235, 1987.

Kikutani, H.; Inui, S.; Sato, R.; Barsumian, E.L.; Owaki, H.; Yamasaki, K.; Kaisho, T.; Uchi-bayashi, N.; Hardy, R.R.; Hirano, T.; Tsunasawa, S.; Sakiyama, F.; Suemura, M. and Kishi-moto, T.: Molecular structure of human lymphocyte receptor for Immunoglobulin E. Cell 47: 657–665, 1986.

Kinashi, T.; Harada, N.; Severinson, E.; Tanabe, T.; Sideras, P.; Konishi, M.; Azuma, C.; Tomi-naga, A.; Bergstedt-Lindqvist, S.; Takahashi, M. et al.: Cloning of complementary DNA encoding T-cell replacing factor and identity with B-cell growth factor II. Nature 324: 70–73, 1986.

Kindred, B. and Shreffler, D.C.: H-2 dependence of co-operation between T and B cells in vivo. J. Immunol. 109: 940–943, 1972.

King, A.C. and Cuatrecasas, P.: Resolution of high and low affinity epidermal growth factor receptors. Inhibition of high affinity component by low temperature, cycloheximide, and phorbol esters. J. Biol. Chem. 257: 3053–3060, 1982.

King, C.A.; Wills, M.R.; Hamblin, T.J. and Stevenson, F.K.: Idiotypic IgM on a B-cell surface requires processing for recognition by anti-idiotypic T cells. Cell Immunol. 147: 411–424, 1993.

King, C.I.; Ottesen, E.A. and Nutman, T.B.: Cytokine regulation of antigen-driven immunoglobulin production in filarial parasite infections in humans. J. Clin. Invest. 85: 1810–1815, 1990.

King, C.L.; Gallin, J.I.; Malech, H.L.; Abramson, S.L. and Nutman, T.B.: Regulation of immunoglobulin production in hyperimmunoglobulin E recurrent infection syndrome by interferon-gamma. Proc. Natl. Acad. Sci. USA 86: 10085–10089, 1989.

Kiniwa, M.; Gately, M.; Gubler, U.; Chizzonite, R.; Fargeas, C. and Delespesse, G.: Recombinant Interleukin-12 suppresses the synthesis of Immunoglobulin E by Interleukin-4 stimulated human lymphocytes. J. Clin. Invest. 90: 262–266, 1992.

Kinnon, C.: Inherited immunodeficiency. Gene Therapy - New Challenges for the Pharmaceutical Industry, London, September 15–16, 1994.

Kino, T.; Hatanaka, H.; Hashimoto, M.; Nishiyama, M.; Goto, T.; Okuhara, M.; Kohsaka, M.; Aoki, H. and Imanaka, H.: FK-506, a novel immunosuppressant isolated from a Streptomyces. J. Antibiotics 40: 1249–1255, 1987.

Kirnbauer, R.; Charvat, B.; Schauer, E.; Koeck, A.; Urbanski, A.; Foerster, E.; Neuner, P.; Assmann, I.; Luger, T.A. and Schwarz, T.: Modulation of intercellular adhesion molecule-1 expression on human melanocytes and melanoma cells: evidence for a regulatory role of Il-6, Il-6, TNF beta, and UBV light. J. Invest. Derm. 98: 320–326, 1992.

Kishimoto, T.; Akira, S. and Taga, T.: Il-6 receptor and mechanism of signal transduction. Int. J. Immunopharm. 14: 431–438, 1992.

Kitamura, T.; Sato, N.; Arai, K. and Miyajima, A.: Expression cloning of the human Il-3 receptor cDNA reveals a shared beta subunit for the human Il-3 and GM-CSF receptors. Cell 66: 1165–1174, 1991.

Klagsbrun, M. and D'Amore, P.A.: Regulators of angiogenesis. Ann. Rev. Physiol. 53: 217–239, 1991.

Klar, D. and Hämmerling, G.J.: Induction of assembly of MHC class I antigens in germ cell testicular cancer. Am. J. Clin. Pathol. 93: 202–207, 1989.

Klaus, G.G.B.; Humphrey, J.H.; Kunkl, A. and Dongworth, D.W.: The follicular dendritic cell: its role in antigen presentation in the generation of immunological memory. Immunol. Rev. 53L, 3, 1980.

Klaus, G.G.B. and Kunkl, A.: The role of T cells in B cell priming and germinal centre development. Adv. Exp. Med. Biol. 149: 743, 1982.

Klaus, G.G.B.; Harnett, M.M. and Rigley, K.P.: G-protein regulation of polyphosphoinositide breakdown in B cells. Proc. of the 2nd Int. Conf. on Lymphocyte Activation N.Y.: Plenum Press, 95–100, 1989.

Klein, B.; Zhang, X.G.; Jourdan, M.; Boiron, J.M.; Portier, M.; Lu, Z.Y.; Wijdenes, J.; Brochier, J. and Bataille R.: Interleukin-6 is the central tumor growth factor in vitro and in vivo in multiple myeloma. Eur. Cytokine Netw. 1: 193, 1990.

Klein, H.; Becher, R.; Lübbert, M.; Oster, W.; Schleiermacher, E.; Brach, M.A.; Soza, L.; Lindemann, A.; Mertelsmann, R. and Herrmann, F.: Synthesis of granulocyte colony stimulating factor and its requirement for terminal divisions in chronic myelogenous leukemia. J. Exp. Med. 171: 1785, 1990.

Klickstein, L.B.: Shapleigh, L. and Goetzl, E.: Lipoxygenation of arachidonic acid as a source of PMN leucocyte chemotactic factors in synovial fluids and tissue in rheumatoid arthritis and spondyloarthritis. J. Clin. Invest. 66: 1166–1170, 1980.

Klickstein, L.B.; Bartow, T.J.; Miletic, V.; Rabson, L.D.; Smith, J.A. and Fearon, D.T.: Identification of distinct C3b and C4b recognition sites in the human C3b/C4b receptor (CR1, CD35) by deletion mutagenesis. J. Exp. Med. 168: 1699–1717, 1988.

Klopstock, A.; Schwartz, J.; Bleiberg, Y.; Adam, A. and Szeinberg, A.: Hereditary nature of the behaviour of erythrocytes in immune adherence-haemagglutination phenomenon. Vox Sang 10: 177–187, 1965.

Knauer, D.J. and Cunningham, D.D.: Protease nexins: cell-secreted proteins which regulate extracellular serine proteinases. Trends Biochem. Sci. 9: 231–233, 1984.

Knauer, K.A.; Kagey-Sobotka, A.; Adkinson, N.F. and Lichtenstein, L.M.: Platelet augmentation of IgE-dependent histamine release from human basophils and mast cells. Int. Arch. Allergy Appl. Immunol. 74: 29–35, 1984.

Knoflach, P.; Müller, C. and Eibel, M.M.: Crohn's disease and intravenous immunoglobulins. Ann. intern. Med. 112: 385, 1990.

Knowles, D.M.; Sullivan, T.J.; Parker, C.W. and Williams, R.C.: In vitro antibody-enzyme conjugates with specific bactericidal activity. J. Clin. Invest. 52: 1443–1452, 1973.

Knuth, A.; Wölfel, T.; Klehmann, E.; Boon, T. and Meyer zum Büschenfelde, K.H.: Cytolytic T-cell clones against an autologous human melanoma: specificity study and definition of three antigens by immunoselection. Proc. Natl. Acad. Sci. USA 86: 2804–2808, 1989.

Knuth, A.; Wölfel, T. and Meyer zum Büschenfelde, K.H.: Cellular and humoral immune responses against cancer: implications for cancer vaccines. Curr. Op. Immunol. 3: 659–664, 1991.

Kobayashi, M.; Fitz, L.; Ryan, M.; Hewick, R.M.; Clark, S.C.; Chang, S.; Loudon, R.; Sherman, F.; Perussia, B. and Trinchieri, G.: Identification and purification of natural killer cell stimulatory factor (NKSF), a cytokine with multiple biologic effects on human lymphocytes. J. Exp. Med. 170: 827–845, 1989.

Kobayashi, S.; Teramura, M.; Sugawara, I.; Oshimi, K. and Mizoguchi, H.: Interleukin-11 acts as an autocrine growth factor for human megakaryoblastic cell lines. Blood 81: 889–893, 1993.

Koch, A.E.; Burrows, J.C.; Haines, G.K.; Carlos, T.M.; Harlan, J.M. and Leibovich, S.J.: Immunolocalization of endothelial and leukocyte adhesion molecules in human rheumatoid and osteoarthritic synovial tissues. Lab. Invest. 64: 313–320, 1991.

Koch, K.C.; Ye, K.; Clark, B.D. and Dinarello, C.A.: Interleukin 4 (Il-4) up-regulates gene and surface Il-1 receptor type I in murine T helper type 2 cells. Eur. J. Immunol. 22: 153–157, 1992.

Kocks, C. and Rajewsky, K.: Stable expression and somatic hypermutation of antibody V regions in B-cell development pathways. Ann. Rev. Immunol. 7: 537, 1989.

Kodama, T.; Freeman, M.; Rohrer, L.; Zabrecky, J.; Matsudaira, P. and Krieger, M.: Type I macrophage scavenger receptor contains alpha-helical and collagen-like coiled coils. Nature 343: 531–535, 1990.

Kölsch, E.; Oberbarnscheidt, J.; Bruner K. and Heuer, J.: The Fc-receptor: its role in the trans-mission of differentiation signals. Immunol. Rev. 49: 61, 1980.

Koenig, J.I.; Snow, K.; Clarke, B.D.; Toni, R.; Cannon, J.G.; Shaw, A.R.; Dinarello, C.A.; Reich-lin, S.; Lee, S.L. and Lechan, R.M.: Intrinsic pituitary interleukin-1β is induced by bacterial lipopolysaccharide. Endocrinology 126: 3053–3058, 1990.

Koenig, J.I.: Presence of cytokines in the hypothalamic-pituitary axis. Prog. Neuro. Endocrin. Immunol. 4: 143–153, 1991.

Koeppen, H.; Singh, S. and Schreiber, H.: Genetically engineered vaccines. Comparison of ac-tive versus passive immunotherapy against solid tumors. Specific Immunotherapy Of Cancer With Vaccines, eds. Bystryn, J.-C.; Ferrone, S.; Livingston, P., The New York Academy of Sciences 690: 244, 1993.

Kohler, H.; Richardson, B.C.; Rowley, D.A. and Smyk, S.: Immune response to phosphorylcho-line. III. Requirement of the Fc portion and equal effectiveness of IgG subclasses in antire-ceptor antibody- induced suppression. J. Immunol. 119: 1979–1986, 1977.

Kohonen-Corish, M,R.J.; King, N.J.L.; Woodhams, C.E. and Ramshaw, I.A.: Immunodeficient mice recover from infection with vaccinia virus expressing interferon-gamma. Eur. J. Immun-ol. 20: 157–161, 1990.

Koike, T.; Itoh, Y.; Ishii, T.; Ito, I.; Takabayashi, K.; Maruyama, N.; Tomioka, H. and Yoshida, S.: Preventive effect of monoclonal anti-L3T4 antibody on development of diabetes in NOD mice. Diabetes 36: 539–541, 1987.

Kolsch, E.K.; Oberbarnscheidt, J.; Bruner, K. and Heuer, J.: The Fc receptor: its role in the trans-mission of differentiation signals. Immunol. Rev. 49: 61–78, 1980.

Koretz, K.; Momburg, F.; Otto, H.F. and Möller, P.: Sequential induction of MHC antigens on autochthonous cells of the ileum affected by Crohn's disease. Am. J. Pathol. 129: 493–502, 1987.

Korholz, D.; Gerdau, S.; Enczmann, J.; Zessack, N. and Burdach, S.: Interleukin 6–induced dif-ferentiation of a human B cell line into IGM-secreting plasma cells is mediated by c-fos. Eur. J. Immunol. 22: 607–610, 1992.

Korsmeyer, S.J.: Bcl-2: a repressor of lymphocyte death. Immunology Today 13: 285, 1992.

Kosco, M.H.: Cellular interactions during the germinal centre response. Res. Immunol. 142: 245, 1991.

Kraal, G.; Weissman, I.L. and Butcher, E.C.: Germinal centre B cells: antigen specificity and changes in heavy chain class expression. Nature 298: 377, 1982.

Kraal, G.; Weismann, I.L. and Butcher, E.C.: Differences in in vivo distribution and homing of T cell subsets to mucosal vs nonmucosal lymphoid organs. J. Immunol. 130: 1097–1102, 1983.

Kraal, G.: Regulation of activity of high endothelial venules. ENII Conf.: Integrated Function of Molecules of the Immune System. Les Embiez, France, 12th-16th May 1993.

Krajci, P.; Solberg, R.; Sandberg, M.; Oyen, O.; Jahnsen, T. and Brandtzaeg, P.: Molecular clo-ning of the human transmembrane secretory component (poly Ig receptor) and its mRNA expression in human tissues. Biochem. Biophys. Res. Commun. 158: 783–789, 1989.

Krammer, P.H.: PO-1 mediated apoptosis in normal and malignant lymphocytes. ENII Conf.: In-tegrated Function of Molecules of the Immune System. Les Embiez, France, 12th-16th May 1993.

Krasagakis, K.; Garbe, C. and Orfanos, C.E.: Cytokines in human melanoma cells: synthesis, autocrine stimulation and regulatory functions - an overview. Melanoma Res. 3: 425–433, 1993.

Krause, D.S. and Deutsch, C.: Cyclic AMP directly inhibits Il-2 receptor expression in human T cells: expression of both p55 and p75 subunits is affected. J. Immunol. 146: 2285, 1991.

Krejci, J.; Pekarek, J.; Johanovsky, J. and Svejcar, J.: Demonstration of inflammatory activity of the supernatant of hypersensitive lymph node cells incubated with high dose of antigen. Immunology 16: 677–684, 1969.

Krensky, A.M.; Clayberger, C.; Reis, C.S.; Strominger, J.L. and Burakoff, S.J.: Specificity of OKT4+ cytotoxic T lymphocyte clones. J. Immunol. 129: 2002, 1982.

Krieger, J.I.; Grammer, S.F.; Grey, H.M. and Chesnut, R.W.: Antigen presentation by splenic B cells: resting B cells are ineffective whereas activated B cells are effective accessory cells for T cell responses. J. Immunol. 135: 2937, 1985.

Krieger, M.: Molecular flypaper and atherosclerosis: structure of the macrophage scavenger re-ceptor. Trends Biochem. Sci. 17: 141–146, 1992.

Krikorian, J.G.; Portlock, C.S.; Cooney, D.P. and Rosenberg, S.A.: Spontaneous regression of non-Hodgkin's lymphoma. A report of nine cases. Cancer 46: 2093–2099, 1980.

Krueger, J.M.; Walter, J.; Dinarello, C.A.; Wolff, S.M. and Chedid, L.: Sleep-promoting effects of endogenous pyrogen-(interleukin-1). Am. J. Physiol. 246: 994, 1984.

Krych, M.; Atkinson, J.P. and Holers, V.M.: Complement receptors. Curr. Opin. Immunol. 4: 8–13, 1992.

Ku, G.; Doherty, N.S.; Wolos, J.A. and Jackson, R.L.: Inhibition of probucol of interleukin-1 secretion and its implication in atherosclerosis. Am. J. Cardiol. 62: 77, 1988.

Kuhlman, M.; Joiner, K. and Ezekowitz, R.A.B.: The human mannose-binding protein functions as an opsonin. J. Exp. Med. 169: 1733–1745, 1989.

Kuhn, R.; Rajewsky, K. and Muller, W.: Generation and analysis of Il-4 deficient mice. Science 254: 707, 1991.

Kummer, U. and Staerz, U.D.: Concepts of antibody-mediated cancer therapy. Cancer Investigation 11: 174–184, 1993.

Kuna, P.; Reddigari, S.R.; Kornfeld, D. and Kaplan, A.P.: Il-8 inhibits histamine release from human basophils induced by histamine-releasing factors, connective tissue activating peptide III, and Il-3. J. Immunol. 147: 1920, 1991.

Kuna, P.; Reddigari, S.R.; Rucinksi, D.; Oppenheim, J.J. and Kaplan, A.P.: Monocyte chemotactic and activating factor is a potent histamine-releasing factor for human basophils. J. Exp. Med. 175: 489, 1992.

Kunkel, S.L.; Spengler, M.; May, M.A.; Spengler, R.; Larrick, J. and Remick, D.: Prostaglandin E2 regulates macrophage-derived tumor necrosis factor. J. Biol. Chem. 263: 5380, 1988.

Kupper, T.; Horowitz, M.; Lee, F.; Robb, R. and Flood, P.M.: Autocrine growth of T cells independent of interleukin 2: identification of interleukin 4 (Il-4, BSF-1) as an autocrine growth factor for a cloned antigen-specific helper T cell. J. Immunol. 138: 4280–4287, 1987.

Kurki, P.; Helve, T.; Dahl, D. and Virtanen, I.: Neurofilament antibodies in systemic lupus erythematosus. J. Rheumat. 13: 69–73, 1986.

Kurrle, R. and Schorlemmer, H.U.: Immunintervention bei Autoimmunerkrankungen. Infektionen und Autoimmunerkrankungen (Internat. Behring Immunologie Symp., 12.-14.11.1992, Frankfurt).

Kuypers, T.W. and Ross, D.: Leukocyte membrane adhesion proteins LFA-1, CR3 and p150,95: a review of functional and regulatory aspects. Res. Immunol. 140: 461–486, 1989.

Kuzuya, T.; Hoshida, S.; Nishida, M.; Kim, Y.; Fuji, H.; Kitabatake, A.; Kamada, T. and Tada, M.: Role of free radicals and neutrophils in canine myocardial reperfusion injury: Myocardial salvage by a novel free radical scavenger, 2–octadecylascorbic acid. Cardiovasc. Res. 23: 323–330, 1989.

Kwaan, H.C.: The plasminogen-plasmin system in malignancy. Cancer Metas. Rev. 11: 291–311, 1992.

Kyle, D.J. and Burch, R.M.: Recent advances toward novel bradykinin antagonists. Drugs of the Future 17: 305–312, 1992.

Lachmann, P.J.; Coombs, R.R. and Fell, H.B.: The breakdown of embryonic (chick) cartilage and bone cultivated in the presence of complement-sufficient antiserum. 3. Immunological analysis. Int. Arch. Allergy Appl. Immunol. 36: 469–485, 1969.

Laiho, M.; Saksela, O.; Andreasen, P.A. and Keski-Oja, J.: Enhanced production and extracellular deposition of the endothelial-type plasminogen activator inhibitor in cultured human lung fibroblasts by transforming growth factor-ß. J. Cell Biol. 103: 2403–2410, 1986.

Laiho, M.; Saksela, O. and Keski-Oja, J.: Transforming growth factor-ß alters plasminogen activator activity in human skin fibroblasts. Exp. Cell Res. 164: 399–407, 1986.

Laiho, M.; Saksela, O. and Keski-Oja, J.: Transforming growth factor-ß induction of type-I plasminogen activator inhibitor. Pericellular deposition and sensitivity to exogenous urokinase. J. Biol. Chem. 262: 17467–17474, 1987.

Laiho, M. and Keski-Oja, J.: Growth factors in the regulation of pericellular proteolysis: A review. Cancer Res. 49: 2533–2553, 1989.

Lambert, M.E.; Ronai, Z.A.; Weinstein, I.B. and Garrels, J.I.: Enhancement of major histocompatibility class I protein synthesis by DNA damage in cultured human fibroblasts and keratinocytes. Molec. Cell. Biol. 9: 847–850, 1989.

Lamki, L.; Kavanagh, J.; Rosenblum, M. and Murray, J.: Radioimmunotherapy of ovarian cancer with intraperitoneal 90Y-B72.3 with and without EDTA scavengers. 8th Int. Hammersmith Meeting, Creece, 1991.

Lamont, A.G.; Sette, A.; Fujinami, R.; Colon, S.M.; Miles, C. and Grey, H.M.: Inhibition of experimental autoimmune encephalomyelitis induction in SJL/J mice by using a peptide with high affinity for IA molecules. J. Immun. 145: 1687–1693, 1990.

Lane, D.P.: Worrying about p53. Current Biol. 2: 5, 1992.

Lange, W.; Brugger, W.; Rosenthal, F.M.; Kanz, L. and Lindemann, A.: The role of cytokines in oncology. Int. J. Cell Cloning 9: 252–273, 1991.

Langley, P.G.; Hughes, R.D. and Williams R.: Coagulation abnormalities in acute liver failure: Antithrombin III supplementation. Biomed. Progress 5: 41, 1992.

Langner, K.D.; Lauffer, L.; Enssle, K.; Oquendo, P.; Kanzy, E.J.; Dickneite, G. and Kurrle, R.: Structural and functional analysis of a TNF receptor-immunoglobulin fusion protein. In: Serono Symposia Publications from Raven Press, vol. 92: New Advances on Cytokines. S. Romagnani, T.R. Mosmann, A.K. Abbas (eds.), 349–354, 1992.

Lantz, M.; Gullberg, U.; Nilsson, E. and Olsson, I.: Characterization in vitro of a human tumor necrosis factor-binding protein. A soluble form of a tumor necrosis factor receptor. J. Clin. Invest. 86: 1396–1442, 1990.

Lapeyre, B.; Mariottini, P.; Mathieu, C.; Ferrer, P.; Amaldi, F.; Amalric, F. and Caizergues-Ferrer, M.: Molecular cloning of Xenopus fibrillarin, a conserved U3 small nuclear ribonucleoprotein recognized by antisera from humans with autoimmune disease. Molec. Cell Biol. 10: 430–434, 1980.

Larson, S.M.; Brown, J.P.; Wright, P.W.; Carrasquillo, J.A.; Hellström, I. and Hellström, K.E.: Imaging of melanoma with I-131–labeled monoclonal antibodies. J. Nucl. Med. 24: 123, 1983.

Larsson-Sciard, E.L.; Spetz-Hagberg, A.L.; Casrouge, A. and Kourilsky, P.: Analysis of T cell receptor Vß gene usage in primary mixed lymphocyte reactions: evidence for directive usage by different antigen-presenting cells and Mls-like determinants on T cell blasts. Eur. J. Immunol. 20: 1223–1229, 1990.

Last-Barney, K.; Homon, C.A.; Faanes, R.B. and Merluzzi, V.J.: Synergistic and overlapping activities of tumor necrosis factor-µ and Il-1. J. Immunol. 141: 527, 1988.

Laszlo, G. and Dickler, H.B.: IL-4 induces loss of B lymphocyte Fc-gammaRII ligand binding capacity. J. Immunol. 141: 3416, 1988.

Laszlo, J.; Buckley, C.E. and Amos, C.B.: Infusion of isologous immune plasma in chronic lymphocytic leukemia. Blood 31: 104, 1986.

Lauder, I. and Ahern, E.W.: The significance of lymphocytic infiltration in neuroblastoma. Br. J. Cancer 26: 321–330, 1972.

Laurent, G.; Frankel, A.E.; Hertler, A.A.; Schlossmann, D.M.; Casellas, P. and Jansen, F.K.: Treatment of leukemia patients with T101 ricin a chain immunotoxins, in Frankel, AE (ed): Immunotoxins, Boston, Kluwer, 483, 1988.

Law, S.K.A.; Dodds, A.W. and Porter, R.R.: A comparison of the properties of two classes C4A and C4B of the human complement component C4. EMBO J. 3: 1819–1823, 1984.

Lawrence, D.A.; Pircher, R. and Jullien, P.: Conversion of a high molecular weight latent β-TGF from chicken embryo fibroblasts into a low molecular weight active ß-TGF under acidic conditions. Biochem. Biophys. Res. Commmun. 133: 1026–1034, 1985.

Le, J. and Vilcek, J.: Tumour necrosis factor and interleukin 1: Cytokines with multiple overlapping biological activities. Lab. Invest. 56: 234–247, 1987.

Le, P.T.; Lazorick, S.; Whichard, L.P.; Yang, Y.C.; Clark, S.C.; Haynes, B.F. and Singer, K.H.: Human thymic epithelial cells produce Il-6, granulocyte-monocyte-CSF, and leukemia inhibitory factor. J. Immunol. 145: 3310–3315, 1990.

Lea, R.G.; Flanders, K.C.; Harley, C.B.; Manuel, J.; Banwatt, D. and Clark, D.A.: Release of a transforming growth factor (TGF)-beta 2-related suppressor factor from postimplantation murine decidual tissue can be correlated with the detection of a subpopulation of cells containing RNA for TGF-beta 2. J. Immunol. 148: 778–787, 1992.

Leary, A.G.; Wong, G.G.; Clark, S.C.; Smith, A.G. and Ogawa, M.: Leukemia inhibitory factor differentiation-inhibiting activity/human interleukin for DA cells augments proliferation of human hematopoietic stem cells. Blood 75: 1960–1964, 1990.

Leatherbarrow, R.J.; Rademacher, T.W.; Dwek, R.A.; Woof, J.M.; Clark, A.; Burton, D.R.; Richardson, N. and Feinstein, A.: Effector functions of a monoclonal aglycosylated mouse IgG2a: binding and activation of complement component C1 and interaction with human monocyte Fc receptor. Molec. Immun. 22: 407–415, 1985.

Lee, J.; Kunag, W.J.; Rice, G.C. and Wood, W.I.: Characterization of complementary DNA clones encoding the rabbit Il-8 receptor. J. Immunol. 148: 1261–1264, 1992.

Lee, J.C.; Badger, A.M.; Griswold, D.E.; Dunnington, D.; Truneh, A.; Votta, B.; White, J.R.; Young, P.R. and Bender, P.E.: Bicyclic imidazoles as a novel class of cytokine biosynthesis inhibitors. Immunosuppressive and Antinflammatory Drugs, eds. Allison, A.C.; Lafferty, K.J. and Fliri, H., Annals of the New York Academy of Science 696: 149, 1993.

Lee, S.W.; Tsou, A.P.; Chan, H.; Thomas, J.; Petrie, K.; Eugui, E.M. and Allison, A.C.: Glucocorticoids selectively inhibit the transcription of interleukin-1 gene and decrease the stability of Il-1ß mRNA. Proc. Natl. Acad. Sci. USA 85: 1204–1208, 1988.

Lee, Y.-M.; Leiby, K.R.; Allar, J.; Paris, K.; Lerch, B. and Okarma, T.B.: Primary structure of bovine conglutinin, a member of the C-type animal lectin family. J. Biol. Chem. 266: 2715–2723, 1991.

Lehmann, V.; Freudenberg, M.A. and Galanos, C.: Lethal toxicity of lipopolysaccharide and tumor necrosis factor in normal and D-galactosamine-treated mice. J. Exp. Med. 165: 657, 1987.

Leibovich, S.J.; Polverini, P.J.; Shepard, H.M.; Wiseman, D.M.; Shively, V. and Nuseir, N.: Macrophages-induced angiogenesis is mediated by tumor necrosis factor-α. Nature 329: 630–632, 1987.

Leibson, H.J.; Gefter, M.; Zlotnik, A.; Marrack, P. and Kappler, J.W.: Role of gamma-interferon in antibody-producing responses. Nature 309: 799–801, 1984.

Leiferman, K.M.; Ackerman, S.J.; Sampson, H.A.; Haugen, H.S.; Venenice, P.Y. and Gleich, G.J.: Dermal deposition of eosinophil granule major protein in atopic dermatitis: comparison with Onchocerciasis. N. Engl. J. Med. 313: 282, 1985.

Lenschow, D.J.; Zeng, Y.; Thistlewaite, J.R.; Montag, A.; Brady, W.; Gibson, M.G.; Linsley, P.S. and Bluestone, J.A.: Long-term survival of xenogeneic pancreatic islet grafts induced by CTLA4Ig. Science 257: 789–792, 1992.

Lepow, I.H.; Wurz, L.; Ratnoff, O.D. and Pillemer, L.: Studies of the mechanism of inactivation of human complement by plasmin and by antigen-antibody aggregates. J. Immunol. 73: 146–158, 1954.

Lepow, I.H.; Ratnoff, O.D.; Rosen, F.S. and Pillemer, L.: Observation on a proesterase associated with partially purified first component of complement (C'1). Proc. Soc. Exp. Biol. Med. 92: 32–37, 1956.

Lernmark, A.; Freedman, Z.R.; Hofmann, C.; Rubenstein, A.H.; Steiner, D.F.; Jackson, R.L.; Winter, R.J. and Traisman, H.S.: Islet-cell-surface antibodies in juvenile diabetes mellitus. New. Engl. J. Med. 299: 375–380, 1978.

Le Thi Bich Thui, S.C.; Brochier, J.; Fridman, W.H. and Revillard J.P.: Suppression of mitogen induced peripheral B cell differentiation by soluble receptors for Fc IgG released from lymphocytes. Eur. J. Immunol. 10: 894, 1980.

Lett-Brown, M.A.; Thueson, D.O.; Plank, D.E.; Langford, M.P. and Grant, J.A.: Histamine-releasing activity. IV. Molecular heterogeneity the activity from stimulated human thoracic duct lymphocytes. Cell Immunol. 87: 434, 1984.

Leu, R.W.; Kriet, D.; Zhou, A.; Herriott, M.J.; Rummage, J.A. and Shannon, B.J.: Reconstitution of murine resident peritoneal macrophages for antibody-dependent cellular cytotoxicity by homologous serum C1q. Cellular Immunology 122: 48–61, 1989.

Leu, R.W.; Zhou, A.; Rummage, J.A.; Kennedy, M.J. and Shannon, B.J.: Exogenous C1q reconstitutes resident but not inflammatory mouse peritoneal macrophages for Fc receptor-dependent cellular cytotoxicity and phagocytosis. J. Immunol. 143: 3250–3257, 1989.

Levine, A.J.: The p53 tumor suppressor gene and product. Canc. Surv. 12: 59–79, 1992.

Levy, A.P.; Tamargo, R.; Brem, H. and Nathans, D.: An endothelial cell growth factor from the mouse neuroblastoma cell line NB41. Growth Factors 2: 9–19, 1989.

Levy, D.A. and Chen, J.: Healthy IgE-deficient person. N. Engl. J. Med. 283: 541, 1970.

Levy, R. and Miller, R.A.: Tumor therapy with monoclonal antibodies. Fed. Proc. 42: 2650–2656, 1983.

Lewis, A.J.; Glaser, K.B.; Sturm, R.J.; Molnar-Kimber, K.L. and Bansbach, C.C.: Strategies for the development of new antiarthritic agents. Int. J. Immunopharm. 14: 497–504, 1992.

Lhotta, K.; König, P.; Neumayr, H.; Geissler, D. and Dittrich, P.: Renal expression of ICAM-1 in glomerulonephritis. 27th Congress of the European Dialysis and Transplant Association, Vienna, September 5–8, 1990.

Lhotta, K.; Neumayer, H.P.; Joannidis, M.; Geissler, D. and König, P.: Renal expression of intercellular ahesion molecule-1 in different forms of glomerulonephritis. Clinical Science 81: 477–481, 1991.

Lidbury, P.S.; Thiermermann, C.; Korbut, R. and Vane, J.R.: Interaction of endothelins with the endothelium. J. Vasc. Med. Biol. 2: 178 (abstr.), 1990.

Lider, O.; Reshef, T.; Beraud, E.; Ben-Nun, A. and Cohen, I.R.: Anti-idiotypic network induced by T cell vaccination against experimental autoimmune encephalomyelitis. Science 239: 181–183, 1988.

Liebrich, W.; Schlag, P.; Manasterski, M.; Lehner, B.; Stöhr, M.; Möller, P. and Schirrmacher, V.: In vitro and clinical characterisation of a newcastle disease virus-modified autologous tumor cell vaccine for treatment of colorectal cancer patients. Eur. J. Cancer 27: 703–710, 1991.

Lifson, J.D. and Engleman, E.G.: The role of CD4 in normal immunity and HIV infection. Immunol. Rev. 109: 93, 1989.

Lillien, L.E.; Sendtner, M.; Rohrer, H.; Hughes, S.M. and Raff, M.C.: Type-2 astrocyte development in rat brain cultures is initiated by a CNTF-like protein produced by type-1 astrocytes. Neuron 1: 485–494, 1988.

Lin, A.H.; Morton, D.R. and Gorman, R.R.: Acetyl glyceryl ether phosphorylcholine stimulates leukotriene B4 synthesis in human polymorphonuclear leukocytes. J. Clin. Invest. 70: 1058–1065, 1982.

Lin, C.S.; Boltz, R.C.; Siekierka, J.J. and Sigal, N.H.: FK-506 and cyclosporin A inhibit highly similar signal transduction pathways in human T lymphocytes. Cell Immunol. 133: 269–284, 1991.

Lin, C.Y.; Hsu, H.C. and Chian, H.: Improvement of histological and immunological change in steroid and immunosuppressive drug-resistant lupus nephritis by high-dose intravenous gammaglobulin. Nephron 53: 303–310, 1989.

Lin, F.K.; Suggs, S.; Lin, C.H.; Browne, J.K.; Smalling, R.; Egrie, J.C.; Chen, K.K.; Fox, G.M.; Martin, F.; Stabinsky, Z. et al.: Cloning and expression of the human erythropoietin gene. Proc. Natl. Acad. Sci. 82: 7580–7584, 1985.

Lin, H.; Parmacek, M.S.; Morle, G.; Bolling, S. and Leiden, J.M.: Expression of recombinant genes in myocardium in vivo after direct injection of DNA. Circulation 82: 2217–2221, 1990.

Lin, H.S. and Gordon, S.: Secretion of plasminogen activator by bone marrow-derived mononuclear phagocytes and its enhancement by colony-stimulating factors. J. Exp. Med. 150: 231–245, 1979.

Lin, H.Y.; Wang, X.F.; Ng-Eaton, E.; Weinberg, R.A. and Lodish, H.F.: Expression cloning of the TGF-beta type II receptor, a functional transmembrane serine/threonine kinase. Cell 68: 775–785, 1992.

Lindley, I.; Aschauer, H.; Seifert, J.M.; Lam, C.; Brunowsky, W.; Kownatzki, E.; Thelen, M.; Peveri, P.; Dewald, B.; von Tscharner, V. et al.: Synthesis and expression in Escherichia coli of the gene encoding monocyte-derived neutrophil-activating factor: biological equivalence between natural and recombinant neutrophil-activating factor. Proc. Natl. Acad. Sci. 85: 9199–9203, 1988.

Lindsten, T.; June, C.H.; Ledbetter, J.A.; Stella, G. and Thompson, C.B.: Regulation of lymphokine messenger RNA stability by a surface-mediated T cell activation pathway. Science 244: 339–343, 1989.

Lindstrom, P.; Lerner, R.; Palmblad, J. and Patarroyo, M.: Rapid adhesive responses of endothelial cells and of neutrophils induced by leukotriene B4 are mediated by leucocytic adhesion protein CD18. Scand. J. Immunol. 31: 737–744, 1990.

Linscott, W.D.; Ranken, R. and Triglia, R.P.: Evidence that bovine conglutinin reacts with an early product of C3b degradation, and an improved conglutination assay. J. Immunol. 121: 658–664, 1978.

Linsley, P.S.; Bolton-Hanson, M.; Horn, D.; Malik, N.; Kallestad, J.C.; Ochs, V.; Zarling, J.M. and Shoyab, M.: Identification and characterization of cellular receptors for the growth regulator, oncostatin M. J. Biol. Chem. 264: 4282–4289, 1988.

Linsley, P.S.; Brady, W.; Grosmaire, I.; Aruffo, A.; Damle, N. and Ledbetter, J.: Binding of the B cell activation antigen B7 to CD28 costimulates T cell proliferation and Interleukin-1 mRNA accumulation. J. Exp. Med. 173: 721–730, 1991.

Linsley, P.S.; Brady, W.; Urnes, M.; Grosmarie, L.S.; Damle, N.K. and Ledbetter, J.A.: CTLA-4 is a second receptor for the B cell activation antigen B7. J. Exp. Med. 174: 561–570, 1991.

Linsley, P.S.; Wallace, P.M.; Johnson, J.; Gibson, M.G.; Greene, J.L.; Ledbetter, J.A.; Singh, C. and Tepper, M.A.: Immunosuppression in vivo by a soluble form of the CTLA-4 T cell activation molecule. Science 257: 792–794, 1992.

Liszewski, M.K. and Atkinson, J.P.: The role of complement in autoimmunity. In Bigazzi, P., Reichlin, M (eds.): Systemic Autoimmunity, New York, Marcel Dekker, 13–37, 1991.

Littman, B.H.; Dastvan, F.F.; Carlson, P.L. and Sanders, K.N.: Regulation of monocyte/macrophage C2 production and HLA-DR expression by IL-4 (BSF-1) and IFN-gamma. J. Immunol. 142: 520–528, 1989.

Liu, C.-C.; Rafii, S.; Granelli-Piperno, A.; Trapani, J.A. and Young, J.D-E.: Perforin and serine esterase gene expression in stimulated human T cells. Kinetics, mitogen requirements, and effects of cyclosporin A. J. Exp. Med. 170: 2105–2118, 1989.

Liu, F.T.: Molecular biology of IgE-binding protein, IgE-binding factors, and IgE-receptors. Crit. Rev. Immunol. 10: 289, 1990.

Liu, J.; Farmer, J.D.; Lane, W.S.; Friedman, J.; Weissman, I. and Schreiber, S.L.: Calcineurin is a common target of cyclophilin-cyclosporin A and FKBP-FK 506 complexes. Cell 66: 807–815, 1991.

Liu, J.; Modrell, B.; Aruffo, A.; Marken, J.S.; Taga, T.; Yasukawa, K.; Murakami, M.; Kishimoto, T. and Shoyab, M.: Interleukin-6 signal transducer gp130 mediates oncostatin M signaling. J. Biol. Chem. 267: 16763–16766, 1992.

Liu, J.Y.; Joshua, D.E.; Willimas, G.T.; Smith, C.A.; Gordon, J. and MacLennan, I.C.M.: Mechanisms of antigen-driven selection in germinal centres. Nature 342: 929–931, 1989.

Liu, J.Y.; Cairns, J.A.; Holder, M.J.; Abbot, S.D.; Jansen, K.U.; Bonnefoy, J.-Y.; Gordon, J. and MacLennan, I.C.M.: Recombinant 24 kDa CD23 and interleukin-1μ promote the survival of germinal center B cells: evidence for bifurcation in the development of centrocytes rescued from apoptosis. Eur. J. Immunol. 21: 1107, 1991.

Liu, J.Y.; Mason, D.Y.; Johnson, G.D.; Abbot, S.; Gregory, C.D.; Hardie, D.L.; Gordon, J. and MacLennan, I.C.M.: Germinal center cells express bcl-2 protein after activation by signals which prevent their entry into apoptosis. Eur. J. Immunol. 21: 1905, 1991.

Liu, J.Y.; Johnson, G.D.; Gordon, J. and MacLennan, I.C.M.: Germinal centres in T cell dependent antibody responses. Immunology Today 13: 17, 1992.

Liu, M.C.; Proud, D.; Lichtenstein, L.M.; MacGlashan, D.W.; Schleimer, R.P.; Adkinson, N.F.; Kagey-Sobotka, A.; Schulman, E.S. and Plaut, M.: Human lung macrophage-derived histamine-releasing activity is due to IgE-dependent factors. J. Immunol. 136: 2588, 1986.

Livingston, P.O.; Ritter, G. and Calves, M.J.: Antibody response after immunization with the gangliosides GM1, GM2, GM3, GD2 and GD3 in the mouse. Cancer Immun. Immunother. 29: 179–184, 1989.

Livingston, P.O.: Construction of cancer vaccines with carbohydrate and protein (peptide) tumor antigens. Current Opinion in Immunology 4: 624–629, 1992.

Livingston, P.O.: Approaches to augmenting the IgG antibody response to melanoma ganglioside vaccines. Specific Immunotherapy Of Cancer With Vaccines, eds. Bystryn, J.-C.; Ferrone, S. and Livingston, P., The New York Academy of Sciences 690: 204, 1993.

Livingston, P.O.; Calves, M.J.; Helling, F.; Zollinger, W.D.; Blake, M.S. and Lowell, G.H.: GD3/proteosome vaccines induce consistent IgM antibodies against the ganglioside GD3. Vaccine 11: 1199–1204, 1993.

Lloyd, K.O.: Molecular characteristics of tumor antigens. Immunol. Allergy Clin. North Am. 10: 765–779, 1990.

Lloyd, K.O.: Tumor antigens known to be immunogenic in man. Specific Immunotherapy Of Cancer With Vaccines, eds. Bystryn, J.-C.; Ferrone, S. and Livingston, P., The New York Academy of Sciences 690: 50, 1993.

Locksley, R.M.; Heinzel, F.P.; Holaday, B.J.; Mutha, S.S.; Reiner, S.L. and Sadick, M.D.: Induction of Th1 and Th2 CD4+ subsets during murine Leishmania major infection. Res. Immunol. 142: 28, 1991.

Lohde, E.; Luck, M.; Gemperle, P.; Raude, H.; Barzen, G. and Kraas, E.: Quantitative accumulation analysis of the MAb BW 431/26 in human colon cancer after in vivo and ex vivo administration. 8th Int. Hammersmith Meeting, Greece, 1991.

Lolait, S.J.; Lim, A.T.W.; Loh, B.J. and Funder, J.W.: Immunoreactive ß-endorphin in a subpopulation of mouse spleen macrophages. J. Clin. Invest. 73: 277–280, 1984.

London, S.D.; Rubin, D.H. and Cebra, J.J.: Gut mucosal immunization with reovirus serotype 1/L stimulates virus-specific cytotoxic T cell precursors as well as IgA memory cells in Peyer's patches. J. Exp. Med. 165: 830–847, 1987.

Longenecker, B.M.; Reddish, M.; Koganty, R. and MacLean, G.D.: Immune responses of mice and human breast cancer patients following immunization with synthetic Sialyl-Tn conjugated to KLH plus Detox adjuvant. Specific Immunotherapy Of Cancer With Vaccines, eds. Bystryn, J.-C.; Ferrone, S. and Livingston, P., The New York Academy of Sciences 690: 276, 1993.

Longley, R.E.; Gunasekera, S.P.; Faherty, D.; McLane, J. and Dumont, F.: Immunosuppression by discodermolide. Immunosuppressive and Antiinflammatory Drugs, eds. Allison, A.C.; Lafferty, K.J. and Fliri, H., Annals of the New York Academy of Sciences 696: 94, 1993.

Lonky, S.A. and Wohl, H.: Stimulation of human leucocyte elastase by platelet factor 4. Physiologic, morphologic and biomedical effects on hamster lungs in vitro. J. Clin. Invest. 67: 817–826, 1981.

Lopez, A.F.; To, L.B.; Yang, Y.C.; Gamble, J.R.; Shannon, M.F.; Burns, G.F.; Dyson, P.G.; Juttner, C.A.; Clark, S. and Vadas, M.A.: Stimulation of proliferation, differentiation, and function of human cells by primate interleukin 3. Proc. Natl. Acad. Sci. 84: 2761–2765, 1987.

Loppnow, H.; Stelter, F.; Schönbeck, U.; Schlüter, C.; Brandt, E.; Schütt, C. and Flad, H.-D.: LPS-antagonists inhibit LPS-induced activation of vascular endothelial cells: this process is not mediated by mCD14. Immunobiology 189: 1993.

Lord, E.; McAdam, A.; Felcher, A.; Woods, M.; Pulaski, B.; Hutter, E. and Frelinger, J.: Transfection of TGF-ß producing tumors with Il-2 elicits tumor rejection. Specific Immunotherapy of Cancer with Vaccines, Bystryn, J.C.; Ferrone, S. and Livingston, P. (eds)., Annals of the New York Academy of Sciences 690, 1993.

Lotz, M.; Carson, D.A. and Vaughan, J.H.: Substance P activation of rheumatoid synoviocytes: Neural pathway in pathogenesis of arthritis. Science 235: 893–895, 1987.

Lotz, M.; Vaughan, J.H. and Carson, D.A.: Effect of neuropeptides on production of inflammatory cytokines by human monocytes. Science 241: 1218–1221, 1988.

Lotz, M.; Terkeltaub, R. and Villiger, P.M.: Carilage and joint inflammation. Regulation of Il-8 expression by human articular chondrocytes. J. Immunol. 148: 466–473, 1992.

Lotze, M.T.; Carrasquillo, J.A.; Weinstein, J.N.; Bryant, G.J.; Perentesis, P.; Reynolds, J.C.; Mams, L.A.; Eger, R.R.; Keenan, A.M.; Hellström, I.; Hellström, K.E. and Larson, S.M.: Monoclonal antibody imaging of human melanoma. Ann. Surg. 204: 228, 1986.

Lotzova, E.; Savary, C.A. and Herberman, R.B.: Induction of NK cell activity against fresh human leukemia in culture with interleukin 2. J. Immunol. 138: 2718, 1987.

Lovett, D.H.; Haensch, G.M.; Goppelt, M.; Resch, K. and Gemsa, F.: Activation of glomerular mesangial cells by the terminal membrane attack complex of complement. J. Immunol. 138: 2473–2480, 1987.

Lowe, J.A.: Substance P antagonists. Drugs of the Future 17: 1115–1121, 1992.

Lu, H.S.; Clogston, C.L.; Wypych, J.; Fausset, P.R.; Lauren, S.; Mendiaz, E.A.; Zsebo, K.M. and Langley, K.E.: Amino acid sequence and post-translational modification of stem cell factor isolated from buffalo rat liver cell-conditioned medium. J. Biol. Chem. 266: 8102–8107, 1991.

Lucht, W.D.; English, D.K.; Bernard, G.R.; Serafin, W.E. and Brigham, K.L.: Prevention of release of granulocyte aggregants into sheep lung lymph following endotoxemia by N-acetylcysteine. Am. J. Med. Sci. 294: 161–167, 1987.

Luger, T.A.; Wirthe, U. and Kock, A.: Epidermal cells synthesize a cytokine with interleukin-3–like properties. J. Immunol. 134: 915–919, 1985.

Lundberg, C.; Marceau, F. and Hugli, T.E.: C5a-induced hemodynamic and hematologic changes in the rabbit. Am. J. Pathol. 128: 471–483, 1987.

Lundgren, M.; Persson, U.; Larsson, P.; Magnusson, C.; Smith, C.I.E.; Hammarström, L. and Severinson, E.: Interleukin 4 induces synthesis of IgE and IgG4 in human B cells. Eur. J. Immunol. 19: 1311–1315, 1989.

Lurquin, C.; van Pel, A.; Mariamé, B.; De Plaen, E.; Szikora, J.P.; Janssens, C.; Reddehase, M.J.; Lejeune, J. and Boon, T.: Structure of the gene of tumor transplantation antigen P91A. the mutated exon encodes a peptide recognized with Ld by cytolytic T cells. Cell 58: 293–301, 1989.

Lydyard, P.M.; Quartey-Papafio, R.; Bröker, B.; Mackenzie, L.; Jouquan, J.; Blaschek, M.A.; Steele, J.; Petrou, M.; Collins, P.; Isenberg, D. and Youiou, P.Y.: The antibody repertoire of early human B cells. I. High frequency of autoreactivity and polyreactivity. Scand. J. Immunol. 31: 33, 1990.

Lynch, R.G.; Sandor, M.; Waldschmidt, T.J.; Mathur, A.; Schaiff, W.T.; Berg, D.J.; Snapp, K.; Mueller, A.; Robinson, M.G.; Noben, N. and Rosenberg, M.G.: Lymphocyte Fc receptors: expression, regulation and function. Molec. Immun. 27: 1167–1179, 1990.

Lyons, R.M.; Keski-Oja, J. and Moses, H.L.: Proteolytic activation of latent transforming growth factor-ß from fibroblast conditioned medium. J. Cell Biol. 106: 1659–1665, 1988.

Lyons, R.M.; Gentry, L.E.: Purchio, A.F. and Moses, H.L.: Proteolytic processing and activation of latent transforming growth factor-ß. J. Cell Biol. 107: 51A, 1988.

Lyons, R.M. and Moses, H.L.: Transforming growth factors and the regulation of cell proliferation. Eur. J. Biochem. 187: 467–473, 1990.

Macaulay, V.M. and Carney, D.N.: Neuropeptide growth factors. Cancer Investig. 9: 659–673, 1991.

MacDonald, H.R.; Schneider, R.; Lees, R.K.; Howe, R.C.; Acha-Orbea, H.; Festenstein, H.; Zinkernagel. R.M. and Hengartner, H.: T cell receptor Vß use predicts reactivity and tolerance to Mlsa-encoded antigens. Nature 332: 40–45, 1988.

MacDonald, H.R.: Introduction: Mls - a retroviral superantigen. Immunology 4: 285–286, 1992.

MacDonald, S.M.; Schleimer, R.P.; Kagey-Sobotka, A.; Gillis, S. and Lichtenstein, L.M.: Recombinant Il-3 induces histamine release from human basophils. J. Immunol. 142: 3527, 1989.

Mach, J.P.; Forni, M.; Ritschard, J.; Buchegger, F.; Carrel, S.; Widgren, S.; Donath, A. and Albertro, P.: Use and limitations of radiolabeled anti-CEA antibodies and their fragments for photo-scanning detection of human colorectal carcinomas. Oncodevelop. Biol. Med. 1: 49–69, 1980.

Mach, J.P.; Carrel, S.; Forni, M.; Ritschard, J.; Donath, A. and Alberto, P.: Tumor localization of radiolabeled antibodies against carcinoembryonic antigen in patients with carcinoma. A critical evaluation. N. Engl. J. Med. 303: 5, 1980.

Mach, J.P.; Chatal, F.J.; Lubrosco, J.D.; Buchegger, F.; Forni, M.; Ritchard, J.; Berche, C.; Donillard, J.Y.; Carrel, S.; Herlyn, M.; Steplewski, Z. and Koprowski, H.: Tumor localization in patients by radiolabeled monoclonal antibodies against colon carcinoma. Cancer Res. 43: 5593–5600, 1983.

Machold, K.P.; Carson, D.A. and Lotz, M.: Transforming growth factor-β (TGFβ) inhibition of Epstein-Barr virus (EBV)- and Interleukin-4 (Il-4)-induced immunoglobulin production in human B lymphocytes. J. Clin. Immunol. 13: 219, 1993.

Mackay, C.R.; Marston, W.L. and Dudler, L.: Naive and memory T cells show distinct pathways of lymphocyte recirculation. J. Exp. Med. 171: 801–817, 1990.

MacKenzie, A.R.: Immunophilin-binding drugs and their evaluation as antirheumatic agents. Rheumatoid Arthritis, London, UK, June 17–18, 1991.

MacKenzie, A.R.: Immunophilin-binding drugs and their evaluation as antirheumatic agents. Rheumatoid Arthritis Conference Documentation, London, 17.–18. 6. 1991.

MacKie, R.M.: Interferon-alpha for atopic dermatitis. Lancet 1: 1282–1283, 1990.

MacLaren, N.; Muir, A.; Silverstein, J.; Song, Y.-H.; She, J.X.; Krischer, J.; Atkinson, M. and Schatz, D.: Early diagnosis and specific treatment of Insulin-dependent diabetes. Ann. New York Acad. Sci. 696: 342–350, 1993.

MacLennan, I.C.M. and Gray, D.: Antigen-driven selection of virgin and memory B cells. Immunol. Rev. 91: 61, 1986.

MacLennan, I.: Signals involved in B-cell selection and differentiation in follicles. ENII Conf.: Integrated Function of Molecules of the Immune System. Les Embiez, France, 12th-16th May 1993.

Maclouf, J.; Fruteau de Laclos, B. and Borgeat, P.: Stimulation of leukotriene biosynthesis in human blood leukocytes by platelet-derived 12–hydroperoxyicosatetraenoic acid. Proc. Natl. Acad. Sci. USA 79: 6042–6046, 1982.

Maclouf, J.; Henson, P.M. and Murphy, R.C.: Platelet-neutrophil interactions: formation of leukotriene C4 by transcellular metabolism. Blood 70: 354a, 1987.

MacMillan, R.: Beyond willow bard: Is there potential for development of novel anti-inflammatory agents by modulation of the arachidonic acid cascades. Rheumatoid Arthritis, Royal College of Physicians, London, 17./18.6.1991.

Magarian-Blander, J.; Domenech, N. and Finn, O.J.: Specific effective T-cell recognition of cells
transfected with a truncated human mucin cDNA. Specific Immunotherapy of Cancer with
Vaccines, Bystryn, J.C.; Ferrone, S. and Livingston, P. (eds)., Annals of the New York Academy of Sciences 690: 1993.

Maggi, E.; Biswas, P.; Del Prete, G-F.; Parronchi, P.; Macchia, D.; Simonelli, C.; Emmi, L.; De
Carli, M.; Tiri, A.; Ricci, M. and Romagnani, S.: Accumulation of Th2–like helper T cells in
the conjunctiva of patients with vernal conjuctivitis. J. Immunol. 146: 1169, 1992.

Mahoney, K.H. and Heppner, G.H.: FACS analysis of tumor-associated macrophage replication:
differences between metastatic and nonmetastatic murine mammary tumors. J. Leukocyte
Biol. 41: 205–211, 1987.

Maier, W.P.; Gordon, D.S.; Howard, R.F.; Saleh, M.N.; Miller, S.B.; Lieberman, J.D. and Wood-
lee, P.M.: Intravenous immunoglobulin therapy in systemic lupus erythematosus-associated
thrombocytopenia. Arthritis. Rheum. 33: 1233–1239, 1990.

Maillard, J.L.; Pick, E. and Turk, J.L.: Interaction between "sensitized lymphocytes" and antigen
in-vitro. V. Vascular permeability induced by skin-reactive factor. Intern. Arch. Allergy Appl.
Immunol. 42: 50–68, 1972.

Majno, G. and Palade, G.E.: Studies on inflammation-I-the effect of histamine and serotonin on
vascular permeability: an electron microscope study. J. Biophys. Biochem. Cytol. 11:
571–605, 1961.

Makino, K.; Morimoto, M.; Nishi, M.; Sakamoto, S.; Tamura, A.; Inooka, H. and Akasaka, K.:
Proton nuclear magnetic resonance study on the solution conformation of human epidermal
growth factor. Proc. Natl. Acad. Sci. 84: 7841–7845, 1987.

Malamitsi, J.; Skarlos, D.; Fotiou, S.; Papakostas, P.; Aravantinos, G.; Vassilarou, D.; Taylor-Papadimitriou, J.; Koutoulidis, K.; Hooker, G.; Snook, D. and Epenetos, A.A.: Intracavitary use
of two radiolabeled tumor-associated monoclonal antibodies. J. Nucl. Med. 29: 1910–1915,
1988.

Malech, H.L. and Gallin, J.I.: Neutrophils in human diseases. N. Engl. J. Med. 317: 687–694,
1987.

Malefty, R.D.; Abrams, W.J.; Bennett, B.; Figdor, C.G. and DeVries, J.E.: Interleukin 10 (Il-10)
inhibits cytokine synthesis by human monocytes: an autoregulatory role of Il-10 produced by
monocytes. J. Exp. Med. 174: 1209–1220, 1991.

Malhotra, R. and Sim, R.B.: Chemical and hydrodynamic characterization of the human leukocyte receptor for complement subcomponent C1q. Biochem. J. 262: 625–631, 1989.

Malik, A.B.: The role of platelets in the control of vascular endothelial barrier function. Int. Conf.
on: The platelet in health & diseases. Royal College of physicians, London, 1992.

Malik, N.; Kallestad, J.C.; Gunderson, N.L.; Austin, S.D.; Neubauer, M.G.; Ochs, V.; Marquardt,
H.; Zarling, J.M.; Shoyab, M.; Wei, C.M. et al.: Molecular cloning, sequence analysis, and
functional expression of a novel growth regulator, oncostatin M. Mol. Cell Biol. 9:
2847–2853, 1989.

Malizia, E.; Andreucci, G.; Paolucci, D.; Crescenzi, F.; Fabbri, A. and Fraioli, F.: Electroacupuncture and peripheral ß-endorphin and ACTH levels. Lancet 8: 535–536, 1979.

Malkin, D.; Li, F.P.; Strong, L.C.; Fraumeni, J.F.J.; Nelson, C.E.; Kim, D.H.; Kassel, J.; Gryka,
M.A.; Bischoff, F.Z.; Tainsky, M.A. et al.: Germ line p53 mutations in a familial syndrome of
breast cancer, sarcomas, and other neoplasms. Science 250: 1233–1238, 1990.

Mantovani, A.; Wang, J.M.; Balotta, C.; Abdeljalil, B. and Bottazzi, B.: Origin and regulation of
tumor-associated macrophages: the role of tumor-derived chemotactic factor. Biochem. Biophys. Acta 865: 59–67, 1986.

Mantovani, A.; Bottazzi, B.; Colotta, F.; Sozzani, S. and Ruco, L.: The origin and function of
tumor-associated macrophages. Immunology Today 13: 265, 1992.

Mao, C.; Merlin, G.; Ballotti, R.; Metzler, M. and Aguet, M.: Rapid increase of the human IFN-
gamma receptor phosphorylation in response to human IFN-gamma and phorbol myristate
acetate. Involvement of different serine/threonine kinases. J. Immun. 145: 4257–4264, 1990.

Marcus, A.J.; Weksler, B.B.; Jaffe, E.A. and Broekman, M.J.: Synthesis of prostacyclin from platelet-derived endoperoxides by cultured human endothelial cells. J. Clin. Invest. 66: 979–986,
1980.

Marcus, A.J.; Broekman, M.J.; Safier, L.B.; Ullman, H.L.; Islam, N.; Serhan, C.N.; Rutherford, L.E.; Korchak, H.M. and Weissmann, G.: Formation of leukotrienes and other hydroxy acids during platelet-neutrophil interactions in vitro. Biochem. Biophys. Res. Commun. 109: 130–137, 1982.

Marcus, A.J.; Safier, L.B.; Ullman, H.L.; Broekman, M.J.; Islam, N.; Oglesby, T.D.; Gorman, R.R. and von Schacky, C.: Platelet neutrophil interactions in the eicosanoid pathway. In: Oppenheim, J.J. and Jacobs, D.M. (eds.) Leukocytes and Host Defense, Alan R. Liss, New York, 365–371, 1986.

Marguette, C.; Ban, E.; Fillon, G. and Haour, F.: Receptors for interleukin 1, 2 and 6 (Il-1α and β, Il-2, Il-6) in mouse, rat and human pituitary. Neuroendocrinology 52: 48, 1990.

Marley, G.M.; Doyle, L.A.; Ordónez, J.V.; Sisk, A.; Hussain, A. and Chiu, Y.R.-W.: Potentiation of interferon induction of class I major histocompatibility complex antigen expression by human tumor necrosis factor in small cell lung cancer cell lines. Cancer Res. 49: 6232–6236, 1989.

Maron, R.; Zerubavel, R.; Friedman, A. and Cohen, I.R.: T lymphocyte line specific for thyroglobulin produces or vaccinates against autoimmune thyroiditis in mice. J. Immunol. 131: 2316–2322, 1983.

Marquardt, H.; Todaro, G.J.; Henderson, L.E. and Oroszlan, S.: Purification and primary structure of a polypeptide with multiplication-stimulating activity from rat liver cell cultures. Homology with human insulin-like growth factor II. J. Biol. Chem. 256: 6859–6865, 1981.

Marquadt, H.; Hunkapiller, M.W.; Hood, L.E. and Todaro, G.J.: Rat transforming growth factor type I: structure and relationship to epidermal growth factor. Science 223: 1079–1082, 1984.

Marrack, P. and Kappler, J.: The staphylococcal enterotoxins and their relatives. Science 248: 705, 1990.

Marshall, J.S. and Bell, E.B.: Induction of an auto-anti-IgE response in rats. I. Effects on serum IgE concentrations. Eur. J. Immunol. 15: 272–277, 1985.

Marshall, J.S. and Bell, E.B.: Induction of an auto-anti-IgE response in rats. III. Inhibition of a specific IgE response. Immunology 66: 428–433, 1989.

Martin, F.H.; Suggs, S.V.; Langley, K.E.; Lu, H.S.; Ting, J.; Okino, K.H.; Morris, C.F.; McNiece, I.K.; Jacobsen, F.W.; Mendiaz, E.A. et al.: Primary structure and functional expression of rat and human stem cell factor DNAs. Cell 63: 203–211, 1990.

Martin, J.F.: Platelets, Megakaryocytes and nitric oxide in thrombosis and atherosclerosis. Int. Conf. on: The platelet in health & disease. Royal College of physicians, London, 1992.

Martin, S.D. and Springer T.A.: Purified intercellular adhesion molecule-1 (ICAM-1) is a ligand for lymphocyte function-associated antigen 1 (LFA-1). Cell 51: 813–819, 1987.

Martin, S.E. and Martin, W.J.: Interspecies brain antigen detected by naturally occurring mouse anti-brain autoantibody. Proc. natn. Acad. Sci. USA 72: 1036–1040, 1983.

Martin, W.J. and Kachel, D.L.: Reduction of neutrophil-mediated injury to pulmonary endothelial cells by dapsone. Am. Rev. Respir. Dis. 131: 544–547, 1985.

Mary, D.; Aussel, C.; Ferrua, B. and Fehlmann, M.: Regulation of interleukin-2 synthesis by cAMP in human T cells. J. Immunol. 139: 1179, 1987.

Massague, J.; Cheifetz, S.; Endo, T. and Nadal-Ginard, B.: Type β transforming growth factor is an inhibitor of myogenic differentiation. Proc. Natl. Acad. Si. USA 83: 8206–8210, 1986.

Massague, J.: The TGF-beta family of growth and differentiation factors. Cell 49: 437–438, 1987

Massague, J.: Receptors for the TGF-beta family. Cell 69: 1067–1070, 1992.

Masucci, M.G.; Gavioli, R.; De Campos-Lima, P.E.; Zahng, Q.-J.; Trivedi, P. and Dolcetti, R.: Transformation-associated Epstein-Barr virus antigens as targets for immune attack. Specific Immunotherapy Of Cancer With Vaccines, eds. Bystryn, J.-C.; Ferrone, S. and Livingston, P., The New York Academy of Science 690: 86, 1993.

Masuda, A.; Longo, D.L.; Kobayashi, Y.; Appela, E.; Oppenheim, J.J. and Matsushima, K.: Induction of mitochondrial manganese superoxide dismutase by interleukin-1. FASEB J. 2: 2087–2091, 1988.

Masuda, M.; Motoji, T.; Oshimi, K. and Mizoguchi, H.: Interleukin-7 and its effects on leukemia and lymphoma cells. Leukemia and Lymphoma 5: 231–235, 1991.

Masui, T.; Wakefield, L.M.; Lechner, J.F.; LaVeck, M.A.; Sporn, M.B. and Harris, C.C.: Type β transforming growth factor is the primary differentiation-inducing serum factor for normal human bronchial epithelial cells. Proc. Natl. Acad. Sci. USA 83: 2438–2442, 1986.

Mathe, G.; Loc, T. and Bernard, J.: Effect sur la leucemie 1210 de la souris d'un combinaison par diazotation d'A-methopterine et de gamma-globulines de hamsters porteurs de cell leucemie par heterograffe. C. Acad. Sci. (Paris) 246: 1626, 1958.

Matsuda, T.; Martinelli, G.P. and Osler, A.G.: Studies on immunosuppression by cobra venom factor. II. On responses to DNP-Ficoll and DNP-Polyacrylamide. J. Immunol. 121: 2048–2051, 1978.

Matsuda, T.; Hirano, T. and Kishimoto, T.: Establishment of interleukin 6 (IL-6)/B cell stimulatory factor 2 (BSF-2)-dependent cell line and prevention of anti-IL-6/BSF-2 monoclonal antibodies. Euro. J. Immunol. 18: 951, 1988.

Matsue, H.; Cruz, P.D.; Bergstresser, P.R. and Takashima, A.: Cytokine expression by epidermal cell subpopulations. J. Invest. Dermatol. 99: 42, 1992.

Matsumoto, A.K.; Kopicky-Burd, J.; Carter, R.H.; Tuveson, D.A.; Tedder, T.F. and Fearon, D.T.: Intersection of the complement and immune systems: A signal transduction complex of the B lymphocyte-containing complement receptor type 2 and CD19. J. Exp. Med. 173: 55–64, 1991.

Matter, B.; Zukoski, C.F.; Killen, D.A. and Ginn, E.: Transplanted carcinoma in an immunosuppressed patient. Transplantation 9: 71–74, 1970.

Mattes, M.J.; Thomson, T.M.; Old, L.J. and Lloyd, K.O.: A pigmentation-associated, differentiation antigen of human melanoma defined by a precipitating antibody in human serum. Int. J. Cancer 32: 717–721, 1983.

Maul, G.G.; French, B.T.; van Venrooij, W.J. and Jiminez S.A.: Topoisomerase I identified by scleroderma 70 antisera; enrichment of topoisomerase I at the centromere in mouse mitotic cells before anaphase. Proc. natn. Acad. Sci. USA 83: 5145–5149, 1986.

May, C.D. and Remigio, L.: Observations on high spontaneous release of histamine from leukocytes in vitro. Clin. Allergy 12: 229, 1982.

May, G.R.; Crook, P.; Moore, P.K. and Page, C.P.: The role of nitric oxide as an endogenous regulator of platelet and neutrophil activation within the pulmonary circulation of the rabbit. Br. J. Pharmacol. 102: 759–763, 1991.

May, G.R.; Paul, W.; Crook, P.; Butler, K.D. and Page, C.P.: The pharmacological modulation of thrombin-induced cerebral thromboembolism in the rabbit. Br. J. Pharmacol. 106: 133–138, 1992.

Mayumi, M.; Kawabe, T.; Nishioka, H.; Tanaka, M.; Kim, K.M.; Heike, T.; Yodoi, J. and Mikawa, H.: Interferon and (2'-5') oligoadenylate enhance the expression of low affinity receptors for IgE (Fc epsilon R2 CD23) on the human monoblast cell line U937. Mol. Immunol. 26: 241–247, 1989.

Mazur, E.M.; Cohen, J.L.; Wong, G.G. and Clark, S.C.: Modest stimulatory effect of recombinant human GM-CSF on colony growth from peripheral blood human megarkaryocyte colony formation. Exp. Hematol. 16: 1128, 1987.

Mazur, P.; Henzel, W.J.; Seymour, J.L. and Lazarus, R.A.: Ornatins: potent glycoprotein IIb-IIIa antagonists and platelet aggregation inhibitors from the leech Placobdella ornata. Eur. J. Biochem. 202: 1073–1082, 1991.

McAdam, A.; Pulaski, B.; Harkins, S.; Hutter, E.; Frelinger, J. and Pohl, C.: Coexpression of Il-2 and y-IFN enhances tumor immunity. Specific Immunotherapy of Cancer with Vaccines, Bystryn, J.C.; Ferrone, S. and Livingston, P. (eds.), Annals of the New York Academy of Sciences 690: 349, 1993.

McCarthy, D.O.; Kluger, M.J. and Vander, A.J.: Suppression of food intake during infection: Is interleukin-1 involved? Am J. Clin. Nutrition 42: 1179–1182, 1985.

McCauliffe, D.P.; Lux, F.A.; Lieu, T.-S.; Sanz, I.; Hanke, J.; Newkirk, M.M.; Bachinski, L.L.; Itoh, Y.; Siciliano, M.J.; Reichlin, M.; Sontheimer, R.D. and Capra, J.D.: Molecular cloning, expression, and chromosome 19 localizatin of a human Ro/SSA autoantigen. J. Clin. Invest. 85: 1379–1391, 1990.

McConkey, D.J.; Nicotera, P.; Hartzell, P.; Bellomo, G.; Wyllie, A.H. and Orrenius, S.: Glucocorticoids activate a suicide process in thymocytes through an elevation of cytosolic calcium concentration. Arch. Biochem. Biophys. 269: 365–370, 1989.

McDonnell, T.J.; Marin, M.C.; Hus, B.; Brisbay, S.M.; McConnell, K.; Tu, S-M.; Campbell, M.L. and Rodriguez-Villanueva, J.: Symposium: Apoptosis/Programmed Cell Death: The bcl-2 oncogene: apoptosis and neoplasia. Radiation Res. 136: 307–312, 1993.

McDougall, C.J.; Ngoi, S.S.; Goldman, I.S.; Godwin, T.; Felix, J.; DeCosse, J.J. and Rigas, B.: Reduced expression of HLA class I and II antigens in colon cancer. Cancer Res. 50: 8023–8027, 1990.

McGregor, J.L.: Potential new anti-thrombotic drugs targeted against platelet adhesion molecules. Int. Conf. on: The platelet in health & disease. Royal College of physicians, London, 1992.

McIntyre, K.W.; Stepan, G.J.; Kolinsky, K.D.; Benjamin, W.R.; Plocinski, J.M.; Kaffka, K.L.; Campen, C.A.; Chizzonite, R.A. and Lilian, P.L.: Inhibition of interleukin 1 (IL-1) binding and bioactivity in vitro and modulation of acute inflammation in vivo by IL-1 receptor antagonist and anti IL-1 receptor monoclonal antibody. J. Exp. Med. 173: 932–939, 1991.

McKenzie, A.N.J.; Culpepper, J.A.; de Waal Malefyt, R.; Briere, F.; Punnonen, J.; Aversa, G.; Sato, A.; Dang, W.; Cocks, B.G.; Menon, S. et al.: Interleukin 13, a T-cell-derived cytokine that regulates human monocyte and B-cell function. Proc. Natl. Acad. Sci. USA 90: 3735–3739, 1993.

McLean, C.S.; Sterlin, J.S.; Mowat, J.; Nash, A.A. and Stanley, M.A.: Delayed type hypersensitivity response to the human papillomavirus type 16 protein in a mouse model. J. Gen. Virol. 74: 239–245, 1993.

McLean, R.H.; Wyatt, R.J. and Julian, B.A.: Complement phenotypes in glomerulonephritis: Increased frequency of homozygous null C4 phenotypes in IgA nephropathy and Henoch-Schönlein purpura. Kidney Int. 26: 855–860, 1984.

McManus, L.M.; Morley, C.A.; Levine, S.P. and Pinckard, R.N.: Platelet activating factor (PAF) induced release of platelet factor 4 (PF4) in vitro and during IgE anaphylaxis in the rabbit. J. Immunol. 123: 2835–2841, 1979.

McMichael, A.: Cytotoxic T lymphocytes and immune surveillance. Cancer Surveys 13: 5, 1992.

McMichael, A.J.; Gotch, F.M.; Noble, G.R. and Beare, P.A.S.: Cytotoxic T-cell immunity to influenza. New Engl. J. Med. 309: 13–17, 1983.

McMillan, R.M. and Foster, S.J.: Leukotriene B4 and inflammatory disease. Agents Actions 24: 114–119, 1988.

Mealy, K.; van Lanschot, J.J.B.; Robinson, B.G.; Rounds, J. and Wilmore, D.W.: Are the catabolic effects of tumor necrosis factor mediated by glucocorticoids? Arch. Surg. 125: 42–47, 1990.

Medof, M.E.; Iida, K.; Mold, C. and Nussenzweig, V.: Unique role of the complement receptor CR1 in the degradation of C3b associated with immune complexes. J. Exp. Med. 156: 1739–1754, 1982.

Medof, M.E. and Oger, J.J-F.: Competition for immune complexes by red cells in human blood. J. Clin. Lab. Immunol. 7: 7–13, 1982.

Medof, M.E. and Nussenzweig, V.: Control of the function of substrate-bound C4b-C3b by the complement receptor CR1. J. Exp. Med. 159: 1669–1685, 1984.

Medof, M.E.; Kinoshita, T. and Nussenzweig, V.: Inhibition of complement activation on the surface of cells after incorporation of decay-accelerating factor (DAF) into their membranes. J. Exp. Med. 160: 1558–1578, 1984.

Medof, M.E.; Walter, E.I.; Roberts, W.L.; Hass, R. and Rosenberry, T.L.: Decay-accelerating factor of complement is anchored to cells by a C-terminal glycolipid. Biochemistry 25: 6740–6747, 1986.

Meeker, T.C.; Lowder, J.; Manoley, D.G.; Miller, R.A.; Thielemans, K.; Warnke, R. and Leby, R.A.: Clinical trial of anti-idiotype therapy for B-cell malignancy. Blood 65: 1349–1363, 1985.

Mega, J.; Bruce, M.G.; Beagle, K.W.; McGhee, J.R.; Taguchi, T.; Pitts, M.; McGhee, M.L.; Bucy, R.P.; Eldridge, J.H.; Mestecky, J. and Kiyono, H.: Regulation of mucosal responses by CD4+ T lymphocytes: Effects of anti-L3T4 treatment on the gastrointestinal immune system. Int. Immunol. 3: 793–805, 1991.

Mehta, J.; Mehta, P.; Lawson, D.L.; Ostrowski, N. and Brigmon, L.: Influence of a selective thromboxane synthetase blocker CGS-13080 on thromboxane and prostacyclin synthesis in whole blood: evidence for synthesis of prostacyclin by leukocytes from platelet-derived endoperoxides. J. Lab. Clin. Med. 106:246–252, 1985.

Meinardus-Hager, G.; Schulze-Osthoff, K. and Sorg, C.: Endothelial activation: inflammatory response and angiogenesis. Biomedical Progress 4: 17, 1991.

Mencia-Huerta, J.M.; Hadji, L. and Benveniste, J.: Release of a slow-reacting substance of anaphylaxis from rabbit platelets. J. Clin. Invest. 6: 1586–1591, 1981.

Mencia-Huerta, J.M.; Hosford, D. and Braquet, P.: Acute and long-term pulmonary effects of platelet-activating factor. J. Clin. Ep. Immunol. 19: 125–142, 1989.

Meneguzzi, G.; Cerni, C.; Kieny, M.P. and Lathe, R.: Immunization against human papillomavirus type 16 tumor cells with recombinant vaccinia viruses expressing E6 and E7. Virology 181: 62–69, 1991.

Menzies, R.; Patel, R.; Hall, N.R.S.; O'Grady, M.P. and Rier, S.E.: Human recombinant interferon alpha inhibits naloxone binding to rat brain membranes. Life Sci. 50: PL227–PL232, 1992.

Merluzzi, V.J.; Faanes, R.B.; Czajkowksi, M.; Last-Barney, K.; Harrison, P.C.; Kahn, J. and Rothlein, R.: Membrane-associated interleukin 1 activity on human U937 tumor cells: stimulation of PGE2 production by human chondrosarcoma cells. J. Immunol. 139: 166, 1987.

Mestecky, J.: The common mucosal immune system and current strategies for induction of immune responses in external secretions. J. Clin. Immunol. 7: 265–276, 1987.

Mestecky, J. and McGhee, J.R.: Immunoglobulin A (IgA): Molecular and cellular interactions involved in IgA biosynthesis and immune response. Adv. Immunol. 40: 153–245, 1987.

Metcalf, D.: Stimulation by human urine or plasma of granulo-poiesis by human marrow cells in agar. Exp. Hematol. 2: 157–173, 1974.

Metcalf, D.: The molecular biology and functions of the granulocyte-macrophage colony-stimulating factors. Blood 67: 257–267, 1986.

Metcalf, D.; Nicola, N.A. and Gearing, D.P.: Effects of injected leukemia inhibitory factor on hematopoietic and other tissues in mice. Blood 76: 50, 1990.

Metcalf, D.: The leukemia inhibitory factor (LIF). Int. J. Cell Clon. 9: 95–108, 1991.

Metcalf, D.; Hilton, D. and Nicola, N.A.: Leukemia inhibitory factor can potentiate murine megakaryocyte production in vitro. Blood 77: 2150–2153, 1991.

Metzger, H.; Alcaraz, G.; Hohman, R.; Kinet, J.P.; Pribluda, V. and Quarto, R.: The receptor with high affinity for immunoglobulin E. Annu. Rev. Immunol. 4: 419, 1986.

Mian, I.S.; Bradwell, A.R. and Olson, A.J.: Structure, function and properties of antibody binding sites. J. Mol Biol. 217: 133–151, 1991.

Michael, J.: The role of digestive enzymes in orally induced immune tolerance. Immunol. Invest. 18: 1049–1054, 1989.

Michalek, S.M.; Moore, R.N.; McGhee, J.R.; Rosenstreich, D.L. and Mergenhagen, S.E.: The primary role of lymphoreticular cells in the mediation of host responses to bacterial endotoxin. J. Infect. Dis. 141: 55–63, 1980.

Miethke, T.; Heeg, K.; Wahl, C. and Wagner, H.: Crosslinked staphylococcal enterotoxin B stimulates CD8+ T cells only in the presence of unlinked costimulator signals. Immunobiol. 183: 433–450, 1991.

Miethke, T.; Wahl, C.; Echtenacher, B.; Krammer, P.; Heeg, K. and Wagner, H.: T cell mediated lethal shock triggered in mice by the superantigen staphylococcal enterotoxin B: Critical role of tumor necrosis factor. J. Exp. Med. 175: 91, 1992.

Mignatti, P.; Tsuboi, R.; Robbins, E. and Rifkin, D.B.: In vitro angiogenesis on the human amniotic membrane: requirement for basic fibroblast growth factor-induced proteinases. J. Cell Bioll 108: 671–682, 1989.

Mihm, M.C.; Soter, N.A;; Dvorak, H.F. and Austen, K.F.: The structure of normal skin and the morphology of atopic eczema. J. Invest. Dermatol. 67: 305, 1976.

Miles, S.A.; Rezai, A.R.; Saazar-Gonzales, J.F.; Meyden M. van der; Stevens, R.H.; Logan, D.M.; Mitszyasu, T.R.T.; Taga, T.; Hirano, T.; Kishimoto, T. and Martinez-Maza, O.: AIDS Kaposi-sarcoma derived cells produce and respond to interleukin-6. Proc. Natl. Acad. Sci USA 87: 4068, 1990.

Miller, D.K.; Calaycay, J.R.; Chapman, K.T.; Howard, A.D.; Kostura, M.J.; Molineaux, S.M. and Thornberry, N.A.: The Il-1ß converting enzyme as a therapeutic target. Immunosuppressive and Antiinflammatory Drugs, eds. Allison, A.C.; Lafferty, K.J. and Fliri, H., Annals of the New York Academy of Sciences 696: 133, 1993.

Miller, R.A.; Maloney, D.G.; Warnke, R. and Levy, R.: Treatment of B-cell lymphoma with monoclonal anti-idiotype antibody. N. Engl. J. Med. 306: 517–522, 1982.

Miller, R.A.; Hart, S.; Samoszuk, M.; Coulter, C.; Brown, S. and Levy, R.: Shared idiotypes expressed by human B-cell lymphomas. N. Engl. J. Med. 321: 851–856, 1989.

Mimura, G.; Kida, K.; Matsuura, N.; Toyota, T.; Kitagawa, T.; Kobayashi, T.; Hibi, I.; Ikeda, Y.; Tuchida, I.; Kuzuya, H. et al.: Immunogenetics of early onset insulin-dependent diabetes mellitus among the Japanese: HLA, Gm, BF, GLO, and organ specific autoantibodies. Diabetes Res. Clin. Pract. 8: 253–262, 1990.

Minami, Y.; Kono, T.; Yamada, K. and Taniguchi, T.: The interleukin-2 receptors: insights into a complex signalling mechanism. Biochimica et Biophysica Acta 1114: 163–177, 1992.

Miraldi, F.D.; Nelson, A.D.; Kraly, C.; Ellery, S.; Landmeier, B.; Coccia, P.F.; Strandjord, S.E. and Cheung, N.K.: Diagnostic imaging of human neuroblastoma with radiolabeled antibody. Radiol. 161: 413–418, 1986.

Misko, I.; Pope, D.; Hütter, R.; Soszynski, T. and Kane, R.: HLA-DR antigen associated restriction of EBV specific cytotoxic T-cell colonies. Int. J. Cancer 33: 239–243, 1984.

Mitchell, M.S.; Harel, W.; Kan-Mitchell, J.; LeMay, L.G.; Goedegebuure, P.; Huang, X.-Q.; Hofman, F. and Groshen, S.: Active specific immunotherapy of melanoma with allogeneic cell lysates. Rationale, results, and possible mechanisms of action. Specific Immunotherapy Of Cancer With Vaccines, eds. Bystryn, J.-C.; Ferrone, S. and Livingston, P., The New York Academy of Sciences 690: 153, 1993.

Mita, S.; Tominaga, A.; Hitoshi, Y.; Sakamoti, K.; Honjo, T.; Akagi, M.; Kikuchi, Y.; Yamaguchi, N. and Takatsu, K.: Characterization of high-affinity receptors for interleukin 5 on interleukin 5–dependent cell lines. Proc. Natl. Acad. Sci. USA 86: 2311–2315, 1989.

Mitropoulou, J.; Becker, H. and Helmke, K.: High-dose-intravenous immunoglobulins in rheumatoid arthritis. Clin. Exp. Rheumatol. 5: 207, 1987.

Mitsuya, H.; Matis, L.; Megson, M.; Bunn, P.; Murray, C.; Mann, D.; Gallo, R. and Broder, S.: Generation of an HLA-restricted cytotoxic T cell line reactive against cultured tumor cells from a patient infected with human T cell leukemia/lymphoma virus. J. Exp. Med. 158: 994–999, 1983.

Miyake, T.; Kung, C.K. and Goldwasser, E.: Purification of human erythropoietin. J. Biol. Chem. 252: 5558–5564, 1977.

Miyauchi, T.; Tomobe, Y.; Shiba, R.; Ishikawa, T.; Yanagisawa, M.; Kimura, S.; Sugishita, Y.; Ito, I.; Goto, K. and Masaki, T.: Involvement of endothelin in the regulation of human vascular tonus. Circulation 81: 1874–1880, 1990.

Miyazawa, K.; Hendrie, P.C.; Mantel, C.; Wood, K.; Ashman, L.K. and Broxmeyer, H.E.: Comparative analysis of signaling pathways between mast cell growth factor (c-kit ligand) and granulocyte-macrophage colony-stimulating factor in a human factor-dependent myeloid cell line involves phosphorylation of Raf-1, GTPase-activating protein and mitogen-activated protein kinase. Exp. Hematol. 19: 1110–1123, 1991.

Miyazono, K.; Okabe, T.; Urabe, A.; Takaku, F. and Heldin, C.H.: Purification and properties of an endothelial cell growth factor from human platelets. J. Biol. Chem. 262: 4098–4103, 1987.

Mizel, S.B.: Interleukin-1 and T cell activation. Immunol. Rev. 63: 51–55, 1982.

Möller, G.: Antibody mediated suppression of the immune response is determinant specific. Eur. J. Immunol. 15: 409, 1985.

Möller, P.; Herrmann, B.; Moldenhauer, G. and Momburg, F.: Defective expression of MHC class I antigens is frequent in B-cell lymphomas of high grade malignancy. Int. J. Cancer 40: 32–39, 1987.

Möller, P.; Momburg, F.; Koretz, K.; Moldenhauer, G.; Herfarth, C.; Otto, H.F.; Haemmerling, G.J. and Schlag, P.: Influence of major histocompatibility complex class I and II antiens on survival in colorectal carcinoma. Cancer Res. 51: 729–736, 1991.

Möller, P.; Koretz, K.; Schlag, P. and Momburg, F.: Frequency and abnormal expression of HLA-A,B,C and HLA-DR molecules, invariant chain, and LFA-3 (CD58) in colorectal carcinoma and its impact on tumor recurrence. Int. J. Cancer 6 (suppl.): 155–162, 1991.

Möller, P. and Hammerling, G.: The role of surface HLA-A,B,C molecules in tumor immunity. Cancer Surveys 13: 104–128, 1992.

Moertel, C.G.; Fleming, T.R.; MacDonald, J.S.; Haller, D.G.; Lawie, J.A.; Goodman, P.J.; Ungerleider, J.S.; Emerson, W.A.; Tormey, D.C. and Glick, J.H.: Levamisole and Fluoroacil for adjuvant therapy of resected colon carcinoma. N. Engl. J. Med. 322: 352–358, 1990.

Moffatt, M.F.; Sharp, P.A.; Faux, J.A.; Young, R.P.; Cookson, W.O.C.M, and Hopkin, J.M.: Factors confounding genetic linkage between atopy and chromosome 11q. Clin. Exp. Allergy 22: 1046–1051, 1992.

Mole-Bajer, J.; Bajer, A.S.; Zinkowski, R.P.; Balczon, R.D. and Brinkley, B.R.: Autoantibodies from a patient with scleroderma CREST recognized kinetochores of the higher plant Haemanthus. Proc. natn. Acad. Sci. USA 87: 3599–3603, 1990.

Moll, U.M.; Lane, B.; Zucker, S.; Suzuki, K. and Nagase, H.: Localization of collagenase at the basal plasma membrane of a human pancreatic carcinoma cell line. Cancer Res. 50: 6995–7002, 1990.

Mollenhauer, E.; Schmidt, R.; Heinrichs, M. and Rittner, C.: Scleroderma: Possible significance of silent alleles at the C4B locus. Arthritis Rheum. 27: 711–712, 1984.

Momand, J.; Zambetti, G.P.; Olson, D.C.; George, D. and Levine, A.J.: The mdm-2 oncogene product forms a complex with the p53 protein and inhibits p43–mediated transactivation. Cell 69: 1237–1245, 1992.

Momberg, F.; Degener, T.; Bacchus, E.; Moldenhauer, G. and Hammerling, G.J.: Loss of HLA-ABC and de novo expression HLA-D in colorectal cancer. Int. J. Cancer 37: 179–184, 1989.

Momburg, F. and Koch, S.: Selective loss of β2–microglobulin mRNA in human colon carcinoma. J. Exp. Med. 169: 309–314, 1989.

Momburg, F.; Neefjes, J.J.; Roelse, J. and Hämmerling, G.J.: The role of proteasome and transporters in antigen presentation. ENII Conf.: Integrated Function of Molecules of the Immune System. Les Embiez, France, 12th-16th May 1993.

Monaco, J.; Cho, S. and Attaya, M.: Transport protein genes in the murine MHC: possible implications for antigen processing. Science 250: 1723–1726, 1990.

Moncada, S.; Gryglewski, R.; Bunting, S. and Vane, J.R.: An enzyme isolated from arteries transforms prostaglandin endoperoxidase to an unstable substance that inhibits platelet aggregation. Nature (London) 263: 663–665, 1976.

Moncada, S.; Palmer, R.J. and Higgs, E.A.: NO: Physiology, pathophysiology an pharmacology. Pharmacol. Rev. 43 (part 2): 109–142, 1991.

Monsky, W.L. and Chen, W.T.: Proteases of cell adhesion proteins in cancer. Cancer Biol. 4: 251–258, 1993.

Montelione, G.T.; Wuethrich, K.; Nice, E.C.; Burgess, A.W. and Scheraga, H.A.: Solution structure of murine epidermal growth factor: determination of the polypeptide backbone chain-fold by nuclear magnetic resonance and distance geometry. Proc. Natl. Acad. Sci. 84: 5226–5230, 1987.

Montesano, R.; Vassalli, J.-D.; Baird, A.; Guillemin, R. and Orci, L.: Basic fibroblast growth factor induces angiogenesis in vitro. Proc. Natl. Acad. Sci. USA 83: 7297–7301, 1986.

Moore, M.D.; Cooper, N.R.; Tack, B.F. and Nemerow, G.R.: Molecular cloning of the cDNA encoding the Epstein-Barr virus/C3d receptor (complement receptor type 2) of human B lymphocytes. Proc. Natl. Acad. Sci. USA 84: 9194–9198, 1987.

Moore, M.W.; Carbone, F.R. and Bevan, J.J.: Introduction of soluble protein into the class I pathway of antigen presentation. Cell 54: 777–785, 1988.

Moqbel, R. and Pritchard, D.I.: Parasites and allergy: evidence for a "cause and effect" relationship. Clin. Exp. Allergy 20: 611, 1990.

Morahan, G.; Allison, J. and Miller, J.F.A.P.: Tolerance of class I histocompatibility antigens expressed extrathymically. Nature 339: 622, 1989.

Moran, P.; Beasly, H.; Gorrel, A.; Martin, E.; Gribling, P.; Fucus, H.; Gillet, N.; Burton, L.E. and Caras, I.W.: Human recombinant soluble decay accelerating factor inhibits complement activation in vitro and in vivo. J. Immunol. 149: 1736–1743, 1992.

Moreland, L.W.; Bucy, R.P.; Tilden, A.; Pratt, P.W.; LoBuglio, A.F.; Khazaeli, M.; Everson, M.P.; Daddona, P.; Ghrayeb, J.; Kilgarriff, C.; Sanders, M.E. and Koopman, W.J.: Use of a chimeric monoclonal anti-CD4 antibody in patients with refractory rheumatoid arthritis. Arthritis and Rheumatism 36: 307, 1993.

Morgan, B.P.; Campbell, A.K.; Luzio, J.P. and Hallett, M.B.: Recovery of polymorphonuclear leucocytes from complement attack. Biochem. Soc. Trans. 12: 779–780, 1984.

Morgan, B.P. and Campbell, A.K.: The recovery of human polymorphonuclear leucocytes from sublytic complement attack is mediated by changes in intracellular free calcium. Biochem. J. 231: 205–208, 1985.

Morgan, B.P.; Dankert, J.R. and Esser, A.F.: Recovery of human neutrophils from complement attack: removal of the membrane attack complex by endocytosis and exocytosis. J. Immunol. 138: 246–253, 1987.

Morgan, B.P.; Daniels, R.H. and Williams, B.D.: Measurement of terminal complement complexes in rheumatoid arthritis. Clin. Exp. Immunol. 73: 473–478, 1988a.

Morgan, B.P.; Daniels, R.H.; Watts, M.J. and Williams, B.D.: In vivo and in vitro evidence of cell recovery from complement attack in rheumatoid synovium. Clin. Exp. Immunol. 73: 467–472, 1988b.

Morgan, B.P.: Non-lethal complement membrane attack on human neutrophils: transient cell swelling and metabolic depletion. Immunology 63: 71–77, 1988.

Morgan, B.P.: Effects of the membrane attack complex of complement on nucleated cells. Current Topics in Microbiology and Immunology, Springer Verlag, Berlin, 178: 1992.

Morgan, D.A.; Ruscetti, F.W. and Gallo, R.: Selective in vitro growth of T-lymphocytes from normal human bone marrow. Science 192: 1007–1009, 1976.

Morgan, E.L. and Weigle, W.O.: Biological activities residing in the Fc region of immunoglobulin. Adv. Immunol. 40: 61, 1987.

Morikawa, K.; Oseko, F. and Morikawa, S.: The suppressive effect of deoxyspergualin on the differentiation of human B lymphocytes maturing into immunoglobulin-producing cells. Transplantation 54: 526–531, 1992.

Morimoto, C. and Schlossman, S.F.: CD26 - A key costimulatory molecule on CD4 memory T cells. The Immunologist 2: 4, 1994.

Moriuchi, J.; Ichikawa, Y.; Tayaka, M.; Shimizu, H.; Tsuji, K.; Wakisaka, A.; Dawkins, R. and Arimori, S.: Association of the complement allele C4AQO with primary Sjögren's syndrome in Japanese patients. Arthritis Rheum. 34: 224–227, 1991.

Morrissey, P.J.; Goodwin, R.G.; Nordan, R.P.; Anderson, D.; Grabstein, K.H.; Cosman, D.; Sims, J.; Lupton, S.; Acres, B. and Reed, S.G. Recombinant interleukin 1, pre-B cell growth factor, has costimulatory activity on purified mature T cells. J. Exp. Med. 169: 707–716, 1989.

Morrison, D.C. and Kline, L.F.: Activation of the classical and properdin pathways of complement by bacterial lipopolysaccarides (LPS). J. Immunol. 118: 362–368, 1977.

Morrow, M.A.; Lee, G.; Gillis, S.; Yancopoulos, G.D. and Alt, F.W.: Interleukin-7 induces N-myc and c-myc expression in normal precursor B lymphocytes. Genes and Dev. 6: 61–70, 1992.

Morton, D.L.; Hoon, D.S.B.; Nizze, J.A.; Foshag, L.J.; Famatiga, E.; Wanek, L.A.; Chang, C.; Irie, C.R.; Gupta, R.K. and Elashoff, R.: Polyvalent melanoma vaccine improves survival of patients with metastatic melanoma. Specific Immunotherapy Of Cancer With Vaccines, eds. Bystryn, J.-C.; Ferrone, S. and Livingston, P., The New York Academy of Sciences 690: 120, 1993.

Moscatelli, D.: High and low affinity binding sites for basic fibroblast growth factor on cultured cells: absence of a role for low affinity binding in the stimulation of plasminogen activator production by bovine capillary endothelial cells. J. Cell Physiol. 131: 123–130, 1987.

Moses, M.A.; Sudhalter, J. and Langer, R.: Identification of an inhibitor of neovascularization from cartilage. Science 248: 1408–1410, 1990.

Mosmann, T.R.; Cherwinski, H.; Bond, M.W.; Giedlin, M.A. and Coffman, R.L.: Two types of murine helper T-cell clone I. Definition according to profiles of lymphokine activities and secreted proteins. J. Immunol. 136: 2348, 1986.

Mosmann, T.R. and Coffman, R.L.: Heterogeneity of cytokine secretion patterns and functions of helper T cells. Adv. Immunol. 46: 111, 1989.

Mosmann, T.R. and Coffman, R.L.: Th1 and Th2 cells: Different patterns of lymphokine secretion lead to different functional properties. Annu. Rev. Immunol. 7: 145–173, 1989.

Mosmann, T.R. and Moore, K.W.: The role of IL-10 in cross-regulation of TH1 and TH2 responses. Immunoparasitol Today 12: 49, 1991.

Moss, D.J.; Rickinson, A.B. and Pope, H.H.: Long term T cell mediated immunity to Epstein-Barr virus in man. I. Complete regression of virus-induced transformation on cultures of seropositive donor leukocytes. Int. J. Cancer 22: 662–668, 1978.

Mostov, K.E.; Friedlander, M. and Blobel, G.: The receptor for transepithelial transport of IgA and IgM contains multiple immunoglobulin-like domains. Nature 308: 37–43, 1984.

Moulds, J.M.; Nickells, M.W.; Moulds, J.J.; Brown, M.C. and Atkinson, J.P.: The C3b/C4b receptor is recognized by the Knups, McCoy, Swain-Langley, and York blood group antisera. J. Exp. Med. 173: 1159–1163, 1991.

Moulds, J.M.; Krych, M.; Holers, V.M.; Liszewski, M.K. and Atkinson, J.P.: Genetics of the complement system and rheumatic diseases. Gene Factors 18: 893, 1992.

Müller, Berghaus, G.: Beziehungen zwischen Komplement und Blutgerinnung. Klin. Wschr. 55: 663–672, 1977.

Müller-Eberhard, H.J.: Complement. Annue Rev. Biochem. 44: 697, 1975

Müller-Eberhard, H.J.: Current trends in complement research. Behring Inst. Mitt. 61: 1, 1977.

Müller-Eberhard, H.J.: Molecular organization and function of the complement system. Annu. Rev. Biochem. 57: 321–347, 1988.

Mueller-Eckhardt, C.; Kuenzlen, E.; Thilo-Korner, D. and Pralle, H.: High-dose intravenous immunoglobulin for post-transfusion purpura. N. Engl. J. Med. 308: 287, 1983.

Mufson, R.A.; Szabo, J. and Eckert, D.: Human Il-3 induction of c-jun in normal monocytes is independent of tyrosine kinase and involves protein kinase C. J. Immunol. 148: 1129–1135, 1992.

Mukaida, N.; Zachariae, C.C.; Gusella, G.L. and Matsushima, K.: Dexamethasone inhibits the induction of monocyte chemotactic-activating factor production by Il-1 or tumor necrosis factor. J. Immunol. 146: 1212–1215, 1991.

Mule, J.J.; Smith, C.A. and Rosenberg, S.A.: Interleukin 4 (B cell stimulatory factor 1) can mediate the induction of lymphokine-activated killer activity directed against fresh tumor cells. J. Exp. Med. 166: 792–798, 1987.

Muller, D.; Quantin, B.; Gesnel, M-C.; Millon-Collard, R.; Abecassis, J. and Breathnach, R.: The collagenase gene family consists of at least four members. Biochem. J. 253: 187–192, 1988.

Muller, W.; Hanauski-Abel, H. and Loos, M.: Biosynthesis of the first component of complement by human and guinea pig peritoneal macrophages: evidence for an independent production of the C1 subunits. J. Immunol. 121: 1578–1584, 1978.

Mulligan, M.S.; Yeh, C.G.; Rudolph, A.R. and Ward, P.A.: Protective effects of soluble CR1 in complement- and neutrophil-mediated tissue damage. J. Immunol. 148: 1479–1485, 1992.

Munker, R.; Gasson, J.; Ogawa, M. and Koeffler, H.P.: Recombinant human TNF induces production of granulocyte-monocyte colony-stimulating factor. Nature 323: 79–82, 1986.

Murakami, S.; Ono, S.; Harada, N.; Hara, Y.; Katoh, Y.; Dobashi, K.; Takatsu, K. and Hamaoka, T.: T-cell-derived factor B151–TRF1/Il-5 activates blastoid cells among unprimed B cells to induce a polyclonal differentiation into immunoglobulin M-secreting cells. Immunology 65: 221–228, 1988.

Murata, J.; Saiki, I.; Makabe, T.; Tsuta, Y.; Tokura, S. and Azuma, I.: Inhibition of tumor-induced angiogenesis by sulfated chitin derivatives. Cancer Res. 51: 22–26, 1991.

Murphy, P.M. and Tiffany, H.L.: Cloning of complementary DNA encoding a functional human interleukin-8 receptor. Science 253: 1280–1283, 1991.

Murphy, G.F.; Radu, A.; Kaminer, M. and Berd, D.: Autologous melanoma vaccine induces inflammatory responses in melanoma metastases: relevance to immunologic regression on immunotherapy. J. Invest. Dermatol. 100: 335–341, 1993.

Murphy, M.P and Morris, R.E.: Brequinar sodium (Dup 785) is a highly potent antimetabolite immunosuppressant that suppresses heart allograft rejection. Med. Sci. Res. 19: 835–836, 1991.

Murphy-Ullrich, J.; Schultz-Cherry, S. and Hook, M.: Transforming growth factor-ß complexes with thrombospondin. Molecular Biology of the Cell 3: 181–188, 1992.

Murray, P.D.; McKenzie, D.T.; Swain, S.L. and Kagnoff, M.F.: Interleukin 5 and interleukin 4 produced by Peyer's path T cells selectively enhance immunoglobulin A expression. J. Immunol. 139: 2669–2674, 1987.

Murray, G.: Experiments in immunity in cancer. Can. med. Ass. J. 79: 249, 1958.

Mussoni, L.; Riganti, M.; Acero, R.; Erroi, A.; Conforti, G.; Mantovani, A. and Donati, M.B.: Macrophages associated with murine tumours express plasminogen activator activity. Int. J. Cancer 41: 227–230, 1988.

Mustoe, T.A.; Pierce, G.F.; Thomason, A.; Gramates, P.; Sporn, M.B. and Deuel, T.F.: Accelerated healing of incisional wounds in rats induced by transforming growth factor-ß. Science (Wash. DC), 237: 1333–1336, 1987.

Muul, L.M.; Spiess, P.J.; Cirector, E.P. and Rosenberg, S.A.: Identification of specific cytolytic immune responses against autologous tumor in humans bearing malignant melanoma. J. Immunol. 138: 989–995, 1987.

Myoken, Y.; Kayada, Y.; Okamoti, T.; Kan, M.; Sato, G.H. and Sato, J.D.: Vascular endothelial cell growth factor (VEGF) produced by A-431 human epidermoid carcinoma cells and identification of VEGF membrane binding sites. Proc. Natl. Acad. Sci. USA 88: 5819–5823, 1991.

Nabozny, G.H.; Cobbold, S.P.; Waldmann, H. and Kong, Y.M.: Suppression in murine experimental autoimmune thyroiditis: in vivo inhibition of CD4+ T-cell-mediated resistance by a nondepleting rat CD4 monoclonal antibody. Cell Immunol. 138: 185–196, 1991.

Nachman, R.L.; Weksler, B. and Fabris, B.: Characterization of human platelet vascular permeability-enhancing activity. J. Clin. Invest. 51: 549–556, 1972.

Nachman, R.L.; Hajjar, K.A.; Silverstein, R.L. and Dinarello, C.A.: Interleukin 1 induces endothelial cell synthesis of plasminogen activator inhibitor. J. Exp. Med. 163: 1595–1600, 1986.

Nadler, J.; Breitmeyer, F. and Coral, N.: Anti B4 blocked ricin immunotherapy for patients with B-cell malignancies: Results of bolus and constant infusion phase I trials. 2nd Int. Symp. on Immunotoxin, Lake Buena Vista, 1990.

Nadler, S.G.; Tepper, M.A.; Schacter, B. and Mazzucco, C.E.: Interaction of the immunosuppressant deoxyspergualin with a member of the Hsp 70 family heat shock proteins. Science 258: 484–486, 1992.

Nadler, S.G.; Cleaveland, J.; Tepper, M.A.; Walsh, C. and Nadeau, K.: Studies on the interaction of the immunosuppressant 15–Deoxyspergualin with heat shock proteins. Immunosuppressive and Antiinflammatory Drugs, eds. Allison, A.C.; Lafferty, K.J. and Fliri, H., Annals of the New York Academy of Sciences 696: 412, 1993.

Nagano, Y.; Mizuochi, T.; Taniguchi, T.; Matsuta, K.; Miyamoto, T. and Kobata, A.: Structural difference of the sugar chains of IgGs purified from sera of patients with Sjörgen syndrome with or without complication of rheumatoid arthritis. Proc. of the XXXth Annual Meeting of Japan Rheumat. Assoc., 1986.

Nagase, H.; Enghild, J.J. and Salvesen, G.: Stepwise activation of the precursor of matrix metalloproteinase 3 (stromelysin) by proteinases and (4–aminophenyl)mercuric acetate. Biochem. 29: 5783–5789, 1990.

Nagata, M.; Hara, T.; Aoki, T.; Mizuno, Y.; Akeda, H.; Inaba, S.; Tsumoto, K. and Ueda, K.: Inherited deficiency of ninth component of complement: an increased risk of meningococcal meningitis. J. Pediatr. 114: 260–264, 1989.

Naito, Y.; Fukata, J.; Shindo, K.; Ebisui, O.; Murakami, N.; Tominaga, T.; Nakai, Y.; Mori, K.; Kastingh, N.W. and Imura, H.: Effects of interleukins on plasma arginine vasopressin and oxytocin levels in conscious, freely moving rats. Biochem. Biophys. Res. Commun. 174: 1189–1195, 1991.

Nakamura, M.; Manser, T.; Pearson, G.D.; Daley, M.J. and Gefter, M.L.: Effector of IFN-gamma on the immune response in vivo and on gene expression in vitro. Nature 307: 381–382, 1984.

Nakamura, H.; Nakanishi, K.; Kita, A. and Kadokawa, T.: Interleukin-1 induces analgesia in mice by a central action. Eur. J. Pharmacol. 149: 49–54, 1988.

Nakane, A.; Minagawa, T. and Kato, K.: Endogenous tumor necrosis factor (cachectin) is essential to host resistance against Listeria monocytogenes infection. Infect. Immun. 56: 2563, 1988.

Nakanishi, K.; Hashimoto, T.; Hiroishi, K.; Matsui, K.; Yoshimito, T.; Morse, H.C.; Furuyama, J.; Hamaoka, T.; Higashino, K. and Paul, W.E.: Demonstration of up-regulated Il-2 receptor expression on an invitro cloned BCL1 subline. J. Immunol. 138: 1817–1825, 1987

Nakanishi, K.; Yoshimoto, T.; Katoh, Y.; Ono, S.; Matsui, J.; Hiroishi, K.; Noma, T.; Honjo, T.; Takatsu, K.; Higashino, K. et al.: Both B151–T cell replacing factor 1 and Il-5 regulate Ig secretion and Il-2 receptor expression on a cloned B lymphoma line. J. Immunol. 140: 1168–1174, 1988.

Nakatsuru, K.; Ohgo, S.; Oki, Y. and Matsukura, S.: Interleukin-1 stimulates arginine vasopressin release from superfused rat hypothalamo-neurohypophyseal complexes independently of cholinergic mechanism. Brain Res. 554: 38–45, 1991.

Namen, A.E.; Schmierer, A.E.; March, C.J.; Overell, R.W.; Park, L.S.; Urdal, D.L. and Mochizuki, D.Y.: B cell precursor growth- promoting activity: purification and characterization of a growth factor active on lymphocyte precursors. J. Exp. Med. 167: 988–1002, 1988.

Nardella, F.A.; Teller, D.C.; Barber, C.B. and Mannik, M.: IgG rheumatoid factors and staphylococcal protein A bind to common molecular region on IgG. J. Exp. Med. 162: 1811, 1985.

Nardella, F.A.; Schröder, A.K.; Svensson, M.-L.; Sjöquist, J.; Barber, C. and Christensen, P.: T15 group A streptococcal Fc receptor bind to the same location on IgG as staphylococcal protein A and IgG rheumatoid factors. J. Immunol. 140: 922, 1987.

Natali, P.G.; Bigotti, A.; Nicotra, M.R.; Viora, M.; Manfredi, D. and Ferrone, S.: Distribution of human class I (HLA-A,B,C) histocompatibility antigens in normal and malignant tissues of nonlymphoid origin. Cancer Res. 44: 4679–4687, 1984.

Natsumeda, Y. and Carr, S.F.: Human type I and II IMP dehydrogenases as drug targets. Immunosuppressive and Antiinflammatory Drugs, eds. Allison, A.C.; Lafferty, K.J. and Fliri, H., Annals of the New York Academy of Sciences 696: 88, 1993.

Naume, B.; Gately, M. and Espevik, T.: A comparative study of Il-12 (cytotoxic lymphocyte maturation factor)-, Il-2- and Il-7-induced effects on immunomagnetically purified CD56+ NK cells. J. Immunol. 148: 2429–2436, 1992.

Nelp, W.B.; Eary, J.F.; Jones, R.F.; Hellström, K.E.; Hellström, I.; Beaumier, P.L. and Krohn, F.A.: Preliminary studies of monoclonal antibody lymphoscintigraphy in malignant melanoma. J. Nucl. Med. 28: 34, 1987.

Nemazee, D.A.: Immune complexes can trigger specific, T cell-dependent autoanti-IgG antibody production in mice. J. Exp. Med. 161: 242, 1985.

Nepon, G.T. and Erlich, H.: MHC class-II molecules and autoimmunity. Annu. Rev. Immunol. 9: 493–525, 1991.

Neuber, K.; Sephan, U.; Franken, J. and Konig, W.: Staphylococcus aureus modifies the cytokine-induced immunoglobulin synthesis and CD23 expression in patients with atopic dermatitis. Immunology 73: 197–204, 1991.

Neufeld, G. and Gospodarowicz, D.: Basic and acidic fibroblast growth factors interact with the same cell surface receptors. J. Biol. Chem. 261: 5631–5637, 1986.

Newberg, M.H.; Ridge, J.P.; Vining, D.R.; Salter, R.D. and Engelhard, V.H.: Species specificity in the interaction of CD8 with the µ3 domain of MHC class I molecules. J. Immunol. 149: 136–142, 1992.

Newburger, J.W.; Takahashi, M. and Burns, J.C.: The treatment of Kawasaki syndrome in autoimmune diseases. Immunology Today 11/11: 383, 1990.

Newman, S.L. and Mikus, L.K.: Deposition of C3b and C3bi onto particulate activators of the human complement system. J. Exp. Med. 161: 1414, 1985.

Newton, R.C.: Effect of interferon on the induction of human monocyte secretion of interleukin-1 activity. Immunology 56: 441, 1985.

Nichols, T.C.; Bellinger, D.A.; Reddick, R.L.; Read, M.S.; Koch, G.G.; Brinkhous, K.M. and Griggs, T.R.: Role of von Willebrand factor in arterial thrombosis: Studies in normal and von Willebrand disease pigs. Circulation 83 (suppl. IV): 56–64, 1991.

Nicholson-Weller, A.; Burge, J.; Fearon, D.T.; Weller, P.F. and Austen, K.F.: Isolation of a human erythrocyte membrane glycoprotein with decay-accelerating activity for C3 convertases of the complement system. J. Immunol. 129: 184–189, 1982.

Nicola, N.A. and Metcalf, D.: Subunit promiscuity among hemopoietic growth factor receptors. Cell 67: 1–4, 1991.

Nicola, N.A.: Receptors for colony-stimulating factors. Br. J. Haematology 77: 133–138, 1991.

Nicosia, R.F. and Bonanno E.: Inhibition of angiogenesis in vitro by Arg-Gly-Asp-containing synthetic peptide. Am. J. Pathol. 138: 829–833, 1991.

Niederhoff, H.; Pernice, W.; Sedlacek, H.H.; Schindera, F.; Schütte, B. and Straßburg, H.-M.: Purpura Schoenlein-Henoch. Dtsch. Med. Wchschr. 44: 1567–1571, 1979.

Niewiaröwski, J.F.: Proteins secreted by the platelets. Thromb. Haemost. 38: 924–938, 1977.

Niitsu, Y.; Watanabe, N.; Sone, H.; Neda, H.; Yamauchi, N. and Urushizaki, I.: Mechanism of the cytotoxic effect of tumor necrosis factor. Jpn. J. Cancer Res. 76: 1193–1197, 1985.

Nilsson, J.; von Euler, A.M. and Dalsgaard, C.J.: Stimulation of connective tissue cell growth by substance P and substance K. Nature 315: 61–63, 1985.

Nishioka, Y.; Sone, S.; Orino, E.; Nii, A. and Ogura, T.: Down-regulation by Interleukin 4 of activation of human alveolar macrophages to the tumoricidal state. Cancer Res. 51: 5526–5531, 1991.

Nister, M.; Hammacher, A.; Mellstroem, K.; Siegbahn, A.; Roennstrand, L.; Westermark, B. and Heldin, C.H.: A glioma-derived PDGF A chain homodimer has different functional activities from a PDGF AB heterodimer purified from human platelets. Cell 52: 791–799, 1989.

Nobile-Orazio, E.; Meucci, N.; Barbieri, S.; Carpo, M. and Scarlato, G.: High-dose intravenous immunoglobulin therapy in multifocal motor neuropathy. Neurology 43: 537–544, 1993.

Noel, P.; Nelson, S.; Bokulic, R.; Bagby, G.; Lippton, H. and Summer, W.: Pentoxifylline inhibits lipopolysaccharide-induced serum tumor necrosis factor and mortality. Abstr. Am. Rv. Respir. Dis. 139: A222, 1989.

Nophar, Y.; Kemper, O.; Brakebusch, C.; Englemann, H.; Zwang, R.; Aderka, D.; Holtmann, H. and Wallach, D.: Soluble forms of tumor necrosis factor receptors (TNF-Rs). The cDNA for the type I TNF-R, cloned using amino acid sequence data of its soluble form, encodes both the cell surface and a soluble form of the receptor. EMBO J. 9: 3269–3278, 1990.

Nordquist, R.; Anglin, H. and Lerner, M.P.: Antibody-induced antigen redistribution and shedding from human breast cancer cells. Science 197: 366, 1977.

Nose, A.; Tsuji, K. and Takeichi, M.: Localization of specificity determining sites in cadherin cell adhesion molecules. Cell 61: 147–155, 1990.

Nossal, G.J.; Abbot, A.P.; Mitchell, J. and Lummus, Z.: Antigens in immunity. XV. Ultrastructural features of antigen capture in primary and secondary lymphoid follicles. J. Exp. Med. 127: 27, 1968.

Novotny, J. and Sharp, K.: Electrostatic field in antibodies and antibody/antigen complexes. Prog. Biophys. molec. Biol. 58: 203–224, 1992.

Nuchtern, J.G.; Bonifacino, J.S.; Biddison, W.E. and Klausner, R.D.: Brefeldin A implicates egress from endoplasmic reticulum in class I restricted antigen presentation. Nature 339: 223–226, 1989.

Nüsslein, H.G.: Die Interleukin-4–induzierte IgE-Sythese. Allergologie 7: 275–279, 1993.

Oblakowski, P.; Bello-Fernandez, C.M.; Reittie, J.R.; Heslop, H.E.; Galatowicz, G.; Veys, P.; Wolkes, S.; Prentice, H.G.; Hazelhurst, G.; Hoffbrand, A.V. and Brenner, M.K.: Possible mechanism of selective killing of myeloid leukemia blasts by lymphokine-activated killer cells. Blood 77: 1996, 1991.

O'Connor-McCourt, M.D. and Wakefield, L.M.: Latent transforming growth factor-ß in serum: a specific complex with α2-marcroglobulin. J. Biol. Chem. 262: 14090–14099, 1987.

Oers, M.H.J. van; Heyden, A.A.P.A.M. and van der Aarden, L.A.: Interleukin-6 (IL-6) in serum and urine of renal transplant recipients. Clin. Exp. Immunol. 71: 314, 1988.

Oettgen, H.F.: Cytokines in clinical cancer therapy. Current Opinion in Immunology 3: 699–705, 1991.

Oganian, S.H. and Schlager, S.I.: Humoral immune killing of nucleated cells: mechanisms of complement-mediated attack and target cell defense. CRC Crit. Rev. Immunol. 1: 165–209, 1981.

O'Garra, A.; Stapleton, G.; Dhar, V.; Pearce, M.; Schumacher, J.; Rugo, H.; Barbis, D.; Stall, A.; Cupp, J.; Moore, K. et al.: Production of cytokines by mouse B cells: B lymphomas and normal B cells produce interleukin 10. Int. Immunol. 2: 821–832, 1990.

Ogawa, M.; Matsuzaki, Y.; Nishikawa, S.; Hayashi, S.; Kunisada, T.; Sudo, T.; Kina, T.; Nakauchi, H. and Nishikawa, S.: Expression and function of c-kit in hemopoietic progenitor cells. J. Exp. Med. 174: 63–71, 1991.

O'Grady, P.; Kuo, M.D.; Baldassare, J.J.; Huang, S.S. and Huang, J.S.: Purification of a new type high-molecular-weight receptor (type-V receptor) of transforming growth-factor-beta (TGF-beta) from bovine liver-identification of the type-V TGF-beta receptor in cultured-cells. J. Biol. Chem. 266: 8563–8589, 1991.

Oh, K.O.; Zhou, Z.; Kim, K.K.; Samanta, H.; Fraser, M.; Kim, Y.J.; Broxmeyer, H.E. and Kwon, B.S.: Identification of cell surface receptors for murine macrophage inflammatory protein-1 alpha. J. Immunol. 147: 2978–2983, 1991.

Ohanian, S.H. and Borsos, T.: Lysis of tumor cells by antibody and complement. II. Lack of correlation between amount of C4 and C3 fixed and cell lysis. J. Immunol. 114: 1292–1295, 1975.

Ohsugi, Y.; Suzuki, S. and Takagaki, Y.: Antitumor and immunosuppressive effects of mycophenolic acid derivatives. Cancer Res. 36: 2923–2927, 1976.

Ohta, M.; Greenberg, J.S.; Anklesaria, P.; Bassols, A. and Massague, J.: Two forms of transforming growth factor-ß distinguished by multipotential haematopietic progenitor cells. Nature (London) 329: 539–541, 1987.

Ohtsuki, M. and Massague, J.: Evidence for the involvement of protein kinase activity in transforming growth factor-beta signal transduction. Mol. Cell Biol. 12: 261–265, 1992.

Oikawa, T.; Shimamura, M.; Ashino-Fuse, H.; Iwaguchi, T.; Ishizuka, M. and Takeuchi, T.: Inhibition of angiogenesis by 15–Deoxyspergualin. J. Antibiotics 44: 1033–1035, 1991.

Oiki, S. and Okada, Y.: C1q induces chemotaxis and K+ conductance activation coupled to increased cytosolic Ca2+ in mouse fibroblasts. J. Immunol. 141: 3177–3185, 1988.

Oka, Y. and Orth, D.N.: Human plasma epidermal growth factor/beta-urogastrone is associated with blood platelets. J. Clin. Invest. 72: 249–259, 1983.

Okada, N.; Harada, R.; Fujita, T. and Okada, H.: Monoclonal antibodies capable of causing hemolysis of neuraminidase-treated human erythrocytes by homologous complement. J. Immunol. 143: 2262, 1988.

Okuda, K.; Sanghera, J.S.; Pelech, S.L.; Kanakura, Y.; Hallek, M.; Griffin, J.D. and Druker, B.J.: Granulocyte-macrophage colony-stimulating factor, interleukin-3, and steel factor induce rapid tyrosine phosphorylation of p42 and p44 MAP kinase. Blood 79: 2880–2887, 1992.

Okuda, Y. and Ogata, H.: The effect of the protease inhibitor FUT-175 on phospholipase A2, complement, prostaglandins and prekallikrein during endotoxin shock. Masui 38: 334–342, 1989.

Oldham, R.K.; Foon, K.A.; Morgan, A.C.; Woodhouse, C.S.; Schroff, R.W.; Abrams, P.G.; Fer, M.; Schoenberger, C.S.; Farrell, M.; Kimball, E. and Sherwin, S.A.: Monoclonal antibody therapy of malignant melanoma: in vivo localization in cutaneous metastasis after intravenous administration. J. Clin. Oncol. 2: 1235–1244, 1984.

Oldham, R.K.; Dillman, R.O.; Birch, R.; Barth, N.; Cohen, R.J.; Minor, D.R.; Maleckar, J.; Ya-nelli, J. and West, W.H.: Treatment of advanced cancer with interleukin-2 (rIl-2) and tumor-derived activated cells (TDAC). Proc. AACR 31: A1586, 1990.

Oliff, A.; Defeo-Jones, D.; Boyer, M.; Martinez, D.; Kiefer, D.; Vuocolo, G.; Wolfe, A. and Socher, S.H.: Tumors secreting human TNF-/cachectin induce cachexia in mice. Cell 50: 555–563, 1987.

Olive, D. and Mawas, C.: Therapeutic applications of anti-CD4 antibodies. Crit. Rev. in Therap. Drug Carriers Syst. 10: 29–63, 1993.

Ollert, M.W.; Frade, R.; Fiandino, A.; Panneerselvam, M.; Petrella, E.C.; Barel, M.; Pangburn, M.R.; Bredehorst, R. and Vogel, C.W.: C3–cleaving membrane proteinase. A new complement regulatory protein of human melanoma cells. J. Immunol. 144: 3862, 1990.

O'Neill, G.J.; Nerl, C.W.; Kay, P.H.; Christiansen, F.T.; McCluskey, J. and Dawkins, R.L.: Complement C4 is a marker for adult rheumatoid arthritis. Lancet 2: 214–, 1982.

Oppenheim, J.J.; Kovacs, E.J.; Matsushima, K. and Durum, S.K.: There is more than one interleukin 1. Immunology Today 7: 45–56, 1986.

Oppenheim, R.W.; Prevette, D.; Yin, Q.W.; Collins, F. and McDonald, J.: Control of embryonic motoneuron survival in vivo by ciliary neurotrophic factor. Science 251: 1616–1618, 1991.

Orchard, M.A.; Kagey-Sobotka, D.; Proud, D. and Lichtenstein, L.M.: A platelet derived supernatant (PDS) releases histamine from human basophils: evidence for interaction with IgE. Thromb. Haemost. 54 (abstr.): 232, 1985.

Orren, A.; Potter, P.C.; Cooper, R.C. and du Toit, E.: Deficiency of the sixth component of complement and susceptibility to Neisseria meningitis infections: studies in 10 families and 5 isolated cases. Immunology 62: 295–306, 1987.

Osborn, L.; Hession, C.; Tizard, R.; Vassallo, C.; Lukowskyi, S.; Chi-Rosso, G. and Lobb, R.: Direct expression and cloning of VCAM-1, a cytosine-induced endothelial protein that binds to lymphocytes. Cell 59: 1203, 1989.

Oster, W.; Cicco, N.A.; Klein, H.; Hirano, T.; Kishimoto, T.; Lindemann, A.; Mertelsmann, R. and Herrmann, F.: Participation of the cytokines interleukin-6, tumor necrosis factor-alpha, and interleukin-1ß secreted by acute myelogenous leukemia blasts in autocrine and paracrine leukemia growth control. J. Clin. Invest. 84: 451, 1989.

Oster, W. and Schulz, G.: Interleukin 3: biological and clinical effects. Int. J. Cell Cloning 9: 5–23, 1991.

Osterland, C.K.; Espinoza, L.; Parker, L.P. and Schur, P.H.: Inherited C2 deficiency and systemic lupus erythematosus: Studies on a family. Ann. Intern. Med. 82: 323–328, 1975.

Ostrand-Rosenberg, S.; Thakur, A. and Clements, V.: Rejection of mouse sarcoma cells after transfection of MHC class II genes. J. Immunol. 144: 4068–4071, 1990.

Otsuka, T.; Miyajima, A.; Brown, N.; Otsu, K.; Abrams, J.; Saeland, S.; Caux, C.; de Waal Malefijt, R.; de Vries, J.; Meyerson, P. et al.: Isolation and characterization of an expressible cDNA encoding human Il-3. Induction of Il-3 mRNA in human T cell clones. J. Immunol. 140: 2288–2295, 1988.

Otter, M.; Kuiper, J.; Bos, R.; Rijken, D.C. and Van Berkel, T.J.C.: Characterization of the inter-action both in vitro and in vivo of tissue-type plasminogen activator (t-PA) with rat liver cells. Effects of monoclonal antibodies to t-PA. Biochem. J. 284: 545–550, 1992.

Otterness, I.G.; Bliven, M.L.; Downs, J.T.; Natoli, E.J. and Hanson, D.C.: Inhibition of inter-leukin 1 synthesis by Tenidap; a new drug for arthritis. Cytokine 3: 277–283, 1991.

Ottesen, S.S.; Kieler, J. and Christensen, B.: Changes in HLA A,B,C expression during sponta-neous transformation of human urothelial cells in vitro. Eur. J. Clin. Oncol. 23: 991–995, 1987.

Owen, N.E. and Villereal, M.L.: Lys-bradykinin stimulated Na+ influx and DNA synthesis in cultured human fibroblasts. Cell 32: 979, 1983.

Owhashi, M. and Heber-Katz. E.: Protection from experimental allergic encephalomyelitis con-ferred by a monoclonal antibody directed against a shared idiotype on rat T cell receptors spe-cific for myelin basic protein. J. Exp. Med. 168: 2153–2164, 1988.

Oxholm, P. and Winther, K.: Thrombocyte involvement in immune inflammatory reactions. Allergy 41: 1–10, 1986.

Oyekan, A.O. and Botting, J.H.: A minimally invasive technique for the study of intravascular platelet aggregation in anaesthetised rats. J. Pharmacol. Meth. 15: 271–277, 1986.

Paccaud, J.P.; Schifferli, J.A. and Baggiolini, M.: NAP-1/Il-8 induces up-regulation of CR1 receptors in human neutrophil leukocytes. Biochem. Biophys. Res. Commun. 166: 187–192, 1990.

Paccaud, J-P.; Carpentier, J-L. and Schifferli, J.A.: Difference in the clustering of complement receptor type 1 (CR1) on polymorphonuclear leukocytes and erythrocytes: effect on immune adherence. Eur. J. Immunol. 20: 283–289, 1990.

Pace, J.L.; Russell, S.W.; Torres, B.A.; Johnson, H.M. and Gray, P.W.: Recombinant mouse gamma interferon induces the priming step in macrophage activation for tumor cell killing. J. Immunol. 130: 2011–2013, 1983.

Page, C.P.; Paul, W. and Morley, J.: An in vivo model for studying platelet aggregation and disaggregation. Thromb. Haemostas. 47: 210–213, 1982.

Page, C.P.: A role for platelet-activating factor and platelets in the induction of bronchial hyper-reactivity. Int. J. Tissue React. 9: 27–32, 1987.

Page, C.P.: The role of platelet-activating factor in asthma. J. Allergy Clin. Immunol. 81: 144–152, 1988.

Palaszynski, E.W. and Ihle, J.N.: Evidence for specific receptors for interleukin 3 on lympho-kine-dependent cell lines established from long-term marrow cultures. J. Immunol. 132: 1872–1878, 1984.

Palmer, R.M.J.; Ferrige, A.G. and Moncada, S.: Nitric oxide release accounts for the biological activity of endothelium-derived relaxing factor. Nature 327: 524–526, 1987.

Pals, S.T.; den Otter, A.; Miedema, F.; Kabel, P.; Keizer, G.D.; Scheper, R.J. and Meijer, C.: Evi-dence that leukocyte function-associated antigen-1 is involved in recirculation and homing of human lymphocytes via high endothelial venules. J. Immunol. 140: 1851–1853, 1988.

Pals, S.T. and Koopman, G.: Role of adhesion receptors in B-cell selection in the germinal center. ENII Conf.: Integrated Function of Molecules of the Immune System. Les Embiez, France, 12th-16th May 1993.

Panneerselvam, M.; Bredehorst, R. and Vogel, C.W.: Immobilized doxorubicin increases the complement susceptibility of human melanoma cells by protecting complement component C3b against inactivation. Proc. Natl. Acad. Sci. USA 83: 9144, 1986.

Panneerselvam, M.; Welt, S.; Old, L.J. and Vogel, C.W.: A molecular mechanism of complement resistance of human melanoma cells. J. Immunol. 136: 2534–2541, 1986.

Panneerselvam, M.; Bredehorst, R. and Vogel, C.W.: Resistance of human melanoma cells against the cytotoxic and complement-enhancing activities of doxorubicin. Cancer Res. 47: 4601, 1987.

Pantel, K.; Schlimok, G.; Kutter, D.; Schaller, G.; Genz, T.; Wiebecke, B.; Backmann, R.; Funke, I. and Reithmuller, G.: Frequent down-regulation of major histocompatibility class I antigen expression on individual micrometastatic carcinoma cells. Cancer Res. 51: 4712–4715, 1991.

Paoletti, E.; Tartaglia, J. and Cox, W.I.: Immunotherapeutic strategies for cancer using poxvirus vectors. Specific Immunotherapy Of Cancer With Vaccines, eds. Bystryn, J.-C.; Ferrone, S. and Livingston, P., The New York Academy of Sciences 690: 292, 1993.

Pappo, J. and Ermak, T.H.: Uptake and translocation of fluorescent latex particles by rabbit Peyer's patch follicle epithelium: A quantitative model for M cell uptake. Clin. Exp. Immunol. 76: 144–148, 1989.

Pardoll, D.M.: New strategies for active immunotherapy with genetically engineered tumor cells. Current Opinion in Immunology 4: 619–623, 1992.

Pardoll, D.M.: Cancer vaccines. TiPS 14: 1993.

Pardoll, D.M.: Genetically engineered tumor vaccines. Specific Immunotherapy Of Cancer With Vaccines, eds. Bystryn, J.-C.; Ferrone, S. and Livingston, P., The New York Academy of Sciences 690: 292, 1993.

Parekh, R.; Kwek, R.A.; Sutton, B.J.; Fernandes, D.L.; Leung, A.; Stanworth, D.; Rademacher, T.W.; Mizuochi, T.; Taniguchi, T.; Matsuta, K.; Takeuchi, F.; Nagano, Y.; Miyamoto, T. and Kobata, A.: Association of rheumatoid arthritis and primary osteoarthritis with changes in the glycosylation pattern. Nature 316: 452–457, 1985.

Parekh, R.; Isenberg, D.; Rook, G.; Roitt, I.; Dwek, R.A. and Rademacher, T.W.: A comparative analysis of disease-associated changes in the galactosylation of serum IgG. J. Autoimmun. 2: 101–104, 1989.

Parekh, R.B.: Oligosaccharides as specific ligands for the LECAM. BFE 8: 746–751, 1991.

Parham, P.: Getting into the groove. Nature 342: 617, 1989.

Parham, P.: The box and the rod. Nature 357: 538, 1992.

Park, L.S.; Friend, D.; Grabstein, K. and Urdal, D.L.: Characterization of the high-affinity cell-surface receptor for murine B-cell-stimulating factor 1. Proc. Natl. Acad. Sci. 84: 1669–1673, 1987.

Park, L.S.; Friend, D.; Sassenfeld, H.M. and Urdal, D.L.: Characterization of the human B cell stimulatory factor I receptor. J. Exp. Med. 166: 476–488, 1987.

Parker, C.J.; Stone, O.L.; White, V.F. and Bernshaw, N.J.: Vitronectin (S protein) is associated with platelets. Br. J. Haematol. 71: 245–252, 1989.

Parker, C.J.: Regulation of complement by membrane proteins: an overview. Current Topics in Microbiology and Immunology, Springer Verlag, Berlin, 178: 1992.

Parnet, P.; Brunke, D.; Goujon, E.; Mainard, J.; Biragyn, A.; Arkins, S.; Dantzer, R. and Kelley, K.: Molecular identification of two types of interleukin-1 receptors in the murine pituitary gland. J. Neuroendocrinol. 5: 213–219, 1993.

Parrillo, J.E.: Septic shock: clinical manifestations, pathogenesis, hemodynamics, and management in a critical care unit. In: Textbook of Critical Care Medicine. Shoemaker, W.C.; Ayres, S.; Grenvik, A. et al. (eds.). Philadelphia, W.B. Saunders, 111–125, 1989.

Parronchi, P.; Tiri, A.; Macchia, D.; de Carli, M.; Biswas, P.; Simonelli, C.; Maggi, E.; del Prete, G.; Ricci, M. and Romagnani, S.: Noncognate contact-dependent B cell Activation can promote IL-4–dependent in vitro human IgE synthesis. J. Immunol. 144: 2102–2108, 1990.

Parronchi, P.; Macchia, D.; Piccinni, M-P.; Biswas, P.; Simonelli, C.; Maggi, E.; Ricci, M.; Ansari, A.A. and Romagnani, S.: Allergen- and bacterial antigen-specific T-cell clones established from atopic donors show a different profile of cytokine production. Proc. Natl. Acad. Sci. USA 88: 4538–4542, 1991.

Partridge, T.A.: Myoblast transfer: a possible therapy for inherited myopathies? Muscle & Nerve 14(3): 197–212, 1991.

Partridge, T.: Neuromuscular disease and the potential applications of gene therapy. Gene Therapy - New Challenges for the Pharmaceutical Industry, London, September 15–16, 1994.

Passwell, J.H. and Laufer, J.: The role of complement proteins in the pathogenesis of disease. Israel J. Med. Sciences 28: 471, 1992.

Pastan, I.H.: Recombinant immunotoxins: new therapeutic agents for cancer treatment. Cancer Detection and Prevention 17: 289–293, 1993.

Pasternack, B.: The prediction of asthma in infantile eczema. J. Pediatr. 66: 164, 1965.

Patel, P.M.; Flemming, C.L.; Russell, S.J.; Gore, M.E.; Eccles, S.A. and Collins, M.K.L.: Cytokine gene transfer as a therapeutic strategy. Human Genetic Therapy, Conf. Documentation, London, 1992.

Patel, K.J.; Aluvihare, V.R. and Neuberger, M.S.: Efficient cross-linked endocytosis and antigen presentation by membrane immunoglobulin is conferred by its µ/ß sheath. ENII Conf.: Integrated Function of Molecules of the Immune System. Les Embiez, France, 12th-16th May 1993.

Patterson, W.P. and Ringenberg, Q.S.: The pathophysiology of thrombosis in cancer. Seminars in Oncology, 17: 140–146, 1990.

Paty, P.S.K.; Sherman, P.F.; Shepard, J.M.; Malik, A.B. and Kaplan, J.E.: Role of adenosine in platelet-mediated reduction in pulmonary vascular permeability. Am. J. Physiol. 262: H771–H777, 1992.

Paul, J.; Conkie, D. and Burgos, H.: Effects of erythropoietin on cell populations and macro-molecular synthesis in foetal mouse erythroid cells. J. Embryol. Exp. Morphol. 29: 453–472, 1973.

Paul, L.; Skanes, V.M.; Mayden, J. and Levine, R.P.: C4–mediated inhibition of immune preci-pitation and differences in inhibitory action of genetic variants. C4A3 and C4B1. Complement 5: 110–119, 1988.

Paul, N. and Ruddle, N.: Lymphotoxin. Annu. Rev. Biochem. 6: 407–438, 1990.

Paul, S.R.; Bennett, F.; Calvetti, J.A.; Kelleher, K.; Wood, C.R.; Ohara, R.M.jr.; Leary, A.C.; Sibley, B.; Clark, S.C.; Williams, D.A. and Yang, Y.C.: Molecular cloning of a cDNA encod-ing interleukin 11, a stromal cell-derived lymphopoietic cytokine. Proc. Natl. Acad. Sci. USA 87: 7512–7516, 1990.

Paul, W.E. and Ohara, J.: B-cell stimulatory factor-I/interleukin 4. Annu. Rev. Immunol. 5: 429, 1987.

Paul, W.E.: Interleukin-4: a prototypic immunoregulatory lymphokine. Blood 77: 1859–1870, 1991.

Pavlath, G.K.; Dhawan, J. and Blau, H.M.: Myoblast-mediated gene therapy. Human Genetic Therapy, Conf. Documentation, London, 1992.

Pavli, P.; Woodhams, C.E.; Doe, W.F. and Hume, D.A.: Isolation and characterization of antigen-presenting dendritic cells from the mouse intestinal lamina propria. Immunoloy 70: 40–47, 1990.

Payan, D.G.; Brewster, D.R. and Goetzl, E.J.: Specific stimulation of human T lymphocytes by substance P. J. Immunol. 131: 1613–1615, 1983.

Payne, L.C.; Weigent, D.A. and Blalock, J.E.: Induction of pituitary sensitivity to interleukin-1: A new function for corticotropin releasing hormone. Biochem. Biophys. Res. Commun. 198: 480–484, 1994.

Peerschke, E.I.B. and Ghebrehiwet, B.: Human blood platelets possess specific binding sites for C1q. J. Immunol. 138: 1537–1541, 1987.

Peerschke, E.I.B.; Malhotra, R.; Ghebrehiwet, B.; Reid, K.B.M.; Willis, A.C. and Slim, R.B.: Isolation of a human endothelial cell C1q receptor (C1q-R). J. Leuk. Biol. 53: 179–184, 1983.

Peerschke, E.I.B. and Ghebrehiwet, B.: Identification and partial characterization of human pla-telet C1q binding sites. J. Immunol. 14: 3505–3511, 1988.

Peerschke, E.I.B. and Ghebrehiwet, B.: Modulation of platelet responses to collagen by C1q receptors. J. Immunol. 144: 221–225, 1990.

Peerschke, E.I.B.; Reid, K.B.M. and Ghebrehiwet, B.: Platelet activation by C1q is accompanied by the induction of alphaIIb/beta3 (GPIIb/IIIa) and expression of procoagulant activity. J. Exp. Med. 178: 579–587, 1993.

Pekelharing, J.M.; Hepp, E.; Kamerling, J.P.; Gerwig, G.J. and Leijnse, B.: Alteration in carbo-hydrate composition of serum IgG from patients with rheumatoid arthritis and from pregnant women. Ann. Rheum. Dis. 47: 91–95, 1988.

Peleman, R.; Wu, J.; Eargene, C. and Delespesse, G.: Recombinant IL-4 suppresses the produc-tion of IFN-gamma by human mononuclear cells. J. Exp. Med. 170: 1751–1757, 1989.

Pellegrino, M.A.; Ferrone, S.; Cooper, N.R.; Dierich, M.P. and Reisenfeld, R.A.: Variation in sus-ceptibility of a human lymphoid cell line to immune lysis during the cell cycle: lack of corre-lation with antigen density and complement binding. J. Exp. Med. 140: 578–590, 1974.

Pene, J.; Rousset, F.; Brière, F.; Chrétien, I.; Bonnefoy, J.Y.; Spits, H.; Yokota, T.; Arai, N.; Arai, K.-I.; Banchereau, J. and de Vries J.E.: IgE production by normal human lymphocytes is in-duced by interleukin 4 and suppressed by interferons and μ and prostaglandin E2. Proc. Natl. Acad. Sci. USA 85: 6880–6884, 1988.

Pene, J.; Rousset, F.; Brière, F.; Paliard, X.; Chrétien, I.; Banchereau, J. and de Vries, J.E.: IgE production by normal human B cells induced by alloreactive T cell clones is mediated by IL-4 and suppressed by IFN-. J. Immunol. 141: 1218–1224, 1988.

Pene, J.; Rousset, F.; Briere, F.; Chrétien, I.; Wideman, J.; Bonnefoy, J.Y. and de Vries, J.E.: Interleukin-5 enhances Interleukin-4 induced IgE production by normal human B cells: the role of soluble CD23 antigen. Eur. J. Immunol. 18: 929–935, 1988.

Pene, J.; Rousset, F.; Briere, F.; Chrétien, I.; Bonnefoy, J.Y.; Spits, H.; Yokota, T.; Arai, N.; Arai, K.-I.; Bachereau, J. and de Vries, J.E.: IgE production by human B cells is induced by IL-4 and suppressed by interferons gamma, alpha and prostaglandin E2. Proc. Natl. Acad. Sci. USA 85: 8166–8170, 1988.

Pene, J.; Rousset, F.; Briere, F.; Chretien, I.; Bonnefoy, J.Y.; Spitz, H.; Yokota, T.; Arai, N.; Arai, K.; Banchereau, J. et al.: IgE production by normal human lymphocytes is induced by interleukin 4 and suppressed by interferon gamma and alpha and prostaglandin E2. Proc. Natl. Acad. Sci. 85: 6880–6884, 1988.

Pene, J.; Chretien, I.; Rousset, F.; Briere, F.; Bonnefoy, J.Y. and De Vries, J.E.: Modulation of Il-4–induced human IgE production in vitro by IFN-gamma and Il-5: The role of soluble CD23 (s-CD23). J. Cell Biochem. 39: 253–264, 1989.

Pennica, C.; Kohr, W.J.; Fendly, B.M.; Shire, S.J.; Raab, H.E.; Borchardt, P.E.; Lewis, M. and Goeddel, D.V.: Characterization of a recombinant extracellular domain of the type 1 tumor necrosis factor receptor: evidence for tumor necrosis factor-alpha induced receptor aggregation. Biochem. 31: 1134–1141, 1992.

Peppel, K.; Crawford, D. and Beutler, B.: A tumor necrosis factor (TNF) receptor-IgG heavy chain chimeric protein as a bivalent antagonist of TNF activity. J. Exp. Med. 174: 1483–1489, 1991.

Pernice, W.; Schmitz, H.; Schindera, F.; Behrens, F. and Sedlacek, H.H.: Antigen-specific detection of immune complexes in patients with Hepatitis B, Influenza A and Rubella. Behring Inst. Mitt. 64: 102–108, 1979.

Pernice, W.; Sodomann, C.P.; Lüben, G.; Seiler, F.R. and Sedlacek, H.H.: Antigen-specific detection of HbsAG-containing immune complexes in the course of Hepatitis B virus infection. Clin. exp. Immunol. 37: 376–380, 1979.

Pernow, B.: Substance P. Acta Physiol. Scand. 29: 1–90, 1953.

Pert, A.; Dionne, R.; Ng, L.; Bragin, E.; Moody, T.W. and Pert, C.B.: Alterations in rat central nervous system endorphins following transauricular electroacupuncture. Brain Res. 224: 83–93, 1981.

Petit-Frere, C.; Duga, B.; Braquet, P. and Mencia-Huerta, M.: Interleukin-9 potentiates the interleukin-4–induced IgE and IgG1 release from murine B lymphocytes. Immunology 79: 146–151, 1993.

Petrak, R.A.; Balk, R.A. and Bone, R.C.: Prostaglandins, cyclo-oxygenase inhibitors, and thromboxane synthesis inhibitors in the pathogenesis of multiple organ failure. Crit. Care Clin. 5: 303–314, 1989.

Peri, G.; Rossi, V.; Taraboletti, G.; Erroi, A. and Mantovani, A.: Ia antigen expression and Il-1 activity in murine tumour-associated macrophages. Immunology 59: 527–533, 1986.

Perussia, B.; Mangoni, L.; Engers, H.D. and Trinchieri, G.: Interferon production by human and murine lymphocytes in response to alloantigens. J. Immunol. 125: 1589–1595, 1980.

Peschel, C.; Paul, W.E.; Ohara, J. and Green, I.: Effects of B cell stimulatory factor-1/interleukin 4 on hematopoietic progenitor cells. Blood 70: 254–263, 1987.

Petroni, K.C.; Shen, L. and Guyre, P.M.: Modulation of human polymorphonuclear leukocyte IgG Fc receptors and Fc receptor-mediated functions by IFN-gamma and glucocorticoids. J. Immunol. 140: 3467–3472, 1988.

Pfeiffer, A. and Herz, A.: Endocrine actions of opioids. Horm. Metab. Res. 16: 386–397, 1984.

Pfeilschifter, J. and Vosbeck, K.: Transforming growth factor $\beta2$ inhibits interleukin-1β and tumor necrosis factor α-induction of nitric oxide synthase in rat renal mesangial cells. Biochem. Biophys. Res. Comm. 175: 372–379, 1991.

Phan, S.H.; Gannon. D.E.; Varani, J.; Ryan, U.S. and Ward, P.A.: Xanthine oxidase activity in rat pulmonary artery endothelial cells and its alteration by activated neutrophils. Am. J. Pathol. 134: 1201–1211, 1989.

Philips, D.R.; Jennings, L.K. and Prasanna, H.R.: Ca2+ mediated association of glycoprotein G (thrombin-sensitive protein, thrombospondin) with human platelets. J. Biol. Chem. 255: 11629–11632, 1980.

Philips, D.R.; Charo, I.F.; Parise, L.V. and Fitzgerald, L.A.: The platelet membrane glycoprotein IIb-IIIa complex. Blood 71: 831–843, 1988.

Philpott, G.W.; Bower, R.J. and Parker, C.W.: Selective iodination and cytotoxicity of tumor cells with an antibody-enzyme conjugate. Surgery 74: 51, 1973.

Philpott, G.W.; Shearer, W.T.; Bower, R.W. and Parker, C.W.: Selective cytotoxicity of hapten-substituted cells with an antibody-enzyme conjugate. J. Immunol. 111: 921–929, 1973.

Philpott, G.W.; Bower, R.J.; Parker, K.L.; Shearer, W.T. and Parker, C.W.: Affinity cytotoxicity of tumor cells with antibody-glucose oxidase conjugates, peroxidase, and arsphenamine. Cancer Res. 34: 2159, 1974.

Philpott, G.W.; Grass, E.H. and Parker, C.W.: Affinity cytotoxicity with an alcohol dehydrogenase-antibody conjugate and allyl alcohol. Cancer Res. 39: 2084, 1979.

Phipps, R.P.; Stein, S.H. and Roper, R.L.: A new view of prostaglandin E regulation of the immune response. Immunol. Today 12: 349, 1991.

Pick, E. and Turk, J.L.: The biological activitites of soluble lymphocyte products. Clin. Exp. Immunol. 10: 1–23, 1972.

Picker, L.J. and Butcher, E.C.: Physiological and molecular mechanisms of lymphocyte homing. Annu. Rev. Immunol. 10: 561–591, 1992.

Pike, L.J.; Bowen-Pope, D.F.; Ross, R. and Krebs, E.G.: Characterization of platelet-derived growth factor-stimulated phosphorylation in cell membranes. J. Biol. Chem. 258: 9383–9390, 1983.

Pirofsky, B.: Autoimmunization and the Autoimmune Hemolytic Anemias, William and Wilkins, Baltimore, MD, 455–478, 1969.

Planck, S.R.; Dang, T.T.; Graves, D.; Tara, D.; Ansel, J.C. and Rosenbaum, J.T.: Retinal pigment epithelial cells secrete interleukin-6 in response to interleukin-1. Invest. Ophth. Vis. Sci. 33: 78–82, 1992.

Plaut, M.; Pierce, J.H.; Watson, C.J.; Hanley-Hyde, J.; Nordan, R.P. and Paul, W.E.: Mast cell lines produce lymphokines in response to cross-linkage of FcRI or calcium ionophores. Nature (London) 339: 64–66, 1989.

Plautz, G.E.; Yang, Z.Y.; Wu, B.Y.; Gao, X.; Huang, L. and Nabel, G.J.: Immunotherapy of malignancy by in vivo gene transfer into tumors. Proc. Natl. Acad. Sci. USA 90: 4645–4649, 1993.

Pober, J.S. and Gimbrone M.A.jr.: Expression of Ia-like antigens by human vascular endothelial cells is inducible in vitro: Demonstration by monoclonal antibody binding and immunoprecipitation. Proc. Natl. Acad. Sci. USA 79: 6641–6645, 1982.

Pober, J.S.; Gimbrone, M.A.jr.; Cotran, R.S.; Reiss, C.S.; Burakoff, S.J.; Fiers, W. and Ault, K.A.: Ia expression by vascular endothelium is inducible by activated T-cells and by human gamma-interferon. J. Exp. Med. 157: 1339–1353, 1983.

Pober, J.S.; Bevilacqua, M.P.; Mendrick, D.L.; Lapierre, L.A.; Fiers, W. and Gimbrone, M.A.jr.: Two distinct monokines, interleukin-1 and tumor necrosis factor, each independently induce biosynthesis and transient expression of the same antigen on the surface of cultured human vascular endothelial cell. J. Immunol. 136: 1680–1687, 1986.

Pober, J.S.: Effects of TNF and related cytokines on human vascular endothelial cells. In: Bock, G.; Marsh, J. (eds): CIBA Foundation Symposium 131: Tumor necrosis factor. Chichester, Wiley, 170–179, 1987.

Pober, J.S.; Lapierre, L.A.; Stolpen, A.H.; Brock, T.A.; Springer, T.A.; Fiers, W.; Bevilacqua, M.P.; Mendrick, D.L. and Gimbrone, M.A.jr.: Activation of cultured human endothelial cells by recombinant lymphotoxin: Comparison with tumor necrosis factor and interleukin-1 species. J. Immunol. 138: 3319–3324, 1987.

Pober, J.S.: Cytokine-mediated activation of vascular endothelium. Am. J. Pathol. 133: 426, 1988.

Pober, J.S. and Cotran, R.S.: Cytokines and endothelial cell biology. Physiological Revies 70: 427–451, 1990.

Pockley, A.G. and Montgomery P.C.: Regulatory role of Interleukin 5 and 6 on immunoglobulin production in clutured rat salivary glands. Immunol. Invest. 21: 103–110, 1992.

Poljak, R.J.: Structure of antibodies and their complexes with antigens. Molec. Immun. 28: 1341–1345, 1991.

Pollack, S.; Cunningham-Rundles, C.; Smithwick, E.M.; Barandum, S. and Good, R.A.: High-dose intravenous gammaglobulin in autoimmune neutrophenia (letter). N. Engl. J. Med. 307: 253, 1982.

Pollanen, P.; Soder, O. and Parvinen, M.: Interleukin-1µ stimulation of spermatogonial proliferation in vivo. Reprod. Fertil. Develop. 1: 85–87, 1989.

Polley, M.J. and Nachman, R.L.: Human complement in thrombin-mediated platelet function. Uptake of the C56–9 complex. J. Exp. Med. 150: 633–645, 1979.

Polley, M.J. and Nachman, R.L.: The human complement system in thrombin-mediated platelet function. In: Gordon, J.L. (ed.) Platelets in Biology and Pathology-2, Elsevier, North Holland Biomedical Press, Oxford, 309–319, 1981.

Polley, M.J. and Nachman, R.L.: Human platelet activation by C3a and C3a des-arg. J. Exp. Med. 158: 603–615, 1983.

Polverini, P.J. and Leibovich, J.: Induction of neovascularization in vivo and endothelial proliferation in vitro by tumor-associated macrophages. Lab. Invest. 51: 635–642, 1984.

Poncet, P.; Matthes, T.; Billecocq, A. and Dighiero, G.: Immunochemical studies of polyspecific natural autoantibodies: charge, lipid reactivity, Fab'2 fragments activity and complement fixation. Molec. Immun. 25: 981–989, 1988.

Ponzoni, M.; Casalaro, A.; Lanciotti, M.; Montaldo, P.G. and Cornaglia-Ferraris, P.: The combination of gamma-interferon and tumor necrosis factor causes a rapid and extensive differentiation of human neuroblastoma cells. Canc. Res. 52: 931–939, 1992.

Popp, W.; Fucik, E.; Kramer, G.; Hainz, R.; Rami, B.; Böck, A.; Herkner, K.; Zwick, H. and Sertl, K.: ICAM-1 in pulmonary health and bronchial hyperresponsiveness. WMW 4: 1992.

Porcel, J.M. and Vergani, D.: Review. Complement and lupus: old concepts and new directions. Lupus 1: 343–349, 1992.

Porcel, J.M. and Vergani, D.: El sistema del complemento: una fascinante cascada biologica. Med. Clin. (Barc.) 100: 428–435, 1993.

Porcelli, S.; Morita, C. and Brenner, M.B.: Non-MHC encoded antigen-presenting molecules. ENII Conf.: Integrated Function of Molecules of the Immune System. Les Embiez, France, 12th-16th May 1993.

Porgador, A.; Tzehoval, E.; Vadai, E.; Feldman, M. and Eisenbach, L.: Immunotherapy via gene therapy: comparison of the effects of tumor cells transduced with the interleukin-2, interleukin-6, or interferon-gamma genes. J. Immunother. Emphasis Tumor Immunol. 14: 191–201, 1993.

Porter, A.G.: The prospects for therapy with tumour necrosis factors and their antagonists. Tibtech 9: 158, 1991.

Postlethwaite, A.E.; Raghow, R.; Stricklin, G.P.; Poppleton, H.; Seyer, J.M. and Kang, A.H.: Modulation of fibroblast functions by interleukin 1: increased steady-state accumulation of type 1 procollagen messenger RNAs and stimulation of other functions but not chemotaxis by human recombinant interleukin 1 µ and ß. J. Cell Biol. 106: 311–318, 1988.

Powell, M.C.; Perkins, A.C.; Pimm, M.V.; Al Jetaily, M.; Wastle, M.L.; Durrant, L.; Baldwin, R.W. and Symonds, E.M.: Diagnostic imaging of gynecologic tumors with the monoclonal antibody 791/36. Am. J. Obstet. Gynecol. 157: 28, 1987.

Prence, E.M.; Dong, J.M. and Sahagian, G.G.: Modulation of the transport of a lysosomal enzyme by PDGF. J. Cell Biol. 110: 319–326, 1990.

Press, O.W.; Eary, J.F.; Badger, C.C.; Martin, P.J.; Appelbaum, F.R.; Levy, R.; Miller, R.; Brown, S.; Nelp, W.B.; Krohn, K.A. et al.: Treatment of refractory non-Hodgkin's radiolabeled MB-1 (anti-CD 27) antibody. J. Clin. Oncol. 7: 1027–1038, 1989.

Pressman, D. and Keighley, G.: The zone of activity of antibodies as determined by the use of radioactive tracers; the zone of an activity of nephrotoxic antikidney serum. J. Immunol. 59: 141, 1948.

Pressman, D. and Korngold, L.: The in vivo localization of anti-Wagner-osteogenic-sarcoma antibodies. Cancer 6: 619, 1953.

Pretolani, M.; Ferrer-Lopez, P. and Vargaftig, B.B.: From anti-asthma drugs to PAF-acether antagonism and back. Biochem. Pharmacol. 38: 1373–1384, 1989.

Price, G.; Brenner, M.K.; Prentice, H.G.; Hoffbrand, A.V. and Newland, A.C.: Cytotoxic effects of tumor necrosis factor and gamma interferon on acute myeloid leukaemia blast cells. Br. J. Cancer 55: 287, 1987.

Prober, J.S.; Bevilacqua, M.P.; Mendrick, D.C.; Lapierre, L.A.; Fiers, W. and Gimbrone, M.A.jr.: Two distinct monokines, interleukin 1 and tumour necrosis factor, each independently induce biosynthesis and transient expression of the same antigen on the surface of cultured human vascular endothelial cells. J. Immuno. 136: 1680–1687, 1986.

Pruitt, S.K.; Baldwin, W.M.; Marsch, H.C.; Ijn, S.S.; Yeh, G.C. and Bollinger, R.R.: Effects of soluble complement receptor type 1 on natural antibody levels during xenograft rejection. Transplant. Proc. 24: 477–478, 1992.

Pukel, C.S.; Lloyd, K.O.; Travassos, L.R.; Dippold, W.G.; Oettgen, H.F. and Old, L.J.: GD3, a prominent ganglioside of human melanoma. Detection and characterization by a mouse monoclonal antibody. J. Exp. Med. 155: 1133–1147, 1982.

Pullen, A.M.; Kappler, J.W. and Marrack, P.: Tolerance to self antigens shapes the T-cell repertoire. Immunol. Rev. 107: 125–139, 1989.

Pullen, A.; Wade, T.; Marrack, P. and Kappler, J.: Identification of the region of T cell receptor β chain that interacts with the self-superantigen Mls-13. Cell 61: 1365–1374, 1990.

Pung, Y.-H.; Vetro, S.W. and Bellanti, J.A.: Use of interferons in atopic (IgE-mediated) diseases. Annals of Allery, 71: 234, 1993.

Punnonen, J.; Aversa, G.; Cocks, B.G.; McKenzie, A.N.J.; Menon, S.; Zurawski, G.; De Waal Malefyt, R. and De Vries, J.E.: Interleukin 13 induces interleukin 4–independent IgG4 and IgE synthesis and CD23 expression by human B cells. Proc. Natl. Acad. Sci. USA 90, 3730–3734, 1993.

Purkerson, J. and Isakson, P.: A two-signal model for regulation of immunoglobulin isotype switching. FASEB J. 6: 3245–3252, 1992.

Puri, R.K. and Rosenberg, S.A.: Combined effects of interferon-alpha and interleukin 2 on the induction of a vascular leak syndrome in mice. Cancer Immunol. Immunother. 28: 267–274, 1989.

Pusztai, L.; Lewis, C.E.; Lorenzen, J. and McGee, J.O.D.: Growth factors: regulation of normal and neoplastic growth. J. Pathol. 169: 191–201, 1993.

Qin, S.; Cobbold, S.; Benjamin, R. and Waldmann H.: Induction of classical transplantation tolerance in the adult. J. Exp. Med. 169: 779–794, 1989.

Quantin, B.; Murphy, G. and Breathnach, R.: Pump-1 cDNA codes for a protein with characteristics similar to those of classical collagenase family. members. Biochem. 28: 5327–5334, 1989.

Quelle, F.W. and Wojchowski, D.M.: Proliferative action of erythropoietin is associated with rapid protein tyrosine phosphorylation in responsive B6SUt.EP cells. J. Biol. Chem. 266: 609–614, 1991.

Quertermous, T.; Runge, M.S. and Haber, E.: Recombinant hybrid immunoglobulin molecules and method of use. IPN WO 90/02338, 1990.

Rae, S.A. and Smith, M.J.H.: The stimulation of lysosomal enzyme secretion from human polymorphonuclear leucocytes by leukotriene B4. J. Pharm. Pharmacol. 33: 616–617, 1981.

Rae, S.A.; Davidson, E.M. and Smith, M.J.H.: Leukotriene B4, an inflammatory mediator in gout. Lancet 2: 1122, 1982.

Rainer, H.; Kovats, E.; Lehmann, H.G.; Micksche, M.; Rauhs, R.; Sedlacek, H.H.; Seidl, W.; Schemper, M.; Schiessel, R.; Schwieger, B. and Wunderlich, M.: Effectiveness of postoperative adjuvant therapy with cytotoxic chemotherapy or immunotherapy in the prevention of recurrence of Duke's B and C colon cancer. In: Recent Results in Cancer Research 79: 41–47, Klein, H.O., ed. Springer, Berlin, 1981.

Räisänen-Sokolowski, A.; Myllärniemi, M. and Häyry, P.: Effect of mycophenolic mophetil (RS61443) on rat aortic allograft arteriosclerosis. Int. Conference on New Trends in Clinical and Experimental Immunosuppression. Geneva, Switzerland, February 10–13, 1994.

Räisänen-Sokolowski, A.; Aho, P.; Tufvesson, G. and Häyry, P.: Mechanism of action of 15–Deoxyspergualin in inhibition of allograft arteriosclerosis in rat aortic transplants. Int. Conference on New Trends in Clinical and Experimental Immunosuppression. Geneva, Switzerland, February 10–13, 1994.

Raisz, L.G.: Sandberg, A.L.; Goodson, J.M.; Simmons, H.A. and Mergenhagen, S.E.: Complement-dependent stimulation of prostaglandin synthesis and bone resorption. Science 185: 787–791, 1974.

Rajka, G.: Major problems in dermatology. In: Rook, A (ed) Atopic dermatitis, vol.3. Saunders, London, 1975.

Rajka, G.: Atopic dermatitis: clinical aspects. In: Rajka, G (ed) Essential aspects of atopic dermatitis. Springer, Berlin, 4–55, 1989.

Ramansee, H.-G.; Kroschewski, R. and Frangoulis, B.: Clonal anergy induced in mature Vβ6 T-lymphocytes on immunizing M1s-1H mice with M1s-1a expressing cells. Nature 339: 541, 1989.

Ramarathinam, L.; Castle, M.; Wu, Y. and Liu, Y.: T cell costimulation by B7/BB1 induces CD8 T cell-dependent tumor rejection: an important role of B7/BB1 in the induction, recruitment, and effector function of antitumor T cells. J. Exp. Med. 179: 1205–1214, 1994.

Ramirez, F. and Di Liberto, M.: Complex and diversified regulatory programs control the expression of vertebrate collagen genes. FASEB J. 4: 1616–1623, 1990.

Ramshaw, I.A.; Andrew, M.E.; Phillips, S.M.; Boyle, D.B. and Coupar, B.E.H.: Recovery of immunodeficient mice from a vaccinia virus/Il-2 recombinant infection. Nature 329: 545–546, 1987.

Ramstedt, U.; Ng, J.; Wigzell, H.; Serhan, C.N. and Samuelsson, B.: Action of novel eicosanoids lipoxin A and B on human natural killer cell cytotoxicity: effects on intracellular cAMP and target cell binding. J. Immunol. 135: 3434, 1985.

Ran, M. and Witz, I.P.: Tumor-associated immunoglobulins. The elution of IgG-2 from mouse tumors. Int. J. Cancer 6: 361–372, 1970.

Randall, R.E. and Young, D.F.: Humoral and cytotoxic T cell responses to internal and external structural proteins of Simian virus 5 induced by immunization with solid matrix antibody and antigen complexes. J. Gen. Virol. 69: 2505, 1987.

Ranges, G.E.; Sriram, S. and Cooper, S.M.: Prevention of type II collagen-induced arthritis by in vivo treatment with anti-L3T4. J. Exp. Med. 162: 1105–1110, 1985.

Ranges, G.E.; Fortin, S.; Barger, M.T.; Sriram, S. and Cooper, S.M.: In vivo modulation of murine induced arthritis. Int. Rev. Immunol. 4: 83–90, 1988.

Rappaport, R.S. and Dodge, G.R.: Prostaglandin E inhibits the production of human interleukin-2. J. Exp. Med. 155: 943, 1982.

Rasmussen, R.; Takatsu, K.; Harada, N.; Takahashi, T. and Bottomly, K.: T cell-dependent hapten-specific and polyclonal B cell responses require release of interleukin 5. J. Immunol. 140: 705–712, 1988.

Ratanachiayavong, S.; Demaine, A.G.; Campbell, R.D. and McGregor, A.M.: Heat shock protein 70 (HSP70) and complement C4 genotypes in patients with hyperthyroid Grave's disease. Clin. Exp. Immunol. 84: 48–52, 1991.

Ratnoff, O.D. and Lepow, I.H.: Some properties of an esterase derived from preparations of the first component of complement. J. Exp. Med. 106: 327–343, 1957.

Ratnoff, O.D.; Pensky, J.; Ogston, D. and Naff, G.B.: The inhibition of plasmin, plasma kallikrein, plasma permeability factor and the C'1r subcomponent of the first component of complement by serum C'1 esterase inhibitor. J. Exp. Med. 129: 315–331, 1970.

Ravetch, J.V. and Kinet, J.P.: Fc receptors. Annu. Rev. Immunol. 9: 457–492, 1991.

Ravindranatz, M.H.; Morton, D.L. and Irie, R.F.: An epitope common to gangliosides 0-acetyl-GD3 and GD3 recognized by antibodies in melanoma patients after active specific immuno-therapy. Cancer Res. 49: 3891–3897, 1989.

Raz, E.; Watanabe, A.; Baird, S.M.; Eisenberg, R.A.; Parr, T.B.; Lotz, M.; Kipps, T.J. and Carson, D.: Systemic immunological effects of cytokine genes injected into skeletal muscle. Proc. Natl. Acad. Sci. USA 90: 4523–4527, 1993.

Razi-Wolf, Z.; Freeman, G.J.; Galvin, F.; Benacerraf, B.; Nadler, L. and Reiser, H.: Expression and function of the murine B7 antigen, the major costimulatory molecule expressed by peritoneal exudate cells. Proc. Natl. Acad. Sci. USA 89: 4210–4214, 1992.

Real, F.X.; Mattes, M.J.; Houghton, A.N.; Oettgen, H.F.; Lloyd, K.O. and Old, L.J.: Class 1 (unique) tumor antigens of human melanoma. Identification of a 90.000 dalton cell surface glycoprotein by autologous antibody. J. Exp. Med. 160: 1219–1233, 1984.

Real, F.X.; Furukawa, K.S.; Mattes, M.J.; Gusik, S.A.; Cordon Cardo, C.; Oettgen, H.F.; Old, L.J. and Lloyd, K.O.: Class 1 (unique) tumor antigens of human melanoma: Identification of unique and common epitopes on a 90–kDa glycoprotein. Proc. Natl. Acad. Sci. USA 85: 3965–3969, 1988.

Rechler, M.M.; Zapf, J.; Nissley, S.P.; Froesch, E.R.; Moses, A.C.; Podskalny, J.M.; Schilling, E.E. and Humbel, R.E.: Interactions of insulin-like growth factors I and II and multiplication-stimulating activity with receptors and serum carrier proteins. Endocrinology 107: 1451–1459, 1980.

Reed, A.M.; Pachman, L. and Ober, C.: Molecular genetic studies of major histocompatibility complex genes in children with juvenile dermatomyositis: Increased risk associated with HLA-DQA1*0501. Hum. Immunol. 32: 235–240, 1991.

Reed, J.C.; Alpers, J.D.; Nowell, P.C. and Hoover, R.G.: Sequential expression of protooncogenes during lectin-stimulated mitogenesis of normal human lymphocytes. Proc. Natl. Acad. Sci. USA 83: 3982–3986, 1986.

Reed, J.C.: Bcl-2 and the regulation of programmed cell death. J. Cell Biol. 124: 1–6, 1994.

Reichlin, M.; Rader, M.; and Harley, J.B.: Autoimmune response to the Ro/SSA particle is directed to the human antigen. Clin. exp. Immun. 76: 373–377, 1989.

Reid, K.B.: Proteins involved in the activation and control of the two pathways of human complement. Biochem. Soc. Trans. 11: 1–12, 1983.

Reinhold, U.; Pawelec, G.; Wehrmann, W.; Herold, M.; Wernet, P. and Kreysel, H.W.: Immunoglobulin E and immunoglobulin G subclass distribution in vivo and relationship to in vitro generation of interferon-gamma and neopterin in patients with severe atopic dermatitis. Int. Arch. Allergy Appl. Immunol. 87: 120–126, 1988.

Reinhold, U.; Wehrmann, W.; Kukel, S. and Kreysel, H.W.: Evidence that defective interferon-gamma production in atopic dermatitis patients is due to intrinsic abnormalities. Clin. Exp. Immunol. 79: 374–379, 1990.

Reinhold, U.; Wehrmann, W.; Kukel, S. and Kreysel, H.W.: Recombinant IFN-gamma in severe atopic dermatitis. Lancet 1: 1282, 1990.

Reimer, G.; Rose, K.M.; Scheer, U. and Tan, E.M.: Autoantibody to RNA polymerase I in scleroderma sera. J. clin. Invest. 79: 65–72, 1987.

Reiter, C.; Kakavand, B.; Rieber, E.P.; Schattenkirchner, M.; Riethmüller, G. and Krüger, K.: Treatment of rheumatoid arthritis with monoclonal CD4 antibody M-T151: clinical results and immunopharmacologic effects in an open study, including repeated administration. Arthritis Rheum. 34: 525–536, 1991.

Reith, A.D.; Ellis, C.; Lyman, S.D.; Anderson, D.M.; Williams, D.E.; Bernstein, A. and Pawson, T.: Signal transduction by normal isoforms and W mutant variants of the Kit receptor tyrosine kinase. EMBO J. 10: 2451–2459, 1991.

Remuzzi, G.: Platelets and renal diseases. Int. Conf. on: The platelet in health & disease. Royal College od physicians, London, 1992.

Renner, C.; Pfreundschuh, M.; Diehl, V. and Pohl, C.: Active specific immunotherapy of Hodgkin's lymphoma by an anti-idiotype vaccine against the Hodgkin-associated CD30 antigen. Specific Immunotherapy Of Cancer With Vaccines, eds. Bystryn, J.-C.; Ferrone, S. and Livingston, P., The New York Academy of Sciences 690: 352, 1993.

Renz, H.; Enssle, K.; Lauffer, L.; Kurrle, R. and Gelfand, E.W.: Inhibition of allergen-induced IgE and IgG1 production by soluble Il-4 receptor (sIL-4R). J. Allergy Clin. Immunol. 91: 234, 1993.

Restifo, N.; Spiess, P.; Karp, S.; Mule J. and Rosenberg, S.: A nonimmunogenic sarcoma transduced with the cDNA for interferon gamma elicits CD8+ T cells against the wild-type tumor: correlation with antigen presentation capability. J. Exp. Med. 175: 1423–1431, 1992.

Rettori, V.; Jurcovicova, J. and McCann, S.M.: Central action of interleukin-1 in altering the release of TSH, growth hormone, and prolactin in the male rat. J. Neurosci. Res. 18: 179–183, 1987.

Reynes, M.; Aubert, J.P.; Cohen, J.H.M.; Audouin, J.; Tricottet, V.; Diebold, J. and Kazatchkine, M.D.: Human follicular dendritic cells express CR1, CR2 and CR3 complement receptor antigens. J. Immunol. 135: 2687–2693, 1985.

Rich, D.P.; Anderson, M.P.; Gregory, R.J.; Cheng, S.H.; Paul, S.; Jefferson, D.M.; McCann, J.D.; Kliner, K.W.; Smith, A.E. and Welsh, M.J.: Expression of cystic fibrosis transmembrane conductance regulator corrects defective chloride channel regulation in cystic fibrosis airway epithelial cells. Nature 347: 358–363, 1990.

Rickinson, A.B.; Moss, D.J.; Allen, D.J.; Wallace, L.E.; Rowe, M. and Epstein, M.A.: Reactivation of Epstein-Barr virus-specific cytotoxic T cells by in vitro stimulation with the autologous lymphoblastoid cell line. Int. J. Cancer 27: 593–601, 1981.

Rickingson, A.; Brooks, J.; Lee, S.; Kurilla, M. and Rowe, M.: Cytotoxic T-cell control of Epstein-Barr virus-positive maligancies. ENII Conf.: Integrated Function of Molecules of the Immune System. Les Embiez, France, 12th-16th May 1993.

Riechmann, L.; Clark, M.; Waldmann, H. and Winter, G.: Reshaping human antibodies for therapy. Nature 332: 323–327, 1988.

Riechmann, L.; Foote, J. and Winter, G.: Expression of an antibody Fv fragment in myeloma cells. J. Mol. Biol. 203: 825–828, 1988.

Riethmüller, G.; Schneider-Gädicke, E. and Johnson, J.P.: Monoclonal antibodies in cancer therapy. Curr. Opin. Immunol. 5: 732–739, 1993.

Rigley, K.P.; Harnett, M.M. and Klaus, G.G.B.: Co-cross-linking of surface immunoglobulin Fc-gamma receptors on B lymphocytes uncouples the antigen receptors from their associated G protein. Eur. J. Immunol. 19: 481, 1989.

Rimoldi, M.T.; Tenner, A.J.; Bobak, D.A. and Jointer, K.A.: Complement component C1q enhances invasion of human mononuclear phagocytes and fibroblasts by trypanosoma cruizi trypomastigotes. J. Clin. Invest. 84: 1982–1989, 1989.

Rincon, M.; Tugores, A.; Lopez-Rivas, A.; Silva, A.; Alonso, M.; De Landazuri, M. and Lopez-Botet, M.: Prostaglandin E2 and the increase of intracellular cAMP inhibits the expression of interleukin 2 receptors in human T cells. Eur. J. Immun. 18: 1791–1796, 1988.

Rittner, C.; Meier, E.M.M.; Stradman, B.; Giles, C.M.; Koechling, R.; Mollenhauer, E. and Kreth, H.W.: Partial C4 deficiency in subacute sclerosing panencephalitis. Immunogenetics 20: 407–415, 1984.

Ritz, J.; Pesando, J.M.; Sallan, S.E.; Clavell, L.A.; Notis-McConarty, J.; Rosenthal, P. and Schlossman, S.F.: Serotherapy of acute lymphoblastic leukemia with monoclonal antibody. Blood 58: 141, 1981.

Ritz, J.; Schmidt, R.E.; Michon, J.; Hercend, T. and Schlossman, S.F.: Characterization of functional surface structures on human natural killer cells. Advances in Immunology 42: 181–211, 1988.

Rivest, S. and Rivier, C.: Central mechanisms and sites of action involved in the inhibitory effects of CRF and cytokines on LHRH neuronal activity. Annals of the New York Academy of Sciences 697: 117, 1993.

Rivest, S. and Rivier, C.: Interleukin-1ß inhibits the endogenous expression of the early gene c-fos located within the nucleus of LHRH neurons and interferes with hypothalamic LHRH release during proestrus in the rat. Brain Res. 613: 132–142, 1993.

Rivier, C. and Vale, W.W.: In the rat, interleukin-1µ acts at the level of the brain and the gonads to interfere with gonadotropin and sex steroid secretion. Endocrinology 124: 2105–2109, 1989.

Rivier, C.: Vale, W. and Brown, M.: In the rat, interleukin-1µ and -ß stimulate adrenocorticotropin and catecholamine release. Endocrinology 125: 3096–3102, 1989.

Rivier, C.: Effect of peripheral and central cytokines on the hypothalamic-pituitary-adrenal axis of the rat. Annals of the New York Academy of Sciences 697: 97, 1993.

Robb, R.J.; Munck, A. and Smith, K.A.: T-cell growth factor receptors: Quantitation, specificity and biological relevance. J. Exp. Med. 154: 1455–1474, 1981.

Robbins, P.D.; Tahara, H.; Mueller, G.; Hung, G.; Bahnson, A.; Zitvogel, L.; Galea-Lauri, J.; Ohashi, T.; Patrene, K.; Boggs, S.S.; Evans, C.H.; Barranger, J.A. and Lotze, M.T.: Retroviral vectors for use in human gene therapy for cancer, Gaucher disease, and arthritis. Annals of the New York Academy of Sciences 716: 72, 1994.

Roberts, A.B.; Sporn, M.B.; Assoian, R.K.; Smith, J.M.; Roche, N.S.: Wakefield, L.M.; Heine, U.I.; Liotta, L.A.; Falanga, V.; Kehrl, J.H. and Fauci, A.S.: Transforming growth factor type-ß: rapid induction of fibrosis and angiogenesis in vivo and stimulation of collagen formation in vitro. Proc. Natl. Acad. Sci. USA 83: 4167–4171, 1986.

Roberts, I.S.; Saunders, F.K. and Boulnois, G.J.: Bacterial capsules and interactions with complement and phagocytes. Biochem. Soc. Trans. 17: 462–464, 1989.

Roberts, P.A.; Morgan, B.P. and Campbell, A.K.: 2–chloroadenosine inhibits complement-induced reactive oxygen metabolite production and recovery of human polymorphonuclear leucocytes attacked by complement. Biochim. Biophys. Res. Commun. 126: 692–697, 1985.

Robinson, C.: Tenidap sodium, Rec. INNM; USAN. Drugs Gut. 15: 898–901, 1990.

Roche, W.R.: Mast cells and tumor angiogenesis: The tumor-mediated release of an endothelial growth factor from mast cells. Int. J. Cancer 36: 721–728, 1985.

Rock, K.L.; Benacerraf, B. and Abbas, A.K.: Antigen presentation by hapten-specific B lymphocytes. I. Role of surface immunoglobulin receptors. J. Exp. Med. 160: 1102–1113, 1984.

Rock, K.L.; Gamble, S.; Rothstein, L.; Gramm, C. and Benacerraf, B.: Dissociation of β2–micro-globulin leads to the accumulation of a substantial pool of inactive class I MHC heavy chains on the cell surface. Cell 65: 611–620, 1991.

Rocklin, R.E. and David, J.: Immediate hypersensitivity. In: Rubenstein, E., Federman, D.D. (eds.) Scientific American Medicine, Scientific American, New York, 1–14, 33–35, 1991.

Roemer, K. and Friedmann, T.: Mechanisms of action of the p53 tumor suppressor and prospects for cancer gene therapy by reconstitution of p53 function. Annals of the New York Academy of Sciences 716: 265, 1994.

Rötzschke, O.; Falk, K.; Deres, K.; Schild, H.; Norda, M.; Metzger, J.; Jung, G. and Rammensee, H.G.: Isolation and analysis of naturally processed viral peptides as recognized by cytotoxic cells. Nature 348: 252–254, 1990.

Rogers, D.F.; Aursudkij, B. and Barnes, P.J.: Effects of tachykinins on mucus secretion in human bronchi in vitro. Eur. J. Pharmacol. 174: 283–286, 1989.

Rohr, G.; Kusterer, K.; Schille, M.; Gladisch, R.; Schwedes, U.; Teuber, J. and Usadel, K.H.: Treatment of Crohn's disease and ulcerative colitis with 7S-immunoglobulin. Lancet 1: 170, 1987.

Rohrer, L.; Freeman, M.; Kodama, T.; Penman, M. and Krieger, M.: Coiled-coil fibrous domains mediate ligand binding by macrophage scavenger receptor type II. Nature 343: 570–572, 1990.

Roifman, C.M.; Wang, G.X.; Freedman, M. and Pan, Z.Q.: Il-7 receptor mediates tyrosine phosphorylation but does not activate the phosphatidylinositol-phospholipase C-gamma 1 pathway. J. Immunol. 148: 1136–1142, 1992.

Rokeach, L.A.; Haselby, J.A.; Meilof, J.F.; Smeenk, R.J.T.; Unnasch, T.R..; Greene, B.M. and Hoch, S.O.: Characterisation of the autoantigen calreticulin. J. Immunol. 147: 3031–3039, 1991.

Rollins, B.J.; Walz, A. and Baggiolini, M.: Recombinant human MCP-1/JE induces chemotaxis, calcium flux, and the respiratory burst in human monocytes. Blood 78: 1112–1116, 1991.

Rollins, B.J. and Sunday, M.E.: Suppression of tumor formation in vivo by expression of the JE gene in malignant cells. Mol. Cell. Biol. 11: 3125–3131, 1991.

Romagnani, S.: Regulation and deregulation of human IgG synthesis. Immunol. Today 11: 316, 1990.

Romagnani, S.: Type 1 T helper and type 2 T helper cells: functions, regulation and role in protection and disease. Int. J. Clin. Lab. Res. 21: 152–158, 1991.

Roman, M.; Axelrod, J.H.; Dai, Y.; Naviaux, R.K.; Friedmann, T. and Verma, I.M.: Circulating human or canine factor IX from retrovirally transduced primary myoblasts and established myoblast cell lines grafted into murine skeletal muscle. Somat. Cell. Mol. Genet. 18: 257–258, 1992.

Romero, P.; Maryansi, J.L.; Corradin, G.; Nussenzweig, R.; Nussenzweig, V. and Zavala, F.: Cloned cytotoxic T cells recognize an epitope in the circumsporozoite protein and protect against malaria. Nature 341: 323–326, 1989.

Romero, R.; Avila C.; Santhanam, U. and Sehgal, P.B.: Amniotic fluid interleukin-6 in preterm labor. J. Clin. Invest. 85: 1392, 1990.

Ronen, D.; Teitz, Y.; Goldfinger, N. and Rotter, V.: Expression of wild-type and mutant p53 proteins by recombinant vaccinia viruses. Nucleic Acids Res. 20: 3435–3441, 1992.

Rong, G.H.; Alessandri, G. and Sindelar, W.F.: Inhibition of tumor angiogenesis by hexuronyl hexosaminoglycan sulfate. Cancer 57: 586–590, 1986.

Roodman, G.D.; Kurihara, N.; Ohsaki, Y.; Kukita, A.; Hosking, D.; Demulder A.; Smith J.F. and Singer, F.R.: Interleukin-6 a potential autocrine/paracrine factor in Paget's disease of the bone. J. Clin. Invest. 89: 46, 1992.

Rooney, I.A. and Morgan, B.P.: Protection of human amniotic epithelial cells (HAEC) from complement-mediated of three complement inhibitory membrane proteins. Immunology 71: 308–311, 1990a.

Rooney, I.A. and Morgan, B.P.: Non-lethal doses of antibody and complement stimulate release of prostaglandin E2 from human amniotic cells in vitro. Biochem. Soc. Trans. 18: 617, 1990b.

Rooney, I.A.; Davies, A.; Griffiths, D.; Williams, J.D.; Davies, M.; Meri, S.; Lachmann, P.J. and Morgan, B.P.: The complement inhibiting protein, protectin (CD59 antigen) is present and functionally active on glomerular epithelial cells. Clin. Exp. Immunol. 83: 251–256, 1991.

Rordorf-Adam, C.; Lazdins, J.; Woods-Cook, K.; Alteri, E.; Henn, R.; Geiger, T.; Feige, U.; Towbin, H. and Erard, F.: An assay for the detection of interleukin-1 synthesis inhibitors: effects of anti-rheumatic drugs. Drugs Exp. Clin. Res. 15: 355–362, 1989.

Rosa, R.; Berissi, H.; Weissenbach, J.; Maroteaux, L.; Fellous, M. and Revel, M.: The β2-micro-globulin mRNA in human Daudi cells has a mutated initiation codon but is still inducible by interferon. EMBO Journal 2: 239–243, 1983.

Rose, T.M. and Bruce, A.G.: Oncostatin M is a member of a cytokine family that includes leu-kemia-inhibitory factor, granulocyte colony-stimulating factor, and interleukin 6. Proc. Natl. Acad. Sci. 88: 8641–8645, 1991.

Rosenbach, T.; Grabbe, J.; Moller, A.; Schwanitz, H.J. and Czarnetzki, B.M.: Generation of leu-kotrienes from normal epidermis and their demonstration in cutaneous disease. Brit. J. Der-matol. 113 (suppl. 28): 157–167, 1985.

Rosenberg, S.A.; Lotze, M.T.; Muul, L.M.; Chang, A.E.; Avis, F.P.; Leitman, S.; Linehan, W.M.; Robertson, C.N.; Lee, R.E.; Rubin, J.T. et al.: A progress report on the treatment of 157 pati-ents with advanced cancer using lympholine-activated killer cells and interleukin-2 or high-dose interleukin-2 alone. N. Engl. J. Med. 316: 889–897, 1987.

Rosenberg, S.A.; Lotze, M.T. and Mule, J.J.: New approaches to the immunotherapy of cancer using Interleukin-2. Ann. Intern. Med. 108: 853–864, 1988.

Rosenberg, S.A.; Packard, B.S.; Aebersold, P.M.; Solomon, D.; Topalian, S.L.; Toy, S.T.; Simon, P.; Lotze, M.T.; Yang, J.C.; Seipp, C.A. et al.: Use of tumor-infiltrating lymphocytes and in-terleukin-2 in the immunotherapy of patients with metastatic melanoma. N. Engl. J. Med. 319: 1676–1680, 1988.

Rosenberg, S.A.; Aebersold, P.; Cornetta, K.; Kasid, A.; Morgan, R.A.; Moen, R.; Karson, E.M.; Lotze, M.T.; Yang, J.C.; Topalian, S.L. et al.: Gene transfer into humans-immunotherapy of patients with advanced melanoma, using tumor-infiltrating lymphocytes modified by retro-viral gene transduction. N. Engl. J. Med. 323: 570–578, 1990.

Rosenfeld, M.A.; Yoshimura, K.; Trapnell, B.C.; Yoneyama, K.; Rosenthal, E.R.; Dalemans, W.; Fukayama, M.; Bargon, J.; Stier, L.E.; Stratford-Perricaudet, L.; Perricaudet, M.; Guggino, W.B.; Pavirani, A.; Lecocq, J.-P. and Crystal, R.G.: In vivo transfer of the human cystic fibro-sis transmembrane conductance regulator gene to the airway epithelium. Cell 68: 153–155, 1992.

Rosenstein, M.; Ettinghausen, S.E. and Rosenberg, S.A.: Extravasation of intravascular fluid mediated by the systemic administration of recombinant interleukin 2. J. Immunol. 137: 1735–1742, 1986.

Rosenthal, A.S. and Shevach E.M.: Function of macrophages in antigen recognition by guinea pig T lymphocytes. J. Exp. Med. 138: 1194–1212, 1973.

Ross, R. and Glomset, J.A.: Atherosclerosis and the arterial smooth muscle cell: proliferation of smooth muscle is a key event in the genesis of the lesions of atherosclerosis. Science 180: 1332–1339, 1973.

Ross, R.: Platelet-derived growth factor. The Lancet 1: 1179–1182, 1989.

Ross, G.D. and Medof, M.E.: Membrane complement receptors specific for bound fragments of C3. Adv. Immunol. 37: 217–267, 1985.

Ross, G.D.: Complement and complement receptors. Curr. Opin. Immunol. 2: 50–62, 1989.

Ross, G.D.: Complement Receptor Type 1. In: Current Topics in Microbiology and Immunolo-gy 178, 1992. Springer, Berlin.

Ross, S.C. and Densen, P.: Complement deficiency states and infections. Epidemiology, patho-genesis and consequences of neisserial and other infections in an immune deficiency. Medici-ne 63: 243–273– 1984.

Rossen, R.D.; Michael, L.H.; Kagiyama, A.; Savage, H.E.; Hanson, G.; Reisberg, M.A.; Moake, J.N.; Kim, S.H.; Self, D.; Weakley, S.; Giannini, E. and Entman, M.L.: Mechanism of com-plement activation after coronary artery occlusion: Evidence that myocardial ischemia in dogs causes release of constituents of myocardial subcellular origin that complex with human C1q in vivo. Circulation Res. 62: 572–584, 1988.

Roszman, T.L. and Brooks, W.H.: Signaling pathways of the neuroendocrine-immune network. In: Neuroimmunoendocrinology, 2nd. rev. edn (ed. Blalock, J.E.), 170–190, 1992. Chemical Immunology, Vol. 52, Karger, Basel.

Roth, R.A.: Structure of the receptor for insulin-like growth factor II: the puzzle amplified. Science 239: 1269–1271, 1988.

Roth, G.J.: Platelets and blood vessels: the adhesion event. Immunology Today 13: 100–105, 1992.

Rousset, F.; de Waal; Malefijt, R.; Slierendregt, B.; Aubry, J.P.; Bonnefoy, J.Y.; Defrance, T.; Banchereau, J. and de Vries, J.E.: Regulation of Fc receptor for IgE (CD23) and class II MHC antigen expression on Burkitt's lymphoma cell lines by human Il-4 and IFN-α. J. Immunol. 140: 2625–2631, 1988.

Rousset, F.; Billaud, M.; Blanchard, D.; Figdor, C.; Lenour, G.M.; Spits, H. and de Vries, J.E.: Il-4 induces LFA-1 and LFA-3 expression on Burkitt's lymphoma cell lines. Requirement of additional activation by phorbol myristate acetate for induction of homotypic cell adhesions. J. Immunol. 143: 1490–1498, 1989.

Rousset, F.; Robert, J.; Andary, M.; Bonnin, J.-P.; Souillet, G.; Chrétien, I.; Briere, F.; Pene, J. and de Vries, J.E.: Shifts in Interleukin-4 and Interferon-gamma production by T cells of patients with elevated serum IgE levels and the modulatory effects of these lymphokines on spontaneous IgE synthesis. J. Allergy Clin. Immunol. 87: 58–69, 1991.

Roux, S.; Steiner, B.; Hadvary, P. and Weller, T.: Selective blockade of the platelet receptor GP-IIb-IIIa by a noncyclic peptidomimetic - effects in in vitro and in vivo thrombus formation. Thromb. Haem. 65: 812, 1991.

Rowe, D.J. and Beverly, P.C.L.: Characterization of breast cancer infiltrates using monoclonal antibodies to human leukocyte antigens. Br. J. Cancer 49: 149–160, 1984.

Rowland-Jones, S.; Gotch, F.; McAdam, S. and Philips, R.: Escape variants of HIV. ENII Conf.: Integrated Function of Molecules of the Immune System. Les Embiez, France, 12th-16th May 1993.

Rubanyi, G.M. and Vanhoutte, P.M.: Hypoxia releases a vasoconstrictor substance from canine vascular endothelium. J. Physiol. (London) 364: 46–56, 1985.

Rubanyi, G.M.: Endothelium-dependent pressure-induced constraction of isolated canine carotid arteries. Amer. J. Physiol. 255: 783–788, 1988.

Rubanyi, G.M.: Potential physiological and pathological significance of endothelins. Drugs of the Future 17: 915–936, 1992.

Ruby, J. and Ramshaw, I.: The antiviral activity of immune CD8+ T cells is dependent on interferon-gamma. Lymphokine Cytokine Res. 10: 353–358, 1991.

Rudd, P.M.; Leatherbarrow, R.J.; Rademacher, T.W. and Dwek, R.A.: Diversification of the IgG molecule by oligosaccharides. Molec. Immun. 28: 1369–1378, 1991.

Rughetti, A.; Turchi, V.; Ghetti, C.A.; Scambia, G.; Panici, P.B.; Roncucci, G.; Mancuso, S.; Frati, L. and Nuti, M.: Human B-cell immune response to the polymorphic epithelial mucin. Cancer Res. 53: 2457–2459, 1993.

Ruiz-Cabello, F.; Klein, E. and Garrido, F.: MHC antigens on human tumors. Immunology Letters 29: 181–190, 1991.

Russell, G.: Bone damage and its revention by drugs. Biochemical Monitoring. Rheumatoid Arthitis, Royal College of Physicians, London, 17./18.6.1991.

Russell, R.G.G.; Boysen, M.; Chapman, K.; Fawthrop, F.; Frazer, A.; Seid, J.; Al-Humidan, A-K.; Rahman, S.; Bentley, H.; Oyajobi, K.; Graveley, R. and Bunning, R.A.D.: The possible roles of cytokines, growth factors and their inhibitors. Osteoarthritis, Current Research and Prospects For Pharmacological Intervention. Russel, R.G.C. and Dieppe, P.A. eds., published by IBC Technical Services Ltd. 1991.

Ryan, U.S.; Schultz, D.R.; Goodwin, J.D.; Vann, J.M.; Selvaraj, M.P. and Hart, M.A.: Role of C1q in phagocytosis of salmonella minnesota by pulmonary endothelial cells. Infection and Immunity 57: 1356–1362, 1989.

Rybak, S.A. and Youle, R.J.: Clinical use of immunotoxins. Immunol. Allergy Clin N. Am. 11: 359, 1991.

Saadat, S.; Sendtner, M. and Rohrer, H.: Ciliary neurotrophic factor induces cholinergic differentiation of rat sympathetic neurons in culture. J. Cell Biol. 108: 1807–1816, 1989.

Sacks, T.; Moldow, C.F.; Craddock, P.R.; Bowers, T.K. and Jacob H.S.: Oxygen radical mediated enothelial cell damage by complement-stimulated granulocytes: an in vitro model of immune vascular damage. J. Clin. Invest. 61: 1161–1167, 1978.

Sadick, M.D.; Heinzel, F.P.; Holaday, B.J.; Pu, R.T.; Dawkins, R.S. and Locksley, R.M.: Cure of murine leishmaniasis with anti-interleukin 4 monoclonal antibody. Evidence for a T cell-dependent, interferon-gamma-independent mechanism. J. Exp. Med. 171: 115, 1990

Sahin, U.; Hartmann, F.; Senter, P.; Pohl, C.; Engert, A.; Diehl, V. and Pfreundschuh, M.: Specific activation of the prodrug Mitomycin phosphate by a bispecific anti-CD30/anti-alkaline phosphatase monoclonal antibody. Cancer Res. 50: 6955, 1990.

Saida, Y.; Ogawa, M.; Kadokura, A.; Fukisawa, R. and Sugisaki, T.: Effects of high-dose gammaglobulin therapy on systemic lupus erythematosus. Jpn. J. Dermatol. 98: 1219–1229, 1988.

Saizawa, K.; Rojo, J. and Janeway, C.A. jr.: Evidence for a physical association of CD4 and the CD3μ:ßT cell receptor. Nature 328: 260, 1987.

Sakai, K.; Sinha, A.; Mitchell, D.J.; Zamvil, S.S.; McDevitt, H.O.; Rothbard, J.B. and Steinman, L.: Involvement of distinct T cell receptors in the autoimmune encephalitogenic response to nested epitopes of myelin basic protein. Proc. Natl. Acad. Sci. USA 85: 8608–8612, 1988.

Saksela, O.; Moscatelli, D.; and Rifkin, D.B.: The opposing effects of basic fibroblast growth factor and transforming growth factor-ß on the regulation of plasminogen activator in capillary endothelial cells. J. Cell Biol. 105: 957–963, 1987.

Salama, A.; Mahn, I.; Neuzner, J.; Graubner, M. and Mueller-Eckhardt, C.: IgG therapy in autoimmune heamolytic anemia of warm type. Blut 48: 391–392, 1984.

Sallusto, F.; Lane, P. and Lanzavecchia, A.: Factors controlling antigen uptake, processing and presentation by human dendritic cell lines in vitro. ENII Conf.: Integrated Function of Molecules of the Immune System. Les Embiez, France, 12th-16th May 1993.

Salmi, M. and Jalkanen, S.: Vascular adhesion protein-1 (VAP-1) - a new homing-associated molecule. ENII Conf.: Integrated Function of Molecules of the Immune System. Les Embiez, France, 12th-16th May 1993.

Salter, R.D.; Norment, A.M.; Chen, B.P.; Clayberger, C.; Krensky, A.M.; Littman, D.R. and Parham, P.: Polymorphism in the μ3 domain of HLA-A molecules affects binding to CD8. Nature 338: 345–347, 1989.

Salter, R.D.; Benjamin, R.J.; Wesley, P.K.; Buxton, S.E.; Garrett, T.P.J.; Clayberger, C.; Krensky, A.M.; Norment, A.M.; Littman, D.R. and Parham, P.: A binding site for the T-cell coreceptor CD8 on the μ3 domain of HLA-A2. Nature 345: 41, 1990.

Saltzman, E.M.; Thom, R.R. and Casnellie, J.E.: Activation of a tyrosine protein kinase is an early event in the stimulation of T lymphocytes by interleukin-2. J. Biol. Chem. 263: 6956–6959, 1988.

Saltzman, E.M.; White, K. and Casnelli, J.E.: Stimulation of the antigen and interleukin-2 receptors on T lymphocytes activates distinct tyrosine protein kinases. J. Biol. Chem. 265: 10138–10142, 1990.

Samanta, A.K.; Oppenheim, J.J. and Matsushima, K.: Interleukin 8 (monocyte-derived neutrophil chemotactic factor) dynamically regulates its own receptor expression on human neutrophils. J. Biol. Chem. 265: 183–189, 1990.

Sambhi, S.K.; Kohonen-Corish, M.R.J. and Ramshaw, I.A.: Local production of tumor necrosis factor encoded by recombinant vaccinia virus is effective in controlling viral replication in vivo. Proc. Natl. Acad. Sci. USA 88: 4025–4029, 1991.

Sampson, H.A. and McCaskill, C.M.: Food hypersensitivity in atopic dermatitis: evaluation of 113 patients. J. Pediatr. 107: 669, 1985.

Sampson, H.A. and MacDonald, S.M.: IgE-dependent histamine-releasing factors. Springer Semin. Immunopathol. 15: 89–98, 1993.

Samuelsson, B.; Goldyne, M.; Granström, E.; Hamberg, M.; Hammarström, S. and Malmsten, C.: Prostaglandin and thromboxanes. Annu. Rev. Biochem. 47: 997–1029, 1978.

Samuelsson, B.: Leukotrienes: mediators of immediate hypersensitivity reactions and inflammation. Science 220: 568, 1983.

Sanders, M.E.; Kopicky, J.A.; Wigley, F.M.; Shin, M.L.; Frank, M.M. and Joiner, K.A.: Membrane attack complex of complement in rheumatoid synovial tissue demonstrated by immunofluorescent microscopy. J. Rheumatol. 13: 1028–1034, 1986.

Sanderson, C.J.; Campbell, H.D. and Young, I.G.: Molecular and cellular biology of eosinophil differentiation factor (interleukin-5) and its effects on human and mouse B cells. Immunol. Rev. 102: 29–50, 1988.

Sanderson, C.J.: The biological role of interleukin-5. Int. J. Cell Cloning 8 (suppl. 1): 147–153, 1990.

Sandford, A.J.; Shirakawa, T.; Moffatt, M.F.; Daniels, S.E.; Ra, C.; Faux, J.A.; Young, R.P.; Namakura, Y.; Lathrop, G.M.; Cookson, W.O.C.M. and Hopkin, J.M.: Localisation of atopy and the β subunit of the high affinity IgE receptor (Fc RI) on chromosome 11q. Lancet 341: 332–334, 1993.

Sandstedt, P.; Kostulas, V. and Larsson, L.E.: Intravenous gammaglobulin for post-encephalitic epilepsy. Lancet II, 8412: 1154, 1984.

Sano, M. and Kitajima, S.: Activation of microtubule-associated protein kinase in PC12D cells in response to both fibroblast growth factor and epidermal growth factor and concomitant stimulation of the outgrowth of neurites. J. Neurochem. 58: 837–844, 1992.

Saperas, E.; Yang, H.; Rivier, C. and Taché, Y.: Central action of recombinant interleukin-1 to inhibit acid secretion in rats. Gastroenterology 99: 1599–1606, 1990.

Sapolsky, R.; Rivier, C.; Yamamoto, G.; Plotsky, P. and Vale, W.: Interleukin-1 stimulates the secretion of hypothalamic corticotropin-releasing factor. Science 238: 522–524, 1987.

Sara, V.R.; Uvnaes-Moberg, K.; Uvnaes, B.; Hall, K.; Wetterberg, L.; Posloncec, B. and Goiny, M.: The distribution of somatomedins in the nervous system of the cat and their release following neural stimulation. Acta Physiol. Scand. 115: 467–470, 1982.

Sarret, Y.; Woodley, D.T.; Grigsby, K.; Wynn, K. and O'Keefe, E.J.: Human keratinocyte locomotion: the effect of selected cytokines. J. Invest. Derm. 98: 12–16, 1992.

Sarfati, M. and Delespesse, G.: Possible role of human lymphocyte receptor for IgE (CD23) or its soluble fragments in the in vitro synthesis of human IgE. J. Immunol. 141: 2195–2199, 1988.

Sariban, E.; Imamura, K.; Luebbers, R. and Kufe, D.: Transcriptional and posttranscriptional regulation of tumor necrosis factor gene expression in human monocytes. J. Clin. Invest. 81: 1506–1510, 1988.

Sasso, E.H.; Barber, C.V.; Nardella, F.A.; Yount, W.J. and Mannik, M.: Antigenic specifities of human monoclonal and polyclonal IgM rheumatoid factors. J. Immunol. 140: 3098, 1988.

Sato, K.; Satoh, T.; Shizume, K.; Yamakawa, Y.; Ono, Y.; Demura, H.; Akatsu, T.; Takahashi, N. and Suda, T.: Prolonged decrease of serum calcium concentration by murine gamma-interferon in hypercalcemic, human tumor (EC-GI)-bearing nude mice. Cancer Res. 52: 444–449, 1992.

Sato, T.A.; Widmer, M.B.; Finkelman, F.D.; Madani, H.; Jacobs, C.A.; Grabstein, K.H. and Maliszewski, C.R.: Recombinant soluble murine Il-4 receptor can inhibit or enhance IgE responses in vivo. J. Immunol. 150: 2717–2723, 1993.

Satoh, T.; Nakafuku, M.; Miyajima, A. and Kaziro, Y.: Involvement of ras p21 protein in signal-transduction pathways from interleukin 2, interleukin 3, and granulocyte/macrophage colony-stimulating factor, but not from interleukin 4. Proc. Natl. Acad. Sci. USA 88: 3314–3318, 1991.

Savill, J.S.; Dransfield, I.; Hogg, N. and Haslett, C.: Vitronectin receptor-mediated phagocytosis of cells undergoing apoptosis. Nature 343: 170–173, 1990.

Sautes, C.; Varin, N.; Hogarth, P.M.; Unkeless, J.C.; Teillaud, C.; Even, J.; Lynch, A. and Fridman, W.H.: Molecular and functional studies of recombinant soluble Fc-gamma receptors. Mol. Immunol. 27: 1201, 1990.

Savage, P.; So, A.; Spooner, R.A. and Epenetos, A.A.: A recombinant single chain antibody interleukin-2 fusion protein. Br. J. Cancer 67: 304–310, 1993.

Scarborough, R.M.; Rose, J.W.; Hsu, M.A.; Phillips, D.R.; Fried, V.A.; Campbell, A.M.; Nannizzi, L. and Charo, I.F.: Barbourin. A GP11b-IIIa-specific integrin antagonist from the venom of Sistrurus m. barbouri. J. Biol. Chem. 266: 9359–9362, 1991.

Scarborough, R.M. et al.: cited by Tuffin, D.P., 1992.

Scolding, N.J.; Houston, W.A.J.; Morgan, B.P.; Campbell, A.K. and Compston, D.A.S.: Reversible injury of cultured rat oligodendrocytes by complement. Immunolgy 67: 441–446, 1989.

Scolding, N.J.; Morgan, B.P.; Houston, W.A.J.; Linington, C.; Campbell, A.K. and Compston, D.A.S.: Vesicular removal by oligodendrocytes of membrane attack complexes formed by activated complement. Nature 339: 620–622, 1989.

Scott, C.D.; Martin, J.L. and Baxter, R.C.: Production of insulin-like growth factor I and its binding protein by adult rat hepatocytes in primary culture. Endorcinology 116: 1094–1101, 1985.

Sears, M.R.; Burrows, B.; Flannery, E.M.; Herbison, G.P.; Hewitt, C.J. and Hollaway, M.D.: Relation between airway responsiveness and serum IgE in children with asthma and in apparently normal children. N. Engl. J. Med. 325: 1067, 1991.

Seder, R.A.; Boulay, J.L.; Finkelman, F.; Barbier, S.; Ben-Sasson, S.Z.; Le Gros, G. and Paul, W.E.: CD8+ T cells can be primed in vitro to produce Il-4. J. Immunol. 148: 1652–1656, 1992.

Sedgwick, J.D.; Holt, P.G. and Turner, K.J.: Production of a histamine-releasing lymphokine by antigen- or mitogen-stimulated human peripheral T cells. Clin. Exp. Immunol. 45: 409, 1981.

Sedlacek, H.H.; Bengelsdorff, H.J. and Seiler, F.R.: Concepts for the therapy of immune complex diseases. Behring Inst. Mitt. 64: 78–95, 1979.

Sedlacek, H.H. and Seiler, F.R.: Prophylaxe und Therapie mit Immunglobulinen: Eine kritische Stellungnahme zur Frage der Immunkomplex-bedingten Entzündungsreaktion. Beitr. Infusionstherapie klin. Ernähr., Karger, Basel, 11: 6–19, 1981.

Sedlacek, H.H.; Gronski, P.; Hofstaetter, T.; Kanzy, E.J.; Schorlemmer, H.U. and Seiler, F.R.: The biological properties of Immunoglobulin G and its split products F(ab')2 and Fab. Klin. Wochenschr. 61: 723–736, 1983.

Sedlacek, H.H, Ring, J.; Weinmann, E.; Guthörlein, G.; Kanzy, E.J.; Gronski, P. and Seiler, F.R.: Fc fragments of human IgG may influence allergic reactions. Int. J. Immunopharm. 9: 635–650, 1987.

Sedlacek, H.H.: Tumor therapy with tumor cells and neuraminidase: cell physiological, immunological and oncological aspects. Contributions to Oncology No. 27, Karger Verlag, 1987.

Sedlacek, H.H.; Schulz, G.; Steinstraesser, A.; Kuhlmann, L.; Schwarz, A.; Seidel, L.; Seemann, G.; Kraemer, H.P. and Bosslet, K.: Monoclonal antibodies in tumor therapy. Contrib. Oncol. Basel, Karger, vol. 32, 1988.

Sedlacek, H.H.; Seemann, G.; Hoffmann, D.; Czech, J.; Lorenz, P.; Kolar, C. and Bosslet, K.: Antibodies as carriers of cytotoxicity. Contributions to Oncology No. 43, Karger Verlag, München, 1992.

Seeger, W.; Suttorp, N.; Helliwig, A. and Bhakdi, S.: Noncytolytic complement complexes may serve as calcium gates to elicit leukotriene B4 generation in human polymorphonuclear leukoytes. J. Immunol. 137: 1286–1293, 1986.

Seemann, G.; Bosslet, K. and Sedlacek, H.H.: Recombinant monoclonal antibodies in tumor therapy. Behring Inst. Mitt. 87: 33–47, 1990.

Segarini, P.R. and Seyedin, S.M.: The high molecular weight receptor to transforming growth factor-ß contains glycosaminoglycan chains. J. Biol. Chem. 263: 8366–8370, 1988.

Segerling, M.S.; Ohanian, S.H. and Borsos, T.: Chemotherapeutic drugs increase killing of tumor cells by antibody and complement. Science 188: 55–57, 1975a.

Segerling, M.S:; Ohanian, S.H. and Borsos, T.: Enhancing effect by metabolic inhibitors on the killing of tumor cells by antibody and complement. Cancer Res. 35: 3195–3203, 1975b.

Seifert, R.A.; Hart, C.E.; Phillips, P.E.; Forstrom, J.W.; Ross, R.; Murray, M.J. and Bowen-Pope, D.F.: Two different subunits associate to create isoform-specific platelet-derived growth facto receptors. J. Biol. Chem. 264: 8771–8778, 1989.

Seigel, L.J.; Harper, M.E.; Wong-Staal, F.; Gallo, R.C.; Nash, W.G. and O'Brien, S.J.: Gene for T-cell growth factor: location on human chromosome 4q and feline chromosome B1. Science 223: 175–178, 1984.

Selvaraj, P.M.; Plunkett, M.L. ; Dustin, M.; Sanders, M.E.; Shaw, S. and Springer, T.A.: The T lymphocyte glycoprotein CD2 binds the cell surface ligand LFA-3. Nature 326: 400–403, 1987.

Semeraro, N.; Montemurro, P.; Conese, M.; Giordano, D.; Stella, M.; Restaino, A.; Cagnazzo, G. and Colucci, M.: Procoagulant activity of mononuclear phagocytes from different anatomical sites in patients with gynecological malignancies. Int. J. Cancer 45: 251–254, 1990.

Sendtner, M.; Kreitzberg, G.W. and Thoenen, H.: Ciliary neurotrophic factor prevents the degeneration of motor neurons after axotomy. Nature 345: 440–441, 1990.

Sendtner, M.; Arakawa, Y.; Stoeckli, K.A.; Kreutzberg, G.W. and Thoenen, H.: Effect of ciliary neurotrophic factor (CNTF) on motoneuron survival. J. Cell Sci. Suppl. 15: 103–109, 1991.

Senger, D.R.; Van de Water, L.; Brown, L.F.; Nagy, J.A.; Yeo, K.T.; Yeo, T.K.; Berse, B.; Jackman, R.W.; Dvorak, A.M. and Dvorak, H.F.: Vascular permeability factor (VPF, VEGF) in tumor biology. Cancer Metast. Rev. 12: 303–324, 1993.

Senter, P.D.; Schreiber, G.J.; Hirschberg, D.L.; Ashe, S.A.; Hellström, K.E. and Hellström, I.: Enhancement of the in vitro and in vivo anti-tumor activities of phosphorylated Mitomycin C and Etoposide derivatives by monoclonal antibody-alkaline phosphatase conjugates. Cancer Res. 49: 5789, 1989.

Senter, P.D.: Activation of prodrugs by antibody-enzyme conjuates: a new approach to cancer therapy. FASEB J. 4: 188, 1990.

Seya, T. and Atkinson, J.P.: Functional properties of membrane cofactor protein of complement. Biochem. J. 264: 581–588, 1989.

Seppa, H.; Grotendorst, G.; Seppa, S. et al.: Platelet-derived growth factor is chemotactic for fibroblasts. J. Cell Biol. 92: 584–588, 1982.

Seyedin, S.M.; Thompson, A.Y.; Bentz, H.; Rosen, D.M.; McPherson, J.M.; Conti, A.; Siegel, N.R.; Galluppi, G.R. and Piez, K.A.: Cartilage-inducing factor-A: apparent identity to transforming growth factor-ß. J. Biol. Chem. 261: 5693–5695, 1986.

Seyedin, S.M.; Segarini, P.R.; Rosen, D.M.; Thompson, A.Y.; Bentz, H. and Graycar, J.: Cartilage, inducing factor-ß is a unique protein structurally and functionally related to transforming growth factor-ß. J. Biol. Chem. 262: 1946–1949, 1987.

Shah, P.C.; Freier, S.; Park, B.H.; Lee, P.C. and Lebenthal, E.: Pancreozymin and secretin enhance duodenal fluid antibody levels to cow's milk proteins. Gastroenterology 83: 916–921, 1983.

Shakib, F. and Stanworth, D.R.: Human IgG subclasses in health and disease (a review). Parts I and II. Ric. Clin. Lab. 10: 463–479, 561–580, 1980.

Shapiro, R.; Riordan, J.F. and Vallee B.L.: Characteristic ribonucleolytic activity of human angiogenin. Biochem. 25: 3527–3532, 1986.

Sharon, P. and Stenson, W.F.: Enhanced synthesis of leukotriene B4 by colonic mucosa in inflammatory bowel disease. Gastroenterology 86: 453–460, 1984.

Sheehan, K.C.; Calderon, J. and Schreiber, R.D.: Generation and characterization of monoclonal antibodies specific for the human IFN-gamma receptor. J. Immun. 140: 4231–4237, 1988.

Sheppard, B.C.; Fraker, D.L. and Norton, J.A.: Prevention and treatment of endotoxin and sepsis lethality with recombinant human tumor necrosis factor. Surgery 106: 156, 1989.

Shero, J.H.; Bordwell, B.; Rothfield, N.F. and Earnshaw, W.C.: High titers of autoantibodies to topoisomerase I (Scl-70) in sera from scleroderma patients. Science 231: 737–740, 1986.

Sherr C.J.: Colony-stimulating factor-1 receptor. Blood 75: 1–12, 1990.

Sherry, B.; Tekamp-Olson, P.; Gallegos, C.; Bauer, D.; Davatelis, G.; Wolpe, S.D.; Masiarz, F.; Coit, D. and Cerami, A.: Resolution of the two components of macrophage inflammatory protein 1, and cloning and characterization of one of those component, macrophage inflammatory protein 1 beta. J. Exp. Med. 168: 2251–2259, 1988.

Shields, J.G.; Armitage, R.J.; Jamieson, B.N.; Beverley, P.C.L. and Callard, R.E.: Increased expression of surface IgM but not IgD or IgG on human B cells in response to IL-4. Immunology 66: 224–227, 1989.

Shimizu, Y.; Newman, W.; Tanaka, Y. and Shaw, S.: Lymphocyte interactions with endothelial cells. Immunology Today 13: 106–112, 1992.

Shindo, K.; Matsumoto, Y.; Hirai, Y.; Sumitomo, M.; Amano, T.; Miyakawa, K.; Matsumura, M. and Mizuno, T.: Measurement of leukotriene B4 in arterial blood of asthmatic patients during wheezing attacks. J. Int. Med. 228: 91–96, 1990.

Shingu, M.; Yoshioka, K.; Nobunaga, M. and Motomatu, T.: C1q binding to human vascular smooth muscle cells mediates immune complex deposition and superoxide generation. Inflammation 13: 561–568, 1989.

Shirazi, Y.; Imagawa, D.K. and Shin, M.L.: Release of leukotriene B4 from sublethally injured oligodendrocytes by terminal complement complexes. J. Neurochem. 48: 271–278, 1987.

Shoenfeld, Y.; Isenberg, D.A.; Rauch, J.; Madaio, M.; Stollar, B.D. and Schwartz, R.S.: Idiotypic cross-reactions of monoclonal human lupus autoantibodies. J. exp. Med. 158: 718–730, 1983.

Shoenfeld, Y.; Rauch, J.; Massicotte, H.; Datta, S.K.; André-Schwarzt, J.; Stollar, B.D. and Schwartz, R.S.: Polyspecificity of monoclonal lupus autoantibodies produced by human-human hybridomas. New Engl. J. Med. 308, 414–420, 1983.

Shows, T.; Eddy, R.; Haley, L.; Byers, M.; Henry, M.; Fujita, T.; Matsui, H. and Taniguchi, T.: Interleukin 2 (IL-2) is assigned to human chromosome 4. Somatic Cell Mol. Genet. 10: 315–318, 1984.

Sica, A.; Wang, J.M.; Colotta, F.; Dejana, E.; Mantovani, A.; Oppenheim, J.J.; Larsen, C.G.; Zachariae, C.O. and Matsushima, K.: Monocyte chemotactic and activating factor gene expression induced in endothelial cells by Il-1 and tumor necrosis factor. J. Immunol. 144: 3034–3038, 1990.

Sideras, P.; Noma, T. and Honjo, T.: Structure and function of interleukin 4 and 5. Immun. Rev. 102: 189–212, 1988.

Sidman, C.L.; Marshall, J.D.; Shultz, L.D.; Gray, P.W. and Johnson, H.M.: Gamma-interferon is one of several direct B cell-maturing lymphokines. Nature 309: 801–804, 1984.

Siebeck, M.; Hoffmann, H.; Weipert, J. and Spannagl, M.: Therapeutic effects of the combination of two proteinase inhibitors in endotoxin shock of the pig. Prog. Clin. Biol. Res. 308: 937–943, 1989.

Siegel, J.P. and Puri, R.K.: Interleukin-2 toxicity. J. Clin. Oncol. 9: 694–704, 1991.

Sigal, N.H.; Siekierka, J.J. and Dumont, F.J.: Observations on the mechanism of action of FK-506: a pharmacologic probe of lymphocyte signal transduction. Biochem. Pharmacol. 40: 2201–2208, 1990.

Sigal, N.H.; Lin, C.S. and Siekierka, J.J.: Inhibition of human T-cell activation by FK-506, rapamycin, and cyclosporine A. Transplant. Proc. 23: 1–5, 1991.

Sikora, K.: Genes, dreams, and cancer. BMJ 308: 1217–1221, 1994.

Sikora, K.; Harris, J.; Hurst, H. and Lemoine, N.: Therapeutic strategies using c-erbB-2 promoter-controlled drug activation. Annals of the New York Academy of Sciences 716: 115, 1994.

Silva, A.T.; Bayson, K.F. and Cohen, J.: Prophylactic and therapeutic effects of a monoclonal antibody to tumor necrosis factor-μ in experimental Gram-negative shock. Infect. Dis. 162: 421, 1990.

Simkin, N.J.; Jelinik, D.F. and Lipsky, P.E.: Inhibition of human B-cell responsiveness by prostaglandin E2. J. Immun. 138: 1074–1081, 1987.

Simmon, D.L.; Walker, C.; Power, C. and Pigott, R.: ICAM, an adhesion ligand of LFA-1, is homologous to the NCAM. Nature 331: 624–627, 1988.

Simmon, D.L.; Walker, C.; Power, C. and Pigott, R.: Molecular cloning of CD 31, a putative intercellular adhesion molecule closely related to CEA. J. Exp. Med. 171: 2147–2152, 1990.

Simpson, R.J.; Moritz, R.L.; Van Roost and Van Snick, J.: Characterization of a recombinant murine interleukin-6: assignment of disulfide bonds. Biochim. Biophys. Res. Commun. 157: 364–372, 1988.

Sims, J.E.; Acres, R.B.; Grubin, C.E.; McMahan, C.J.; Wignall, J.M.; March, C.J. and Dower, S.K.: Cloning the interleukin 1 receptor from human T cells. Proc. Natl. Acad. Sci. 86: 8946–8950, 1989.

Sims, P.J. and Weidmer, T.: Repolarization of the membrane potential of blood platelets after complement damage: evidence for a Ca2+ dependent exocytic elimination of C5b-9 pores. Blood 68: 556–561, 1986.

Sims, P.J.; Faioni, E.M.; Wiedmer, T. and Shattil, S.J.: Complement proteins C5b-9 cause release of membrane vesicles from the platelet surface that are enriched in the membrane receptor for coagulation factor Va and express prothrombinase activity. J. Biol. Chem. 263: 18205–18212, 1988.

Sims, P.J.; Rollins, S.A. and Wiedmer, T.: Regulatory control of complement on blood platelets. Modulation of platelet procoagulant response by a membrane inhibitor of the C5b-9 complex. J. Biol. Chem. 264: 19288–19235, 1989.

Sinclair, N.R.St.C.: Regulation of the immune response. I. Reduction in ability of specific antibody to inhibit longlasting IgG immunological priming after removal of the Fc fragment. J. Exp. Med. 129: 1183–1201, 1969.

Sinclair, N.R.St. C. and Chan, P.I.: Regulation of the immune response. IV. The role of the Fc-fragment in feedback inhibition by antibody. Adv. Exp. Med. Biol. 12: 609–615, 1971.

Sinclair, N.R.St.C. and Panoskaltsis, A.: Interference with Fc signals increases an antibody response by T cell-deprived cultures to a T-dependent antigen. Cell Immunol. 107: 465–470, 1987.

Sinclair, N.R.St.C. and Panoskaltsis, A.: Immunoregulation by Fc signals. A mechanism for self-non-self dicrimination. Immunol. Today 8: 76–79, 1987.

Sinha, A.A.; Brautbar, C.; Szafer, F.; Friedmann, A.; Tzfoni, E.; Todd, J.A.; Steinman, L. and Mc-Devitt, H.O.: A newly characterized HLA-DQ beta allele associated with pemphigus vulgaris. Science 239: 1026–1029, 1988.

Sjoholm, A.G.; Braconier, J.-H. and Soderstrom, C.: Properdin deficiency in a family with fulminant meningococcal infections. Clin. Exp. Immunol. 50: 291–297, 1982.

Skaper, S.D. and Varon, S.: Age-dependent control of dorsal root ganglion neuron survival by macromolecular and low-molecular-weight trophic agents and substratum-bound laminins. Brain Res. 389: 39–46, 1986.

Skerra, A. and Plückthun, A.: Assembly of a functional immunoglobulin Fv fragment in Escherichia coli. Science 240: 1038–1041, 1988.

Skladanowski, A. and Konopa, J.: Adriamycin and daunomycin induce programmed cell death (apoptosis) in tumor cells. Biochem. Pharmacol. 46: 375–382, 1993.

Slifman, N.R.; Adolphson, C.R. and Gleich, G.J.: Eosinophils: biochemical and cellular aspects. In: Middleton E, Reed CE, Ellis EF, Adkinson NF, Yunginger, JW (eds) Allergy: principles and practice. Mosby, St. Louis, 179–205, 1988.

Slovin, S.F.; Lackman, R.D.; Ferrone, S.; Kiely, P.E. and Mastrangelo, M.J.: Cellular immune response to human sarcomas: cytotoxic T cell clones reactive with autologous sarcomas I: development, phenotype, and specificity. J. Immunol. 137: 3042–3048, 1986.

Smedly, L.A.; Tonnesen, M.G.; Sanhaus, R.G.; Haslett, C.; Guthrie, L.A.; Jonston, R.B.; Heson, P.S. and Worthen, G.S.: Neutrophil-mediated injury to endothelial cells. Enhancement by endotoxin and essential role of neutrophil elastase. J. Clin. Invest. 77: 1233–1242, 1986.

Sminia, T.; Twisk, K.; van der Ven, I. and Soesatyo, M.: The uptake of soluble and particulate antigen by the gut. Adv. Exp. Biol. 505–508, 1990.

Sminia, T. and Van der Ende, M.B.: Macrophage subsets in the rat gut: An immunohistochemical and enzyme-histochemical study. Acta Histochem. 90: 43–50, 1991.

Smith, A.G.; Heath, J.K.; Donaldson, D.D.; Wong, G.G.; Moreau, J.; Stahl, M. and Rogers, D.: Inhibition of pluripotential embryonic stem cell differentiation by purified polypeptides. Nature 336: 688–690, 1988.

Smith, C.A. and Rennick, D.M.: Characterization of a murine lymphokine distinct from interleukin-2 and interleukin-3 possessing a T-cell growth factor activity and a mast growth activity that synergizes with Il-3. Proc. Natl. Acad. Sci. USA 83: 1857–1863, 1986.

Smith, C.A.; Davis, T.; Anderson, D.; Solam, L.; Beckmann, M.P.; Jerzy, R.; Dower, S.K.; Cosman, D. and Goodwin, R.G.: A receptor for tumor necrosis factor defines an unusual family of cellular and viral proteins. Science 248: 1019–1023, 1990.

Smith, E.M.; Morrill, A.C.; Meyer, W.J. and Blalock, J.E.: Corticotropin releasing factor induction of leukocyte-derived immunoreactive ACTH and endorphins. Nature 322: 881–882, 1986.

Smith, E.M.; Galin, F.S.; LeBoeuf, R.D.; Coppenhaver, D.H.; Harbour, D.V. and Blalock, J.E.: Nucleotide and amino acid sequence of lymphocyte-derived corticotropin: Endotoxin induction of a truncated peptide. Proc. Natl. Acad. Sci. USA 87: 1057–1060, 1990.

Smith, E.M.: Hormonal activities of cytokines. Chem. Immunol. 52: 154–169, 1992.

Smith, G.M. and Freuler, F.: The measurement of intravascular aggregation by continuous platelet counting. Bibl. Anat. 12: 229–234, 1973.

Smith, L.R.; Brown, S.L. and Blalock, J.E.: Interleukin-2 induction of ACTH secretion: Presence of Il-2 receptor μ-chain-like molecule on pituitary cells. N. Neuroimmunol. 21: 249–254, 1989.

Smith, M.E.; Marsh, S.G.E.; Bodmer, J.G.; Gelsthorpe, K. and Bodmer, W.F.: Loss of HLA-ABC allele products and lymphocyte functioassociated antigen-3 in colorectal neoplasia. Proc. Natl. Acad. Sci. USA 86: 5557–5561, 1989.

Smith, M.J.H. ; Ford-Hutchinson, A.W. and Bray, M.A.: Leukotriene B4: A potential mediator of inflammation. J. Pharm. Pharmacol. 32: 517–518, 1980.

Smith, J.W.; Steiner, A.L. and Parker, C.W.: Human lymphocyte metabolism: effects of cyclic and noncyclic nucleotides on stimulation by phytohemagglutinin. J. clin. Invest. 50: 442–448, 1971.

Smith, K.A.: Interleukin 2: Inception, impact, and implications. Science 240: 1169–1176, 1988.

Smith, K.A.: The interleukin 2 receptor. Annual Review of Cell Biology 5: 397–425, 1989.

Smolenski, L.A.; Kaumaya, P.; Atassi, M.Z. and Pierce, S.K.: Characteristics of peptides which compete for presented antigen-binding sites on antigen-presenting cells. Eur. J. Immunol. 20: 953–960, 1990.

Snapper, C.M. and Paul, W.E.: B cell stimulatory factor-1 (interleukin 4) prepares resting murine B cells to secrete IgG1 upon subsequent stimulation with bacterial lipopolysaccharide. J. Immunol. 139: 10, 1987.

Snapper, C.M. and Paul W.E.: Interferon- and B cell stimulatory factor 1 reciprocally regulate Ig isotpye production. Science 236: 944–947, 1987.

Snapper, C.M.; Finkelman, F.D. and Paul, W.E.: Regulation of IgG1 and IgE production by interleukin 4. Immunol. Rev. 102: 51, 1988.

Snider, D.P. and Segal, D.M.: Efficiency of antigen presentation after antigen targeting to surface IgD, IgM, MHC, Fc-gammaRII, and B220 molecules on murine splenic B cells. J. Immunol. 143: 59, 1989.

Snider, R.M.; Longo, K.P.; Drozda, S.E.; Lowe, III, J.A. and Leeman, S.E.: Effect of CP-96,345, a nonpeptide substance P receptor antagonist, on salivation in rats. Proc. Natl. Acad. Sci. 88: 10042–10044, 1991.

Snyder, D.S. and Unanue, E.R.: Corticosteroids inhibit murine macrophage Ia expression and interleukin 1 production. J. Immunol. 129: 1803–1805, 1982.

Solley, G.O.; Gleich, G.J.; Jordan, R.E. and Schroeter, A.L.: The late phase of the immediate wheal and flare skin reaction: its dependence upon IgE antibodies. J. Clin. Invest. 58: 408, 1976.

Sollid, L.M.; Kvale, D.; Brandtzaeg, P.; Markussen, G. and Thorsby, E.: Interferon-gamma enhances expression of secretory component, the epithelial receptor for polymeric immunoglobulins. J. Immunol. 138: 4303–4306, 1987.

Sondel, P.M.; Hank, J.A.; Kohler, P.C.; Chen, B.P.; Minkoff, D.Z. and Molenda, J.A.: Destruction of autologous human lymphocytes by interleukin 2–activated cytotoxic cells. J. Immunol. 137: 502–511, 1986.

Sonoda, E.; Matsumoto, R.; Hitoshi, Y.; Ishii, T.; Sugimoto, M.; Araki, S.; Tominaga, A.; Yamaguchi, N. and Takatsu, K.: Transforming growth factor β induces IgA production and acts additively with interleukin 5 for IgA production. J. Exp. Med. 170: 1415–1420, 1989.

Sorkin, E.; Stecher, V.J. and Borej, J.F.: Chemotaxis of leucocytes and inflammation. Ser. Haematol. 3: 131, 1970.

Sornasse, T.; Flamand, V.; DeBecker, G.; Bazin, H.; Tielemans, F.; Thielemans, K.; Urbain, J.; Leo, O. and Moser, M.: Antigen-pulsed dendritic cells can efficiently induce an antibody response in vivo. J. Exp. Med. 175: 15, 1992.

Sorvillo, J.M.; Gigli, I. and Pearlstein, E.: The effect of fibronectin on the processing of C1q- and C3b/bi-coated immune complexes by peripheral blood monocytes. J. Immunol. 136: 1023–1026, 1986.

Sotomayor, E.M.; Fu, Y.-X.; Lopez-Cepero, M.; Herbert, L.; Jimenez, J.J.; Albarracin, C. and Lopez, D.M.: Role of tumor-derived cytokines on the immune system of mice bearing a mammary adenocarcinoma. II. Down-regulation of macrophage-mediated cytotoxicity by tumor-derived granulocyte-macrophage colony-stimulating factor. J. Immunol. 147: 2816–2823, 1991.

Souillet, G.; Rousset, F. and de Vries, J.E.: Alpha-Interferon treatment of patient with hyper IgE: syndrome. Lancet i: 1384, 1989.

Soulder, B.M.; Reisinger, E.C.; Koefler, D.; Bitterlich, G.; Wachter, H. and Dierich, M.P.: Complement receptors; another part of entry for HIV. Lancet 2: 271–272, 1989.

Souroujon, M.; White-Scharf, M.E.; André-Schwartz, J.; Gefter, M.L. and Schwartz, R.S.: Preferential autoantibody reactivity of the preimmune B cell repertoire in normal mice. J. Immun. 140: 4173–4179, 1988.

Spalding, D.M. and Griffin, J.A.: Different pathways of differentiation of pre-B cell lines are induced by dendritic cells and T cells from different lymphoid tissues. Cell 44: 507–515, 1986.

Spangelo, B.L.; Judd, A.M.; MacLeod, R.M.; Goodman, D.W. and Isakson, P.C.: Endotoxin-induced release of interleukin-6 from rat medial basal hypothalami. Endocrinology 127: 1779–1785, 1990.

Spangelo, B.L.; Jarvis, W.D.; Judd, A.M. and MacLeod, R.M.: Induction of interleukin-6 release by interleukin-1 in rat anterior pituitary cells in vitro: Evidence for an eicosanoid-dependent mechanism. Endocrinology 129: 2886–2894, 1991.

Spiegelberg, H.L.: Biological activities of immunoglobulins of different classes and subclasses. Adv. Immunol. 19: 259–294, 1974.

Spies, T.; Bresnahan, M.; Bahram, S.; Arnold, D.; Blanck, G.; Mellins, E.; Pious, D. and DeMars, R.: A gene in the major histocompatibility complex class II region controlling the class I antigen presentation pathway. Nature 348: 744–747, 1990.

Spies, T. and DeMars, R.: Restored expression of major histocompatibility class I molecules by gene transfer of a putative peptide transporter. Nature 351: 323–325, 1991.

Spilberg, I.; Mandell, B.; Mehta, J.; Sillivan, T. and Simehowitz, L.: Dissociation of the neutrophil functions of exocytosis and chemotaxis. J. Lab. Clin. Med. 92: 297, 1978.

Spitler, L.E.; del Rio, M.; Khenetigan, A.; Wedel, N.I.; Brophy, N.A.; Miller, L.L.; Harkonen, W.S.; Rosendorf, L.L.; Lee, H.M.; Mischak, R.P. et al.: Therapy of patients with malignant melanoma using a monoclonal anti-melanoma antibody-ricin A chain immunotoxin. Cancer Res. 47: 1717–1723, 1987.

Spitler, L.E.: Clinical studies: Solid tumors, in Frankel AE (ed): Immunotoxins. Boston, Kluwer, 493, 1988.

Spits, H.; Yssel, H.; Takebe, Y.; Arai, N.; Yokota, T.; Lee, F.; Arai, K.; Banchereau, J. and de Vries, J.E.: Recombinant IL-4 promotes the growth of human T cells. J. Immunol. 135: 1142–1147, 1987.

Spits, H.; Yssel, H.; Paliard, X.; Kastelein, R.; Figdor, D. and de Vries, J.E.: IL-4 inhibits IL-2 mediated induction of human lymphokine activated killer cells, but not the generation of antigen specific cytotoxic T lymphocytes in mixed leucocyte cultures. J. Immunol. 141: 29–36, 1988.

Sporn, M.B.; Roberts, A.B.; Shull, J.H.; Smith, J.M., Ward, J.M. and Sodek, J.: Polypeptide transforming growth factors isolated from bovine sources and used for wound healing in vivo. Science (Wash. DC) 219: 1329–1331, 1983.

Sporn, M.B. and Robert, A.B.: Peptide growth factors are multifunctional. Nature 332: 217–219, 1988.

Spragg, R.G.; Hisnhaw, D.B.; Hyslop, P.A.; Shraufstatter, I.U. and Cochrane C.G.: Alterations in adenosine triphosphate and energy charge in cultured endothelial and P388D1 cells after oxidant injury. J. Clin. Invest. 76: 1471–1476, 1985.

Spranger, M.: Lindholm, D.; Bandtlow, C.; Heumann, R.; Grahn, H.: Naher-Noe, M. and Thoenen, H.: Regulation of nerve growth factor (NGF) synthesis in the rat central nervous system.: Comparison between the effects of interleukin-1 and various growth factors in astrocyte cultures and in vivo. Eur. J. Neurosci. 2: 69–76, 1990.

Sprengers, E.D. and Kluft, C.: Plasminogen activator inhibitors. Blood 69: 381–387, 1987.

Springer, G.F.; Desai, P.R.; Tegtmeyer, H.; Spencer, B.D. and Scanlon, E.F.: Pancarcinoma T/Tn antigen detects human carcinoma long before biopsy does and its vaccine prevents breast carcinoma. Specific Immunotherapy Of Cancer With Vaccines, eds. Bystryn, J.-C.; Ferrone, S. and Livingston, P., The New York Academy of Sciences 690: 355, 1993.

Springer, T.A.: Adhesion receptors of the immune system. Nature 346: 425–434, 1990.

Sriram, S.; Topham, D.J. and Carroll, L.: Haplotype-specific suppression of experimental allergic encephalomyelitis with anti-IA antibodies. J. Immunol. 139: 1485–1489, 1987.

Suba, E.A. and Csako, G.: C1q (C1) receptor on human platelets: Inhibition of collagen-induced platelet aggregation by C1q (C1) molecules. J. Immunol. 117: 304–309, 1976.

Subramanyam, M.; Gutheil, W.G.; Bachovchin, W.W. and Huber, B.T.: Mechanism of HIV-1 tat induced inhibition of antigen-specific T cell responsiveness. J. Immunol. 150: 2544–2553, 1993.

Suda, T.; O'Garra, A.; MacNeil, I.; Fischer, M.; Bond, M.W. and Zlotnik, A.: Identification of a novel thymocyte growth-promoting factor derived from B cell lymphomas. Cell. Immunol. 129: 228–240, 1990.

Sugisaki, T.; Shiwachi, S.; Yonekura, M. et al.: High-dose intravenous gammaglobulin for membranous nephropathy (MN), membranoproliferative glomerulonephritis (MPGN) and lupus nephritis (LN). Fed. Proc. 41: 2467, 1982.

Sugita, T.; Ueno, M.; Furukawa, O.; Murakami, T.; Takata, I. and Tosa, T.: Effect of a novel anti-rheumatic drug, TA-383, of type II collagen-induced arthritis - suprressive effect of TA-383 on Interleukin-6 production. Int. J. Immunopharmac. 15: 515–519, 1993.

Sullivan, D.A.; Bloch, K.J. and Allansmith, M.R.: Hormonal influence on the secretory immune system of the eye: androgen control of secretory component production by the rat exorbital gland. Immunology 52: 239–246, 1984.

Sullivan, D.A.; Bloch, K.J. and Allansmith, M.R.: Hormonal influence on the secretory immune system of the eye: androgen regulation of secretory component levels in rat tears. J. Immun. 132: 1130–1135, 1984.

Sullivan, D.A. and Allansmith, M.R.: Hormonal influence on the secretory immune system of the eye: androgen modulation of IgA levels in tears of rats. J. Immun. 134: 2978–2982, 1985.

Sullivan, D.A.; Colgy, E.B.; Kann, L.E.; Allansmith, M.R. and Wira, C.R.: Production and utilization of a mouse monoclonal antibody to rat IgA: identification of gender-related differences in the secretory immune system. Immun. Invest. 15: 311–318, 1986.

Sullivan, D.A. and Allansmith, M.R.: Hormonal influence on the secretory immune system of the eye: endocrine interactions in the control of IgA and secretory component levels in tears of rats. Immunology 60: 337–343, 1987.

Sullivan, D.A.: Influence of the hypothalamic-pituitary axis on the androgen regulation of the ocular secretory immune system. J. steroid Biochem. 30: 429–433, 1988.

Sullivan, D.A. and Allansmith, M.R.: The effect of aging on the secretory immune system of the eye. Immunology 63: 403–410, 1988.

Sullivan, D.A.; Hann, L.E. and Vaerman, J.P.: Selectivity, specificity and kinetics of the androgen regulation of the ocular secretory immune system. Immun. Invest. 17: 183–194, 1988.

Sullivan, D.A. and Hann, L.E.: Hormonal influence on the secretory immune system of the eye: endocrine impact on the lacrimal gland accumulation and secretion of IgA and IgG. J. steroid Biochem. 34: 253–262, 1989.

Sullivan, G.W.; Patselas, T.N.; Redick, J.A. and Mandell, G.L.: Enhancement of chemotaxis and protection of mice from infection. Trans. Assoc. Am. Physicians 97: 337–345, 1984.

Sullivan, G.W.; Carper, H.T.; Novick, W.J.jr. and Mandell, G.L.: Inhibition of the inflammatory action of IL-1 and TNF on neutrophil function by pentoxifylline. Infect. Immun. 56: 1722–1729, 1988.

Sultan, Y.; Kazatchkine, M.D.; Maisonneuve, P. and Nydegger, U.E.: Anti-idiotypic suppression of autoantibodies to factor VIII (anti-haemophilic factor) by high-dose intravenous gamma-globulin. Lancet 2: 765–768, 1984.

Sumner, W.C. and Foraker, A.G.: Spontaneous regression of human melanoma. Clinical and experimental studies. Cancer 13: 179, 1960.

Surh, C.D.; Roche, T.E.; Danner, D.J.; Ansari, A.; Coppel, R.L.; Prindiville, T.; Dickson, E.R. and Gershwin, M.E.: Antimitochondrial autoantibodies in primary biliary cirrhosis recognize cross-reactive epitope(s) on protein X and dihydrolipoamide acetyltransferase of pyruvate dehydrogenase complex. Hepatology 10: 127–133, 1989.

Suttorp, N.; Seeger, W.; Zinsky, S. and Bhakdi, S.: Complement complex C5b-8 induces PgI2 formation in cultured endothelial cells. Am. J. Physiol. 253: C13–21, 1987a.

Suttorp, N.; Seeger, W.; Zucker-Reimann, J.; Roka, L. and Bhakdi, S.: Mechanism of leukotriene generation in polymorphonuclear leukocytes by staphylococcal alpha-toxin. Infect Immun. 55: 104–110, 1987b.

Suzuki, H. and Hashiwagi, H.: Molecular biology of cytokine effects on vascular endothelial cells. Int. Rev. Exp. Path. 32: 95–148, 1991.

Suzuki, K.; Enghild, J.J.; Morodomi, T.; Salvesen, G. and Nagase, H.: Mechanisms of activation of tissue procollagenase by matrix metalloproteinase 3 (stromelysin). Biochem. 29: 10261–101270, 1990.

Suzuki, S.; Argraves, W.W.; Arai, H.; Languino, L.F.; Pierschbacher, M.D. and Ruoslahti, E.: Amino acid sequence of the vitronectin receptor alpha subunit and comparative expression of adhesion receptor mRNAs. J. Biol. Chem. 262: 14050–14058, 1987.

Svennevig, J.L.; Lunde, O.C.; Holter, J. and Bjorgsvik, D.: Lymphoid infiltration and prognosis in colorectal carcinoma. Br. J. Cancer 49: 375–377, 1984.

Swain, S.L.; Dutton, R.W.; McKenzie, D.; Helstrom, H. and English, M.: Role of antigen in the B cell response. Specific antigen and the lymphokine Il-5 synergize to drive B cell lymphoma proliferation and differentiation to Ig secretion. J. Immunol. 140: 4224–4230, 1988.

Swain, S.L.: Regulation of the development of distinct subsets of CD4+ T cells. Res. Immunol. 142: 14, 1991.

Swanson, L.W.; Sawchenko, P.E. and Lind, R.W.: Regulation of multiple peptides in CRF parvocellular neurosecretory neurons: implications for the stress response. In: Progress in Brain Research, Vol. 68 (eds Hokfert, T.; Fuxe, K. and Pernow, B.), 169–190, 1986. Elsevier, New York.

Sweetser, M.T.; Morrison, L.A.; Braciale, V.L. and Braciale, T.J.: Recognition of pre-processed endogenous antigen by class I but not class II MHC-restricted T cells. Nature 342: 180–182, 1989.

Sykora, K.W.; Kolitz, J.; Szabo, P.; Grzeschik, K.H.; Moore, M.A. and Mertelsmann, R.: Human interleukin 2 gene is located on chromosome 4. Cancer Invest. 2: 261–265, 1984.

Szakal, A.K. and Manna, M.G.jr.: The ultrastructure of antigen localization and viruslike particles in mouse spleen germinal centers. Exp. Mol. Pathol. 8: 75, 1968.

Szakal, A.K.; Kosco, M.H. and Tew, J.G.: A novel in vivo follicular dendritic cell-dependent icosome mediated mechanism for delivery of antien to antigen processing cells. J. Immunol. 140: 341, 1988.

Szakal, A.K.; Kosco, M.H. and Tew, J.G.: Microanatomy of lymphoid tissue during humoral immune responses. Structure function relationship. Ann. Rev. Immunol. 7: 91, 1989.

Szende, B.; Lapis, K.; Redding, T.W.; Srkalovic, G. and Schally, A.V.: Growth inhibition of MXT mammary carcinoma by enhancing programmed cell death (apoptosis) with analogs of LH-RH and somatostatin. Breast Cancer Research and Treatment 14: 307–314, 1989.

Schade, U.F.: Pentoxifylline increases survival in murine endotoxin shock and decreases formation of tumor necrosis factor. Circ. Shock 31: 171–181, 1990.

Schall, T.J.; Jongstra, J.; Dyer, B.J.; Jorgensen, J.; Clayberger, C.; Davis, M.M. and Krensky, A.M.: A human T cell-specific molecule is a member of a new gene family. J. Immunol. 141: 1018–1025, 1988.

Schall, T.J.; Lewis, M.; Koller, K.J.; Lee, A.; Rice, G.C.; Wong, G.H.; Gatanage, T.; Granger, G.A.; Lentz, R.; Raab, H. et al.: Molecular cloning and expression of a receptor for human tumor necrosis factor. Cell 61: 361–370, 1990.

Scharf, S.; Friedmann, A.; Brautbar, C.; Szafer, F.; Steinman L,; Horn, G.; Gyllenstein, U. and Erlich H.A.: HLA class II allelic variation and susceptibility in pemphigus vulgaris. Proc. Natl. Acad. Sci. USA 85: 3504–3508, 1988.

Scheppler, J.A.; Nicholson, J.K.A.; Swan, D.C.; Ahmed-Ansari, A. and McDougal, J.S.: Down-modulation of MHC-I in a CD4+ T cell line, CEM-E5, after HIV-1 infection. J. Immunol. 143: 2858–2866, 1989.

Schifferli, J.A.; Ng, Y.C. and Peters, D.K.: The role of complement and its receptor in the elimination of immune complexes. N. Engl. J. Med. 315: 488–495, 1986.

Schifferli, J.A.: The classical pathway of complement prevents the formation of insoluble antigen-antibody complexes: biological implications. Immunol. Lett. 14: 225–228, 1986/1987.

Schifferli, J.A.; Ng, Y.C.; Estreicher, J. and Walport, M.J.: The clearance of tetanus toxoid/antitetanus toxoid immune complexes from the circulation of humans. Complement- and erythrocyte complement receptor 1–dependent mechanisms. J. Immunol. 140: 899–904, 1988.

Schifferli, J.A.; Ng, Y.C.; Paccaud, J-P. and Walport, M.J.: The role of hypocomplementaemia and low erythrocyte complement receptor type 1 numbers in determining abnormal immune complex clearance in humans. Clin. Exp. Immunol. 75: 329–335, 1989.

Schilling, T.; Krüger, C.; Stelter, F.; Schletter, J.; Fan, X.; Witt, S.; Grunwald, U.; Dietz, H. and Schütt, C.: LPS activation of CD14–negative human monocytes is mediated by soluble CD14. Immunobiology 189: 187, 1993.

Schimpff, R.M.; Donnadieu, M. and Gautier, M.: Somatomedin activity measured as sulphation factor in culture media from normal human liver and connective tissues explants. Effects of human growth hormone. Acta Endocrinol. 98: 24–28, 1981.

Schirrmacher, V.; Schlag, P.; Liebrich, W.; Patel, B.T. and Stoeck, M.: Specific immunotherapy of colorectal carcinoma with Newcastle-disease virus-modified autologous tumor cells prepared from resected liver metastasis. Specific Immunotherapy Of Cancer With Vaccines, eds. Bystryn, J.-C.; Ferrone, S. and Livingston, P., The New York Academy of Sciences 690: 364, 1993.

Schlager, S.I.; Ohanian, S.H. and Borsos, T.: Inhibition of antibody-complement mediated killing of tumor cells by hormones. Cancer Res. 36: 3672–3677, 1976.

Schleef, R.R.; Bevilacqua, M.P.; Sawdey, M.; Gimbrone, M.A. and Loskutoff, D.J.: Cytokine activation of vascular endothelium. Effects on tissue-type plasminogen activator and type I plasminogen activator inhibitor. J. Biol. Chem. 263: 5797–5803, 1988.

Schlesinger, M.; Nave, Z.; Levy, Y.; Slater, P.E. and Fishelson, Z.: Prevalence of hereditary properdin, C7 and C8 deficiencies in patients with meningococcal infections. Clin. Exp. Immunol. 81: 423–427, 1990.

Schmaier, A.H.; Smith, P.M. and Colman, R.W.: Platelet C1 inhibitor: a secreted alpha-granule protein. J. Clin. Invest. 75: 242–250, 1985.

Schmitt, M.; Jänicke, F. and Graeff, H.: Tumor-associated proteases. Fibrinolysis 6: 3–26, 1992.

Schnabl, E.; Stockinger, H.; Majdic, O.; Gaugitsch, H.; Lindley, I.J.; Maurer, D.; Hajek-Rosenmayr, A. and Knapp, W.: Activated human T lymphocytes express MHC class I heavy chains not associated with ß2–microglobulin. J. Exp. Med. 171: 1431–1442, 1990.

Schneider, P.M.; Carroll, M.C.; Alper, C.A.; Rittner, C.; Whitehead, A.S.; Yunis, E.J. and Colten, H.R.: Polymorphism of the human complement C4 and steroid 21–hydroxylase genes. Restriction fragment length polymorphism revealing structural deletion, homoduplications and size variants. J. Clin. Invest. 78: 650–657, 1986.

Schönermark, S.; Rauterberg, E.W.; Shin, M.L.; Löke, S.; Roelcke, D. and Hänsch, G.M.: Homologous species restriction in lysis of human erythrocytes: a membrane-derived protein with C8-binding capacity functions as an inhibitor. J. Immunol. 136: 1772, 1986.

Schönharting, M.M. and Schade, U.F.: The effect of pentoxifylline in septic shock – New pharmacologic aspects of an established drug. J. Med. 20: 97–105, 1989.

Schor, A.M. and Schor, S.L.: Tumor angiogenesis. J. Pathol. 141: 385–413, 1983.

Schorlemmer, H.-U.; Kanzy, E.J.; Lauffer, L. and Kurrle, R.: Immunosuppressive therapy of experimental autoimmune diseases like SLE and rheumatoid arthritis by recombinant Il-1 recpetor. Inf. Conf. on Cellular and Molecular Aspects of Self-Reacitivity and Autoimmune Diseases, Taormina, Italy, June 7–12, 1992.

Schrader, J.W.; Clark-Lewis, I.; Crapper, R.M. and Wong, G.W.: P-cell stimulating factor: characterization, action on multiple lineages of bone-marrow-derived cells and role in oncogenesis. Immun. Rev. 76: 79–104, 1983.

Schrader, J.W.: The panspecific hemopoietin of activated T lymphocytes (interleukin-3). Ann. Rev. Immunol. 4: 205–230, 1986.

Schrader, C.E.; George, A.; Kerlin, R.L. and Cebra, J.J.: Dendritic cells support production of IgA and other non-IgM isotypes in clonal microculture. Int. Immunol. 2: 563–570, 1990.

Schreiber, A.B.; Winkler, M.E. and Erynck, R.: Transforming growth factor α: a more potent angiogenic mediator than epidermal growth factor. Science 232: 1250–1253, 1986.

Schreiber, R.D.; Farrar, M.A.; Hershey, G.K. and Fernandez-Luna, J.: The structure and function of interferon-gamma receptors. Int. J. Immunopharm. 14: 413–419, 1992.

Schreiber, S.L.: Chemistry and biology of the immunophilins and their immunosuppressive ligands. Science 251: 283–287, 1991.

Schrezenmeier, H. and Fleischer, B.: A regulatory role for the CD4 and CD8 molecules in T cell activation. J. Immunol. 141: 398–403, 1988.

Schrier, P.L.; Bernards, R.; Vaessen, R.T.M.J.; Houweling, A. and van der Eb, A.J.: Expression of class I major histocompatibility antigens switched off by highly oncogenic adenovirus 12 in transformed rat cells. Nature 305: 771–775, 1983.

Schroeder, J.M.; Mrowietz, U.; Morita, E. and Christophers, E.: Purification and partial biochemical characterization of a human monocyte-derived, neutrophil-activating peptide that lacks interleukin 1 activity. J. Immunol. 139: 3474–3483, 1987.

Schulman, E.S.; Liu, M.C.; Proud, D.; MacGlashan, D.W.; Lichtenstein, L.M. and Plaut, M.: Human lung macrophages induce histamine release from basophils and mast cells. Am. Rev. Respir. Dis. 131: 230, 1985.

Schultz, D.C.; Bazel, S.; Wright, L.M.; Tucker, S.; Lange, M.K.; Tachovsky, T.; Longo, S.; Niedbala, S. and Alhedeff, J.A.: Western blotting and enzymatic activity analysis of Cathepsin D in breast tissue and sera of patients with breast cancer and benign breast disease and of normal controls. Cancer Res. 54: 48–54, 1994.

Schulz, G.; Cheresh, D.A.; Varki, N.M.; Yu, A.; Staffileno, L.K. and Reisfeld, R.A.: Detection of ganglioside GD2 in tumor tissues and sera of neuroblastoma patients. Cancer Res. 44: 5914–5920, 1984.

Schumacher, T.N.M.; deBruijn, M.L.H.; Vernie, L.N.; Kast, W.M.; Melief, C.J.; Neefjes, J.J. and Ploegh, H.L.: Peptide selection by MHC class I molecules. Nature 350: 703–706, 1991.

Schumaker, V.N.; Phillips, M.L. and Hanson, D.C.: Dynamic aspects of antibody structure. Molec. Immun. 28: 1347–1360, 1991.

Schwander, J.C.; Hauri, C.; Zapf, J. and Froesch, E.R.: Synthesis and secretion of insulin-like growth factor and its binding protein by the perfused rat liver: dependence on growth hormone status. Endocrinology 113: 297–305, 1983.

Schwartz, R.H.: A cell culture model for T lymphocyte clonal anergy. Science 248: 1349–1356, 1990.

Schwartz, R.H.: Cositmulation of T lymphocytes: the role of CD28, CTLA-4, and B7/BB1 in interleukin-2 production and immunotherapy. Cell 71: 1065–1068, 1992.

Schwartz, S.A.; Gordon, K.E.; Johnston, M.V. and Goldstein, G.W.: Use of intravenous immune globulin in the treatment of seizure disorders. J. Allergy Clin Immunol. 84: 603–607, 1989.

Schweigerer, L.; Neufeld, G.; Friedman, J.; Abrahamn, J.A.; Fiddes, J.C. and Gospodarowicz, D.: Capillary endothelial cells express basic fibroblast growth factor, a mitogen that promotes their own growth. Nature 325: 257–259, 1987.

Stadler, B.M.; Stämpfli, M.R.; Miescher, S.; Furukawa, K. and Vogel, M.: Biological activities of anti-IgE antibodies. Int. Arch. Allergy Immunol. 102: 121–126, 1993.

Stanislawski, M.; Rousseau, V.; Goavec, M. and Ito, H.: Immunotoxins containing glucose oxidase and lactoperoxidase with tumoricidal properties: in vitro killing effectiveness in a mouse plasmacytoma cell model. Cancer Res. 49: 5497–5504, 1989.

Stanisz, A.M.; Befus, D. and Bienenstock, J.: Differential effects of vasoactive intestinal peptide, substance P, and somatostatin on immunoglobulin synthesis and proliferation by lymphocytes from Peyer's patches, mesenteric lymph nodes, and spleen. J. Immun. 136: 152–156, 1986.

Stanley, S.I.; Bishoff, J. and Davie J.M.: Antigen induced rheumatoid factors: protein and carbohydrate antigens induce different rheumatoid factor responses. J. Immunol. 139: 2936, 1987.

Starnes, H.F.jr.; Pearce, M.K.; Tewari, A.; Yim, J.H.; Zou, J.C. and Abrams, J.S.: Anti-IL-6 monoclonal antibodies protect against lethal Escherichia coli infection and lethal tumor necrosis factor-α challenge in mice. Immunology 145: 4185, 1990.

Stassin, V.; Coulie, P.; Birshtein, B.; Secher, D. and Van Snick, J.: Determinants recognized by murine rheumatoid factors: molecular localization using a panel of mouse myeloma variant immunoglobulins. J. Exp. Med. 158: 1763, 1983.

Staunton, D.E.; Dustin, M.L. and Springer T.A.: Functional cloning of ICAM-2 a cell adhesion ligand for LFA-1 homologous to ICAM-1. Nature 339: 61–64, 1989.

Steele-Perkins, G.; Turner, J.; Edman, J.C:; Hari, J.; Pierce, S.B.; Stover, C.; Rutter, W.J. and Roth, R.A.: Expression and characterization of a functional human insulin-like growth factor I receptor. J. Biol. Chem. 263: 11486–11492, 1988.

Steinman, L.; Rosenbaum, J.T.; Sriram, S. and McDevitt, H.O.: In vivo effects of antibodies to immune response gene products: prevention of experimental allergic encephalitis. Proc. Natl. Acad. Sci. USA 78: 7111–7114, 1981.

Steinman, L.: The use of monoclonal antibodies for treatment of autoimmune disease. J. Clin. Immunol. 10: 30S, 1990.

Steinman, R.M.; Kaplan, G.; Whitmaner, M.D. and Cohn, Z.A.: Identification of a novel cell type in peripheral lymphoid organs of mice. V. Purification of spleen dendritic cells, new surface markers, and maitenance in vitro. J. Exp. Med. 149: 1–16, 1979.

Steinman, R.M.; Gutchinov, B.; Witmer, M.D. and Nussenzweig, M.C.: Dendritic cells are the principal stimulators of the primary mixed leukocyte reaction in mice. J. Exp. Med. 157: 613–627, 1983.

Steinman, R.M.: Contrasting potential roles of dendritic cells during HIV-1 infection. ENII Conf.: Integrated Function of Molecules of the Immune System. Les Embiez, France, 12th–16th May 1993.

Steinman, R.: Features and functions of different components of the dendritic cell system. ENII Conf.: Integrated Function of Molecules of the Immune System. Les Embiez, France, 12th–16th May 1993.

Stelter, F.; Dietz, H.; Krüger, C.; Grunwald, U.; Bufler, P.; Schilling, T.; Witt, S.; Engelmann, H. and Schütt, C.: Functional characterization of recombinant CD14 expressed in L929 mouse fibroblasts. Immunobiology 189: 1993.

Stephan, R.N.; Saizawa, M.; Conrad, P.J.; Dean, R.E.; Geha, A.S. and Chaudry, I.H.: Depressed antigen presentation function and membrane IL-2 activity of peritoneal macrophages after laparotomy. Surgery 102: 147–150, 1987.

Steplewski, Z.; Chang, T.H.; Herlyn, M. and Koprowski, H.: Release of monoclonal antibody-defined antigens by human colorectal carcinoma and melanoma cells. Cancer Res. 41: 2723, 1981.

Sterio, M.; Gebauer, E.; Vucicevic, G.; Zalisevskij, G.; Felle, D. and Kolarov, N.: Intravenöses Immunglobulin bei der Behandlung von malignen Epilepsien bei Kindern. Wiener klin. Wochschr. 102: 230–233, 1990.

Stern, A.S.; Podlaski, F.J.; Hulmes, J.D.; Pan, Y.C.E.; Quinn, P.M.; Wolitzky, A.G.; Familletti, P.C.; Stremlo, D.L.; Truitt, T.; Chizzonite, R. and Gately, M.K.: Purification to homogeneity and partial characterization of cytotoxic lymphocyte maturation factor from human B-lymphoblastoid cells. Proc. Natl. Acad. Sci. USA 87: 6808–6812, 1990.

Stern, J.B. and Smith K.A.: Interleukin 2 induction of T cell G1 progression and c-myb expression. Science 233: 203–206, 1986.

Stetler, D.A.; Rose, K.M.; Wenger, M.E.; Berlin, C.M. and Jacob, S.T.: Anti-protein kinase NII antibodies in rheumatic autoimmune diseases. J. biol. Chem. 259: 2077–2079, 1984.

Stetler-Stevenson, W.G.; Krutzsch, H.C. and Liotta, L.A.: Tissue inhibitor of metalloproteinases (TIMP-2). A new member of the metalloproteinase inhibitor family. J. Biol. Chem. 264: 17374–17378, 1989.

Stevens, J.H.; O'Hanley, P.; Shapiro, J.M.; Mihm, F.G.; Satoh, P.S.; Collins, J.A. and Raffin, T.A.: Effects of anti-C5a antibodies of the adult respiratory distress syndrome in septic primates. J. Clin. Invest. 77: 1812–1816, 1986.

Stevenson, F.K. and Hawkins, R.E.: Molecular vaccines against cancer. The Immunologist 2: 16, 1994.

Stifler, W.C.: A twenty-one year follow-up of infantile eczema. J. Pediatr. 66: 166, 1965.

Stollar, B.D.: Reaction of systemic lupus erythematosus sera with histone fractions and histone-DNA complexes. Arthritis Rheum. 14: 485–492, 1971.

Stollar, D.; Levine, L.; Lehrer, H.I. and Van Vunakis, H.: The antigenic determinants of denatured DNA reactive with lupus erythematosus serum. Proc. natn. Acad. Sci. USA 48: 874–880, 1962.

Stollar, B.D.: Autoantibodies and autoantigens: a conserved system that may shape a primary immunoglobulin gene pool. Molec. Immunol. 28: 1399–1412, 1991.

Stoppelli, M.P.; Verde, P.; Grimaldi, G.; Localtelli, E.K. and Blasi, F.: Increase in urokinase plasminogen activator mRNA synthesis in human carcinoma cells is a primary effect of the potent tumor-promoter phorbol myristate acetate. J. Cell Biol. 102: 1235–1244, 1986.

Strasser, T. and Schiffl, H.: Leukotriene B4 is involved in hemodialysis-associated neutropenia. Biochim. Biophys. Acta 1046: 326–329, 1990 and Tridon, A.; Albuiswson, E.; Deteix, P. et al.: Leukotriene B4 in hemodialysis. Artif. Organs 14: 387–398, 1990.

Strauch, U.G.; Lifka, A.; Berlin, A.; Briskin, M.J.; Clements, J.; Weissman, I.L.; Butcher, E.C. and Holzmann, B.: Binding to the mucosal vascular addressin MAdCAM-1 reveals distinct functions of integrins LPAM-1 (µ4ß1) and VLA-4 (µ4ß1) in lymphocyte homing. ENII Conf.: Integrated Function of Molecules of the Immune System. Les Embiez, France, 12th-16th May 1993.

Stribling, R.; Brunette, E.; Liggitt, D.; Gaensler, K. and Debs, R.: Aerosol gene delivery in vivo. Proc. Natl. Acad. Sci. USA 89: 11277–11281, 1992.

Strieter, R.M.; Remick, D.G.; Ham, J.M.; Colletti, L.M.; Lynch, J.P. and Kunkel, S.L.: Tumor necrosis factor-alpha gene expression in human blood. J. Leukoc. Biol. 47: 366, 1990.

Strony, J.; Phillips, M.; Brands, D.; Moake, J. and Adelman, B.: Aurintricarboxylic acid in a canine model of coronary artery thrombosis. Circulation 81: 1106–1114, 1990.

Sturmhöfel, K. and Hämmerling, G.J.: Reconstitution of H-2 class I expression by gene transfection decreases susceptibility to natural killer cells of an EL4 class I loss variant. Europ. J. Immunol. 20: 171–177, 1990.

Taga, T.; Lawanishi, Y.; Hardy, R.R.; Hirano, T. and Kishimoto, T.: Receptors for B cell stimulatory factor 2. Quantitation, specificity, distribution, and regulation of their expression. J. Exp. Med. 166: 967–981, 1987.

Taga, T.; Hibi, M.; Hirata, Y.; Yamasaki, K.; Yasukawa, K.; Matsuda, T.; Hirano, T. and Kishimoto, T.: Interleukin (IL)-6 triggers the association of its receptor (IL-6R) with a possible signal transduction transducer, gp130. Cell 58: 573, 1989.

Tai, T.; Paulson, J.C.; Cahan, L.D. and Irie, R.F.: Ganglioside GM2 as a human tumor antigen (OFA-I-1). Proc. Natl. Acad. Sci. USA 80: 5392–5396, 1985.

Tai, T.; Cahan, L.D.; Tsuchida, T.; Saxton, R.E.; Irie, R.F. and Morton, D.L.: Immunogenicity of melanoma-associated gangliosides in cancer patients. Int. J. Cancer 35: 607–612, 1985.

Takahashi, M.; Takahashi, S., Brade, V. and Nussenzweig, V.: Requirements for the solubilization of immune aggregates by complement. The role of the classical pathway. J. Clin. Invest. 62: 349–358, 1978.

Takahasi, T.; Yamaguchi, T.; Kitamura, K.; Suzuyama, H.; Honda, M.; Yokota, T.; Kotanagi, H.; Takahashi, M. and Hashimoto, Y.: Clinical application of monoclonal antibody-drug conjugates for immunotargeting chemotherapy of colorectal carcinoma. Cancer 61: 881, 1988.

Takao, T.; Tracey, D.E.; Mitchell, W.M. and De Souza, E.B.: Interleukin-1 receptors in mouse brain: Characterization and neuronal localization. Endocrinology 127: 3070–3078, 1990.

Takao, T.; Mitchell, W.M.; Tracey, D.E. and De Souza, E.B.: Identification of interleukin-1 receptors in mouse testis. Endocrinology 127: 251–258, 1990.

Takao, T.; Culp, S.G.; Newton, R.C. and De Souza, E.B.: Type I interleukin-1 receptors in mouse brain-endocrine-immune axis labelled with 125I recombinant human interleukin-1 receptor antagonist. J. Neuroimmunol. 41: 51–60, 1992.

Takatsu, K.; Kikuchi, Y.; Takahashi, T.; Honjo, T.; Matsumoto, M.; Harada, N.; Yamaguchi, N. and Tominaga, A.: Interleukin 5, a T-cell-derived B-cell differentiation factor also induces cytotoxic T lymphocytes. Proc. Natl. Acad. Sci 84: 4234–4238, 1987.

Takatsu, K.; Tominaga, A.; Harada, N.; Mita, S.; Matsumoto, M.; Takahashi, T.; Kikuchi, Y. and Yamaguchi, N.: T cell-replacing factor (TRF)/interleukin 5 (Il-5): molecular and functional properties. Immun. Rev. 103: 107–135, 1988.

Takeichi, M.: Cadherin cell adhesion receptors as a morphogenetic regulator. Science 251: 1451–1455, 1991.

Takeshita, K.; Yamagishi, I.; Harada, M.; Otomo, S.; Nakagawa, T. and Mizushima, Y.: Immunological and anti-inflammatory effects of chlarithromycin: inhibiton of interleukin 1 production of murine peritoneal macrophages. Drugs Exp. Clin. Rec. 15: 4025–4031, 1989.

Talal, N.: Lessons from autoimmunity. Specific Immunotherapy Of Cancer With Vaccines, eds. Bystryn, J.-C.; Ferrone, S. and Livingston, P., The New York Academy of Sciences 690: 19, 1993.

Tamaru, T. and Brown, W.R.: IgA antibodies in rat bile inhibit cholera toxin-induced secretion in ileal loops in situ. Immunology 55: 579–583, 1985.

Tan, H.P.; Lebeck, L.K. and Nehlsen-Cannarella, S.L.: Regulatory role of cytokines in IgE-mediated allergy. J. Leukocyte Biol. 52: 115, 1992.

Tan, L.K.; Shops, R.J.; Oi, V.T. and Morrison, S.L.: Influence of the hinge region on complement activation, C1q binding, and segmental flexibility in chimeric human immunoglobulins. Proc. natn. Acad. Sci. USA 87: 162–166, 1990.

Tanaka, K.; Isselbacher, K.; Khouvy, G. and Jay, G.: Reversal of oncogenesis by the expression of a major histocompatibility complex class I gene. Science 228: 26–30, 1985.

Tanaka, T.; Danno, K.; Ikai, K. and Imamura, S.: Effects of substance P and substance K on the growth of cultured keratinocytes. J. Invest. Dermatol. 90: 399, 1988.

Tanaka, T.; Camerini, D.; Seed, B.; Torimoto, Y.; Dang, N.H.; Kameoka, J.; Dahlberg, H.N.; Schlossman, S.F. and Morimoto, C.: Cloning and functional expression of the T cell activation antigen CD26. J. Immunol. 149: 481–486, 1992.

Tannock, I.F. and Hayashi, S.: The proliferation of capillary endothelial cells. Cancer Res. 32: 77, 1972.

Tao, M. and Levy, R.: A novel vaccine for B cell lymphoma: idiotype/granulocyte-macrophage colony stimulating factor fusion protein. Nature 362: 755–758, 1993.

Tao, M.-H. and Morrison, S.L.: Studies of a glycosylated chimeric mouse-human IgG. J. Immun. 143: 2595–2601, 1989.

Tarkowski, A.; Czerkinsky, C. and Nilsson, L.-A.: Detection of IgG rheumatoid factor secreting cells in autoimmune MRL/1 mice: a kinetic study. Clin. Exp. Immunol. 58: 7, 1984.

Tartaglia, L.A. and Goeddel, D.V.: Two TNF receptors. Immunol. Today 13: 151–153, 1992.

Tashjian, A.H.J.; Voelkel, E.F.; Lazzaro, M.; Singer, F.R.; Roberts, A.B.; Derynck, R.; Winkler, M.E. and Levine, L.: μ and ß human transforming growth factors stimulate prostaglandin production and bone resorption in cultured mouse calvaria. Proc. Natl. Acad. Sci. USA 82: 4535–4538, 1985.

Tate, R.M. and Repine, J.E.: Neutrophils and the adult respiratory distress syndrome. Am. Rev. Respir. Dis. 128: 552–559, 1983.

Tausk, F. and Gigli, I.: The human C3b receptor: function and role in human diseases. J. Invest. Dermatol. 94: 141–145, 1990.

Taylor, C.W. and Hersh, E.M.: Use of recombinant cytokines in cancer therapy. Cytokines in health and diseases, 433, 1992.

Taylor, H.P. and Immock, N.J.: Mechanism of neutralization of influenza virus by secretory IgA is different from that of monomeric IgA or IgG. J. Exp. Med. 161: 198–209, 1985.

Taylor, S. and Folkman, J.: Protamine is an inhibitor of angiogenesis. Nature 297: 307–312, 1982.

Taylor-Papadimitriou, M.; Stewart, L.; Burchell, S. and Beverley, P.: The polymorphic epithelial mucin as a target for immunotherapy. Specific Immunotherapy Of Cancer With Vaccines, eds. Bystryn, J.-C.; Ferrone, S. and Livingston, P., The New York Academy of Sciences 690: 69, 1993.

Tedder, T.F.; Clement, L.T. and Cooper, M.D.: Expression of C3d receptors during human B cell differentiation: Immunofluorescence analysis with the HB-5 monoclonal antibody. J. Immunol. 133: 678–683, 1984.

Tedesco, F.: Complement deficiencies: the eighth component. Prog. Allergy 39: 295–306, 1986.

Teitell, M.; Mescher, M.F.; Olson, C.A.; Littman, D.R. and Kronenberg, M.: The thymus leukemia antigen binds human and mouse CD8. J. Exp. Med. 174: 1131–1138, 1991.

Teng, N.N.H.; Kaplan, H.S.; Hebert, J.M.; Moore, C.; Douglas, H.; Wunderlich, A. and Braude, A.I.: Protection against gram-negative ybacteremia and endotoxemia with human monoclonal IgM antibodies. Proc. Natl. Acad. Sci. USA 82: 1790–1794, 1985.

Tenner, A.J. and Cooper, N.R.: Identification of types of cells in human peripheral blood that bind C1q. J. Immunol. 126: 1174–1179, 1981.

Tenner, A.J. and Cooper, N.R.: Stimulation of a human polymorphonuclear leukocyte oxidative response by the C1q subunit of the first complement component. J. Immunol. 128: 2547–2552, 1982.

Tenner, A.J.; Young, R.; Malbran, A.; Fauci, A.S. and Ambrus, J.L.: In vitro modulation of B cell immunoglobulin (Ig) synthesis by the C1q subcomponent of complement. Fed. Proc. 46: 1195, 1987.

Tenner, A.J.; Robinson, S.L.; Borchelt, J. and Wright, J.R.: Human pulmonary surfactant protein (SP-A), a protein structurally homologous to C1q, can enhance FcR- and CR1–mediated phagocytosis. J. Biol. Chem. 264: 13923–13928, 1989.

Tenner, A.J.: Functional aspects of the C1q receptors. Behring Inst. Mitt. 93: 241–253, 1993.

Tepper, M.A.; Hoeger, P.H.; Geha, R.S. and Nadler, S.G.: Mechanism of action of Deoxyspergualin. Int. Conference on New Trends in Clinical and Experimental Immunosuppression. Geneva, Switzerland, February 10–13, 1994.

Tepper, R.; Pattengale, P. and Leder, P.: Murine Interleukin-4 displays potent anti-tumor activity in vivo. Cell 57: 503–512, 1989.

Teramura, M.; Katahira, J.; Hishino, S.; Motoji, T.; Oshimi, K. and Mizoguchi, H.: Clonal growth of human megakaryocyte progenitors in serum-free cultures: effect of recombinant human interleukin 3. Exp. Hematol. 16: 843, 1988.

Teramura, M.; Kobayashi, S.; Hoshino, S.; Oshimi, K. and Mizoguchi, H.: Interleukin-11 enhances human megarkaryocytopoiesis in vitro. Blood 79: 327–331, 1992.

Ternynck, T. and Avrameas, S.: Murine natural monoclonal autoantibodies: a study of their polyspecificities and their affinities. Immun. Rev. 94: 99–112, 1986.

Teumer, J.; Lindahl, A. and Green, H.: Human growth hormone in the blood of athymic-mice grafted with cultures of hormone-secreting human keratinocytes. FASEB J 4: 3245–3249, 1990.

te Velde, A.A.; Huijbens, R.J.F.; de Vries, J.E. and Figdor, C.G.: Interleukin-4 (IL-4) inhibits secretion of IL-1ß, tumor necrosis factor alpha and IL-6 by human monocytes. Blood 76: 1392–1398, 1990.

te Velde, A.A.; Rousset, F.; Peronne, C.; De Vries, J.E. and Figdor, C.G.: IFN-alpha und IFN-gamma have different regulatory effects on Il-4–induced membrane expression of Fc epsilon RIIb and release of soluble Fc epsilon RIIb by human monocytes. J. Immunol. 144: 3052–3059, 1990.

Tew, J.G. and Mandel, T.E.: Prolonged antigen half-life in the lymphoid follicles of specifically immunized mice. Immunology 37: 69, 1979.

Tew, J.G.; Kosco, M.H.; Burton, G.F. and Szakal, A.K.: Follicular dendritic cells as accessory cells. Immunol. Rev. 117: 185, 1990.

Thiel, M.; Bardenheuer, H. and Peter, K.: Interaction of pentoxifylline (PTX) and adenosine (ADO) in the inhibition of superoxide anion production of human polymorphonuclear leukocytes (PMNL). Abstr. 2nd Int. Congress on the Immune Consequences of Trauma, Shock, and Sepsis: Mechanisms and Therapeutic Approaches. March 6–9, 1991. Munich, FRG.

Thiel, S. and Reid, K.B.M.: Structures and functions associated with the group of mammalian lectins containing collagen-like sequences. FEBS Lett. 250: 78–84, 1989.

Thiemermann, C.; May, G.R.; Page, C.P. and Vane, J.R.: Endothelin-1 inhibits platelet aggregation in vivo: a study with 111–indium-labelled platelets. Br. J. Pharmacol. 99: 303–308, 1990.

Thomas, H.: New horizons in cancer therapy. Drugs of Today 28: 311–331, 1992.

Thomas, J.A.; Hotchin, N.A.; Allday, M.J.; Amlot, P.; Rose, M.; Yacoub, M. and Crawford, D.H.: Immunohistology of Epstein-Barr virus-associated antigens in B cell disorders from immuno-compromised individuals. Transplantation 49: 944–953, 1990.

Thompson, H.S.G. and Staines, N.A.: Could specific oral tolerance be a therapy for autoimmune disease? Immun. Today 11: 396–299, 1990.

Thompson, R.C.; Dripps, D.J. and Eisenberg, S.P.: Interleukin-1 receptor antagonist (Il-1ra) as a probe and as a treatment for Il-1 mediated disease. Int. J. Immunopharmac. 14: 475–480, 1992.

Thompson-Snipes, L.; Dhar, V.; Bond, M.W.; Mosmann, T.R.; Moore, K.W. and Rennick, D.M.: Interleukin 10: a novel stimulatory factor for mast cells and their progenitors. J. Exp. Med. 173: 507–510, 1991.

Thomson, W.; Sanders, P.A.; Davis, M.; Davidson, J.; Dyer, P.A. and Grennan, D.M.: Complement C4B-null alleles in Felty's syndrome. Arthritis Rheum. 31: 984–989, 1988.

Thorsen, S.; Fogh, K.; Broby-Johnsen, U. and Sondergaard, J.: Leukotriene B4 in atopic dermatitis: Increased skin levels and altered sensitivity of peripheral blood T-cells. Allergy 4S: 457–463, 1990.

Thyphronitis, G.; Tsokos, G.C.; June, C.H.; Levine, A.D. and Finkelman, F.D.: IgE secretion by Epstein-Barr virus-infected purified human B lymphocytes is stimulated by IL-4 and suppressed by interferon-gamma. Proc. Natl. Sci. USA 86: 5580–5584, 1989.

Tobias, P.S.; Mathison, J.C. and Ulevitch, R.J.: A family of lipopolysaccharide binding proteins involved in responses to gram-negative sepsis. J. Biol. Chem. 263: 13479–13481, 1988.

Todaro, G.J.; Fryling, C. and DeLarco, J.E.: Transforming growth factors produced by certain human tumor cells: polypeptides that interact with epidermal growth factor receptor. Proc. Natl. Acad. Sci. USA 77: 5258–5262, 1980.

Todd, J.A.; Bell, J.I. and McDevitt, H.O.: A molecular basis for genetic susceptibility to insulin dependent diabetes mellitus. Trends Genet. 4: 129–134, 1988.

Tomasi, T.B.: Regulation of the mucosal IgA response - an overview. Immunol. Invest. 18: 1–15, 1989.

Tominaga, A.; Matsumoto, M.; Harada, N.; Takahashi, T.; Kikuchi, Y. and Takatsu, K.: Molecular properties and regulation of MRNA expression for murine T cell-replacing factor/Il-5. J. Immunol. 140: 1175–1181, 1988.

Tominaga, A.; Takaki, S.; Koyama, N.; Katoh, S.; Matsumoto, R.; Migita, M.; Hitoshi, Y.; Hosoya, Y.; Yamauchi, S.; Kanai, Y. et al.: Transgenic mice expressing a B cell growth and differentiation factor gene (interleukin 5) develop eosinophilia and autoantibody production. J. Exp. Med. 173: 429–437, 1991.

Tomita, Y.; Matsumoto, Y.; Nishiyama, T. and Fujiwara, M.: Reduction of major histocompatibility complex class-I antigens on invasive and high-grade transitional cell carcinoma. J. Pathol. 162: 157–164, 1990.

Tomlinson, S.: Complement defense mechanisms. Curr. Opin. Immun. 5: 83–89, 1993.

Torbohm, I.; Schonermark, M.; Wingen, A.M.; Berger, B.; Rother, K. and Hansch, G.M.: C5b-8 and C5b-9 modulate the collagen release of human glomerular epithelial cells. Kidney Int. 37: 1098–1104, 1990.

Torimoto, Y.; Dang, N.H.; Vivier, E.; Tanaka, T.; Schlossman, S.F. and Morimoto, C.: Coassociation of CD26 (dipeptidyl peptidase IV) with CD45 on the surface of human T lymphocytes. J. Immunol. 147: 2514–2517, 1991.

Touw, I.; Pouwels, K.; Van Agthoven, T.; van Gurp, R.; Budel, L.; Hoogerbrugge, H.; Delwel, R.; Goodwin, R.; Namen, A. and Loewenberg, B.: Interleukin-1 is a growth factor of precursor B and T acute lymphoblastic leukemia. Blood 75: 2097–2101, 1990.

Townsend, A.; Ohlen, C.; Bastin, J.; Ljunggren, H.G.; Foster, L. and Kärre, K.: Association of class I major histocompatibility heavy and light chains induced by viral peptides. Nature 340: 443–448, 1989.

Townsend, A.; Elliott, T.; Cerundolo, V.; Foster, L.; Barber, B. and Tse, A.: Assembly of MHC class I molecules analyzed in vitro. Cell 62: 285–295, 1990.

Townsend, S.E. and Allison, J.P.: Tumor rejection after direct costimulation of CD8 positive T-cells by B7 transfected melanoma cells. Science 259: 368–370, 1993.

Tracey, K.J.; Beutler, B.; Lowry, S.F.; Merryweather, J.; Wolpe, S.; Milsark, I.W.; Hariri, R.J.; Fahey, T.D.; Zentella, A.; Albert, J.D. et al.: Shock and tissue injury induced by recombinant human cachectin. Science 234: 470–474, 1986.

Tracey, K.J.; Fong, Y.; Hesse, D.G.; Manogue, K.R.; Lee, A.T.; Kuo, G.C.; Lowry, S.F. and Cerami, A.: Anti-cachectin/TNF monoclonal antibodies prevent septic shock during lethal bacteraemia. Nature 330: 662, 1987.

Tracey, D.E. and De Souza, E.B.: Identification of interleukin-1 receptors in mouse pituitary cell membranes and AtT-20 pituitary tumor cells. Soc. Neurosci. Abstr. 14: 1052, 1988.

Tracey, K.J.; Vlassara, H. and Cerami, A.: Cachectin/tumour necrosis factor. Lancet 1: 1122–1126, 1989.

Traylor, T.d. and Hogan, E.L.: Gangliosides of human cerebral astrocytomas. N. Neurochem. 34: 126–131, 1980.

Treisman, J.; Higuchi, C.M.; Thompson, J.A.; Gillis, S.; Lindgren, C.G.; Kern, D.E.; Ridell, S.R.; Greenberg, P.D. and Fefer, A.: Enhancement by interleukin 4 of interleukin 2 or antibody-induced proliferation of lymphocytes from interleukin 2-treated cancer patients. Cancer Res. 50: 1160–1167, 1990.

Trier, J.S.: Structure and function of intestinal M cells. In "Molecular Immunology. I. Basic principles". Gastroenterology Clinics of North America. Vol. 20, No. 3, 531–547, Saunders, Philadelphia, 1991.

Trinchieri, G. and Perussia, B.: Immune interferon a pleiotropic lymphokine with multiple effects. Immunology Today 6: 131–136, 1985.

Triozzi, L.; Martin, E.W.; Gochnour, D. and Aldrich, W.: Phase Ib trial of a synthetic β human chorionic gonadotropin vaccine in patients with metastatic cancer. Specific Immunotherapy Of Cancer With Vaccines, eds. Bystryn, J.-C.; Ferrone, S. and Livingston, P., The New York Academy of Sciences 690: 358, 1993.

Tsai, M.; Takeishi, T.; Thompson, H.; Langley, K.E.; Zsebo, K.M.; Metcalfe, D.D.; Geissler, E.N. and Galli, S.J.: Induction of mast cell proliferation, maturation, and heparin synthesis by the rat c-kit ligand, stem cell factor. Proc. Natl. Acad. Sci. USA 88: 6382–6386, 1991.

Tschopp, J.; Peitsch, M.C.; Polzar, B. and Mannherz, H.G.: Nuclear DNA degradation during apoptosis. ENII Conf.: Integrated Function of Molecules of the Immune System. Les Embiez, France, 12th-16th May 1993.

Tse, S.-K. and Cadee, K.: The interaction between interstitial mucus glycoproteins and enteric infections. Parasitol. Today 7: 163–172, 1991.

Tsokos, G.C.; Kinoshita, T.; Thyphronitis, G.; Patel, A.D.; Dickler, H.B. and Finkelman, F.C.: Interactions between murine B lymphocyte surface membrane molecules. Loaded but not free receptors for complement and the Fc portion of IgG co-cap independently with cross-linked surface Ig. J. Immunol. 144: 239–243, 1990.

Tsoukas, C.D., and Lambris, J.D.: Expression of CR2/EBV receptors on human thymocytes detected by monoclonal antibodies. Eur. J. Immunol. 18: 1299–1302, 1988.

Tsuchiya, N.; Endo, T.; Matsuta, K.; Yoshinoya, S.; Aikawa, T.; Kosuge, E.; Takeuchi, F.; Miyamoto, T. and Kobata, A.: Effects of galactose depletion from oligosaccharide chains on immunological activities of human IgG. J. Rheumat. 16: 285–290, 1989.

Tsuda, H.; Sawada, T.; Kawakita, M. and Takatsuki, K.: Mode of action of erythropoietin (Epo) in an Epo-dependent murine cell line. II. Cell cycle dependency of Epo action. Exp. Hematol. 17: 218–222, 1989.

Tsuji, K.; Lyman, S.D.; Sudo, T.; Clark, S.C. and Ogawa, M.: Enhancement of murine hematopoiesis by synergistic interactions between steel factor ligand for c-kit interleukin-11 and other early acting factors in culture. Blood 79: 2855–2860, 1992.

Tuddenham, E.G.D.: Hemophilia, Molecular Genetics. Encyclopedia of Human Biology 4: 151, 1991.

Tuffin, D.P.: Platelet glycoproteins as targets for anti-platelet drugs. Int. Conf. on: The platelet in health & disease. Royal College of Physicians, London, 1992.

Tune, B.M.; Hsu, C.Y.; Bieber, M.M. and Teng, N.N.H.: Effects of anti-lipid A human monoclonal antibody on lipopolysaccharide-induced toxicity to the kidney. J. Urol. 141: 1463–1466,1989.

Turka, L.A.; Linsley, P.S.; Lin, H.; Brady, W.; Leiden, J.M.; Wei, R.-Q.; Gibson, M.L.; Zheng, X.-G.; Myrdal, S.; Gordon, D.; Bailey, T.; Bolling, S.F. and Thompson, C.B.: T-cell activation by the CD28 ligand B7 is required for cardiac allograft rejection in vivo. Proc. Natl. Acad. Sci. USA, 89: 11102–11105, 1992.

Tzeng, D.Y.; Deuel, T.F.; Huang, J.S. and Boehner, R.L.: Platelet-derived growth factor promotes human peripheral monocyte activation. Blood 66: 179–183, 1985.

Uchibayashi, N.; Kikutani, H.; Barsumian, E.L.; Hauptmann, R.; Schneider, F.J.; Schwenden-wein, R.; Summergruber, W.; Spevak, W.; Maurer-Fogy, I.; Suemura, M. and Kishimoto, T.: Recombinant soluble Fc epsilon receptor II (Fc epsilon RIII CD23) has IgE binding activity but no B cell growth promoting activity. J. Immunol. 142: 3901–3908, 1989.

Uehara, A.; Okumura, T.; Kitamori, S.; Takasugi, Y. and Namiki, M.: Interleukin-1: A cytokine that has potent antisecretory and anti-ulcer actions via the central nervous system. Biochem. Biophys. Res. Commun. 173: 585–590, 1990.

Uher, F. and Dickler, H.B.: Cooperativity between B lymphocyte membrane molecules: in-dependent ligand occupancy and cross-linking of antigen receptors and Fc receptors down-regulates B lymphocyte function. J. Immunol. 137: 3124, 1986.

Uhr, J.W. and Bauman, J.B.: Antibody formation. I. The suppression of antibody formation by passively administered antibody. J. Exp. Med. 113: 935–957, 1961.

Uhr, J.W. and Möller G.: Regulatory effect of antibody on the immune response. Adv. Immunol. 8: 81, 1968.

Ullrich, A.; Coussens, L.; Hayflick, J.S.; Dull, T.J.; Gray, A.; Tam, A.W.; Lee, J.; Yarden, Y.; Libermann, T.A.; Schlessinger, J. et al.: Human epidermal growth factor receptor cDNA sequence and aberrant expression of the amplified gene in A431 epidermoid carcinoma cells. Nature 309: 418–425, 1984.

Ulmer, A.J.; Mattern, T.; Feller, A.C.; Heymann, E. and Flad, H.D.: CD26 antigen is a surface dipeptidyl peptidase IV (DPPIV) as characterized by monoclonal antibodies clone TII-19-4-7 and 4ELIC7. Scand. J. Immunol. 31: 429–435, 1990.

Ulmer, J.B.; Donnelly, J.J.; Parker, S.E.; Rhodes, G.H.; Felgner, P.L.; Dwarki, V.J.; Gromkow-ski, S.H.; Deck, R.R.; DeWitt, C.M.; Friedman, A.; Hawe, L.A.; Leander, K.R.; Martinez, D.; Perry, H.C.; Shiver, J.W.; Montgomery, D.L. and Liu, M.A.: Heterologous protection against influenza by injection of DNA encoding a viral protein. Science 259: 1745–1749, 1993.

Ulsperger, E.; Rainer, H.; Locker, G.; Vetterlein, M.; Schiessel, R.; Hofbauer, F.; Armbruster, C.; Depisch, D.; Politzer, P.; Dinstl. K.; Wagner, O.; Wunderlich, M.; Waldhör, T. and Schulte-Hermann, R.: Adjuvant vaccination in colorectal carcinoma. Specific Immunotherapy Of Can-cer With Vaccines, eds. Bystryn, J.-C.; Ferrone, S. and Livingston, P., The New York Academy of Sciences 690: 360, 1993.

Umezawa, H.; Kondo, S.; Iinuma, H.; Kunimoto, S.; Ikeda, H.; Iwasawa, H.; Ikeda, D. and Takeuchi, T.: Structure of an antitumor antibiotic, spergualin. J. Antibiotics 34: 1622–1623, 1981.

Underwood, J.C.: Lymphoreticular-cell infiltration in human tumors: Prognostic and histological implications. A review. Br. J. Cancer 30: 538–548, 1974.

Unkeless, J.C.; Scigliano, E. and Freedman, V.H.: Structure and function of human and murine receptors for IgG. Annu. Rev. Immunol. 6: 251–281, 1988.

Unnasch, T.R.; Gallin, M.Y.; Soboslay, P.T.; Erttmann, K.D. and Greene, B.M.: Isolation and characterisation of expressing cDNA clones encoding antigens of onchocerca volvulus infec-tive larvae. J. Clin. Invest. 82: 262–269, 1988.

Uno, H. and Hanifin, J.: Epidermal Langerhans cells and chronic lesions of atopic dermatitis observed by L-dopa. J. Invest. Dermatol. 75: 52, 1980.

Uotila, P. and Vapaatalo, H.: Synthesis, pathways and biological implications of eicosanoids. Ann. Clin. Res. 16: 226, 1984.

Uotila, P.: Inhibition of prostaglandin E2 formation and histamine action in cancer immuno-therapy. Cancer Immunol Immunother. 37: 251–254, 1993.

Urban, J.L.; Horvath, S.J. and Hood, L.: Autoimmune T cells: Immune recognition of normal and variant peptide epitopes and peptide-based therapy. Cell 59: 257–271, 1989.

Usuba, O.; Fujii, Y.; Miyoshi, I.; Naiki, M. and Senda, F.: Establishment of a human monoclonal antibody to Hanganutziu-Deicher antigen as a tumor-associated carbohydrate antigen. Jpn. J. Cancer Res. 79: 1340–1348, 1988.

Usuki, K.; Heldin, N.E.; Miyazono, K.; Ishikawa, F.; Takuku, F.; Westermark, B. and Heldin, C.H.: Production of platelet-derived endothelial cell growth factor by normal and transformed human cells in culture. Proc. Natl. Acad. Sci USA 86: 7427–7431, 1989.

Valent, P.J.; Besemer, J.; Kishi, K.; Kaltenbrunner, R.; Kuhn, B.; Maurer, D.; Lechner, K. and Bettelheim, P.: IL-3 promotes basophilic differentiation of KU812 cells through high affinity binding sites. J. Immunol. 145: 1885, 1990.

Valente, W.A.; Vitti, P.; Rotella, C.M.; Vaughan, M.M.; Aloj, S.M.; Grollman, E.F.; Ambesi-Impiombato, F.S. and Kohn, L.D.: Antibodies that promote thyroid growth. A distinct population of thyroid-stimulating autoantibodies. New Engl. J. Med. 309: 1028–1034, 1983.

Vallé, A.; Zuber, C.E.; Defrance, T.; Djossou, O.; De Rie, M. and Banchereau, J.: Activation of human B lymphocytes through CD40 and interleukin 4. Eur. J. Immunol. 19: 1453–1467, 1989.

Van Damme, J.; Van Beeumen, J.; Conings, R.; Decock, B. and Billiau, A.: Purification of granolocyte chemotactic peptide/interleukin-8 reveals N-terminal sequence heterogeneity similar to that of beta-thromboglobulin. Eur. J. Biochem. 181: 337–344, 1989.

Van Damme, J.: Interleukin-8 and related molecules. In: Thompson, A. ed. The Cytokine Handbook, London: Academic Press, 201–214, 1991.

Van den Dobbelsteen, G.P.J.M.; Brunekreef, K.; Sminia, T. and van Rees, E.P.: Effect of mucosal and systemic immunization with pneumococcal polysaccharide type 3, 4 and 14 in rat. Scand. J. Immunol. 36: 661–669, 1992.

van den Eynde, B.; Hainaut, P.; Herin, M.; Knutz, A.; Lemoine, C.; Weynants, P.; van der Bruggen, P.; Fauchet, R. and Boon, T.: Presence on a human melanoma of multiple antigens recognized by autologous CTL. Int. J. Cancer 44: 634–640, 1989.

van den Eynde, B.; Lethé, B.; van Pel, A.; de Plaen, E. and Boon, T.: The gene coding for a major tumor rejection antigen of tumor P815 is identical to the normal gene of synthetic DBA/2 mice. J. Exp. Med. 173: 1373–1384, 1991.

Van der Bruggen, P.; Traversari, C.; Chomez, P.; Lurquin, C.; de Plaen, E.; Van den Eynde, B.; Knutz, A. and Boon, T.: A gene encoding an antigen recognized by cytolytic T lymphocytes on a human melanoma. Science 254: 1643–1647, 1991.

van der Bruggen, P. and van den Eynde, B.: Molecular definition of tumor antigens recognized by T lymphocytes. Curr. Op. Immunol. 4: 608–612, 1992.

van der Graaf, F.; Koedam, A.; Griffin, J.H. and Bouma, B.N.: Interaction of human plasma kallikrein and its light chain with C1 inhibitor. Biochemistry 22: 4860–4866, 1983.

Van der Lubbe, P.A.; Reiter, C.; Riethmüller, G.; Sanders, M.E. and Breedveld, F.C.: Treatment of rheumatoid arthritis (RA) with chimeric CD4 monoclonal antibody. Arthritis Rheum. 34: 89, 1991.

van der Meché, F.G.A.; Schmitz, P.I.M. and the Dutch Guillain Barré Study Group: A randomized trial comparing intravenous immunoglobulin in plasma exchange in Guillain Barré syndrome. N. Engl. J. Med. 326: 1123–1129, 1992.

Van der Poll, T.: Cytokines and their inhibition in septicaemia. Br. J. Intens. Care 99–110, 1992.

Van Der Rest, M. and Garrone, R.: Collagen family of proteins. FASEB J. 5: 2814–2823, 1991.

Van der Zee, J.S.; Van Swieten, P. and Aalberse, R.C.: Inhibiton of complement activation by IgG4 antibodies. Clin. Exp. Immunol. 64: 415–422, 1986.

van de Winkel, J.G.J. and Anderson, C.L.: Biology of human immunoglobulin G Fc receptors. J. Leukocyte Biol. 49: 511–524, 1991.

Van Doorn, P.A.; Brand, A.; Strengers, P.F.W.; Meulstee, J. and Vermeulen, M.: High-dose intravenous immunogloublin treatment in chronic inflammatory demyelinating polyneuropathy: a double-blind, placebo-controlled, crossover study. Neurology 40: 209–212, 1990.

Van Dyne, S.; Holers, V.M.; Lubilin, D.M. and Atkinson, J.P.: The polymorphism of the C3b/C4b receptor in the normal population and in patients with systemic lupus erythematosus. Clin. Exp. Immunol. 68: 570–579, 1987.

Vane, R.J.; Anggard, E.E. and Botting, R.M.: Regulatory functions of the vascular endothelium. N. Engl. J. Med. 323: 27–36, 1990.

Van Engelen, B.G.M.; Renier, W.O.; Weemaes, C.M.R. and Strengers, P.F.W.: Treatment of idiopathic West- and Lennox epilepsy with intravenous immunoglobulins. Acta Neurol. Scand. 133: 25, 1990.

Van Furth, R.: Current view on the mononuclear phagocyte system. Immunobiology 161: 178–185, 1982.

Vánky, F.; Roberts, T.; Klein, E. and Willems, J.: Auto-tumor immunity in patients with solid tumors: participation of CD3 complex and MHC class I antigens in the lytic interaction. Immunol. Letters 16: 21–26, 1987.

Vánky, F.; Stuber, G.; Rotstein, S. and Klein, E.: Auto-tumor recognition following in vitro induction of MHC antigen expression on solid tumors: stimulation of lymphocytes and generation of cytotoxicity against the original MHC-antigen-negative tumor cells. Cancer Immunol. Immunoth. 28: 17–21, 1989.

Vánky, F.; Wang, P.; Patarroyo, M. and Klein, E.: Expression of the adhesion molecule ICAM-1 and major histocompatibility complex class I antigens on human tumor cells is required for their interaction with autologous lymphocytes in vitro. Cancer Immunol. Immunoth. 31: 19–27, 1990.

Van Loghem, E.: Allotypic markers. Monogr. Allergy 19: 40–51, 1986.

van Loon, A.P.G.M.; Ozmen, L.; Fountoulakis, M.; Kania, M.; Haiker, M. and Garotta, G.: High-affinity receptor for interferon-gamma (IFN-gamma), a ubiquitous protein occurring in different molecular forms on human cells: blood monocytes and eleven different cell lines have the same IFN-gamma receptor protein. J. Leukocyte Biol. 49: 462–473, 1991.

Van Noesel, C.J.M.; Lankester, A.C. and van Lier, R.A.W.: Dual antigen recognition by B cells. Immunology Today 14: 8, 1993.

Vannucchi, A.M.; Frossi, A. and Rafanelli, D.: In vivo stimulation of megakaryocytopoiesis by granulocyte-macrophage colony-stimulating factor. Blood 76: 1473, 1990.

Van Rijckevorsel-Harmant, K.; Delire, M. and Ruequoy-Ponsar, M.: Treatment of idiopathic West and Lennox-Gastaut syndromes by intravenous administration of human polyvalent immunoglobulins. Euro. Arch. Psychiatr. Neurol. Sci. 236: 119, 1986.

Van Rijckevorsel-Harmant, K. and Delire, M.: Intravenous immunoglobulins in the treatment of intractable epilepsy. Neurologia et Psychiatria 11: 93, 1988.

Van Rijckevorsel-Harmant, K.; Delire, M.; Sindie, C.J.M.; Chalon, M.P. and Harmant, J.: Intravenous immunoglobulins in intractable epilepsy. Advances in Epileptology 17: 336, 1989.

Van Rijthove, A.W.A.M.; Dijkmans, B.A.L.; Goeithe, H.S.; Boers, M. and Cats, A.: Long term cyclosporine therapy in rheumatoid arthritis. J. Rheum. 18: 19–23, 1991.

Van Rooijen, N.: Antigen processing and presentation in vivo: The microenvironment as a crucial factor. Immunol. Today 11: 436–439, 1990.

Van Snick, J.; Cayphas, S.; Vink, A.; Uyttenhove, C.; Coulie, P.G.; Rubira, M.R. and Simpson, R.J.: Purification and NH2–terminal amino acid sequence of a T-cell-derived lymphokine with growth factor activity for B-cell hybridomas. Proc. Natl. Acad. Sci 83: 9679–9683, 1986.

Van Snick, J.; Cayphas, S.; Szikora, J.P.; Renauld, J.C.; van Roost, E.; Boon, T. and Simpson, R.J.: cDNA cloning of murine interleukin-HP1: homology with human interleukin 6. Eur. J. Immunol. 18: 193–197, 1988.

Van Snick, J. and Coulie P.: Rheumatoid factors and secondary immune responses in the mouse. Eur. J. Immunol. 13: 890, 1983.

Van Wart, H.E. and Birkedal-Hansen, H.: The cysteine switch: A principal of regulation of metalloproteinase activity with potential applicability to the entire matrix metalloproteinase gene family. Proc. Natl. Acad. Sci. USA 87: 5578–5582, 1988.

Van Zeben, D.; Giphart, M.J.; Christiansen, F.T.; Hoetjer, M.; Meyer, E.C. and Breedveld, F.C.: Properdin factor B and complement factor C4 allotypes in rheumatoid arthritis: Results of a follow-up study. Hum. Immunol. 33: 148–151, 1992.

Varani, J.; Fligiel, S.E.G.; Till, G.O.; Kunkel, R.G.; Ryan, U.S. and Ward, P.A.: Pulmonary endothelial cell killing by human neutrophils. Possible involvement of hydroxyl radical. Lab. Invest. 53: 665–674, 1985.

Varesio, L.; Herberman, R.B.; Gerson, J.M. and Holden, H.T.: Suppression of lymphokine production by macrophages infiltrating murine virus-induced tumors. Int. J. Cancer 24: 97–102, 1979.

Varga, L.; Alper, C.A.; Zam, Z. and Fuest, G.: Decreased inhibition of immune precipitation by sera with the C2 B allotype. Clin. Immunol. Immunopath. 59: 65–71, 1991.

Venter, J.C.; Fraser, C.M. and Harrison, L.C.: Autoantibodies to B2–adrenergic receptors: a possible cause of andrenergic hyporesponsiveness in allergic rhinitis and asthma. Science 207: 1361–1363, 1980.

Vercelli, D.; Jabara, H.H.; Lee, W.; Woodland, N.; Geha, R.S. and Leung, D.Y.M.: Human recombinant IL-4 induces Fc R2/CD23 on normal human monocytes. J. Exp. Med. 167, 1401, 1988.

Vercelli, D.; Jabara, H.H.; Arai, K. and Geha, R.S.: Induction of human IgE synthesis requires IL-4 and T/B cell interactions involving the T cell receptor/CD3 complex and MHC class II antigens. J. Exp. Med. 169: 1295–1307, 1989.

Versteeg, R.; Noordermeer, I.A.; Krüse-Wolters, M.; Ruiter, D.J. and Schrier, P.I.: c-myc down-regulates class I HLA expression in human melanomas. EMBO J. 7: 1023–1029, 1988.

Versteeg, R.; van der Minne, C.; Plomp, A.; Sijts, A.; van Leeuven, A. and Schrier, P.: N-myc expression switched off and class I human leukocyte antigen expression switched on after somatic cell fusion of neuroblastoma cells. Mol. Cell. Biol. 10: 5416–5423, 1990.

Vezina, C.; Kudelsi, A. and Sehgal, S.N.: Rapamycin (AY-22, 989), a new antifungal antibiotic. I. Taxonomy of the producing Streptomycetes and isolation of the active principle. J. Antibiotics 28: 721–726, 1975.

Vieira, P.; de Waal-Malefyt, R.; Dang, M.N.; Johnson, K.E. and Kastelein, R.: Isolation and expression of human cytokine synthesis inhibitory factor cDNA clones: homology to Epstein-Barr virus open reading frame BCRFI. Proc. Natl. Acad. Sci. USA 88: 1172–1176, 1991.

Vijayasaradhi, S.; Bouchard, B. and Houghton, A.N.: The melanoma antigen gp75 is the human homologue of the mouse b (brown) locus gene product. J. Exp. Med. 171: 1375–1380, 1990.

Vik, D.P. and Fearon, D.T.: Cellular distribution of complement receptor type 4 (CR4): expression on human platelets. J. Immunol. 138: 254–258, 1987.

Villinger, P.M.; Cronin, M.T.; Amenomori, T.; Wachsman, W. and Lotz, M.: IL-6 production by human T-lymphocytes. J. Immunol. 146: 550, 1991.

Vladutiu, A.O. and Steinman, L.: Inhibition of experimental autoimmune thyroiditis in mice by anti-I-A antibodies. Cell Immunol. 109: 169–180, 1987.

Vlasselaer van, P.; Punnonen, J. and DeVries J.E.: Transforming growth factor-ß directs IgA switching in human B cells. J. Immunol. 148: 2062–2067, 1992.

Vlodavsky, I.; Eldor, A.; Haimovitz-Friedman, A.; Matzner, Y.; Ishai-Michaeli, R.; Lider, O.; Naparstek, Y.; Cohen, I.R. and Fuks, Z.: Expression of heparanase by platelets and circulating cells of the immune system: possible involvement in diapedesis and extravasation. Invasion Metastasis 12: 112–127, 1992.

Vogel, S.N.; Douches, S.D.; Kaufman, E.N. and Neta, R.: Induction of colony stimulating factor in vivo by recombinant interleukin 1 alpha and recombinant tumor necrosis factor alpha 1. J. Immunol. 138: 2143–2148, 1987.

Vogel, C.W.: Complement, a biologic effector mechanism for tumor cell killing. Immunol. Allergy Clin. N. Am. 11: 277, 1991.

Vogelstein, B. and Kinzler, K.W.: p53 function and dysfunction. Cell 70: 523–526, 1992.

Vogt, W.: Anaphylatoxins: possible roles in disease. Complement Inflamm. 3: 177–188, 1986.

Voisin, G.A.: Role of antibody classes in the regulatory facilitation reaction. Immunol. Rev, 49: 3, 1980.

Von Boehmer, H.: Thymic selection: a matter of life and death. Immunology Today 13: 454, 1992.

von der Heide, R.H. and Hunt, S.V.: Does the availability of either B cells or CD4+ cells limit germinal centre formation. Immunol. 69: 487, 1990.

von Kempis, J.; Torbohm, I.; Schonermark, M.; Jahn, B.; Seitz, M. and Hansch, G.M.: Effect of the late complement components C5b-9 and of platelet-derived growth factor on the prostaglandin release of human synovial fibroblast-like cells. Int. Arch. Allergy Appl. Immunol. 90: 248–255, 1989.

von Knebel-Doeberitz, M.; Koch, S.; Drzonek, H. and zur Hausen, H.: Glucocorticoid hormones reduce the expression of major histocompatibility class I antigens on human epithelial cells. Eur. J. Immunol. 20: 35–40, 1990.

von Ritter, C.; Grisham, M.B. and Granger, D.N.: Sulfasalazine metabolites and dapsone attenuate formyl-methionyl-leucyl-phenylalanine-induced mucosal injury in rat ileum. Gastroenterology 96: 811–816, 1989.

Voss, S.D.; Robb, R.J.; Weil-Hillman, G.; Hank, J.A.; Sugamura, K.; Tsudo, M. and Sondel, P.M.: Increased expression of the interleukin 2 (IL-2) receptor ß chain (p70) on CD56+ natural killer cells after in vivo IL-2 therapy. p70 expression does not alone predict the level of intermediate affinity IL-2 binding. J. Exp. Med. 172: 1101–1114, 1990.

Waaler, E.: On the occurrence of a factor in human serum activating the specific agglutination of sheep blood corpuscles. Acta Path. Microbiol. Scand. 17: 172–188, 1940.

Wagemaker, G.; Burger, H.; Van Gils, F.C.; van Leen, R.W. and Wielenga, J.J.: Interleukin-3. Biotherapy 2: 337–345, 1990.

Wagner, H.; Heeg, K. and Miethke T.: T cell mediated lethal shock induced by bacterial superantigens. Behring Inst. Mitt. 91: 46–53, 1992.

Wahl, S.M.; Hunt, D.A.; Wakefield, L.M.; McCartney-Francis, N.; Wahl, L.M.; Roberts, A.B. and Sporn, M.B.: Transforming growth factor-beta (TGF-ß) induces monocyte chemotaxis and growth factor production. Proc. Natl. Acad. Sci. USA 84: 5788–5792, 1987.

Wahl, W.L.; Plautz, G.E.; Fox, B.A.; Nabel, G.J.; Shu, S. and Chang, A.E.: Generation of therapeutic T lymphocytes after in vivo transfection of tumor with a gene encoding allogeneic Class I Major Histocompatibility Complex antigen. Surg. Forum 43: 476–478, 1992.

Wakefield, L.M.; Smith, D.M.; Masui, T.; Harris, C.C. and Sporn, M.B.: Distribution and modulation of the cellular receptor for transforming growth factor-ß. J. Cell Biol. 105: 965–975, 1987.

Waldmann, T.A. and Strober, W.: Metabolism of immunoglobulins. Prog. Allergy 13: 1–110, 1969.

Waldor, M.K.; Sriram, S.; McDevitt, H.O. and Steinman, L.: In vivo therapy with monoclonal anti-I-A-antibody suppresses immune responses to acetylcholine receptor. Proc. Natl. Acad. Sci. USA 80: 2713–2717, 1983.

Waldor, M.K.; Sriram, S.; Hardy, R.; Herzenberg, L.A.; Lanier, L.; Lim, M. and Steinman, L.: Reversal of experimental allergic encephalomyelitis with monoclonal antibody to a T-cell subset marker. Science 22: 415–417, 1985.

Walker, C.M.; Moody, D.J.; Stites, D.P. and Levy, J.A.: CD8+ lymphocytes can control HIV infection in vitro by suppressing virus replication. Science 234: 1563–1566, 1986.

Wallace, J.L.; Keenan, C.M.; MacNaughton, W.K. and McKnight, G.W.: Comparison of the effects of endothelin-1 and endothelin-3 on the rat stomach. Eur. J. Pharmacol. 167: 41–47, 1989.

Wallach, D.; Fellous, M. and Revel, M.: Preferential effect of gamma interferon on the synthesis of HLA antigens and their mRNAs in human cells. Nature 299: 833–836, 1982.

Wallack, M.K.; McNally, K.R.; Leftheriotis, E.; Seigler, H.; Balch, C.; Wanebo, H.; Bartolucci, A.A. and Bash, J.A.: A southeastern cancer study group phase I/II trial with vaccinia melanoma oncolysates. Cancer 57: 649–655, 1986.

Wallack, M.K. and Sivanandham, M.: Clinical trials with VMO for melanoma. Specific Immunotherapy Of Cancer With Vaccines, eds. Bystryn, J.-C.; Ferrone, S. and Livingston, P., The New York Academy of Sciences 690: 178, 1993.

Wallis, R.S.; Fayen, J.; Wiblin, T.S.; Fujiwara, H. and Ellner, J.J.: Direct mitogenic properties of Interleukin-1. J. Lab. Med. 117: 234–240, 1991.

Walport, J.J. and Lachmann, P.J.: Erythrocyte complement receptor type 1, immune complexes, and the rheumatic diseases. Arthritis Rheum. 31: 153–158, 1988.

Walther, Z.; May, L.T. and Sehgal, P.B.: Transcriptional regulation of the interferon-beta 2/B cell differentiation factor BSF-2/hepatocyte-stimulating factor gene in human fibroblasts by other cytokines. J. Immunol. 140: 974–977, 1988.

Walz, A.: NAP-1/IL-8 and related chemotactic cytokines. Rheumatoid Arthritis, Royal College of Physicians, London, 17./18.6.1991.

Wang, B.; Rieger, A.; Kilgus, O.; Ochiai, K.; Maurer, D.; Fodinger, D.; Kinte, J.-P. and Stingl, G.: Epidermal Langerhans cells from normal human skin bind monomeric IgE via Fc RI. J. Exp. Med. 175: 1353, 1992.

Wang, B.; Ugen, E.; Srikantan, V.; Agadjanyan, M.G.; Dang, K.; Refaeli, Y.; Sato, A.I.; Williams, W.V. and Weiner, D.B.: Gene inoculation generates immune responses against human immunodeficiency virus type I. Proc. Natl. Acad. Sci. USA 90: 4156–4160, 1993.

Wang, B.; Boyer, J.; Srikantan, V.; Coney, L.; Carrano, R.; Phan, C.; Merva, M.; Dang, K.; Agadjanyan, M.; Gilbert, L.; Ugen, K.E.; Williams, W.V. and Weiner, D.B.: DNA inoculation induces neutralizing immune responses against human immunodeficiency virus type 1 in mice and nonhuman primates. DNA Cell Biol. 12: 799–806, 1993.

Wang, H.-M. and Smith K.A.: The interleukin 2 receptor: Functional consequences of its bimolecular structure. J. Exp. Med. 166: 1055–1069, 1987.

Wang, J.M.; Cianciolo, G.J.; Snyderman, R. and Mantovani, A.: Coexistence of a chemotactic factor and a retroviral P15E-related chemotaxis inhibitor in human tumor cell culture supernatants. J. Immunol. 137: 2726–2732, 1986.

Wang, J.M.; Griffin, J.D.; Rambaldi, A.; Chen, Z.G. and Mantovani, A.: Induction of monocyte migration by recombinant macrophage colony-stimulating factor. J. Immunol. 141: 575–579, 1988.

Wang, X.F.; Lin, H.Y.; Ng-Eaton, E.; Downward, J.; Lodish, H.F. and Weinberg, R.A.: Expression cloning and characterization of the TGF-beta type III receptor. Cell 67: 797–805, 1991.

Wank, R.; Schendel, D.J.; O'Neill, G.J.; Riethmueller, G.; Held, E. and Feucht, H.E.: Rare variant of complement C4 is seen in high frequency in patients with primary glomerulonephritis. Lancet. 1: 872–874, 1984.

Ward, B.G.; Mather, S.J.; Hawkins, L.R.; Crowther, M.E.; Shepherd, J.H.; Granowska, M.; Britton, K.E. and Slevin, M.L.: Localization of radioiodine conjugated to the monoclonal antibody HMFG-2 in human ovarian carcinoma: assessment of intravenous and intraperitoneal routes of administration. Cancer Res. 47: 4719, 1987.

Ward, P.A.; Till, G.O.; Kunkel, R. and Beauchamp, C.: Evidence for role of hydroxyl radical in complement and neutrophil-dependent tissue injury. J. Clin. Invest. 72: 789–801, 1983.

Ward, P.: Role of ELAM in inflammation in vivo. Abstr. 2nd. Int. Congress on the Immune Consequences of Trauma, Shock, and Sepsis: Mechanisms and Therapeutic Approaches. March 6–9, 1991. Munich, FRG.

Ward, P.A.; Warren, J.S.; Varani, J. and Johnson K.J.: PAF, cytokines, toxic oxygen products and cell injury. Molec. Aspects Med. 12: 169–174, 1991.

Warner, T.D.; Mitchel, J.A.; de Nucci, G. and Vane, J.R.: Endothelin-1 and endothelin-3 release EDRF from isolated perfused arterial vessels of the rat and rabbit. J. Cardiovasc. Pharmacol. 13: 85–88, 1989.

Warner, T.D.; de Nucci, G. and Vane, J.R.: Rat endothelin is a vasodilator in the isolated perfused mesentery of the rat. Eur. J. Pharmacol. 159: 325–326, 1989.

Warren, H.S.; Danner, R.L. and Munford, R.S.: Sounding board: Anti-endotoxin monoclonal antibodies. New Engl. J. Med. 326: 1153–1157, 1992.

Warren, J.S.; Mandel, D.M.; Johnson, K.J. and Ward, P.A.: Evidence for the role of platelet-activating factor in immune complex vasculitis in the rat. J. Clin. Invest. 83: 669–678, 1989.

Warren J.S.; Yabroff, K.R.; Remick, D.G.; Kunkel, S.L.; Chensue, S.W.; Kunkel, R.G.; Johnson, K.J. and Ward, P.A.: Tumor necrosis factor participates in the pathogenesis of acute immune complex alveolitis in the rat. J. C.in. Invest. 84: 1873–1882, 1989.

Warren, J.S.; Yabroff, K.R.; Mandel, D.M.; Johnson, K.J. and Ward, P.A.: Role of

Watanabe, Y.; Kuribayashi, K.; Miyatake, S.; Nishihara, K.; Nakayama, E.; Taniyama, T. and Sakata, T.: Exogenous expression of mouse interferon gamma cDNA in mouse neuroblastoma C1300 cells results in reduced tumorigenicity by augmented anti-tumor immunity. Proc. Natl. Acad. Sci. USA 86: 9456–9460, 1989.

Watt, A.G. and House, A.K.: Colonic carcinoma: A quantitated assessment of lymphocyte infiltration at the periphery of colonic tumors related to prognosis. Cancer 41: 279–282, 1978.

Webster, E.L. and De Souza, E.B.: Corticotropin-releasing factor receptors in mouse spleen: Identification, autoradiographic localization, and regulation by divalent cations and guanine nucleotides. Endocrinology 122: 609–617, 1988.

Weinberg, A.D.; Whitham, R.; Swain, S.L.; Morrison, W.J.; Wyrick, G.; Hoy, C.; Vandenbark, A.A. and Offner, H.: Transforming growth factor-beta enhances the in vivo effector function and memory phenotype of antigen-specific T helper cells in experimental autoimmune encephalomyelitis. J. Immunol. 148: 2109–2118, 1992.

Weiner, L.M.; O'Dwyer, J.; Kitson, J.; Comis, R.L.; Frankel, A.E.; Bauer, R.J.; Konrad, M.S. and Groves, E.S.: Phase I evaluation of an anti-breast carcinoma monoclonal antibody 260F9-recombinant Ricin A chin immunoconjugate. Cancer Res. 49: 4062, 1989.

Weis, J.J.; Toothaker, L.E.; Smith, J.A.; Weis, J.H. and Fearon, D.T.: Structure of the human B lymphocyte receptor for C3d and the Epstein-Barr virus and relatedness to other members of the family of C3/C4 binding proteins. J. Exp. Med. 167: 1047–1066, 1988.

Weisman, H.F.; Bartow, T.; Leppo, M.K.; Marsh, H.C.jr.; Carson, G.R.; Concino, M.F.; Boyle, M.P.; Roux, K.H.; Weisfeldt, M.L. and Fearon, D.T.: Soluble human complement receptor type 1: in vivo inhibitor of complement suppressing post-ischemic myocardial inflammation and necrosis. Science 249: 146–151, 1990.

Weissbarth, E.; Sedlacek, H.H.; Seiler, F.R.; Fricke, M. and Deicher, H.: Release of 3H-Serotonin and endogenous β-thromboglobulin from human platelets by immune complexes. Behring Inst. Mitt. 64: 121–126, 1979.

Weisz-Carrington, P.; Roux, M.E.; McWilliams, M.; Phillips Quagliata, J.M. and Lamm, M.E.: Hormonal induction of the secretory immune system in the mammary gland. Proc. Natn. Acad. Sci. USA 75: 2928–2932, 1978.

Weksler, B. and Coupal, C.E.: Platelet dependent generation of chemotactic activity in serum. J. Exp. Med. 137: 1419–1430, 1973.

Wells, D.J. and Goldspink, G.: Age and sex influence expression of plasmid DNA directly injected into mouse skeletal muscle. FEBS Lett. 306: 203–205, 1992.

Wells, D.J.: Improved gene transfer by direct plasmid injection associated with regeneration in mouse skeletal muscle. FEBS Lett. 332: 179–182, 1993.

Welsh, C.H.; Lien, D.; Worthen, S. and Weil, J.V.: Pentoxifylline decreases endotoxin-induced pulmonary neutrophil sequestration and extravascular protein accumulation in the dog. Am. Rev. Respir. Dis. 138: 1106–1114, 1988.

Wendling, D.; Wijdenes, J.; Racadot, E. and Morel-Fourrier, B.: Therapeutic use of monoclonal anti-CD4 antibody in rheumatoid arthritis. J. Rheumatol. 18: 325–327, 1991.

Wendling, D.; Wijdenes, J. and Racadot, E.: Therapeutic use of a monoclonal, anti-CD4 antibody in refractory rheumatoid polyarthritis. Preliminary results. Rev. Rheum. Mal. Osteo-Articulaires, 58: 13, 1991.

Wenzel, R.; Bone, R.; Fein, A.; Quenzer, R.; Schentag, J.; Gorelick, K.J.; Wedel, N.I. and Perl, T.: Results of a second double-blind, randomized, controlled trial of antiendotoxin antibody E5 in gram-negative sepsis. In: program and abstracts of the 31st Interscience Conference on Antimicrobial Agents and Chemotherapy, Chicago, September 29–October 2, 1991. Washington, D.C.: American Society for Microbiology 31: 294, 1991.

Wenzel, R.P.: Anti-endotoxin monoclonal antibodies - a second look. New Engl. J. Med. 326: 1151, 1992.

Wetzler, M.; Talpaz, M.; Lowe, D.G.; Baiocchi, G.; Gutterman, J.U. and Kurzrock, R.: Constitutive expression of leukemia inhibitory factor RNA by human bone marrow stromal cells and modulation by Il-1, TNF-alpha, and TGF-beta. Exp. Hematol. 19: 347–351, 1991.

Wheeler, A.P.; Hardie, W.D. and Bernard, G.: Studies of an antiendotoxin antibody in preventing the physiologic changes of endotoxemia in awake sheep. Am. Rev, Respir. Dis. 142: 775–781, 1990.

White, M.V.; Igarashi, Y.; Emery, B.E.; Lotze, M.T. and Kaliner, M.A.: Effects of in vivo administration of interleukin-2 (Il-2) and Il-4, alone and in combination, on ex vivo human basophil histamine release. Blood 79: 1491–1495, 1992.

White, J.; Herman, A.; Pullen, A.M.; Kubo, R.; Kappler, J.W. and Marrack, P.: The V beat-specific superantigen staphylococcal enterotoxin B: stimulation of mature T cells and clonal deletion in neonatal mice. Cell 56: 27–35, 1989.

White, M.V.; Yoshimura, T.; Hook, W.; Kaliner, M.A. and Leonard, E.J.: Neutrophil attractant/activation protein-1 (NAP-1) causes human basophil histamine release. Immunol. Lett. 22: 151, 1989.

Whiteside, T.L.; Miescher, S.; Hurlimann, J.; Moretta, L. and Von Fliedner, V.: Clonal analysis and in situ characterization of lymphocytes infiltrating human breast carcinomas. Cancer Immunol. Immunother. 23: 169–178, 1986.

Whiteside, T.L.; Heo, D.S.; Takagi, S. and Herberman, R.B.: Tumor-infiltrating lymphocytes from human solid tumors: Antigen-specific killer T lymphocytes or activated natural killer lymphocytes. In: Stevenson, H.C., ed., Adoptive Cellular Immunotherapy of Cancer. New York: Marcel Dekker, 139–157, 1989.

Whiteside, T.L.; Jost, L.M. and Herberman, R.B.: Tumor-infiltrating lymphocytes. Potential and limitations to their use for cancer therapy. Crit. Rev. Oncol./Hematol. 12: 25–47, 1992.

Wiederrecht, G.; Lam, E.; Hung, S.; Martin, M. and Sigal, N.: The mechanism of action of FK-506 and Cyclosporin A. Immunosuppressive and Antiinflammatory Drugs, eds. Allison, A.C.; Lafferty, K.J. and Fliri, H., Annals of the New York Academy of Sciences 696: 9, 1993.

Wiedmer, T.; Esmon, C.T. and Sims, P.J.: Complement proteins C5b-9 stimulate procoagulant activity through platelet prothrombinase. Blood 68: 875–880, 1986.

Wiedmer, T.; Esmon, C.T. and Sims, P.J.: On the mechanism by which complement protein C5b-9 increases platelet prothrombinase activity. J. Biol. Chem. 261: 14587–14592, 1986.

Wierenga, E.A.; Snoek, M.A.; de Giroot, C.; Chrétien, I.; Bos, J.D.; Jansen, H.M. and Kapsenberg, M.L.: Evidence for compartmentalization of functional subsets of CD4+ T lymphocytes in atopic patients. J. Immunol. 144: 4651–4656, 1990.

Wieser, M.; Bonifer, M.R.; Oster, W.; Lindemann, A.; Mertelsmann, R. and Hermann, F.: IL-4 induces secretion of CSF for ganulocytes and CSF for macrophages by peripheral blood monocytes. Blood 73: 1105–1108, 1989.

Wilkstrand, C.J.; Longee, D.C.; McLendon, R.E.; Fuller, G.N.; Friedman, H.S.; Fredman, P.; Svennerholm, L. and Bigner, D.D.: Lactotetraose series ganglioside 3',6'-isoLD11 in tumors of central nervous and other systems in vitro and in vivo. Cancer Res. 53: 120–126, 1993.

Williams, R.S.; Johnston, S.A.; Riedy, M.; Devit, M.J.; McElligott, S.G. and Sanford, J.C.: Introduction of foreign genes into tissues of living mice by DNA-coated microprojectiles. Proc. Natl. Acad. Sci. USA 88: 2726–2730, 1991.

Wilson, B.S.; Imai, K.; Natali, P.G. and Ferrone, S.: Distribution and molecular characterization of a cell surface and a cytoplasmic antigen detectable in human melanoma cells with monoclonal antibodies. Int. J. Cancer 28: 293–300, 1981.

Wilson, J.G.; Ratnoff, W.D.; Schur, P.H. and Fearon, D.T.: Decreased expression of the C3b/C4b receptor (CR1) and the C3d receptor (CR2) on B lymphocytes and of CR1 on neutrophils of patients with systemic lupus erythematosus. Arthritis Rheum. 29: 739–747, 1986.

Wilson, R.E.; Hager, E.B.; Hampres, C.L.; Corson, J.M.; Merrill, J.P. and Murray, J.E.: Immunologic rejection of human cancer transplanted with a renal allograft. N. Engl. J. Med. 278: 479–483, 1968.

Williams, D.E.; Eisenman, J.; Baird, A.; Rauch, C.; Van Ness, K.; March, C.J.; Park, L.S.; Martin, U.; Mochizuki, D.Y.; Boswell, H.S. et al.: Identification of a ligand for the c-kit proto-oncogene. Cell 63: 167–174, 1992.

Williams, T.M.; Fox, K.R. and Kant, J.A.: Interleukin-2: Basic biology and therapeutic use. Hemat. Pathol. 5: 45–55, 1991.

Wintzer, H.-O.; Benzing, M. and von Kleist, S.: Lacking prognostic significance of β2–microglobulin, MHC class I and class II antigen expression in breast carcinomas. Br. J. Cancer 62: 289–295, 1990.

Wira, C.R.; Hyde, E.; Sandoe, C.P.; Sullivan, D. and Spencer, S.: Cellular aspects of the rat uterine IgA response to estradiol and progesterone. J. Steroid Biochem. 12: 451–459, 1980.

Wira, C.R.; Sullivan, D.A. and Sandoe, C.P.: Estrogen-mediated control of the secretory immune system in the uterus of the rat. Ann. N.Y. Acad. Sci. 409: 534–551, 1983.

Wira, C.R. and Sullivan, D.A.: Estradiol and progesterone regulation of immunoglobulin A and G and secretory component in cervicovaginal secretions of the rat. Biol. Reprod. 32: 90–95, 1985.

Wira, C.R. and Colgy, E.M.: Regulation of secretory component by glucocorticoids in primary cultures of rat hepatocytes. J. Immun. 134: 1744–1748, 1985.

Wiseman, C.; Presant, C.; Rao, R. and Smith, J.: Clinical responses to intralymphatic whole-cell melanoma vaccine augmented by in vitro incubation with alpha-Interferon. Specific Immunotherapy of Cancer with Vaccines, Bystryn, J.C.; Ferrone, S. and Livingston, P. (eds)., Annals of the New York Academy of Sciences 690: 388, 1993.

Witte, O.N.: Steel locus defines new multipotent growth factor. Cell 63: 5–6, 1990.

Wölfel, T.; Klehmann, E.; Müller, C.; Schütt, K.H.; Meyer zum Büschenfelde, K.H. and Knuth, A.: Lysis of human melanoma cells by autologuos cytolytic T cell clones. Identification of human histocompatibility leukocyte antigen A2 as a restriction. Element for three different antigens. J. Exp. Med. 170: 797–810, 1989.

Wofsy, D. and Seaman, W.E.: Reversal of advanced murine lupus in NZB/NZW F1 mice by treatment with monoclonal antibody to L3T4. J. Immunol. 138: 3247–3253, 1987.

Wolf, G.T.; Hudson, J.L.; Peterson, K.A.; Miller, H.L. and McClatchey, K.D.: Lymphocyte subpopulations infiltrating squamous carcinomas of the head and neck: Correlations with extend of tumor and prognosis. Otolaryngol Head Neck Surg. 95: 142–151, 1986.

Wolf, S.F.; Temple, P.A.; Kobayashi, M.; Young, E.; Dicig, M.; Lowe, L.; Dzialo, R.; Fitz, L.; Ferenz, C.; Hewick, R.M.; Kelleher, K.; Herrmann, S.H.; Clark, S.C.; Azzoni, L.; Chan, S.H.; Trinchieri, G. and Perussia, B.: Cloning of cDNA for natural killer cell stimulatory factor, a heterodimeric cytokine with multiple biologic effect on T and natural killer cells. J. Immunol. 146: 3074–3081, 1991.

Wolff, J.A.; Malone, R.W.; Williams, P.; Chong, W.; Acsadi, G.; Jani, A. and Felgner, P.L.: Direct gene transfer into mouse muscle in vivo. Science 247: 1465–1468, 1990.

Wolff, J.A.; Ludtke, J.A.; Acsadi, G.; Williams, P. and Jani, A.: Long-term persistence of plasmid DNA and foreign gene expression in mouse muscle. Human Mol. Genet. 1: 363–369, 1992.

Wolff, S.M.: Biological effects of bacterial endotoxin in man. J. Infect. Dis. 128: 259–264, 1973.

Woll, P.J.: Neuropeptide growth factors and cancer. Br. J. Cancer 63: 459–475, 1991.

Woloski, B.M.R.N.J.; Smith, E.M.; Meyer, W.J.; Fuller, G.M. and Blalock, J.E.: Corticotropin-releasing activity of monokines. Science 230: 1035–1037, 1985.

Wolpe, S.D.; Davatelis, G.; Sherry, B.; Beutler, B.; Hesse, D.G.; Nguyen, H.T.; Moldawer, L.L.; Nathan, C.F.; Lowry, S.F. and Cerami, A.: Macrophages secrete a novel heparin-binding protein with inflammatory and neutrophil chemokinetic properties. J. Exp. Med. 167: 570–581, 1987.

Wolpe, S.D. and Cerami, A.: Macrophage inflammatory proteins 1 and 2: members of a novel superfamily of cytokines. FASEB J. 147: 2565–2573, 1989.

Woltering, E.A.; Barrie, R.; O'Dorisio, T.M.; Arce, D.; Ure, T.; Cramer, A.; Holmes, D.; Robertson, J. and Fassler, J.: Somatostatin analogues inhibit angiogenesis in the chick chorio-allontoic membrane. J. Surg. Res. 50: 245–251, 1991.

Wong, G.G.; Witek, J.; Temple, P.A.; Wilkens, K.M:; Leary, A.C.; Luxenberg, D.P.; Jones, S.S.; Brown, E.C.; Kay, R.M.; Orr, E.C.; Shoemaker, C.; Golde, D.W.; Kaufman, R.J.; Hewick, R.M.; Wang, E.A. and Clark, S.C.: Human GM-CSF: Molecular cloning of the complementary DNA and purification of the natural and recombinant proteins. Science 228: 810, 1985.

Wong, G.G.; Witek-Giannotti, J.S.; Temple, P.A.; Kriz, R.; Ferenz, C.; Hewick, R.M.; Clark, S.C.; Ikebuchi, K. and Ogawa, M.: Stimulation of murine hemopoietic colony formation by human Il-6. J. Immunol. 140: 3040–3044, 1988.

Wong, G.H.; Clark-Lewis, I.; McKimm-Brschkin, L.; Harris, A.W. and Schrader, J.W.: Interferon-gamma induces enhanced expression of Ia and H-2 antigens on B lymphoid, macrophage, and myeloid cell lines. J. Immunol. 131: 788–793, 1983.

Wong, G.H.W.; Elwell, H.H.; Oberley, L.W. and Goeddel, D.V.: Manganous superoxide dismutase is essential for cellular resistance to cytotoxicity of tumor necrosis factor. Cell 58: 923–931, 1989.

Wong, H.L.; Wilson, D.E.; Jenson, J.C.; Familletti, P.C.; Stremlo, D.L. and Gately, M.K.: Characterization of a factor(s) which synergizes with recombinant Interleukin 2 in promoting allogeneic human cytolytic T-lymphocyte responses in vitro. Cell Immunol. 111: 39–54, 1988.

Woodbury, R.G.; Brown, J.P.; Yeh, M.Y.; Hellström, I. and Hellström, K.E.: Identification of a cell surface protein, p97 in human melanomas and certain other neoplasms. Proc. Natl. Acad. Sci. USA 77: 2183–2187, 1980.

Wooley, J.C.; Cone, R.D.; Tartof, D. and Chung, S.Y.: Small nuclear ribonucleoprotein complexes of Drosophila melanogaster. Proc. natn. Acad. Sci. USA 79: 6762–6766, 1982.

Wooley, P.H.; Luthra, H.S.; Lafuse, W.P.; Huse, A.; Stuart, J.M. and David, C.S.: Type II collagen-induced arthritis in mice. III. Suppression of arthritis by using monoclonal and polyclonal anti-Ia-antisera. J. Immunol. 134: 2366–2374, 1985.

Wraith, D.C. and Askonas, B.A.: Induction of influenza A virus cross-reactive cytotoxic T cells by a nucleoprotein/haemagglutin preparation. J. Gen. Virol. 66: 1327, 1985.

Wright, S.D.; Tobias, P.S.; Ulevitch, R.J. and Ramos, R.A.: Lipopolysaccharide (LPS) binding protein opsonizes LPS-bearing particles for recognition by a novel receptor on macrophages. J. Exp. Med. 170: 1231–1241, 1989.

Wright, S.D.; Ramos, R.A.; Tobias, P.S.; Ulevitch, R.J. and Mathison, J.C.: CD14, a receptor for complexes of lipopolysaccharide (LPS) and LPS binding protein. Science 249: 1431–1433, 1990.

Wu, C.; Wilson, J. and Wu, G.: Targeting genes: delivery and persistent expression of a foreign gene driven by mammalian regulatory elements in vivo. J. Biol. Chem. 264: 16985–16987, 1989.

Wu, G.Y.; Wilson, J.M.; Shalaby, F.; Grossman, M.; Shafritz, D.A. and Wu, C.H.: Receptor-mediated gene delivery in vivo. J. Biol. Chem. 266, 14338–14324, 1991.

Wyllie, A.H.; Kerr, J.F.R. and Currie, A.R.: Cell death: The significance of apoptosis. Int. Rev. Cytology 68: 251–306, 1980.

Wyllie, A.H.; Morris, R.G.; Smith, A.L. and Dunlop, D.: Chromatin cleavage in apoptosis: association with condensed chromatin morphology and dependence on macromolecular synthesis. J. Pathol. 142: 67, 1984.

Wyllie, A.H.: Apoptosis and the regulation of cell numbers in normal and neoplastic tissues: an overview. Cancer Metas. Rev. 11: 95–103, 1992.

Xia, W.; Fearon, D.T.; Moore, F.D.; Schoen, F.J.; Ortiz, F. and Kirkman, R.I.: Prolongation of guinea pig cardiac xenograft survival in rats by soluble human complement recptor type 1. Transplant. Proc. 24:479–480, 1992.

Xiang, Z.Q.; Spitalnik, S.; Tran, M.; Wunner, W.H.; Cheng, J. and Ertl, H.C.J.: Vaccination with a plasmid vector carrying the rabies virus glycoprotein gene induces protective immunity against rabies virus. Virology 1994, in press.

Yamaguchi, H.; Furukawa, K.; Fortunato, S.R.; Livingston, P.O.; Lloyd, K.O.; Oettgen, H.F. and Old, L.J.: Cell-surface antigens of melanoma recognized by human monoclonal antibodies. Proc. Natl. Acad. Sci. USA 84: 2416–2420, 1987.

Yamaguchi, H.; Furukawa, K.; Fortunato, S.R.; Livingston, P.O.; Lloyd, K.O.; Oettgen, H.F. and Old, L.J.: Human monoclonal antibody with dual GM2/GD2 specificity derived from an immunized melanoma patient. Proc. Natl. Acad. Sci. USA 87: 3333–3337, 1990.

Yamasaki, K.; Taga, T.; Hirata, Y.; Yawata, H.; Kawanishi, Y.; Seed, B.; Hirano, T. and Kishimoto, T.: Cloning and expression of the human interleukin-6 (BSF-2/IFNß2) receptor. Science 241: 825, 1988.

Yanagihara, Y.; Sarfati, M.; Marsh, D.; Nutman, T. and Delespesse, G.: Serum levels of IgE-binding factor (soluble CD23) in diseases associated with elevated IgE. Clin. Exp. Allergy 20: 395–401, 1990.

Yanagisawa, J.; Kurihara, H.; Kimura, S.; Tomobe, Y.; Kobayashi, M.; Mitsui, Y.; Yazaki, Y.; Goto, K. and Masaki, T.: A novel potent vasoconstrictor peptide produced by vascular endothelial cells. Nature (London) 332: 411–415, 1988.

Yang, D.C.; Dang, C.V. and Arnett, F.C.: Rat liver histidyl-tRNA synthetase. Purification and inhibition by the myositis-specific anti-Jo-1 autoantibody. Biochem. Biophys. Res. Commun. 120: 15–21, 1984.

Yang, S.Y.; Denning, S.M.; Mizuno, S.; Dupont, B. and Haynes, B.F.: A novel activation pathway for mature thymocytes. Costimulation of CD2 (T,p50) and CD28 (T,p44) induces autocrine interleukin 2/interleukin 2 receptor-mediated cell proliferation. J. Exp. Med. 168: 1457–1468, 1988.

Yao, S.-N. and Kurachi, K.: Expression of human factor IX in mice after injection of genetically modified myoblasts. Proc. Natl. Acad. Sci. USA 89: 3357–3361, 1992.

Yap, K.L. and Ada, G.L.: Transfer of specific cytotoxic T lymphocytes protects mice inoculated with influenza virus. Nature 273: 238–240, 1978.

Yarden, Y.; Escobeo, J.A.; Kuang, W.J.; Yang-Feng, T.L.; Daniel, T.O.; Tremble, P.M.; Chen, E.Y.; Ando, M.E.; Harkins, R.N.; Francke, U. et al.: Structure of the receptor for platelet-derived growth factor helps define a family of closely related growth factor receptors. Nature 323: 226–232, 1986.

Yeh, C.G.; Marsh, H.C.; Carson, G.R.; Berman, I.; Concino, M.F.; Scesney, S.M.; Kuestner, R.E.; Skibbens, R.; Donahue, K.A. and Ip, S.H.: Recombinant soluble human complement receptor type 1 inhibits inflammation in the reversed passive arthus reaction in rats. J. Immunol. 146: 250–256, 1991.

Yodoi, J.; Adachi, M.; Teshipawara, K.; Masuda, T. and Fridman, W.H.: T cell hybridoma coexpressing Fc receptors for different isotypes. I. Reciprocal regulation of Fc gamma R and Fc alpha R expression by IgA and interferon. Immunology 48: 551–559, 1983.

Yokota, T.; Coffman, R.L.; Hagiwara, H.; Rennick, D.M.; Takebe, Y.; Yokota, K.; Gemmell, L.; Shrader, B.; Yang, G.; Meyerson, P. et al.: Isolation and characterization of lymphokine cDNA clones encoding mouse and human IgA-enhancing factor and eosinophil colony-stimulating factor activities: relationship to interleukin 5. Proc. Natl. Acad. Sci. 84: 7388–7392, 1987.

Yokota, A.; Kikutani, H.; Tanaka, T.; Saot, R.; Barsumian, E.L.; Suemura, M. and Kishimoto, T.: Two species of human Fc receptor II (Fc-RII/CD23): tissue-specific and IL-4–specific regulation of gene expression. Cell 55: 611–618, 1988.

Yokota, A.; Yukawa, K.; Yamamoto, A.; Sugiyama, K.; Suemura, M.; Tashiro, Y.; Kishimoto, T. and Kikutani, H.: Two forms of the low-affinity Fc receptor for IgE differentially mediate endocytosis and phagocytosis: identification of the critical cytoplasmic domain. Proc. Natl. Acad. Sci. USA 89: 5030–5034, 1992.

Yokota, T.; Otsuka, T.; Mosmann, T.; Banchereau, J.; Defrance, T.; Blanchard, D.; de Vries, J.E.; Lee, F. and Arai, K.: Isolation and characterization of a human interleukin cDNA clone, homologous to mouse B cell stimulatory factor 1, that expresses B cell-stimulatory activities. Proc. Natl. Acad. Sci. USA 83: 5894–5898, 1986.

Yoshida, S.; Akizuki, M.; Mimori, T.; Yamagata, H.; Inada, S. and Homma, M.: The precipitating antibody to an acidic nuclear protein antigen, the Jo-1, in connective tissue diseases. Arthritis Rheum. 26: 604–611, 1983.

Yoshida, T.; Muramatsu, H.; Muramatsu, T.; Sakomoto, H.; Katoh, O.; Sugimura, T. and Terada, M.: Differential expression of two homologous and clustered oncogenes, Hst1 and Int-2, during differentiation of F9 cells. Biochem. Biophys. Res. Commun. 157: 618–625, 1988.

Yoshimura, T.; Matsushima, K.; Tanaka, S.; Robinson, E.A.; Appella, E.; Oppenheim, J.J. and Leonard, E.J.: Purification of a human monocyte-derived neutrophil chemotactic factor that has peptide sequence similarity to other host defense cytokines. Proc. Natl. Acad. Sci. 84: 9233–9237, 1987.

Yoshimura, A. and Lodish, H.F.: In vitro phosphorylation of the erythropoietin receptor and an associated protein, pp130. Mol. Cell. Biol. 12: 706–715, 1992.

Yoshizawa T.; Shinmi, O.; Giaid, A.; Yanagisawa, M.; Gibson, S.J.; Kimura, S.; Uchiyama, Y.; Polak, J.M.; Masaki, T. and Kanazawa, I.: Endothelin: a novel peptide in the posterior pituitary system. Science 247: 462–464, 1990.

Young, K.R.; Amburs, J.L.; Malbran, A.; Fauci, A.S. and Tenner, A.J.: Complement subcomponent C1q stimulates Ig production by human lymphocytes. J. Immunol. 146: 3356–3364, 1991.

Young, L.S.; Gascon, R.; Alam, S. and Bermudez, L.E.M.: Monoclonal antibodies for treatment of gram-negative infections. Rev. Infect. Dis. 11: S1564–S1571, 1989.

Young, L.S.; Dawson, C.W.; Brown, K.W. and Rickinson, A.B.: Identification of a human epithelial cell surface protein sharing an epitope with the C3d/Epstein-Barr virus receptor molecule of B lymphocytes. Int. J. Cancer 43: 786–794, 1989.

Young, L.; Alfieri, C.; Hennessey, K.; Evans, H.; O'Hara, C.; Anderson, K.C.; Ritz, J.; Shapiro, R.S.; Rickinson, A.; Kieff, E. and Cohen, J.I.: Expression of Epstein-Barr virus transformation-associated genes in tissues of patients with EBV lymphoproliferative disease. N. Engl. J. Med. 321: 1080–1085, 1989.

Young, P.R.; Karanutilake, C. and Zygas, A.P.: Binding of cathepsin D to the mannose receptor on rat peritoneal macrophages. Biochim. Biophys. Acta Mol. Cell. Res. 1095: 1–4, 1991.

Yu, H. and Schultz, R.M.: Relationship between secreted urokinase plasminogen activator activity and metastatic potential in murine B16 cells transfected with human urokinase sense and antisense genes. Cancer Res. 50: 7623–7633, 1990.

Zabel, P.; Schade, F.U: and Schlaak, M.: Pentoxifyllin – Ein Synthesehemmer für Tumornekrose-Faktor-alpha. Immun. Infekt. 20: 80–83, 1992.

Zachariae, C.O.C.; Anderson, A.O.; Thompson, H.L.; Appella, E.; Mantovani, A.; Oppenheim, J.J. and Matsushima, K.: Properties of monocyte chemotactic and activating factor (MCAF) purified from a human fibrosarcoma cell line. J. Exp. Med. 171: 2177–2182, 1990.

Zachary, I.; Woll, P.J. and Rozengurt, E.: A role for neuropeptides in the control of cell proliferation. Devel Biol. 124: 295–308, 1987.

Zalcberg, I.; Silveira, A.V. and Möller, G.: Regulation of the antibody response to sheep erythrocytes by monoclonal IgG antibodies. Eur. J. Immunol. 17: 1343, 1987.

Zalman, L.S.; Wood, L.M. and Müller-Eberhard, H.J.: Isolation of a human erythrocytes membrane protein capable of inhibiting expression of homologous complement transmembrane channels. Proc. Natl. Acad. Sci. USA 810: 6975, 1986.

Zamvil, S.S.; Mitchell, D.J.; Morre, A.C.; Kitamura, K.; Steinman, L. and Rothbard, J.B.: T-cell epitope of the autoantigen myelin basic protein that induces encephalomyelitis. Nature 324: 258–260, 1986.

Zamvil, S.S.; Mitchell, D.J.; Powell, M.B.; Sakai, K.; Rothbard, J.B. and Steinman, L.: Multiple discrete encephalitogenic epitopes of the autoantigen myelin basic protein include a determinant for I-E class II-restricted T cells. J. Exp. Med. 168: 1181–1186, 1988.

Zapf, J. and Froesch, E.R.: Insulin-like growth factors/somatomedins: structure, secretion, biological actions and physiological role. Hormone Res. 24: 121–130, 1986.

Zarling, J.M.; Shoyab, M.; Marquardt, H.; Hanson, M.B.; Lioubin, M.N. and Todaro, G.J.: Oncostatin M: a growth regulator produced by differentiated histiocytic lymphoma cells. Proc. Natl. Acad. Sci. USA 83: 9739–9743, 1986.

Zatloukal, K.; Wagner, E.; Cotten, M.; Phillips, S.; Plank, C.; Steinlein, P.; Curiel, D.T. and Birnstiel, M.L.: Transferrinfection: A highly efficient way to express gene constructs in eukaryotic cells. Antisense Strategies, eds. Baserga, R. and Denhardt, D.T., Annals of the New York Academy of Sciences 660: 136–153, 1992.

Zahn, X.; Bates, B.; Hu, X.G. and Goldfarb, M.: The human FGF-5 oncogene encodes a novel protein related to fibroblast growth factors. Mol. Cell Biol. 8: 3487–3495, 1988.